# Animal Nutrition
## and
# Immunity

# Animal Nutrition
## and
# Immunity

**DV Reddy**

BVSc, MVSc (Animal Science), PhD (Animal Nutrition)

Ex-Dean, Professor and Head
Department of Animal Nutrition
Rajiv Gandhi Institute of Veterinary Education and Research
Puducherry (UT)
India

## Oxford & IBH Publishing Co. Pvt. Ltd.
New Delhi
(*A Unit of* CBS Publishers & Distributors Pvt Ltd)

# CBS Publishers & Distributors Pvt Ltd

New Delhi • Bengaluru • Chennai • Kochi • Kolkata • Mumbai
Bhopal • Bhubaneswar • Hyderabad • Jharkhand • Nagpur • Patna
Pune • Uttarakhand • Dhaka (Bangladesh) • Kathmandu (Nepal)

**Animal Nutrition and Immunity**

**ISBN:** 978-93-89396-26-3

Copyright © Author and Publisher

**First Edition: 2020**

**OXFORD & IBH**
New Delhi
(A Unit of CBS Publishers & Distributors Pvt Ltd)

Published by Satish Kumar Jain and produced by Varun Jain for
**Oxford & IBH Publishing Co. Pvt. Ltd.** under an imprint of
**CBS Publishers & Distributors** Pvt Ltd
4819/XI Prahlad Street, 24 Ansari Road, Daryaganj, New Delhi 110 002, India.
Ph: 23289259, 23266861, 23266867   Fax: 011-23243014   Website: www.cbspd.com
e-mail: delhi@cbspd.com; cbspubs@airtelmail.in.

*Corporate Office:* 204 FIE, Industrial Area, Patparganj, Delhi 110 092
Ph: 011-4934 4934          Fax: 011-4934 4935          e-mail: publishing@cbspd.com;     publicity@cbspd.com

**Branches**

• **Bengaluru:** Seema House 2975, 17th Cross, K.R. Road, Banasankari 2nd Stage, Bengaluru 560 070, Karnataka
  Ph: +91-80-26771678/79          Fax: +91-80-26771680          e-mail: bangalore@cbspd.com
• **Chennai:** 7, Subbaraya Street, Shenoy Nagar, Chennai 600 030, Tamil Nadu
  Ph: +91-44-26260666, 26208620          Fax: +91-44-42032115          e-mail: chennai@cbspd.com
• **Kochi:** 68/1534, 35, 36, Power House Road, Opp. KSEB, Kochi 682018, Kerala
  Ph: +91-484-4059061-65          Fax: +91-484-4059065          e-mail: kochi@cbspd.com
• **Kolkata:** No. 6/B, Ground Floor, Rameswar Shaw Road, Kolkata-700014 (West Bengal), India
  Ph: +91-33-2289-1126, 2289-1127, 2289-1128          e-mail: kolkata@cbspd.com
• **Mumbai:** 83-C, Dr E Moses Road, Worli, Mumbai-400018, Maharashtra
  Ph: +91-22-24902340/41          Fax: +91-22-24902342          e-mail: mumbai@cbspd.com

**Representatives**

| | | | | | |
|---|---|---|---|---|---|
| • Bhopal | 0-8319310552 | • Bhubaneswar | 0-9911037372 | • Hyderabad | 0-9885175004 |
| • Jharkhand | 0-9811541605 | • Nagpur | 0-9421945513 | • Patna | 0-9334159340 |
| • Pune | 0-9623451994 | • Uttarakhand | 0-9716462459 | | |
| • Dhaka (Bangladesh) | 01912-003485 | • Kathmandu (Nepal) | 977-9818742655 | | |

*Printed at* Mudrak, Noida, UP

# Preface

Animals are biological transformers of feedstuffs to produce high-quality animal foods and fibres (e.g. wool) for consumers. Animal nutrition is an interesting, dynamic and challenging discipline in biological sciences. Nutrition today has evolved toward an integrated science unifying many aspects related to biological science, with recent trends in increased accumulation of knowledge and technology in the nutrition, biochemistry and molecular biology of tissues, cells and genes of animal species. Thus nutrition is a foundational subject in livestock and poultry production as well as the rearing and health of companion and zoo animals.

We live in a potentially hostile world filled with a bewildering array of infectious agents that would very happily use animals as rich sanctuaries for propagating their "selfish genes" had the animals not developed a series of effective defence mechanisms. It is these defence mechanisms that can establish a state of immunity against infection. The science of immunology arose from the study of resistance to infection. Immune system is a defence mechanism.

Immunity is a complex physiological system that requires all nutrients for proper functioning. Nutrients needs are greater during the infection (i.e. pathogen invasion) because nutrients are important for synthesis and secretion of signalling molecules, cell proliferation, free radical generation; all these are needed to protect the host. Therefore, optimum nutrition has an increasing role to play in the development of effective immunity in the animal system as well as resistance against disease organisms. Nutrients have been found to contribute immunity and immune responses in several ways. Correct nutrition can reduce infectious diseases by enhancing cell-tissue integrity and optimising defence mechanisms of the immune system. A fully functional immune system is a requirement of a healthy life in modern animal production. Deficiency of nutrient(s) is liable to hinder the functioning of some biochemical reactions in tissue cells, which in turn affects the defensive mechanism; that is lack of any nutrient would impair the immune response.

I found there is no textbook that deals with infection, inflammation, immunity and nutrition for veterinary students. Further, the gut microbiome has emerged as a critical regulator of animal physiology. Dysbiosis (deleterious changes to the composition or number of gut bacteria) is associated with intestinal inflammation and reduced integrity of the gut barrier, which in turn may facilitate 'the set in' of disease processes (due to translocation of microbial metabolites into blood circulation). Hence maintaining or promoting intestinal health is of crucial importance for optimal production efficiency, overall health and promoting the welfare of our production animals. All these aspects found a place in this textbook *Animal Nutrition and Immunity*.

The book has subject matter in eleven chapters. The book begins with 'immune system, nutrition and animal productivity' followed by 'components of immune system and nutrients for their development'. Chapters 3, 4 and 5 detail extensively on 'prooxidants and antioxidants', 'oxidative stress combating potential of plant phenols' and 'immunomodulatory nutrients to support gut health'. Immunity related aspects of amino acids, fatty acids, selenium and vitamin D are substantially dealt in Chapters 7–9 of the book. Ageing and immune system and transition phase and immune system are the subject matter of Chapters 10 and 11, respectively.

Curriculum is something that is to be dynamic and changes often because of the innovative procedures that come in and the research that has happened. Mindful of keeping the curriculum dynamic, Veterinary Council of India (VCI) revised the minimum standards of veterinary education (MSVE) recently in 2016 for BVSc & AH students. Similarly, Indian Council of Agricultural Research (ICAR) constituted Broad Subject Matter Area (BSMA) committees in September 2017 (first one was in 2008) for "Restructuring of Master's and PhD curriculum and syllabi" to be completed soon. BSMA committee on Livestock Production Technology & Products Management (AGB, animal nutrition, LPM, LPT and poultry science) has Dr SP Tiwari, Chairman, and Dr AK Pattanaik, convener. I am sure this textbook will be immensely useful to all UG and PG students as a guide and resource book in furnishing cutting-edge information.

Face is index of the mind. Applying the same analogy, contents of the book are given elaborately.

Writing a textbook is different from writing a scientific review and in order to enable easy readability, references to cite all statements and all the evidences have become a casualty. However, many bibliographic references are given chapter-wise in addition to those mentioned in the text itself for further details on the subject. To the several authors of excellent review articles from whom I have learnt so much and whose information and evidence I have used so freely, I express my gratitude. I have acknowledged the sources of all information in the form of figures and tables. I take this opportunity to offer my apologies to any copyright holder(s) whose rights may unwittingly have been infringed.

With a strong belief in 'Work is Worship' dictum, most of my waking time is devoted to thinking of (1) the subject matter needed to veterinary students and (2) how best it is presented to them for easy readability and comprehension. I consider myself as an eternal reader of diverse sources with an eye on 'nutrition' word. It is my habit to go to professional libraries during my visits to places far and wide to see our friends and relatives. This helped to enrich myself with the latest happenings in the subject.

Writing of my textbooks had been possible only with the divine power, besides hard work, determination and dedication. The same applies to the present text as well. I am thankful to the publishers for their encouragement and meticulous planning in publication of the textbook.

I sincerely invite the readers, my well-wishers and subject experts to feel free and write their frank opinions, critical comments and constructive suggestions. All this will help me to further improve the text in subsequent revisions.

**DV Reddy**

# Contents

# Immune System, Nutrition and Animal Productivity

## NUTRITION AND IMMUNITY IN FARM ANIMALS

### Interaction of Nutrition and Infection

World Health Organisation's monograph entitled 'Interactions of Nutrition and Infection' by Professor Nevin Scrimshaw is the authentic report (published in 1968) to quote that infections worsen nutritional status and poor nutrition weakens immunity to infections. Now, it is common knowledge that poorly nourished animals are more susceptible to infectious diseases. Undernutrition, as well as imbalanced nutrition, impairs the immune system, resulting in less effective protection of the host from viral and bacterial infections. Most of the defence mechanisms are impaired in protein-energy malnutrition (PEM). High-energy intake and high-fat diet (through relative protein deficiency) can influence immune functions. In addition, the effects of infection may have a greater impact on the host when nutrition is imbalanced. Poor nutritional status, therefore, has a synergistic association with infectious disease: infection predisposes to undernutrition and the undernourished state is susceptible to the risk of infection.

Nutritional status of the host can influence the occurrence of various infectious diseases. Several studies indicated that host's nutrition has an important impact on the cell-mediated immune reactions and complement. Impaired nutrition tends to decrease resistance to infection. Nutritional deficiency apparently increases the severity of infection by viral, bacterial, fungal or parasitic pathogens. Supplementation of the diet with higher than the recommended levels of nutrients has been shown to enhance certain aspects of immune function in humans and animals and to increase resistance to infectious diseases.

### Nutrition and Immunocompetence

The immune system and its intricate functions play a critical role in the relationship between infection and malnutrition. This applies to all life stages of animals but especially susceptible are very young and very old animals.

### Immunocompetence

Animals are born with some temporary immunity derived from maternal antibodies. Their cellular system is not yet fully differentiated but is in an active stage of development. When the immune system is able to respond to antigens with the formation of antibodies, the host is called immunocompetent.

The ability of the animal to withstand infectious diseases caused by bacteria, virus or protozoa depends upon the **integrity of immune system**. Proper functioning of the immune system depends upon the availability of nutrients, the precursors of cell growth and activity. The immuneresponsive effects of various nutrients are observed at much higher levels than those actually recommended for optimum production. Improved nutritional status has a profound effect on immunity, disease susceptibility, illness severity and mortality. Let us know the relevance of resistance and resilience.

## Resistance

Resistance to infectious diseases has many facets. Some varieties of viruses, bacteria, protozoa, helminths, etc. are infectious to some species of host animals but not to others. Well-nourished animals can withstand larger numbers of pathogens. Integrity of skin, mucosa, skin pH, stomach pH, bronchial cleansing all play a part in resistance. The chemical attack of microorganisms by enzymes and reactive molecules in tears, saliva, mucous and digestive juices also plays a significant role.

## Resilience

Resilience is the ability of a person/animal to recover quickly from a setback, such as an illness. Coping with disease is a timely process as its recovery from (sub)clinical disease. Quick recovery and short duration of susceptibility are best. Feeding, as opposed to fasting, shortens the recovery period of hospital patients. Enhancing feed intake helps to shorten recovery time from infectious diseases.

## Nutrition and Immunity

Exploring the possibility to stimulate the immune system of healthy animals by nutritional means is an interesting area of research. By improving health of the animals, the need for antibiotic therapy in animal production will decrease. Thus, high-health livestock will provide safe food. Since food animals generally are short-lived as a matter of economics, the effects of proper functioning of the immune system on longevity, cardio-vascular disease, cancer and diseases of old age are considered less important. For companion animals, however, these aspects are extremely interesting since allergy, asthma, autoimmune diseases, cardiovas-cular diseases and cancers are diagnosed frequently and may have their roots in dis-orders of the immune system.

Nutrition has important implications on immunity and incidence of disease, as it has an impact on every physiological process in the body. Only in recent years the specific mechanisms by which nutrients affect immu-nity became apparent. In fact, majority of organisms encountered by an animal on a daily basis do not cause disease under normal circumstances as they are readily detected and eliminated by the innate immune system.

## Effective Innate Immunity

The cellular component of innate immunity identifies pathogens by their presentation of distinct 'pathogen-associated molecular patterns' (PAMPs; Janeway et al, 2005). Specifically, pathogens contain molecules not typically found in mammalian cells and via this strategy, cells of the innate system are able to recognise invading pathogens. Examples of molecules associated with pathogens that are recognised by innate cells include lipotechoic acid, double-stranded RNA, CpG DNA sequences and unusual sugar residues (e.g. mannans) among others. Binding of PAMPs to toll-like receptors (TLRs) initiates killing mechanisms by the neutrophils and macro-phages. In all, it is estimated that the innate immune system recognises approximately $10^3$ molecular patterns.

## Energy and Nutrient needs for Immunity

1. **Energy needs:** Activation of physiological processes within the animal in response to an immunological challenge is necessary for its survival. Accordingly the associated energy cost is incurred by the animal, which reduces the overall productivity potential. Indeed, creating and maintaining a febrile response alone is very energy intensive. It has been estimated that there is approximately a 10–15% increase in

energy usage for every degree of body temperature increase associated with an immune response. Additional energy, above and beyond that necessary for the febrile response, is required for processes such as increased production of inflammatory cytokines, acute phase proteins (APP) and antibody formation.

Shizgal and Martin (1988) reported that sepsis in humans resulted in a 44% increase in energy requirement. Appropriately one would expect that severe infections in non-ruminants and ruminants (e.g. mastitis, metritis) incur additional cost. In an effort to compensate for these direct energy requirements and in an effort to conserve energy, animals will display various behavioural responses such as increased sleep, decreased social activity, decreased sexual behaviour and decreased foraging. Further, there are various metabolic changes that occur relative to gluco-corticoid and norepinephrine activity, which take place in an effort to liberate energy in response to illness. All these behaviour and metabolic responses help the animal to conserve energy. However, they have an overall negative impact on productivity. Information on the precise energetic requirements of immunity in ruminant animals is lacking.

2. **Nutrients needs:** In non-ruminants, essential amino acids, linoleic acid (n-6 fatty acid), vitamins A, E, C, $B_6$, $B_{12}$ and folic acid and microminerals zinc, copper, iron and selenium affect one or more indices of immunity (Calder and Kew, 2002). Vitamin E and zinc received the maximum attention as immunostimulatory nutrients. Forsberg et al. (2010) reviewed the published literature on how specific nutrients benefit the immune system of ruminant livestock. It may be assumed that, at tissue level, nutrients will have similar effects on immunity in ruminants as in non-ruminants. Perhaps dietary sources of the immunostimulatory B-vitamins ($B_6$, $B_{12}$ and folic acid), vitamin C and essential amino acids are less important in ruminants as these are

either endogenously synthesised (e.g. vitamin C) or provided by rumen microorganisms (e.g. B vitamins, amino acids).

## Factors which Alter the Immune Response: Infection and Nutrition

Infection can cause malnutrition and hence deficiencies of several nutrients. Severe malnutrition leads to impaired immune function. Infection and undernutrition are the interrelated major causes of disease and mortality in the developing world (Calder and Jackson, 2000). This statement can also be applied for animals, especially very young and very old ones kept under unhygienic conditions.

Effective protection against invasion of the host by microorganisms requires an intact skin and intact linings of organs that are in contact with the outer world. Since cell turnover rate in these linings is high, nutrients for cell replication and cell growth must be available liberally. The immune response to infection involves a vast increase in cell replication due to the production of acute phase proteins (APP), immunoglobulins and messenger molecules such as cytokines and eicosanoids. An appropriate supply of nutrients is needed to optimise the response.

Cytokines released during inflammation or at an active state of the immune system have an appetite depressant action. Low feed intake of sick animals is the result. Thus immune system activation leads to less growth and less efficient feed utilisation (Sauber and Stahly, 1996).

Another component of the response to infection is the chemical destruction of foreign material (pathogen) by reactive oxygen species (ROS). Protection of the host from the oxidative damage requires sufficient anti-oxidant mechanisms, including antioxidant enzymes that require Fe, Zn, Cu, Mn, Se as active components, antioxidant vitamins such as vitamins C and E and glutathione. Thus, the host needs a supply of a range of nutrients to maintain protection against infective agents and to mount a successful immune response, if infected. Deficiencies of some vitamins and minerals impair immunity and disease resistance (Langseth, 1999; Calder and Jackson, 2000).

## How do Individual Nutrients Affect Immune Function?

A general mechanism by which nutrients support the immune system is via provision of antioxidants. Immune cells activation is characterised by production of high levels of ROS that are used, in part, to kill the ingested pathogens. Immune cell membranes, by themselves, are rich in polyunsaturated fatty acids (PUFA), which are susceptible to ROS-mediated damage (Chew and Park, 2004). Nutrients with antioxidant properties, there-fore, support immunity. These antioxidant nutrients are dealt in detail in Chapter 3.

## Exploration of Alternative Nutritional Strategies to Augment Immunity

In addition to providing adequate amounts of all essential nutrients, other opportunities need to be explored for augmentation of immune functions. As knowledge of the innate and adaptive aspects of immunity has developed, so has knowledge of alternative nutritional strategies to benefit immunity. For example, the gastrointestinal tract is lined with Toll-like receptors (TLRs) that monitor the presence of PAMPs (Harris et al, 2006) and it follows, therefore, that it may be possible to elicit changes in immunity through provision of PAMPs or their facsimiles (exact repro-ductions of PAMPs) in the rations of livestock.

Provision of prebiotics and probiotics in the diet has potential to support immune system. It is possible that this form of nutritional supplementation includes Toll-like receptor signalling in the gastrointestinal tract and thus benefits the immune system (Harris et al, 2006). See Chapter 5 for a detailed description on them.

## IMMUNONUTRITION

It has been known for a long-time that nutrients can influence the host defence by exerting an effect on immune and inflam-matory parameters and thereby modulating the immune function of the body as a major therapeutic strategy for many diseases. That is how the term immunonutrition came into existance.

## Immunonutrition Concept

Immunonutrition concept was originated as early as in 1960, while studying altered immune functions in human patients with malabsorption. This concept may be applied to any situation in which a supply of specific nutrients is used to modify inflammatory or immune responses.

## What is Immunonutrition?

The potential to modulate the activity of immune system by interventions with specific nutrients is termed immunonutrition. Food or feed enriched with nutrients known to be involved in protein synthesis, immuno-stimulation or antioxidant systems are used. For example, immunonutrition has been reported to improve the immune status of preoperative cancer patients, thereby reducing complications and length of hospital stay. Nutrients arginine, eicosapentenoic acid (EPA), docosahexaenoic acid (DHA) and nucleotides can enhance the immune cell responses in cancer patients treated by radiochemotherapy. By modulating the gene expression of immune cells, immunonutrition could make it easier for the organism to adapt to the systemic inflammation and oxidative stress induced by radiochemotherapy (J. Talvas et al, 2015).

The purpose of immunonutrition is to enhance disease resistance. The net effect on the animal is measurable in terms of disease incidence and severity, growth rate and feed use efficiency. Effects on isolated aspects of the immunological response usually cannot be used to predict the net effect on animals under conventional husbandry conditions. Therefore, most animal studies with immunomodulating products rely more on measures of animal performance and disease than on immune parameters.

## Nutritional Modulation of Immune System

Immunomodulation (manipulation of immune system) is one of the most important alternatives as a supportive therapy or to induce natural resistance in animals. It may augment or decrease the magnitude of immune responsiveness. The augmentation of immune response is known as "immunostimulation" or "immunopotentiation". The decrease in responsiveness is termed "immunosuppression". Several compounds are being used as "immunopotentiators or immunostimulants". The use of immunostimulants might be a way to overcome stress-induced immunosuppression and to readjust the immune function to a 'normal' level.

## General Goals of Immune Modulation

The general goals of immune modulation are to enhance cellular defence mechanisms (phagocytosis, chemotaxis, antigen recognition, immune cell proliferation), to maintain mucosal barrier/haemodynamics, to modulate inflammatory response (microcirculation, cytokine response, nitric oxide), to minimise morbidity (infections, pneumonia, deep vein thrombosis), to minimise loss of lean body mass, to decrease antibiotic use, to decrease hospital stay, to decrease intensive care unit (ICU)/ventilator days and to decrease mortality.

Several studies have been conducted in experimental animals and humans over the last two decades with some nutrients, which may modify immune and inflammatory response. These nutrients act independently of their usual nutritional properties and need to be administered in higher doses for them to act as immunonutrients than required.

## How to Develop Strong Immune System? How to nourish it?

A strong immune system improves disease resistance. Many metabolic responses resulting from stress and oxidative damage can be deleterious to disease resistance. Several infectious diseases (especially of viral origin) and mycotoxins in the feed cause "immuno-suppression".

As research in the area of nutritional immunology has increased, it is becoming apparent that nutrient needs for immunity are different from those for growth or skeletal muscle tissue accretion. Research workers in the field of poultry science carried out studies evaluating the nutritional effects on the immune system in avian models. With the advent of ban on "antibiotic growth promoters in feed" in several European Union countries, many nutritionists have implemented dietary strategies that may improve bird health without 'antibiotics-in feed'

M.T. Kidd of Department of Poultry Science, Mississipi State University, USA (Proceedings of the 4th Mid-Atlantic Nutrition Conference, 2006) dealt the nutrition × immunology interrelationships in broilers. Will optimising a nutrient minimum for heightened immunity in 'least cost formulation' result in a healthier flock with better resistance to disease and less mortality? This was the question asked during experimentation. Indeed, immunological techniques (*in vivo* mitogen stimulation and antibody responsiveness) for data capture are quite expensive. Many practical nutritionists had shown interest and asked Dr. Kidd to identify immunity techniques that can be used in the field. Unfortunately, most nutritionists are not trained as immunologists and most immunologists are not trained as nutritionists.

## Determining the Nutrient Needs of Immune System

Determining the total amount of a nutrient required for a particular process of the immune system is complicated by several factors. These include (1) all tissue types contain a resident population of leukocytes and (2) some leukocytes are migrating in and out of tissues and within body fluids, as they constantly monitor and survey for invading pathogens. Because of this flux of leukocytes, the immune system is not centralised and static but rather diffuse and dynamic. Hence the classical "feed and weigh" approaches for determining the nutrient needs and requirements of the immune system are not applicable. Therefore, the nutrient requirements for the immune system are not known in any species to date (Humphrey, 2005).

Nutritional immunologists have primarily focused on the use of nutrients as direct modulators of the immune system, and little attention has been devoted to the actual nutrient needs of the immune system. Like all tissues and cell types, the immune system requires a supply of nutrients to meet its metabolic need. Determining the nutrient needs of the immune system is particularly important for those processes of the immune system, where nutrient supply is most critical. The magnitude of the biological cost in maintaining the immune system depends on the kind of cytokines and the class of immunoglobulins, as related to the activation of complement factors causing inflammation.

A well-developed immune system and optimal immune responsiveness remain important for the welfare and high productivity of livestock and poultry. These qualities can only be obtained by maintaining good health status, since it might reduce the nutrient demand by the gut-associated immune system. Therefore a lot of energy is invested in prophylactic measures such as vaccination and chemoprophylaxis against infectious diseases. But still, the adequate supply of balanced feed is equally important.

### The Immunoreactivity Might be Modulated by Nutritional Factors

Some nutritional factors can modulate the immunoreactivity at the intestinal associated lymphoid tissue, providing protection against bacterial adhesion. There might be additional effects by specific combinations of these additives.

- Immune reactivity can be modulated by nutritional interventions such as alterations in minerals, vitamins (A, D, E, K), arginine, essential fatty acids or other substances (e.g. oligosaccharides).
- The ratio of dietary n-3 to n-6 fatty acids determines the type and rate of eicosanoid production in leukocytes and accessory cells and modulates the immune response, such as macrophage activity.
- Feed restriction has beneficial effects on protection against infections (by *Escherichia coli* and *Eimeria tenella*), which are mediated by a reduction in arachidonic acid metabolites and most probably by modulation of some immune responses.
- The $1,25\text{-}(OH)_2D_3$ has also been attributed with immunomodulatory capacities by regulating lymphocyte proliferation, differentiation of monocytes and secretion of typical cytokines.
- Vitamin A seems to have similar influences on the immune system as vitamin D, as receptors of vitamins A and D are similar and interact with each other.
- The nutrients usually implicated in immunocompetence are vitamin E and selenium. Furthermore, vitamin E and selenium may modulate animal health by their antioxidative properties resulting in a lower oxidative stress.
- Dietary *L*-carnitine supplementation appears to exert an immunomodulatory effect on antigen-specific total IgG and IgG responses in growing chickens.

### Alternative to Antibiotics and Drugs in Feed: Immunomodulators

In order to reduce or remove antibiotics and other prophylactic drugs in feed, there has been a major search for immunomodulators, which could be administered in feed. However, although some substances have promising potential, the problem of passing undamaged gastrointestinal tract and traversing the intestinal/mucosal barrier remains a question. The mucosa-associated lymphoid tissue with its phagocytic M-cells (Fig. 1.1) seems to play an important role especially for particles and macromolecules. Microfold or M cells are present in Peyer's patches in small intestine. See page 223 of Amino Acids and Immunity Chapter 6.

Nutrients with immunomodulating properties include arginine, glutamine, sulphur amino acids, nucleotides, omega-3 fatty acids, probiotics and prebiotics, glutathione, ornithine, α-ketoglutarate, taurine. Feeds contain a number of immunomodulators including β-glucans and arabino (rhamno)galactans of plant, fungal, yeast or microbial origin, saponins and phenolic derivatives. Beta-glucans are taken up by M-cells in the gut and stimulate macrophages as well as the complement system. Thus selected feed ingredients may enhance or modulate immune response.

## β-glucans as Immunomodulators

Beta-glucans are known as 'biological response modifiers' due to their ability to activate the immune system. The main target of beta-glucans appears to be the monocytes/macrophages, neutrophils and natural killer cells, mediated by 'cell membrane receptors'

(Szabo et al, 1996) (Figs 1.1 and 1.2). Studies with animals have documented significant health benefits from using immune modulating β-1,3/1,6-glucan (from yeast cell walls) as a feed ingredient to protect animals against microorganisms (Williams et al, 1996).

Structural elements of bacteria, such as lipopolysaccharides (LPS; also called endotoxins) are among the most potent immunostimulants. However, they are also very toxic. They cause inflammation, resulting in fever, reduced appetite and impaired performance of animals. β-1,3/1,6-glucan enhances the production of the anti-inflammatory IgA. It down regulates the activity of the pro-inflammatory cytokines (PIC; TNF-α, IL-1, IL-6), which are produced when macrophages are activated by lipopolysaccharides. The immune stimulating activity of different oligosaccharides (e.g. mannanoligosaccharides (MOS) and β-1,3/1,6-glucan products) may vary greatly depending on the degree of branching of the molecule (Fig. 1.2).

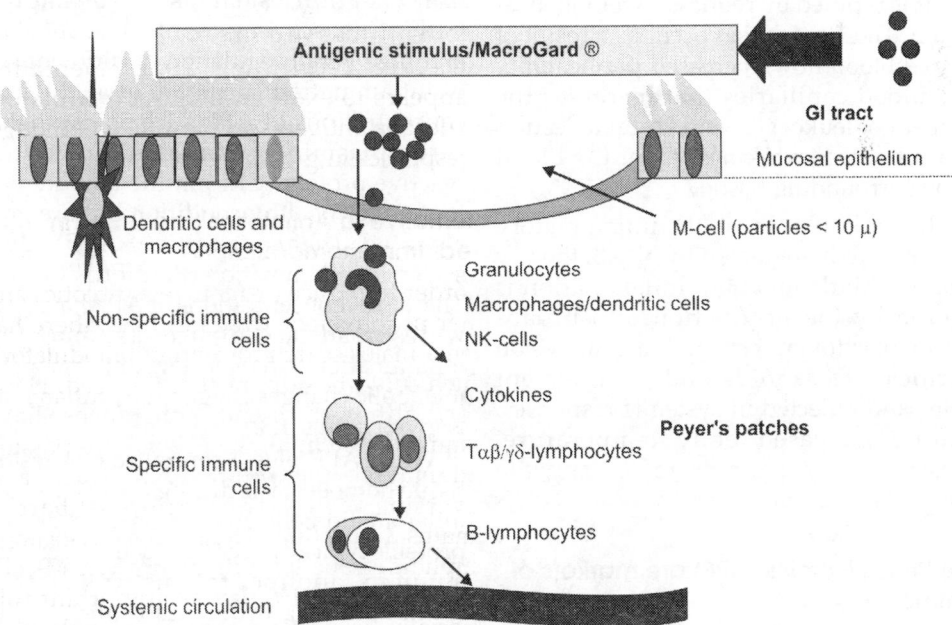

**Fig. 1.1:** The immune cells in the gut and interactions with particles/antigens or immunostimulants (Szabo et al, 1996).

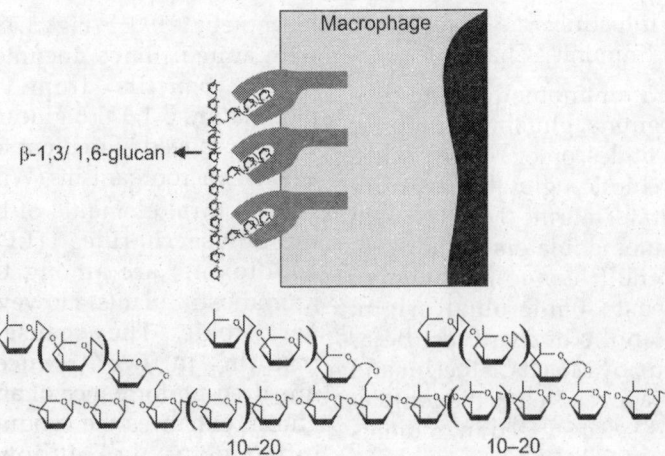

**Fig. 1.2:** Macrophages have special receptors for β-1,3/1,6-glucans (including chemical structure) (Szabo et al, 1996)

## INFECTION AND INFLAMMATORY RESPONSE

### General Significance of Inflammation and its Regulation

Inflammation is the normal, protective and usually temporary response of the innate immune system to eliminate the invading pathogens and toxins and to repair damaged tissue. It is typified by redness, swelling, heat and pain. These responses occur as a result of increased blood flow, increased permeability across blood capillaries that increases the movement of leukocytes and large molecules (e.g. antibodies, cytokines) from the blood into the surrounding tissue.

At the molecular level, the inflammatory process is mainly regulated by NFκB, the key regulator of inflammation. Inflammation is triggered by the production of a broad-spectrum of cytokines, chemokines, adhesion molecules, eicosanoids and complement proteins and reflected in systemic responses, including increased body temperature, increased heart rate and decreased appetite (Bradford et al, 2015).

### Acute Phase Proteins (APP) are markers of inflammation

Acute phase response (APR) occurs mainly in the liver which is one important secondary response to inflammation. This is mainly triggered by pro-inflammatory cytokines (PIC) such as interleukin (IL)-6, IL-1, tumour necrosis factor-α (TNF-α) or IL-1β. Acute phase response is characterised by an increased production of more than 200 acute-phase proteins (APP). APPs play major roles in several aspects of systemic reaction to inflammation, such as opsonisation of pathogens, scavenging of toxic substances and the overall regulation of different stages of inflammation (Ceciliani et al, 2012). The concentrations of APP such as haptoglobin, ceruloplasmin, serum amyloid A and C-reactive protein (CRP) in the blood are very low under healthy condition but are greatly elevated (hence positive APP) during systemic inflammation (Bradford et al, 2015). Therefore, concentrations of APP have gained widespread acceptance as markers of inflammation. An overview of hormonal and metabolic changes triggered by inflammation is given in Fig. 1.3.

While APP play a central role in restoring tissue homoeostasis during the early phase of inflammation, the production of several other proteins typically secreted by the liver such as albumin, apolipoproteins, transferrin or retinol-binding protein is reduced (hence negative APP) during inflammation. The amino acids (from muscle protein breakdown) are utilised partially for gluconeogenesis and the production of APP (Ceciliani et al, 2012).

## Metabolic Alterations

Metabolic alterations are imperative to meet the extraordinary energetic costs of increasing body temperature (fever) and expanding immune responses. These metabolic alterations are regulated in the hypothalamus during a pro-inflammatory condition. The aim is to shift energy and amino acids towards metabolic responses that support the immune system.

i. **Increased proteolysis in skeletal muscle** during inflammation is mediated by an activation of the ubiquitin proteasome

system (UPS). The activation of the UPS is mainly due to increased concentrations of glucocorticoids as a result of the activation of the hypothalamic-pituitary axis in the brain during pro-inflammatory conditions. Cytokines such IL-1, IL-6 or TNF-α are also able to directly activate the UPS in skeletal muscle. Further, they inhibit the anabolic effects of insulin on skeletal muscle (Klasing and Johnstone, 1991). Increased glucocorticoid secretion stimulates gluconeogenesis to supply immune cells with fuels. Many immune cells, such as neutrophils and macrophages, rely heavily on glucose to meet their increased metabolic demands during inflammation (Bradford et al, 2015).

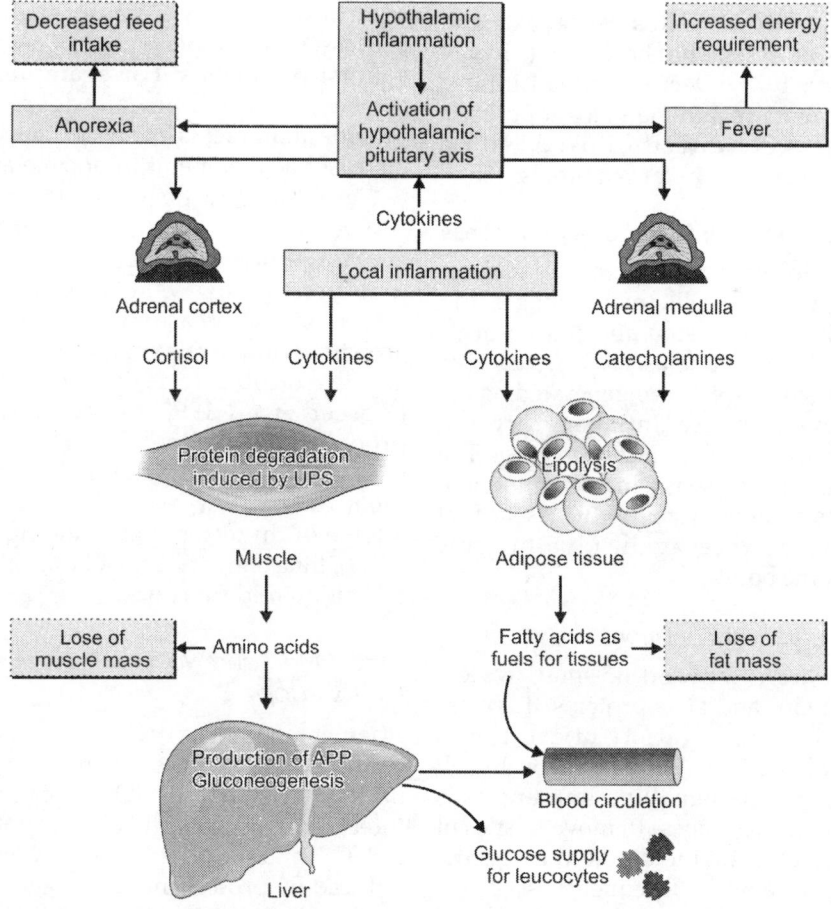

**Fig. 1.3:** A Simplified overview of the hormonal and metabolic changes triggered by inflammation (*Source*: D.K. Gessner et al, 2017).

ii. **An increased rate of lipolysis**, induced by an increased secretion of catecholamines— a process that is also controlled in the hypothalamus—is another metabolic alteration. This aims to supply the body with metabolic fuels to meet the higher energy need.

## Anorexia

Anorexia is negatively linked with animal performance. The loss of appetite in sick animals is an organised, evolved strategy that facilitates recovery. Systemic inflammation causes a shift of the anabolic–catabolic balance towards catabolism meaning that animals have a lower requirement of energy and nutrients for anabolic processes. Indeed, it has been shown that survival of infected animals is positively related to anorexia and weight loss, at least in the short-term (Murray and Murray, 1979). Decreased feed intake, increased energy requirement, loss of muscle and fat mass are directly linked with a reduced performance in farm animals.

## Immune Response—Inflammatory Response

Consequent to entry of pathogen (i.e. disease challenge), immune cells (macrophages and neutrophils) get activated and free radicals [reactive oxygen species (ROS), reactive nitrogen species (RNS)] are generated as the first immune response. Inflammatory response is a reflection of immune response. The inflammatory response is a major component of the innate immune system, which is the first line of the defence against pathogenic invasion of the body.

### Cytokines and their Functions

Cytokines are composed of small water-soluble proteins and glycoproteins. They are produced in a wide variety of cell types, including blood cells. They function in cell signalling, such as signalling immune cells (e.g. T cells, macrophages) to move to sites of infection. Each cytokine binds to a specific 'cell-surface receptor'; subsequent cascades of intracellular signalling then alter cell functions, including up-regulation and/or

down-regulation of genes or transcription factors.

Pro-inflammatory cytokines (PIC; e.g. IL-1, TNF-$\alpha$, IL-6, IL-8 and INF-$\alpha$) are produced. Other inflammatory chemicals include histamine and bradykinins are also released. The concentrations of acute phase proteins (APP) such as C-reactive protein (CRP) increase in the plasma. They regulate the production of inflammatory cytokines. Their concentration in plasma is elevated during chronic inflammatory state. That is why they are referred as positive APP (posAPP).

**Effects of cytokine production:** The production of cytokines initiates events that assist the body in warding off a bacterial or viral invasion. In this direction, nutrients are repartitioned away from normal metabolic processes to pathways that bolster defence against pathogens. For example, there is increased muscle protein degradation to provide amino acids for energy metabolism to increase body temperature and metabolic rate.

Cytokines can influence the endocrine system by modifying the release of hormones affecting hormone receptors or secondary messenger pathways. For example, TNF-$\alpha$ results in a decrease in responsiveness to growth hormone releasing hormone (GHRH) and thyrotropin releasing hormone (TRH) (Elasser et al, 1997); hence growth and productivity decline. GHRH functions in release of growth hormone and prolactin from the pituitary, whereas TRH stimulates the release of thyrotropin stimulating hormone (TSH), thus regulating metabolic rate, growth and all thyroid functions.

### Nitric Oxide and Nuclear Transcription Factor Kappa B

Another inflammatory chemical is nitric oxide (NO), which is synthesised from L-arginine by nitric oxide synthase (NOS). This enzyme has three forms: neuronal (nNOS), endothelial cell (ecNOS) and inducible forms (iNOS). iNOS is induced by pro-inflammatory agents such as bacterial endotoxins (e.g. bacterial lipopoly-saccharide, LPS) and the cytokines. Enhanced formation of NO following induction of iNOS is a component of inflammation. Cytokine stimulation of iNOS involves stimulated production of nuclear transcription factor kappa B (NFκB).

NFκB is a transcription factor (transcription is transfer of genetic code from DNA to produce RNA) that is involved in the stimulation of synthesis of acute phase proteins (APP). NFκB binds to a number of gene promoters in the nucleus and activates transcription of genes involved in the inflammatory response. NFκB is also involved in the expression of cytokines and other factors necessary for immunologic expression. It exists in an inactive form in the cytosol and upon activation, it is translocated to the nucleus via cytokines such as IL-1 produced in inflammatory events.

## Inflammatory Response and Consequences of Pro-inflammatory Activity

i. **Host cell damage:** During disease challenges, the first immune response of the animal involves generation of free radicals (e.g. superoxide anion is produced by a one-electron reduction of molecular oxygen) by macrophages and neutrophils to kill the pathogen. In acute and chronic inflammation, the production of superoxide is increased such that it overwhelms the capacity of superoxide dismutase (SOD) to remove it. Superoxide has beneficial effects in fighting pathogenic invasion. But it also reacts with NO to produce peroxynitrite, which has pro-inflammatory activity. These reactive oxygen species (ROS) are effective not only in destroying invading pathogens but also cause host cell damage. Thus host pathology is an inevitable consequence of disease fighting by the immune system.

ii. **Reduction in feed intake:** An invariable effect of pro-inflammatory activity in fighting disease is a reduction in feed intake. About 70% of the decrease in growth rate that accompanies an inflammatory response is due to reduced feed intake, while 30% is due to inefficiencies in nutrient absorption and metabolism. Dantzer (2001) coined the term 'cytokine-induced sickness behaviour' to describe the non-specific symptoms of infection and inflammation that include weakness, malaise, listlessness, inability to concentrate, depression, lethargy and anorexia. IL-1 is an important cytokine for the induction of sickness behaviour. In animals with subclinical infection, the changes may be subtle, but there can be a reduction in feed intake and a shift in the partitioning of dietary nutrients away from skeletal muscle accretion to metabolic responses that support the immune system (Johnson, 1997).

iii. **Production of inflammatory eicosanoids:** The $PG_2$ series and $TX_2$ series of eicosanoids are inflammatory agents produced in response to immunostimulation. They are synthesised by the cyclooxygenase (COX) pathway. There are two major COX isoenzymes, COX1 and COX2. See Figs 7.4 and 7.7 in Chapter 7.

## Anti-inflammatory Drugs and Dietary Supplements

a. Aspirin and other non-steroidal anti-inflammatory drugs (NSAID) inhibit COX enzyme activity.

b. *Yucca schidigera* products, which are used as feed additives, inhibit NO formation and have anti-inflammatory activity (Marzocco et al, 2004) and inhibit COX activity (Wenzig et al, 2008). Yucca contains resveratrol, a polyphenolic anti-inflammatory agent (Oleszek et al, 2001). Resveratrol, also abundant in grape skins and red wine, inhibits COX enzymes and NO formation.

c. Omega-3 fatty acids have anti-inflammatory properties when provided in optimal proportions with omega-6 fatty acids. Both n-3 and n-6 fatty acids are precursors of eicosanoids, including prostaglandins (PG), thromboxanes (TX) and leukotrienes (LT). The n-6 fatty acids produce eicosanoids that have (pro-) inflammatory properties, while the eicosanoids synthesised from the n-3 series of fatty acids (EPA, DHA) have anti-inflammatory properties (Simopoulos, 2002). The inflammatory properties of n-6 fatty acids are attributed to arachidonic acid. EPA competitively inhibits the production of inflammatory prostaglandins and leukotrienes by competing as a substrate for COX enzymes and 5-lipoxygenase (Simopoulos, 2002).

In dogs, n-3 fatty acids are used as dietary supplements to control inflammatory responses. Dietary supplements of cod liver oil, a source of n-3 fatty acids, reduce the severity of rheumatoid arthritis in humans (Galarraga et al, 2008).

## Immune Stimulation/Activation and Animal Performance

Stimulation of the immune system can be a negative factor in livestock and poultry production because nutrients are diverted from growth to formation of immune-components such as cytokines, acute phase proteins and antibody proteins. The result is a negative effect on growth even if the immune system is responding to a mild or slight pathogenic threat. The main factor responsible for growth inhibition, as mentioned earlier, is a depression in feed intake associated with an inflammatory response (Klasing, 1988).

## Rationale Behind Segregated Early Weaning

The segregated early weaning (SEW at 14–17 days of age) system of pig production was developed to avoid the growth-depressing effects of an immune response. The SEW system is based on weaning the piglets while maternal antibody protection is at its peak and then moving the piglets to an isolated and clean housing facility to prevent disease exposure and activation of the immune system. For the first 2–3 weeks of life, the baby pig has passive immunity obtained via maternal antibodies in the mother's colostrum. However, this immunity is limited only to the antigens to which the mother was exposed prior to farrowing.

This SEW system minimises the young pigs' exposure to diseases (antigens), which also minimises the activation of their immune system. Activation of the immune system by exposure to antigens reduces growth performance of the pig, because nutrients are diverted from growth to the synthesis of cytokines and other components of the immune system. Thus, preventing the activation of pig's immune system by minimising its exposure to antigens result in more efficient nutrient utilisation for growth.

Pigs raised in the SEW system have higher amino acid requirements (because of higher lean muscle) than conventionally reared pigs and the diets should contain protein sources with highly digestible amino acids (Bergstrom et al, 1997). The advantages of the SEW system are maintained throughout the entire growth period with increased growth rate, feed conversion efficiency and carcass leanness.

## Effects of Immune System Activation on Nutrient Metabolism

Nutritional effects of cytokine production and the mechanisms by which pro-inflammatory cytokines inhibit growth are summarised by several workers (Johnson, 1997; Johnson et al, 1997 and Klasing, 1988). Energy, protein, lipid, carbohydrate and mineral metabolism are all negatively impacted.

## Repartitioning of Nutrients

The repartitioning of nutrients may be a defence mechanism against invading pathogens: (i) For example, a pathogen challenge causes a shift in iron from transferrin in the extracellular fluids to intracellular ferritin. Decreased plasma iron lowers the proliferation and virulence of pathogens. Lactoferrin is a glycoprotein in milk that has antimicrobial and anti-inflammatory properties (Wu et al, 2007) by virtue of its ability to scavenge free iron, thus depriving microbes of this nutrient. (ii) In poultry, biotin is sequestered bound to avidin during an inflammatory response, preventing bacteria from acquiring biotin. Providing extra water-soluble vitamins to poultry undergoing disease challenge may actually be providing nutrients to the pathogens rather than to the host.

Various endocrine hormones and cytokine signals participate in redirecting nutrient use away from growth-related processes to immune function during disease stress (Elasser et al, 1997). According to Elasser et al. (1997), 'In an intricate interplay, hormones and cytokines regulate, modify and modulate each other's production and tissue interactions to alter metabolic priorities.' Dietary protein and energy intakes affect blood patterns of hormones and cytokines after disease challenge. Growth hormone has a regulatory role on cytokine production during disease stress (Elasser et al, 1997).

## Association Between Inflammatory/ Immunologic Disorders and Metabolic Disorders

Infections of the mammary gland (mastitis) and uterus (metritis) are common sources of inflammation in lactating dairy cows, particularly near the periparturient period (Waldron et al, 2006). Hence, there may be associations between immunologic disorders and metabolic problems such as ketosis and milk fever. To investigate this possibility, Waldron et al. (2006) produced experimental mastitis by administering *E. coli* LPS into the mammary tissue of early-lactation cows. Acute mastitis did not induce ketosis, but rather increased glucose synthesis by the liver and decreased plasma non-esterified fatty acids (NEFA) and ketone bodies. However, acute mastitis induced by LPS markedly depressed plasma calcium (Waldron et al, 2003) suggesting a possible association of milk fever with mastitis.

## Anti-inflammatory Effects of Growth Promoter Antibiotics

Antibiotics have been used at sub-therapeutic concentrations (below the minimum inhibitory concentration for pathogens) as antimicrobial growth promoters (AGP) for many years. Despite their widespread use, their mode of action in promoting growth has not been conclusively identified. Klasing (1988) proposed that antibiotics may alter intestinal microflora to reduce the production of immunogens that provoke an immune response. Antibiotics may thus act by reducing the microbial burden of the animal, providing greater nutrient availability for growth. It is well known that the antibiotic growth response is greater in a dirty environment than in a hygienic one, supporting the hypothesis that microbial burden is involved.

Niewold (2007) refutes the hypothesis that the intestinal microflora depresses growth and proposed that AGP have a target that is not the intestinal microflora. Antibiotics have been demonstrated to inhibit intestinal inflammatory activity, such as production of pro-inflammatory cytokines and ROS. Niewold (2007) has proposed a new explanation for the antibiotic growth response based on anti-inflammatory activity. At least four major mechanisms have been proposed to explain AGP-mediated growth enhancement:

1. AGP inhibit intestinal microbes that produce immunogens (substances that elicit an immune response), thus reducing the metabolic costs of the innate immune system (Klasing, 1988).
2. AGP reduce growth-depressing metabolites such as ammonia and bile acid degradation products produced by microbes.
3. AGP reduce microbial use of nutrients.
4. AGP enhance the uptake and utilisation of nutrients due to thinning of the intestinal mucosa.

Thus Niewold (2007) concludes that AGP inhibit intestinal inflammation reducing the acute phase response and obviating a shift in nutrients away from growth. Intestinal inflammation leads to an accumulation of inflammatory cells in the mucosa leading to a thicker intestinal wall. The thinner intestinal wall when AGP are fed is consistent with reduced inflammation.

## MECHANISMS OF NUTRIENT IMMUNOMODULATION; CRITICAL PERIODS AND NUTRIENT PRIORITY OF IMMUNE SYSTEM DEVELOPMENT

### Mechanisms of Nutrient Immunomodulation

A substance that modulates the immune response is immunomodulator. Nutrition can influence an animal's ability to mount an immune response and resist infectious diseases. Therefore, it is important for nutritionists to understand the mechanisms of nutrient immunomodulation.

The majority of nutritional immunology research has examined the impact of nutrition on immunity. The major mechanisms responsible for this immunomodulation have been identified (Table 1.1) and are discussed briefly below.

**Mechanism 1:** Nutrients can regulate the immune response directly by altering leukocyte communication pathways and the transcription profile of many genes involved in the coordination of immune responses. Polyunsaturated fatty acids are perhaps the best example of nutrients that directly regulate the immune response, since they alter signal transduction pathways and regulate gene expression. Fatty acids located within the plasma membranes are utilised as substrates for the generation of signalling molecules involved in directing cellular responses. Changing the fatty acid composition of leukocyte plasma membranes can alter the types of communication molecules produced (see Chapter 6 Fatty acids and Immunity) and the ability of the immune system to eliminate certain pathogens.

For example, the types of communication molecules produced from n-3 and n-6 fatty acids can alter resistance to infectious diseases. Feeding increased levels of n-3 fatty acids to chicken improves the primary antibody response titer, decreases the release of IL-1 from macrophages and alters the expression of cytokine genes.

Fat-soluble vitamins are direct modulators of leukocytes. Vitamin E enhances antibody titers, lymphocyte proliferation and alters the type of immune response elicited by altering the production of inflammatory cytokine genes in chickens. In general, the immuno-modulatory properties of these nutrients are achieved when their levels in the diet are included beyond their requirement for growth.

**Mechanism 2:** Nutrients also modulate immunity by minimising the severity of pathology caused by the killing compounds synthesised and released by leukocytes upon exposure to pathogens. Since many of these killing molecules are reactive oxygen species (ROS), the antioxidant vitamins E and C and selenium play an important role in minimising pathology associated with free radical damage. This explains why the requirement for some antioxidants is greater during an inflammatory response.

**Mechanism 3:** The gut is the largest lymphoid tissue in the body and therefore

**Table 1.1:** Mechanisms of nutrient immunomodulation (*Adapted from* Humphrey and Klasing, 2004)

| Sl. No. | Mechanism | Examples |
|---------|-----------|----------|
| 1. | Modulating signal transduction and immunity genes in leukocytes | PUFAs, vitamins A, D and E |
| 2. | Protecting against immunopathology | Antioxidants |
| 3. | Influencing intestinal dynamics | Fibre, prebiotics, probiotics |
| 4. | Influencing hormonal milieu | Feeding regime, glucocorticoids |
| 5. | Denying critical nutrients to pathogens | Iron (mammals); biotin (birds) |
| 6. | Substrate for the immune system | Amino acids, trace minerals, water soluble vitamins |

represents an attractive target for modulating immunity. Gut-associated lymphoid tissue (GALT) is the immune system within the gastrointestinal tract (GIT) located in the lymphoid tissue. GALT can be modulated by feeding supplements of live microorganisms, i.e. probiotics, or complex carbohydrates that stimulate the growth of certain microorganisms, i.e. prebiotics. Feeding probiotics and prebiotics (synbiotics) has resulted in improved gut health and increased enteric and systemic immune responses to specific pathogens. Though the exact mechanism of how probiotics and prebiotics alter immunity is unclear, their use has been shown to improve humoral, cellular and innate immunity. A better understanding of the mechanisms responsible for their immunomodulatory effects is needed.

**Mechanism 4:** An animal's hormonal profile is influenced by the feeding regime along with the nutrient density of the diet. Changes in the hormonal profile influence immunity, since leukocytes have a number of these hormone receptors expressed on their plasma membrane. Plasma glucocorticoid levels increase in response to feed restriction and fasting and this hormone has dramatic effects on developing lymphocytes. The glucocorticoid corticosterone increases the rate of apoptosis of developing B and T lymphocytes and also alters the cytokine profile to promote cell-mediated immunity over humoral immunity.

**Mechanism 5:** Some nutrients are the limiting substrates for pathogen survival. In mammals, iron is the first limiting one for pathogen growth and during times of infection this metal is sequestered by iron binding proteins in an attempt to limit microbial growth. A shift in iron from transferrin in the extracellular fluids to intracellular ferritin decreases plasma iron level. Iron may not be the first limiting nutrient for microbes in all species. It has been shown that biotin is first limiting and iron is second limiting for the growth of *Salmonella typhimurium*. In birds the sequestered biotin is bound to avidin. Thus

pathogenic bacteria are prevented from acquiring biotin.

**Mechanism 6:** The immune system requires a supply of nutrients sufficient to meet its metabolic needs. Inadequate supply of those nutrients can result in impairment in immunity and increase susceptibility to infectious diseases. This has been well-documented by examining the effect of nutrient deficiencies on the immune system. For example, a zinc deficient diet reduces the number of developing T lymphocytes, leading to decreased peripheral T lymphocytes and compromised T lymphocyte mediated immunity (Fraker, 2000). Much less is known, however, when considering the amount of a nutrient that is sufficient or required for a particular process of the immune system, such as the development of lymphocytes.

*1. Immune System Development in Chicken*

a. **Periods of critical nutrient need: Adaptive immunity:** The adaptive immune system consists of B and T lymphocytes. They generate antigen specificity through the development of their antigen receptors within primary immune tissues. In chickens, B lymphocytes develop their antigen specificity in the 'bursa' and T lymphocytes develop their antigen specificity in the 'thymus'. Consequently, lymphocyte development within primary immune tissues is crucial for adaptive immunity, since these events produce antigen-specific and immunocompetent B and T lymphocytes. Development of both B and T lymphocytes is initiated during embryogenesis and continues posthatch. These progenitor cells undergo rapid proliferative and gene rearrangement events within their respective organs in order to produce their lymphocyte population.

For the adaptive immune system, an uninterrupted and sufficient supply of nutrients is critical for developing lymphocytes within primary immune tissues. Nutrient supply is particularly critical between embryonic day 15 to six weeks posthatch in chicken for developing B lymphocytes and embryonic day 6.5 to three weeks posthatch for developing T lymphocytes.

*Contrasts in the development of B and T lymphocytes reflect in timing of critical nutrient supply:* The different periods of critical nutrient need between B and T lymphocytes is primarily related to the contrasts in their development.

i. The majority of T lymphocyte development occurring *in ovo* suggests that embryonic nutrition may contribute more than posthatch nutrition to the development of T lymphocytes. Furthermore, the thymus produces a sufficient quantity and diversity of T lymphocytes for cell-mediated immunity during embryogenesis, since removing the thymus at hatch does not eliminate cell-mediated immunity in later life.

ii. The majority of B lymphocyte development occurring posthatch suggests that posthatch nutrition may contribute more than *in ovo* nutrition to the development of B lymphocytes. The majority of B lymphocyte production by the bursa occurs posthatch and removal of the bursa at hatch permanently impairs humoral immunity. Consequently, it is crucial that developing B and T lymphocytes receive an uninterrupted supply of nutrients. Regarding timing of supply, **uninterrupted nutrient supply for T lymphocytes may be most critical during embryogenesis, while uninterrupted nutrient supply for B lymphocytes may be most critical posthatch.**

*Production of effector cells/memory lymphocytes: Lymphocyte activation:* This is another period of critical nutrient need when lymphocytes encounter their cognate antigen. The lymphocytes specific to the pathogen begin to proliferate rapidly within specialised regions of secondary immune tissue to produce effector cells

responsible for the elimination of the specific pathogen (Goldsby et al, 2003). These proliferative events last for several days after initial contact with antigen. Memory lymphocytes are also produced during this process and are responsible for the rapid adaptive immune response observed upon repeated exposure to the same antigen. Therefore, lymphocyte activation is another period of critical need as these antigen specific cells expand their numbers to fend off the invading pathogen.

b. **Periods of critical nutrient need: Innate immunity:** The innate immune system is responsible for protecting the host during the initial stages of infection. The innate immune system consists of constitutive defences, such as phagocytic cells, epithelial barriers, secretions and preformed protective molecules, which act as barriers to pathogen invasion. Cells of the innate immune system do not undergo proliferative events (unlike lymphocytes) within primary immune tissues and all dividing cells are functional (Goldsby et al, 2003). This suggests that the development of the innate immune system may not be a critical period of nutrient need, especially compared to that of developing lymphocytes.

*Activation of innate immune system is a critical period:* Upon activation, however, the innate immune system becomes anabolic, resulting in the synthesis and secretion of protective proteins and killing compounds that function to eradicate the invading pathogen. The synthesis of these protective proteins, such as acute phase proteins (APP) by the liver, and killing compounds, such as nitric oxide (NO) by macrophages, require additional nutrients. Therefore, activation of the innate immune system is a critical period of nutrient need. The innate immune system has no immunological memory to antigens, so repeat antigen exposure results in an innate immune response similar in magnitude to the initial response. Consequently, the nutrient need for the activated innate immune system will be similar for each encounter with the same antigen.

## 2. Nutrient Priority of the Immune System

Allocation of nutrients to tissues is dependent upon the physiological state of the animal. Tissues differ in their priority for nutrients based upon their metabolic rate (Hammond, 1944), yet the position of the immune system within this nutrient priority scheme is only speculative (Fig. 1.4) (Humphrey, 2005). As mentioned earlier, there are certain periods where nutrient supply is critical for the proper development and function of the immune system. The immune system must be able to acquire nutrients at the appropriate times and amounts to ensure protective immunity.

**Mechanisms to Ensure Nutrient Supply:** One mechanism of ensuring nutrient supply to meet these metabolic needs is through unique changes in the types and amounts of nutrient transporter expression. Nutrient transporters permit substrate specific uptake and can be used as a marker for evaluating a tissue's ability to acquire a specific nutrient. For example, **the bursa has a greater ability to obtain lysine and arginine than the thymus.** Furthermore, **developing lymphocytes contain exclusively high affinity lysine and arginine transporters** that allow for the transport of these essential amino acids at maximum velocity. These types of comparisons will allow for the identification of components of the immune system that are most susceptible to nutrient supply.

## 3. Critical Substrates for the Immune System

While all essential nutrients are critical for the immune system, some essential and even nonessential nutrients appear to be of

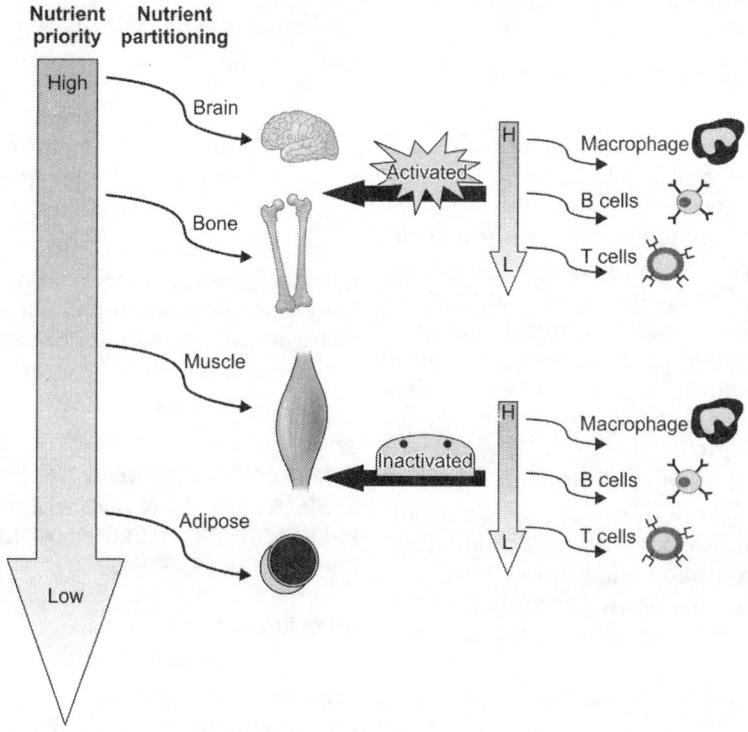

**Fig. 1.4:** Priority of nutrient use by various tissues based upon their metabolic rate (*Adapted from* Hammond, 1944). On the right side are proposed sites where the immune system and leukocyte populations are thought to reside within the nutrient priority framework during both activated and inactivated states

particular importance for cells of the immune system. The identification of these critical nutrients has stemmed from an understanding of their metabolism in various leukocyte populations. In chickens, nutrient metabolism in leukocytes has not been well characterised, while the critical nutrients for cells of the immune system have been identified in the context of mammalian metabolism.

There are major differences in the metabolism of certain nutrients between chickens and mammals, e.g. arginine and glucose, which are of particular importance to cells of the immune system and this may have implications for avian immunity. Nonetheless, the immune system appears to have a critical need for nutrients that produce important metabolites involved in immunological processes. Some examples of metabolic products generated from amino acid and energy substrates that are important for the immune system are discussed briefly here.

## Amino Acid substrates—Arginine and Cysteine

Chickens are uricotelic and have a dietary requirement for arginine. In addition to being used as a substrate for protein synthesis, arginine can be metabolised to produce nitric oxide (NO) and polyamines. Nitric oxide is involved in inflammatory responses, while polyamines are involved in wound healing. In mammals, arginine plays an integral role in the development of B lymphocytes and also regulates the signalling ability of T lymphocytes.

Cysteine can be metabolised to produce glutathione (GSH). GSH is one of the major intracellular antioxidants and its production is regulated by the availability of cysteine. GSH production increases during periods of inflammation (Malmezat et al, 2000); consequently a greater proportion of cysteine metabolism is directed toward GSH synthesis. GSH plays an important role in leukocyte function and these cells have a strong ability to obtain cysteine.

## Energy Substrates—Glucose and Glutamine

Energy metabolism is of particular importance to lymphocytes since their development and activation involve rapid proliferation. Cells of the innate immune system also have an energy demand, though this is assumed to be not of the same magnitude as lymphocytes. Leukocytes primarily utilise glucose and glutamine as an energy source (Ardawi and Newsholme, 1985).

Glucose is the fuel of choice for lymphocytes and in mammals glucose is actually an essential nutrient for lymphocytes. Glucose is also important for generating reducing equivalents through the pentose phosphate pathway. These reducing equivalents are essential for producing killing compounds involved in the macrophage respiratory burst. Second to glucose, glutamine is also a major energy substrate for leukocytes.

Glutamine metabolism can also (like glucose) generate reducing equivalents necessary for the production of ROS. Glutamine conversion to glutamate may also aid in the transport of amino acids, since glutamate is a substrate for many amino acid transport exchange systems (Aledo, 2004).

Identifying and determining the nutrient needs of the immune system is important, since this information will allow nutritionists to formulate diets that contain nutrients in appropriate levels, which are optimum for immunocompetence.

## INTERACTIONS BETWEEN THE IMMUNE SYSTEM, NUTRITION AND ANIMAL PRODUCTIVITY; NUTRITIONAL MODULATION OF IMMUNE RESPONSE

### Introduction

The interactions between nutrition and immunity are particularly important to animal growth and productivity (Fig. 1.5). The immune system can influence animal growth by altering (1) metabolic homeostasis and

(2) the efficiency and rate at which nutrients are used for growth and other productive processes. For example, nutrition modulates the immune system and immune responses modulate nutritional needs. Understanding the interaction between nutrition and immune responses allows animal producers and nutritionists to develop and implement feeding strategies that maximise animal productivity and welfare, while minimising the incidence of infectious diseases (Humphrey, 2005). Such feeding strategies ultimately reduce the cost of animal products to the consumers.

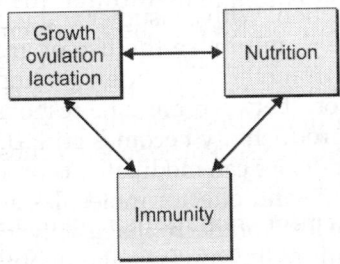

**Fig. 1.5:** Nutrition interacts with the physiological processes involved in immune function, growth and reproduction

### Genetic Selection and Productivity

It is known that many immune responses are associated with decreased growth and productivity. It has been reported that intense genetic selection for higher growth potential led to greater susceptibility to infectious disease. This negative correlation between immunity and productivity has been observed in several research studies. Selection for a high antibody response to 'sheep red blood cells (SRBC)' over 24 generations resulted in a 15% decrease in growth rate (Yang et al, 2000). Conversely, selecting chickens or turkeys for high growth rates has resulted in impaired immunocompetence and disease resistance and altered pro-inflammatory cytokine (PIC) release (Bayyari et al, 1997; Li et al, 1999). This situation demands the need for nutritional approaches to optimise immunocompetence.

### The Systemic Immune Response in Brief

*Recognition of the Pathogen*

The immune system functions to recognise the presence of macromolecules of non-self origin. Lymphocytes primarily recognise protein antigens through their 'cell surface receptors' (e.g. membrane bound immunoglobulin), while phagocytes (such as macrophages and neutrophils) recognise lipid and carbohydrate antigens through their 'surface pattern receptors'. Antigen recognition results in leukocyte activation, cytokine secretion and the engagement of effector mechanisms directed at removal of the pathogen. The PICs act as communication molecules between immune cells and other cells of the body. Secretion of these cytokines occurs rapidly and reaches systematically relevant levels within a few hours after an infectious challenge; they act locally to regulate the immune response. Anti-inflammatory regulators counterbalance the pro-inflammatory cytokines. In addition, some dietary factors can regulate the production of PIC and anti-inflammatory regulators.

### Nutrient Repartitioning

Immune system is capable of repartitioning of nutrients for cell proliferation and effector molecule production. In a homeorhetic response driven by elevated systematic levels of PIC, nutrients are redirected from anabolic pathways (related to growth, skeletal muscle accretion or reproduction) towards pathways that bolster defence against pathogens. For example, nutrient repartitioning results in an increased rate of protein turnover, which leads to increased body temperature and basal metabolic rate. In addition, accelerated protein degradation may augment host defence by increasing proteosome activity and, therefore, enhancing expression of peptide fragments from intracellular proteins on MHC class II molecules. This process permits greater detection of intracellular pathogens and is illustrative of the heightened vigilance and activity of the immune system induced by a generalised stress state.

In some tissues, such as skeletal muscle, increased proteolysis is not matched by augmented protein synthesis causing decreased tissue accretion that is manifested as impaired growth in young animals or negative nitrogen balance in mature animals. Nutrient repartitioning occurs not only with protein and amino acids, but also with virtually every other essential nutrient.

## Effect of an Immune Response on Animal Productivity

1. **Lesser performance:** An immune response can affect production by way of altering metabolism, altering hormone production, inducing pathology, etc. mechanisms (Klasing and Johnstone, 1991). Sick animals grow slower and less efficiently, miss ovulations, or produce less milk. Major component for lesser productivity is due to the cost of immune response *per se*.

2. **Appetite depressing effect:** The immune response causes an overall change in the metabolism and behaviour of an animal. One of the most devastating impacts of this metabolic perturbance on animal performance is decreased feed intake (Johnson, 1998). The appetite depressing effect has been attributed to the effects of the pro-inflammatory cytokines. By altering the hormonal profile of an animal, an immune response can effectively reduce growth rates and reproductive performance (McCann et al, 1998). Clearly, the immune response can be quite detrimental to production systems where weight gain is critical for profitability.

3. **Damage to the host tissue:** The immune response can also inflict damage to host tissue and this pathology is often necessary to eliminate pathogen. For example, during the innate immune response, macrophages are activated to destroy invading pathogens. The macrophages respond to cytokines and other effector molecules by producing antimicrobial factors, including reactive oxygen species and proteases. These mediators effectively destroy invading pathogens. While doing so, damage to host tissue inevitably results as a consequence of disease.

## Good Management and Feeding Practices Minimise the Incidence of Infectious Diseases

Farm management systems, therefore, are geared toward minimising the incidence of infectious diseases through practices such as vaccination and rigorous biosecurity programmes. Feeding growth-promoting levels of antibiotics diminishes challenges from opportunistic and commensal bacteria and consequently improves rates and efficiencies of production. With consumer and legislative pressure to minimise the use of antibiotic growth promoters, an understanding of the connections between immune responses and animal productivity becomes critical. Nutritional strategies can modulate the production of cytokine and effector molecules and thus affect the level of macrophage activation and tissue pathology. However, the elimination of disease is the only mechanism by which this pathology can be completely prevented.

## Effect of an Immune Response on Nutrient Requirements of the Animal

Most research on nutrient requirements of animals is conducted in government-approved facilities that have the appropriate levels of sanitation and pathogen exclusion,which cannot be accomplished in the 'real-world-field' conditions. Consequently, the minimal nutrient requirements summarised in the various National Research Council (NRC) and ICAR or ARC publications may not be relevant to on-farm conditions, where there is a prevalence of sub-clinical infection and hence pathogenic challenges are frequent. Clearly, it is of practical importance to understand the impact of these challenges on nutrient requirements.

The immune system must compete with growth and reproductive processes for nutrients and is a component of the maintenance costs of an animal. When the immune system is engaged in defence against a pathogen, its nutrient demands are increased. Those nutrients are used as substrates for the clonal proliferation of responding lymphocytes, the production of antibodies and the hepatic secretion of acute phase proteins (APP). Among these processes, production of APP quantitatively appears to be the most nutritionally demanding process. The immune system development, maintenance and use require nutrients and these nutrients must ultimately originate from the diet.

Understanding the impact of infection on nutrient requirements is complicated by the fact that each disease strain inflicts its own unique pathologies that have differing consequences for nutrient requirements. For example, organisms that cause enteric pathology might be expected to have a large impact on digestion and absorption of nutrients, while the organisms that inflict liver or kidney damage disproportionately impact nutrient metabolism. Hence, it is necessary to divide the impact of infection on nutrient requirements into two components: (1) effects due to specific pathology and (2) effects due to the response of the immune system to the pathogen.

The immune response to a pathogen can affect the nutrition of animals by altering digestion, absorption, metabolism and excretion of nutrients, thus affecting substrate availability and dietary requirements.

Components of the immune response increase nutrient use, such as the anabolic components of the immune response (e.g. clonal proliferation of lymphocytes, recruitment of new myeloid cells, and antibody synthesis) as well as APP production by the liver.

Metabolism of a specific nutrient may be altered as a consequence of the immune response. For example, retinol is transported in the blood bound to retinol binding protein (RBP). During an immune response, the synthesis of RBP is dramatically reduced, resulting in decreased retinol in the blood (Rosales et al, 1996). In this situation, transport of a nutrient is altered as a consequence of the acute phase response (APR).

In addition, an immune response can increase the need for some substrates. For example, the energetic cost of fever. Pathogen invasion, phagocytosis, inflammation increases body temperature (e.g. shivering), which increases rates of biochemical reactions. Increased cellular utilisation of ATP due to futile cycling also needs some substrates.

Lower rates of productivity during disease also results in decreased nutrient needs. For example, it has been observed lower lysine requirements during a simulated infectious challenge in growing pigs and chickens.

Some nutrients (e.g. antioxidants) are metabolised in greater amounts during an immune response. Accordingly dietary requirements during the disease state may increase. Many effector mechanisms used by the immune system generate large amounts of reactive oxygen species (ROS). Antioxidants (such as ascorbic acid and vitamin E) protect macromolecules against damage from these ROS. It is evident that the requirements for these antioxidant nutrients are greater during an inflammatory response than the levels required by healthy animals. However, the level of nutrient intake is decreased during an immune response because of appetite depression and in turn less feed intake. Therefore, it may be necessary to increase nutrient intake prior to a disease challenge or vaccination.

Further, immune response affects absorption of carotenoids (responsible for pigmentation of meat and eggs) during aflatoxicosis or coccidiosis in the chicken.

## Nutritional Modulation of Immune Response

The immune response can be modulated by nutrition in several ways:
1. Nutrients provide substrates for proliferation of immune cells and effector molecules. On this basis, the nutritional status of

an animal can dramatically affect the degree of immune cell proliferation and/or effector molecule production.

2. Nutritional status of the developing embryo has profound effects on the development of its immune system.

3. Invading pathogens rely on the host for supply of many nutrients to activate the immune system. Therefore, nutrient deficiency or excess can affect the ability of a pathogen to replicate *in vivo*.

4. In addition, nutrients can be effective as substrates for inter- and intra-cellular communication and their availability may be critical for an effective immune response.

5. The pattern of nutrient intake may affect the endocrine system, which then modulates magnitude, type and/or duration of the immune response.

## Immune System Development Process

The time period during which immune cells differentiate and populate the tissues of the body is relatively long compared to other developmental processes and this process extends well beyond birth. In fact, the high rate of cell proliferation in combination with the complexity of regulatory control over the developmental events is unmatched in any other tissue of the neonate. These developmental processes require a complex series of highly regulated cellular differentiation steps followed by deletion of self-reacting clones of lymphocytes that might cause autoimmunity.

For this reason, a chronic deficiency of virtually any required nutrient during the period of immune system development has negative impacts on immunocompetence. Vitamins A and D are some examples. In general these nutrients are required for regulating cell differentiation. Hence their deficiency is particularly detrimental to the development of immunocompetence.

## Immune System Activation

Nutrition affects not only the development of the immune system, but also the immune response to disease. The resting immune system is probably not very nutritionally demanding, as it contains some of the most inactive cells of the body (e.g. resting lymphocytes). However, activation of the immune system results in some of the most metabolically active and rapidly proliferating cells of the body. This sudden burst of activity is tightly regulated and critical decisions are made at this time regarding the threshold for a response, the magnitude of the response and the types of cells recruited for the response. Nutrients are important in supplying the substrates needed for this rapid rate of cell proliferation and the secretion of effector molecules.

In fact, the pro-inflammatory response orchestrates metabolic changes, such as skeletal muscle catabolism, which provide a source of nutrients for these processes even when dietary intake is insufficient. That means immune system is capable of repartitioning nutrients for cell proliferation and effector molecule production. Similarly, repartitioning of some nutrients occurs as a defence mechanism against invading pathogens.

## Increased Pathogenicity Due to Nutrient Excess

Some nutrients serve as substrates for pathogens and support their proliferation and virulence, e.g. iron. The PIC released during a pathogen challenge mediate a shift in iron from transferrin in the extracellular fluids to ferritin in intracellular locations (Weinberg, 1998). This change decreases the amount of iron available to pathogens and decreases their virulence. In neonatal pigs, excecssive amounts of iron provided through the diet or via injection enhance the proliferation of several types of pathogen (Knight et al, 1983). In birds, biotin is the example.

## Increased Pathogenicity Due to Nutrient Deficiency

A nutrient deficiency may also directly affect pathogens. In mice, a selenium deficiency has been demonstrated to provide a host environment in which a non-virulent strain of coxsackievirus may mutate and become virulent (Beck, 2000). The mechanism for this change in the viral genome seems to be related to antioxidant status, as vitamin E deficiency resulted in similar observations.

## Nutrients that Modulate the Immune Response

1. Many nutrients are directly involved in, or regulate, the intracellular and intercellular communication of leukocytes (Grimble, 1998), i.e. these nutrients modulate communication networks within the immune system. These include vitamins A, D and E, minerals such as iron, volatile fatty acids like butyrate (Klasing and Leshchinsky, 2000).

2. Type of dietary PUFA consumed by an animal is reflected in the PUFA content of cellular membranes in monogastric animals. As PUFAs are precursors for eicosanoid synthesis, including prostaglandins and leukotrienes, the PUFA content of cellular membranes affects the types and amounts of eicosanoids released during an immune response. This change in regulatory environment is reflected in the type of immune response that predominates during an infectious challenge and in the outcome of the infection.

   **Omega-3 PUFA:** Feeding n-3 PUFAs of marine origin, primarily eicosapentaenoic acid (EPA; 20:5 n-3) and docosahexaenoic acid (DHA; 22:6 n-3), results in decreased production of $PGE_2$. Supplementation of EPA results in increased production of $PGE_3$, a less biologically active molecule than $PGE_2$, while enrichment with DHA causes suppression of $PGE_2$ formation via cyclooxygenase inhibition (Chapkin et al, 2000).

   In addition, n-3 PUFAs from marine sources have been shown to reduce IL-12 and IFN-γ release causing a shift from T-helper 1 (Th1) towards Th2 responses. This modulation of the immune response causes increased susceptibility to infections that are controlled by a strong Th1 response, such as *Listeria*, but an increase in resistance controlled by a strong Th2 response, such as *E. coli* sepsis (Fritsche et al, 2000).

   In chickens, feeding diets supplemented with n-3 PUFA significantly decreased the incidence of septicaemia by 25%, but resulted in a 24% increase in the incidence of tumours (Klasing and Leshchinsky, 2000).

3. **Vitamin E:** Reactive oxygen species are responsible for activating transcription factors, such as NFκB, which are involved in the regulation of viral gene expression, cytokine synthesis and the acute inflammatory reactions. Vitamin E and other antioxidants can inhibit the activation of these transcription factors, thus affecting the magnitude of the immune response. In addition to this role, vitamin E can affect arachidonic acid metabolism, thereby affecting the immune response in a similar manner to PUFAs.

## Hormonal Profile Modulates the Immune Response

The amount of diet fed, the pattern of feeding (e.g. single meal versus *ad libitum*) and the ratio between protein and energy in the diet influence the hormone production. The hormonal profile in turn modulates the immune response via leukocytes, which have receptors for hormones including glucocorticoids, insulin, glucagon, growth hormone and thyroxin (Berczi et al, 1998). For example, feeding protocols that result in periods of overconsumption of feed impair both cell-mediated and humoral indices of immunity (Klasing, 1988). Often, feeding regimens that restrict feed intake below voluntary levels result in better immunocompetence and enhanced disease resistance (BoaAmponsem et al, 1997).

# 2

# Immune System and Nutrients for Immune Cell Development

## THE IMMUNE SYSTEM AND ITS COMPONENTS

*"Part of the secret of success in life is to eat what you like and let the food fight it out inside."* — *Mark Twain*

### Introduction

In feeding 'Ruminant Animals' it is said "Feed the Rumen Microbes, they in turn Feed the host Ruminant Animal". The same analogy may be applied in the treatment for all diseases taking phagocytes in the place of rumen microbes. Little elaboration gives better clarity. Phagocytes do need nutrients to grow and maintain vigour. "Feed the Phagocytes, they in turn Protect the animal to start with".

Nature has provided white corpuscles (phagocytes), a natural means of devouring and destroying all disease germs. Hence one genuine scientific treatment for all diseases is to stimulate the phagocytes. "Stimulate the phagocytes; the stimulated phagocytes devour the disease; the patient recovers".

Phagocytes can attack, engulf and dispose of small pathogens like bacteria (intracellular killing), and they can attack other pathogens by attaching themselves from the outside and killing them (extracellular killing), some of which may need the assistance of antibodies.

Hippocrates recognised as early as 370 BC that poorly nourished people are more susceptible to infectious diseases because of the recorded fact of associations between famine and epidemics of infectious diseases. Hence nutrients play a pivotal role in boosting the immune system.

### Cycle of Nutrition, Immunity and Infection

In general, undernutrition impairs the immune system and suppresses immune functions that are fundamental to host protection against disease-causing organism. Undernutrition can be due to insufficient intake of energy and macronutrients and/or due to deficiencies in specific micronutrients (vitamins and minerals) or due to imbalanced nutrient intake. Thus, it has been recognised for many years that **nutrient deficiency states are associated with an impaired immune response.** Such situations also lead to increased susceptibility to infectious diseases. In turn, infection can affect the status of several nutrients, thus setting up a vicious cycle of 'undernutrition, compromised immune function and infection'.

Each nutrient has a distinct range of intakes over which it supports optimal immune function. Lowering the level of nutrient below this range or increasing it in excess of the range can impair immune function. Thus, the functioning of the immune system is influenced by nutrients consumed as normal components of the diet and appropriate nutrition is required in order for the host to maintain adequate immune defences towards bacteria, viruses, fungi, parasites and prions. It is also now recognised that immune dysfunction plays a role in the events that follow trauma, burns or major surgery.

## External Environment—Necessity for Immune System

**The environment surrounding us is crowded with organisms, both visible and invisible to the naked eye.** As they enter into the body of living beings some cause harm resulting in infection and disease, while others establish beneficial relationships with the host. The organisms that get into the body and do harm of some kind vary in magnitude from those visible to (1) the naked eye like worms or helminthes, to ones largely visible only (2) under microscopy including fungi, protozoa, bacteria and viruses, to others not seen (3) like prions. All such organisms are referred to as **'pathogens'**.

**To parasitic microorganisms, the animal body represents an extremely attractive environment and a resource for nutrients.** Consequently, all living organisms are under the constant threat of overwhelming attack by viruses, bacteria, prions and parasites. Microorganisms evolve more rapidly than animals so that the nature of the microbiological threat to livestock is changing constantly as exposure to new or variant organisms occurs. To combat this potentially devastating threat, evolution has provided animals with a highly sophisticated, flexible and potent immune system, which is able to protect them against rapidly evolving microorganisms. Hence exposure to external environment activates the immune system to combat the pathogens and thus, the animal becomes resilient.

## The Immune System

Animal defence against various diseases depends on the efficacy of the immune system responsible for elimination of pathogens. This protective capacity is based on the effective immune system, which is considered to be an important determinant of animal health and well-being. In that sense, a remarkable ability of components of the immune system to distinguish between self and non-self is a great achievement of animal evolution. See this aspect later under the topic on 'the immune system is a two-edged sword'. Immune system activation in response to pathogens involving both innate and adaptive immunity is a double-edged sword.

## Three Layers of Immune System

The animal body has a range of defence mechanisms to tackle the pathogens that gain entry. The immune system is organised in layers of increasing specificity designed to protect the host from pathogens. The first line of defence is the ability of the host to prevent entry of the pathogen (physical barriers or external defences) and the next response is mediated by the host's natural or innate immunity. If the pathogen crosses these obstacles, the host has the ability to resist infection and disease by resorting to adaptive immunity.

### 1. Physical Barriers to Infectious Agents or Pathogens

The first line of defence is the physical barrier, including skin and endothelial cells. Natural physical barriers to pathogens are a simple yet effective means of defence. In this respect, intact skin provides a major physical barrier that is generally impermeable to most infectious agents. Sweat glands and sebaceous glands in the skin seem ideal as potential points of entry for infectious agents. However, most bacteria fail to enter due to (1) the low pH, (2) the lactic acid and fatty acids in sweat and sebaceous secretions and (3) the direct inhibitory effects of various secretions of the glands and their potent antimicrobial proteins, such as lysozymes, lactoferrins, defensins and peroxides. If, the continuity of the skin is disrupted or broken, it allows the entry of pathogens resulting in the risk of infection. (4) The mucous membrane linings of hollow viscera such as the respiratory, intestinal and urogenital tracts have mucous secretions, which can trap and immobilise bacteria and thereby prevent adherence and colonisation of epithelial surfaces. Further, the 'moving cilia' of the mucous membrane along with the mucous secretion can expel the entrapped organisms.

The immune response to microorganisms is divided into two categories: innate (natural, non-specific) immunity and adaptive (acquired, specific) immunity, although these categories overlap: Innate immunity is most universal. Innate immune response is inflexible and provides a rapid first line of defence until the development of more powerful and flexible adaptive immunity. The innate and adaptive immune systems are not independent; the innate immune response probably influences the character of the adaptive response and the adaptive immune response harnesses innate effector mechanisms, such as phagocytes (Fearon and Locksley, 1996). Figure 2.1, shows the general scheme of the immune system that depicts several connected ones related to immunity.

## 2. Innate (Natural, Nonspecific) Immunity

If any pathogen gains entry, the innate immune system initiates an immediate immune response upon recognising the molecules patterns of pathogens. It acts through neutrophil granulocytes, monocytes/macrophages and natural killer (NK) cells that release inflammatory mediators and humoral factors including collectins, C-reactive proteins and interferons (Beutler, 2004; Li et al, 2007).

Innate immunity is encoded in the germline and there is no memory effect, with re-exposure to the same pathogen eliciting the same response. Innate immunity is directed against molecular structure of microorganisms [e.g. bacterial lipopolysaccharides (LPS) and teichoic acid] that are essential for microbial survival. The major cells of innate immunity (phagocytic macrophages, dendritic cells and neutrophils) possess pathogen receptors (on their cell surface) specific for common bacterial surface molecules. Engagement of these receptors triggers phagocytosis and destruction of the microorganisms (Fig. 2.3).

## 3. Acquired or Adaptive Immunity

Most organisms survive through innate immune mechanisms alone, but vertebrates have evolved an additional system for pathogen recognition and elimination that

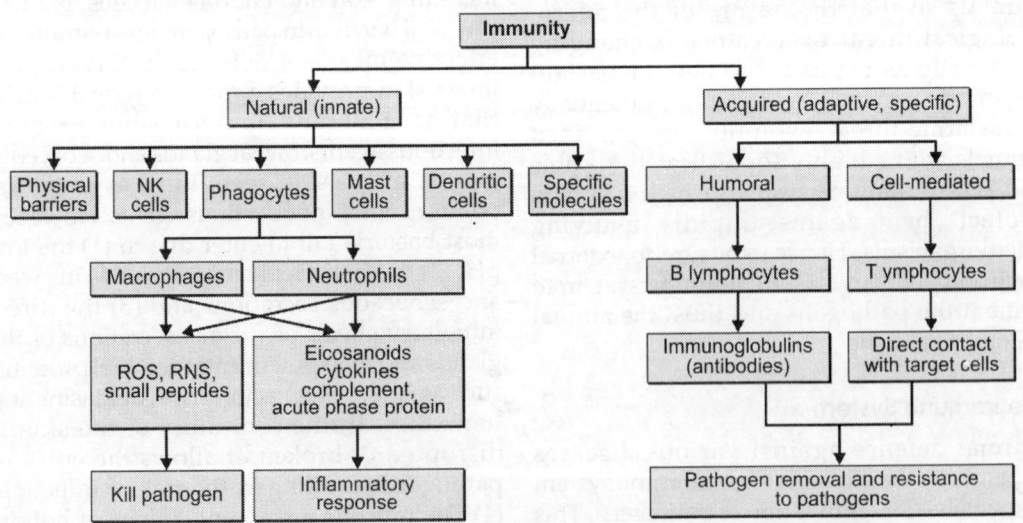

**Fig. 2.1:** General scheme of the immune system (*Adapted from* Surai 2002)

consists of T and B lymphocytes and humoral factors. This system is called the adaptive immune system (Calder, 2006). Acquired immunity involves the specific recognition of molecules (antigens) on an invading pathogen that distinguish it as being foreign to the host. **It is referred to as adaptive because it allows the body to 'tailor-make' recognition molecules adapted to the pathogens it encounters.** Very highly specific recognition along with the development of immunological memory is the hallmark of adaptive immunity. The adaptive system is slow to respond, with the memory providing a relatively rapid response on subsequent exposure to the agent or pathogen. The adaptive system is flexible and vigorous but regulated.

Immune system is also categorised into only two, innate and adaptive with the salient points as mentioned here.

| Categories of the immune system | |
| --- | --- |
| *Innate immunity* | *Adaptive immunity* |
| Non-specific or generic response | Antigen-specific response |
| Immediate following exposure (minutes) | Delayed following exposure (days) |
| Physical and mechanical barriers | No physical/mechanical barriers |
| Cellular and soluble factors | Cellular and soluble factors |
| No immune memory Inflammation | Immunological memory Antibody response (vaccines) |

Traditional teaching in immunology tells us that antigen-specific recall responses are the realm of adaptive immunity. However, over the past decade, there has been increasing evidence and interest in the concept of innate immune memory.

## Functional Consequence of T cell and B cell Circulation

**Lymphocytes (B and T)** affect the acquired or adaptive form of immunity. All lymphocytes arise from bone marrow stem cells. B lymphocytes undergo further development and maturation in the bone marrow in mammals (bursa of Fabricius in birds) before being released into the circulation, while T lymphocytes undergo differentiation and selection within the thymus. **The lymphoid system** is the term used to describe the total mass of lymphocytes in the body. Some of the lymphocytes are circulating, while others are located in organs such as the lymph nodes, spleen, tonsils, Peyer's patches in the intestine, in the foetus and in organs such as the liver and thymus.

**From the bloodstream, lymphocytes can enter peripheral lymphoid organs,** which include lymph nodes, the spleen, mucosal lymphoid tissue and gut-associated lymphoid tissue (GALT) (tonsils, adenoids, appendix and the Peyer's patches of the small intestine). Immune responses occur largely in these lymphoid organs, which are highly organised to promote the interaction of cells and invading pathogens.

Peripheral lymphoid organs are highly anatomically and functionally organised to facilitate interactions between migrating lymphocytes and antigens transported from the tissues. Lymphocytes, which do not encounter antigen, re-enter the bloodstream by way of efferent lymphatics and the thoracic duct. The functional consequence of this T cell and B cell circulation is that all of the body tissues are under continuous immunological surveillance for invading pathogens.

## Interactions Between Natural and Adaptive Immunity

When a lymphocyte antigen receptor engages its complementary antigen (i.e. entry of pathogen), the lymphocytes are attracted to the site by the chemicals called chemokines (special type of cytokines), lymphocytes cease migration, enlarges and rapidly proliferates so that, within 3–5 days, there are a large number of 'effector cells', each specific for the initiating antigen. This antigen-driven clonal expansion accounts for the characteristic delay of several days before adaptive immune responses become effective. Some of the 'effector cells' generated by clonal expansion are very long-living. They are the basis of immunological memory that is characteristic of adaptive immunity.

The interactions between natural and adaptive immunity are presented in (Fig. 2.2) for better comprehension and grasp. These two parts of the immune system work together through direct cell contact and through interactions involving such chemical mediators as cytokines and chemokines.

The adaptive immunity is characterised by high plasticity to recognise up to $10^{11}$ distinct structures and is tightly regulated to turn on or off a response aiming in eradication of pathogens but not destruction of self. In the healthy animal, resistance to infection relies on a balance between the natural and adaptive immunity. Interaction between the different immune cell types that make up these components of host defence is carried out by the relative mix of cytokines, hormone-like proteins, as well as other communicating molecules (Castle, 2000).

The innate immune response, reacts to the invader initially and acts directly to eliminate it by phagocytosis or through activities of complement. Cytokines regulate this response and also act on the liver, skeletal muscle, adipose tissue and brain changing their metabolism and stimulating various responses. The cytokines also interact with T lymphocytes (Fig. 2.2).

## Phagocytosis

Phagocytosis is the ability of some circulating cells that migrate during an inflammatory response to ingest foreign agents or pathogens such as bacteria. It is a complex process resulting in the ingestion and subsequent killing or digestion of these pathogens (Fig. 2.3). The principal phagocytes are neutrophils and macrophages and others include dendritic cells, mast cells and natural killer cells.

Some pathogenic microorganisms have evolved mechanisms (e.g. bacterial capsules) to evade the innate immune response; such ones are usually eliminated by the adaptive immune response.

## Monocytes/Macrophages

Monocytes represent another important cell type in innate immunity. They migrate into the infected tissue shortly after neutrophils where they differentiate into macrophages. Macrophages are critical in innate and adaptive immune responses. They can engulf

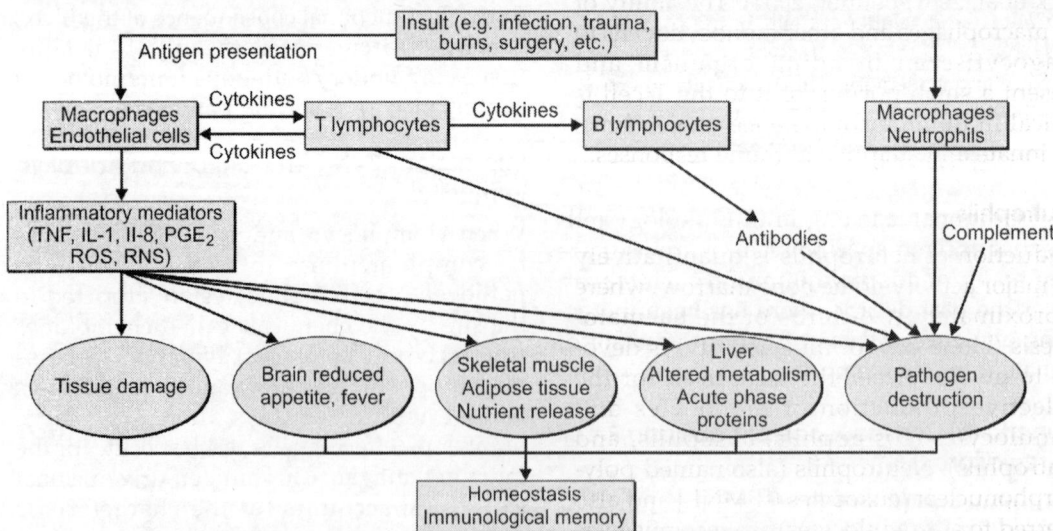

**Fig. 2.2:** The natural and adaptive immunity interactions (*Adapted from* Calder, 2001)

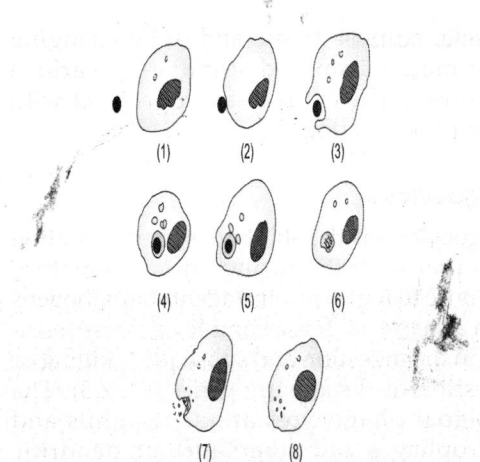

**Fig. 2.3:** Stages in the process of phagocytosis: (1) Chemotactic attraction and movement towards the pathogen; (2) Attachment to the cell wall, possibly assisted by complement or antibody; (3) Phagocytosis and ingestion of the pathogen; (4) Lysosomes coming into contact; (5) 'Forming phagolysosomes'; (6) Killing and digestion; (7) Release of degradation products; (8) Remains digested by enzymes inside the cell

and kill microbes and through the elaboration of chemotactic cytokines (signalling proteins). Macrophages also recruit other myeloid cells to the site of infection. Macrophages can also function as non-professional antigen-presenting cells and interact with T lymphocytes to modulate adaptive immune responses (Birk et al, 2001; Beutler, 2004). The ability of the macrophages and other monocytic cells to phagocytise an invading organism and present a small portion of it to the T cell is critical in immunocompetence, which links the innate and adaptive immune responses.

## Neutrophils

Production of neutrophils is quantitatively the major activity of the bone marrow, where approximately two-thirds of the haematopoiesis (blood-cell-forming activity) is devoted to myelopoiesis, the term used for the collective production of monocytes and granulocytes (eosinophils, basophils, and neutrophils). Neutrophils (also named polymorphonuclear leukocytes ([PMNL] and also referred to as granulocytes) are recognised as an essential part of the innate immune response. Neutrophils are indispensable for defence against intruding pathogens, particularly bacteria and fungi. After an invasion of pathogens, neutrophils migrate into the infected sites and provide the first line of host defence by phagocytosis and oxidative burst. The killing of these organisms in phagosomes is mediated by: (i) fusion with lysosomes (granules) liberating cytotoxic proteins, peptides and enzymes into the phagolysosome (Fig. 2.3) and (ii) activation of a membrane-bound NADPH-oxidase producing superoxide anions ($O_2^-$) that in turn, are metabolised into hydrogen peroxide and other reactive oxygen species (ROS). The cells use these mechanisms both inside the phagolysosome and outside the cell. In the latter process, the fusion of granules (degranulation) and activation of NADPH oxidase localise at the plasma membrane.

Neutrophils display potent antimicrobial functions including phagocytosis, degranulation and neutrophil extracellular trap (NET) (See page 42). "Neutrophils are a homogenous population of short-lived cells" is the outdated dogma (Silvestre-Roig et al., 2019)[1]. Data from the past decade have revealed that neutrophils may also exert immunoregulatory functions, as well as displaying phenotypic and functional plasticity due to their diversity in health and disease. They are generated in great number in the bone marrow and circulate in blood as dormant cells. Neutrophils, once believed, are directly eliminated in the marrow, liver and spleen after circulating for less than one day. Now, they are known to redistribute into multiple tissues with poorly understood kinetics. Now, it is said that the half-life of neutrophils in circulation is about 5 days. Such a short lifespan is compensated by a high turnover rate $10^{10}$ to $10^{11}$ of neutrophils being replaced everyday. In simple terms, neutrophils that are produced in the bone marrow (from stem cells) proliferate and differentiate to mature neutrophils fully equipped with an armoury of granules (the hallmark of granulocytes), which are stores of proteins that can kill microbes and digest tissues.

Recently, neutrophils have also been implicated in immune regulation. C/EBPa and PU.1 are both essential transcription factors necessary for terminal granulocy-topoiesis. PU.1 is absolutely required for myeloid lineage commitment. The balance between PU.1 and C/EBPa and Gfi-1 expression determines the differentiation into the granulocyte or the monocytic pathways. The transcription factor Gfi-1(growth factor independent-1) is necessary for neutrophil differentiation (The reader may refer Borregaard [2010] Neutrophils from Marrow to Microbes, Immunity, 33, 657–670, for greater details).

**Signals generated by microbes and resident macrophages at sites of infection activate the local endothelial cells:** If microorganisms have successfully overcome the physical barriers provided by the skin and mucous membranes and gained access to tissues, signals generated by microbes and resident macrophages at sites of infection activate the local endothelial cells, which capture the bypassing neutrophils and guide them across the endothelial cell lining. Here the neutrophils are activated and tuned for the subsequent interaction with microbes. Once in the tissues, neutrophils kill micro-organisms by microbicidal agents liberated from granules or generated by metabolic activation. It has been clear now that neutrophils may extend their antimicrobial activity beyond life of the neutrophil. Formation of neutrophil extracellular traps (NETs) is an alternative to death by necrosis or apoptosis. Thus, neutrophils can extrude strands of DNA with bactericidal proteins attached that act as extracellular traps for microorganisms (Borregaard 2010).

Neutrophils that have migrated into tissues are more active as phagocytic cells than blood neutrophils (Sorensen et al, 2001) and activate a transcriptional programme that results in generation of several chemokines, including IL-8 and Groa (Scapini et al, 2000, 2005) that recruit additional inflammatory cells.

## Dendritic Cell

Dendritic cells are the most important and efficient (professional) antigen-presenting cells (APC) because of their ability to capture, process and present antigen to T cells. Thus dendritic cells serve to bridge the innate immune system to the adaptive immune system. They are mandatory for the initiation of a primary immune response against a new pathogen.

Dendritic cells (DCs) are generated in the bone marrow but are subsequently widely distributed throughout the tissues, typically in association with epithelial surfaces. Dendritic cells can be divided into 2 subsets: myeloid (mDCs) and plasmacytoid (pDCs) dendritic cells. The mDCs (also known as conventional DCs) facilitate adaptive T cell responses, partly through Toll-like receptor (TLR)-induced IL-12 production. The pDCs are the main producers of type I interferon in response to viral infection.

In peripheral tissues, 'immature' dendritic cells act as sentinels, constantly sampling the surrounding tissues for pathogens. Immature dendritic cells accumulate foreign antigens in their surroundings by micropinocytosis of soluble antigens and phagocytosis of particulate antigens and microorganisms. Because of these processes, dendritic cells can initiate immune responses with pico- and nanomolar concentrations of antigens, compared with the micromolar concentrations required by non-professional antigen-presenting cells, such as B cells and macrophages. So **DCs emerge as key players for the immune system**.

Typically, DCs recognise a wide range of 'danger signals' both from invading microbes and injured host cells through binding either pathogen-associated molecular patterns (PAMPs) or damage-associated molecular pattern molecules (DAMPs) to specialised pattern recognition receptors (PRRs) (Durai and Murphy, 2016). The principal task of the immune system is to distinguish between foreign antigen and self or 'harmless' antigen. DCs perform this complex task, which is indispensable to regulate the delicate balance between immunity and tolerance.

Both dendritic cells and non-professional antigen-presenting cells, such as macrophages and B cells, are able to initiate secondary (memory) responses against reinfecting organisms.

## Mast Cells

Mast cells (MCs) originate from progenitor cells in the bone marrow, which move through the circulation and become mature MCs after homing to different organs under the influence of the local microenvironment (Ribatti, 2016). MC progenitors enter the blood and exit into tissues by transendothelial migration and are undetectable in the blood. Mast cells participate in the acute inflammatory response by releasing a range of chemicals (such as histamine, leukotrienes) to mobilise leukocytes. They increase the delivery of complement and antibodies to initiate and promote the inflammatory response and the subsequent phagocytosis by other cells and may be considered as a component of the immune system (Bachelet et al, 2006).

Mast cells are localised in connective tissues and are more numerous near the boundaries between the external environment and the internal milieu including the skin, the respiratory tract, the gastrointestinal tract and the conjunctiva. In the gastrointestinal tract, MCs represent 1–5% of mononuclear cells in the lamina propria of the mucosa and in the submucosa. They are also found inside the epithelium and deep in the muscle and serosal layers. The gastrointestinal MCs perform their biological functions, releasing mediators as amines (histamine, serotonin), cytokines, proteases, lipid mediators (leukotrienes, prostaglandins) and heparin (Rizzi et al, 2016).

## Complement

Complement is the principal humoral mediator of innate immunity during the host's attack on the pathogen. The liver produces a variety of proteins, collectively known as "complement", which are able to bind to pathogens and thereby mark those pathogens for destruction.

## Natural Killer Cells

Natural killer (NK) cells are large granular lymphocytes that are essential for maintaining the innate immune response and host defence against viral infections and tumour cells. Natural killer cells produce and secrete very potent immunoregulatory cytokines, particularly interferon-γ, which increases cell reactivity and activates macrophages (Justo et al, 2003).

NK cells are the founding members of the innate lymphocyte family, initially recognised more than 40 years ago for their ability to kill tumour targets without prior sensitisation across MHC (MHC I) haplotypes. Work over the last decade has discovered and confirmed the existence of NK cells with antigen-specific memories, which had previously been considered a unique property of T and B cells. Finding that "innate" natural killer cells possessed T cell-like immune memory is an unprecedented discovery that rocked our understanding of the divide between innate and adaptive immunity. Wight et al, (2018) have demonstrated that Ly49 receptors on natural killer cells, which engage the class I antigen-presenting platform on target cells, are critical components of adaptive natural killer cell memory. Adaptive natural killer (NK) cell memory represents a new frontier in immunology.

In most cases, the innate/natural system provides adequate protection from an infection. In cases where the innate immune system is "breached", the acquired (antibody-mediated) system becomes activated. Thus, the three layers of immune system protect the animal (see page 25).

## Inflammation is the Earliest Reaction to an Infection—Appearance of Acute Phase Proteins

White blood cells or leukocytes (in particular neutrophils and macrophages) are immediately attracted to the point at which the infective agent gained entry (after breaching the physical barriers). These phagocytes are the principal cells of innate immunity. The speed of action is rapid, occurring within minutes to hours of the entry of the pathogen. The specificity of recognition is broad and across the board in innate immunity system. Phagocytes secret cytokines. These stimulate liver to produce acute phase proteins (APP). Certain characteristic changes occur in the tissues attacked by the infective agents and these changes constitute **inflammation.** The features of tissue inflammation are redness, warmth, swelling, pain and loss of function.

Many tissue products are released in response to and as a result of the entry of infectious agents. These products include cytokines (interleukins IL-1, IL-6 and TNF-$\alpha$), leukotrienes, histamine, bradykinin, serotonin, prostaglandins, several hormones, reaction products of the complement system and the blood clotting system (fibrinogen). These are responsible for tissue inflammation. Blood flow to the region of tissue injury is increased and leukocytes are attracted. Inflammation is the earliest reaction to an infection, which is accompanied by fever and acute illness characterised by the appearance of APPs or **acute phase reactants.** These acute phase proteins include protease inhibitors, ceruloplasmin, haptoglobin, C-reactive protein (CRP), serum amyloid A protein and acid glycoprotein. The levels of APPs rise in the circulation, while the levels of normal plasma proteins (albumin, transferring and lipoproteins) are reduced. Based on their rise and fall, APPs are named as positive APPs and negative APPs, respectively. The raised CRP in the blood is often a useful sign of an acute infection.

## The Immune System is a Two-edged Sword

The extremely potent and toxic biological mechanisms of the immune system can destroy not only threatening microorganisms but also body tissues. Usually, the tissue destruction and inflammation associated with the eradication of a microbiological threat are acceptable and functionally insignificant. However, in several diseases, e.g. tuberculosis, the immunologically associated tissue destruction and inflammation are harmful, the effect on the individual animal may be devastating.

It is because of their potential to destroy tissues, the 'effector mechanisms of the immune system' are very tightly regulated. Failure of these regulatory mechanisms leads to 'the impact of immune system' being inappropriately directed against body tissues and the development of **autoimmune diseases,** such as rheumatoid arthritis, multiple sclerosis in human beings. If immune responses are directed against innocuous targets, such as allergens or transplanted organs, the resulting immunologically mediated tissue damage and inflammation are the basis of **allergy** and **transplant rejection.**

## Adaptive (Acquired, Specific) Immunity

Two types of adaptive (acquired, specific) immunity occur in the body: humoral immunity and cell-mediated immunity.

### 1. Humoral Immunity

Protection against certain infections can be transferred by serum. This is called humoral immunity and is **mediated by circulating immunoglobulins** (Ig). This humoral immunity is conducted exclusively by B lymphocytes. B lymphocytes are characterised by their ability to produce antibodies or immunoglobulins (Igs), which confer antigen specificity to the acquired immune system. B lymphocytes carry these immunoglobulins that are capable of binding an antigen directly on their cell surface. These B lymphocytes are called **memory cells** and are responsible for the rapid secondary response that occurs to a subsequent exposure to the same antigen. The process of antigen activation of the B lymphocytes may be dependent on T cells (T-dependent) or independent of T cells (Ti antigens).

**Immunoglobulins—five major classes of immunoglobulins:** Immunoglobulins are gamma globulins, constitute about 20% of the circulating plasma proteins. Immunoglobulins are made up of four polypeptide chains—two identical long or heavy chains and two identical short or light chains attached to form a Y-shaped molecule. Each of the two heavy chains is linked to the other and to a light chain by disulphide bonds, giving a roughly Y-shaped molecule.

There are five major classes of immunoglobulins: IgA, IgD, IgG, IgM and IgE, each of which elicits different components of the humoral immune response. Antibodies work in several ways to combat invading pathogens. They can 'neutralise' toxins or microorganisms by binding to them and preventing their attachment to host cells and they can activate complement proteins in plasma, which in turn promote the destruction of bacteria by phagocytes.

IgG is the most important and it constitutes 75% of serum immunoglobulins. It is active both in the blood and in tissue spaces and even crosses the placental barrier, thus conferring immunity to the foetus and newborn. IgM is the largest molecule and can immobilise and agglutinate bacteria. Its large size does not allow it to get out of the bloodstream or cross the placenta. IgA is adapted to function at the mucosal surfaces of hollow organs such as the gut, lungs and urogenital tract, while IgE present in trace amounts and is prominent during allergies. IgD is mainly found on B lymphocytes and is involved in their activation pathway.

**Effector functions of immunoglobulins:** Antibodies bind to bacteria by the amino-terminal antigen-binding sites. Such binding effectively neutralises toxins and microorganisms. Antibodies bound to bacteria are also able to activate a series of plasma proteins that promote phagocytosis and can also directly destroy bacteria. Since, they have binding sites both for an antigen and for receptors on phagocytic cells, antibodies can

also promote the interaction of the two components by forming physical 'bridges', a process known as **opsonisation.**

Phagocytes form part of the innate immune system and possess very limited antigen-specific receptors. The type of phagocytic cell bound by the antibody will be determined by the antibody class: macrophages and neutrophils are specific for IgM and IgG, while eosinophils are specific for IgE. In this way, **antibodies are a form of communication between the acquired and the innate immune response.**

### 2. Cell-Mediated Immunity

Antibodies are highly effective against extracellular pathogens, but they have very limited potency against intracellular pathogens, such as viruses and certain bacteria. T cells, however, are particularly effective against intracellular pathogens, because of their ability to identify infected cells and then mount and coordinate an effective cell-mediated immune response. To meet this end, T cell possesses antigen-specific T cell receptor (TCR) molecules on its surface. Unlike B cell immunoglobulin molecules, T cell receptor is always surface-bound. In contrast to B cells, T cells are only able to recognise (with their TCR) the processed antigens displayed on the surface of an antigen presenting cell (APC). Indeed, the antigen is processed intracellularly by APC into short peptides; linear epitopes of 8 to 20 amino acids long, which associate intracellularly with MHC molecules.

**T cells are divided into two groups: T-helper (Th) (or CD4+T) cells and cytotoxic T-lymphocytes (CTLs) (or CD8+T cells).** T cells can either help other cells to eliminate microbes (CD4+T cells) or kill the infected cells (CD8+T cells). Th or TH cells produce cytokines to help the other T and B cells to grow and divide and grow and divide themselves to produce more cells to fight future infections. CTLs are responsible for destroying pathogen infected cells. Pathogens can be phagocytosed and digested and the digested pieces of pathogens are presented on the surface of the antigen-presenting cell to Th cells. The Th cells may then stimulate clonal expression of a B cell lineage, which then secrete antibodies.

## B and T Cells—Resting Phase and Active Phase

In resting phase T lymphocytes are very similar to B lymphocytes. Upon activation B cells form large plasma cells, while T cells enlarge slightly and begin to secret cytokines (Th cells) and other toxic molecules (cytotoxic T cells) that have effects on other target cells over a short range with no antigen specificity. The cytokines may activate B cells and macrophages. The cytotoxic T cells (CTLs) function to kill the cells harbouring intracellular pathogens.

## Major Histocompatibility Complex (MHC)

The MHC is a large complex of genes that encode the major histocompatibility glycoproteins. These MHC molecules will (on subsequent expression on the cell membrane of the APC) present the epitope to the T cell. The T cell-dependent B-lymphocyte activation is through major histocompatibility complex molecules. These large-surface glycoproteins are present in some form on every nucleated cell and there are two structural variants: class I MHC molecules and class II MHC molecules, which present different types of antigen to the T lymphocytes. Class I MHC molecules are expressed by all nucleated cells and present antigens that are expressed intracellularly (e.g. viral antigens and certain bacterial antigens). Class II MHC molecules occur in antigen presenting cells (APCs), usually a macrophage, B cells and professional APCs (e.g. dendritic cells); present extracellular antigens (e.g. bacterial proteins). MHC-pathogen-peptide complexes are very stable and are expressed on the cell surface.

To help distinguish the two MHC-peptide complexes, another set of surface molecules

on the T cells is needed. These surface markers are named as per the internationally recognised system of 'CD' (cluster of differentiation) numbers - **CD8+T cells** and **CD4+T cells**, respectively, for class I MHC and class II MHC. They are also referred to as CTLs and Th or T helper cells, respectively.

## Effector T Cells Effectively Counteract Viral Infections

**Effector T cells** emerge from parent T cells. Effector CD8+T cells (also known as cytotoxic T lymphocytes, CTLs) play a vital role in counteracting viral infections,which are intracellular and almost completely hidden from the humoral immune response. CD8+T cells proliferate to form a clone of CTLs, which can directly lyse cells infected with virus. These CD8+T cells are ineffective in eliminating certain intracellular bacteria, fungi and parasites that are not neutralised by destruction of their host cell. These microorganisms are also resistant to the humoral immune response. These resistant organisms are neutralised by effector CD4+T cells.

## Effector CD4+T Cells are Commonly Known as T-helper (Th) cells

These effector CD4+T cells are generated by MHC class II-restricted presentation of peptide by APCs. Class II MHC molecules are recognised by CD4+T cells, which proliferate and activate B lymphocytes. **CD4+ Th-cell differentiation** can be biased towards a type 1(Th1) or type 2 (Th2) response. The Th1-biased immune responses are characterised by IgG production and activation of macrophages, while the Th2-biased immune responses result in IgE secretion and eosinophilia and are seen in helminthic infections and allergic diseases.

## Humoral Immunity Versus Cell-mediated Immunity

Humoral immunity is mediated by B lymphocytes, while cell-mediated one is largely the function of T lymphocytes. B lymphocytes operate largely in the extracellular fluid spaces of the body, while T lymphocytes cater to the intracellular compartment. They interact with each other and depend on the innate immune systems (phagocytes, complement, etc.) to dispose of the foreign agent or molecule.

Humoral immunity deals with extracellular pathogens. However, some pathogens, particularly viruses, but also some bacteria, infect individuals by entering cells. These intracellular pathogens escape humoral immunity and are dealt with by cell-mediated immunity, which is conferred by T lymphocytes.

The important difference with respect to humoral immunity is that while B lymphocytes produce antibodies (immunoglobulins) that can travel throughout the body and can act for weeks, the cell-mediated immune defence is the direct result of T lymphocytes and their cytokines acting directly although transiently. Dendritic cells may also help in taking the pathogen to the T cells. As with innate immunity, the targeted migration of T cells is aided by chemokines and other molecules.

**The adaptive immune mechanism** is thus reliant on both B and T lymphocytes, and their response to a pathogen is powerful, flexible, antigen specific and demonstrates immunological memory. B cells on activation initiate clones, which secrete antibodies that are effective largely against extracellular agents such as bacteria and help neutralise their toxins. Th cells or CD4+T cells interact with B cells and macrophages to direct an antigen-specific immune response, mediated through antibodies and cytokines to help neutralise the invading pathogen rather than directly neutralising the invading pathogen.

## Communication within the Immune System: Cytokines

Cytokines are soluble proteins secreted by the cells of the immune system and are mainly released in response to invasion by foreign agents. They lack any direct pathogen recognition or attack or disposal role. They act on cells of the immune system to modulate their activity. Even non-immune cells and tissues such as fibroblasts, endothelial cells also can produce cytokines under certain circumstances. Communication within the acquired immune system and between the innate and acquired system is brought about by direct cell-cell contact involving adhesion molecules and by the production of chemical messengers, which send signals from one cell to another. Cytokines are the chief among these chemical messengers. Cytokines can be divided into interleukins, tumour necrosis factors, interferons, colony-stimulating factors and transforming growth factors.

They are now increasingly designated as 'interleukins' meaning 'between white cells'– obviously referring to their principal function for communication between white blood cells. Interleukins are growth factors targeted to cells of haemopoietic origin. More than 30 interleukins are known. **The majority of interleukins are synthesised by helper CD4+T lymphocytes, as well as through monocytes and macrophages.**

## Activities of Cytokines

Each cytokine can have multiple activities (several beneficial and non-beneficial) on different cell types. Cytokines act by binding to specific receptors on the cell surface and thereby induce changes in growth, development or activity of the target cell. Cytokines are involved in promoting inflammatory responses, cell differentiation and proliferation, as well as movement and inhibition. They also form a special group of antiviral particles called interferons. Cytokines can increase vascular permeability and thus allow movement of immunoglobulins, complements and leukocytes to the site of infection.

## Infection—Innate Immune Response— Production of Cytokines

Inflammation is the earliest reaction to an infection. It is typified by redness, swelling, heat and pain. It occurs as a result of increased blood flow, increased permeability across blood capillaries which permit large molecules (e.g. complement, antibodies, cytokines) to leave the bloodstream and cross the endothelial wall and increased movement of leukocytes from the bloodstream into the surrounding tissue. Thus, inflammation is an integral part of the innate immune response.

Tumour necrosis factor (TNF)-α, interleukin (IL)-1 and IL-6 (pro-inflammatory cytokines) are among the most important cytokines produced by monocytes and macrophages. These cytokines have wide spread metabolic effects on the body. They activate neutrophils, monocytes and macrophages to initiate bacterial and tumour cell killing; increase adhesion molecule expression on the surface of neutrophils and endothelial cells; and stimulate T- and B-lymphocyte proliferation. Thus, TNF-α, IL-1 and IL-6 are mediators of both natural and acquired immunity and are an important link between them.

Production of appropriate amounts of TNF-α, IL-1 and IL-6 is clearly important in response to infection. However, inappropriate production or overproduction can be dangerous, and these cytokines particularly, TNF-α, are implicated in causing some of the pathological responses that occur in chronic inflammatory conditions (e.g. rheumatoid arthritis, psoriasis).

The components of innate and adaptive immunity may be enlisted as follows for better clarity (Table 2.1).

## How Does the Immune System Works?

Having studied so many things about the immune system and its components, let us see, briefly, how it works. When an infection occurs or when an antigen enters the body, it is trapped by the macrophages in lymphoid organs. The phagocytic cells (the first line of defence) that are guarding the body by constant patrolling engulf and digest the foreign substances. However, the partially digested antigens (i.e. processed antigen) with antigenic epitopes attach to lymphocytes (B and T cells). All this series of reactions carried

out by the immune system in the body against the foreign invader is referred to as the **immune response.** T-helper (Th) cells play a key role in the immune response (Fig. 2.4).

This is brought out through the participation of antigen presenting cell (APC), usually a macrophage. Receptors of Th cell (CD4+T cells or T helper cells) bind to class II MHC-antigen complex displayed on the surface of APC. APC secretes interleukin-1, which activates the Th cell. This activated Th cell actively grows and divides to produce clones of Th cells. All the Th cells possess receptors that are specific for the MHC-antigen complex. This facilitates triggering of immune response in an exponential manner. The Th cells secrete interleukin-2 that promotes the proliferation of cytotoxic T lymphocytes or CTLs to attack the infected cells through cell-mediated immunity.

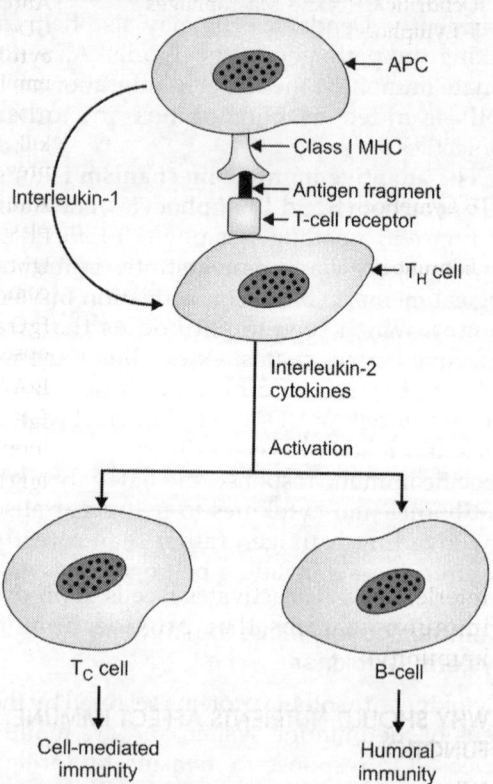

**Fig. 2.4.** Role of T helper cells in immune response (APC, antigen presenting cell; Th,T helper cell; Tc, cytotoxic T cell)

**Table 2.1:** The components of innate and adaptive immunity

| Components of innate immunity | |
| --- | --- |
| *Factor* | *Main Functions* |
| Physical barriers | Block and trap microbes (skin, tears, mucus) |
| Pattern Recognition Receptors | Surveillance and activation of innate immune responses |
| Complement | Bacteriolytic and facilitates phagocytosis |
| Cytokines | Pro-inflammatory and immunoregulatory |
| Oxylipids (prostaglandins, leukotrienes) | Pro-inflammatory and pro-resolving |
| Endothelial Cells | Regulates leukocyte migration and activation |
| Neutrophils | Phagocytosis and production of ROS |
| Macrophages | Phagocytosis; production of cytokines |
| Dendritic Cells | Phagocytosis; link innate and adaptive immunity |
| Natural Killer Cells | Target and help to eliminate infected host cells |
| **Components of adaptive immunity** | |
| Major Histocompatibility Complex | Recognises self from non-self |
| Dendritic Cells and Macrophages | Antigen presentation cells |
| T Lymphocytes | CD4+T Cells or T helper Cells (Th1, Th2, Th17, Treg); produce cytokines that regulate innate and adaptive immunity; immunoglobulin isotype switching |
| | CD8+ T Cells or cytotoxic T lymphocytes (CTLs); attack and kill, cells that express foreign antigens (virus-infected) T Cells; prevalent at mucosal surfaces |
| B Lymphocytes | Antigen presentation; differentiate into antibody-producing plasma cells |
| Immunoglobulins (antibodies) | IgM is the largest and first produced; role in agglutination and complement activation |
| | IgG concentration is high in sera and is important for opsonisation |
| | IgA is found at mucosal surfaces and has anti-viral function |
| | IgE is associated with allergic reactions and parasitic infections |
| | IgD non-secreted regulatory molecule |

Interleukin-2 also activates B cells to produce immunoglobulins that provide humoral immunity.

## WHY SHOULD NUTRIENTS AFFECT IMMUNE FUNCTION?

When malnutrition is present, the overall development and expression of the immune responses significantly get impaired. Similarly, the ageing process affects nutrient needs and the immune responses in an interactive fashion. What roles nutrients play in immune function?

## Nutrients are Primary Factors in the Regulation of the Immune Response

- Both macronutrients and micronutrients derived from the diet affect 'immune system function' through actions at several levels in the gastrointestinal tract, thymus, spleen, regional lymph nodes and immune cells of the circulating blood (Chandra, 1997; Wallace et al, 2000; Cunningham-Rundles, 2001).

- Effects at one level of nutrient may be opposed or modified at another level. Thus, the development of an experimental approach capable of revealing critical interactions requires study of more than one aspect of immune function.

- The effect of any single nutrient is dependent upon concentration, interactions with other key nutrients, host genetic expression and internal environmental conditions.

- In situation of nutrient imbalance, duration of the altered condition and age of the host are also often critical factors (Cunningham-Rundles, 2002).

- Nutrients affect specific immune-cell types differently through influencing intrinsic cell function and by influencing cell-cell interactions. Much of the critical action appears to occur in the local microenvironment during the response to antigen.

The immune system has been divided into **an innate system** and **an adaptive immune system**. Adaptive immunity is further characterised based on cell type as B cells of the humoral immune system and T cells of the cellular immune system.

### Age and Immune Response

Age of the host or developmental stage is often a critical variable. Antigen-specific humoral and cellular immunity are central to the adaptive immune response and these are generated in the adult host. In contrast, neonates and infants rely primarily on innate immunity, specifically complement, maternal antibody, circulating mediators of the inflammatory response and phagocytes.

### Significant T cell Differentiation

It is increasingly clear now that significant T cell differentiation does occur inde-

pendently of the thymus, e.g. in the gastrointestinal tract. Current studies also show that the innate immune system, mediated by such cells as natural killer (NK) and NK T cells, monocytes and dendritic cells, influences the nature of cytokine production by the adaptive immune system. This occurs through secretion of cytokines by innate immune cells into the microenvironment (Devereux, 2002).

The effect of the microenvironment is to drive the immune response towards either a T-helper type 1 (Th1) or a T-helper type 2 (Th2) response (Devereux, 2002). Micronutrients, such as trace elements and vitamins, are present in the local environment and have important regulatory effects on adaptive immune-cell function. For example, the trace element zinc supports a Th1 response, whereas vitamin A appears to produce a Th2 response. Thus, the new immunology provides a more fluid representation of a potentially evolving process that presents as a defined pattern according to an environmental dynamic rather than a static programme that is derived from fixed cellular characteristics.

### Methods to Assess Immunological Functions

When analysing data related to immunomodulating properties of various nutrients, it is necessary to pay special attention to methods used to assess immunological functions. Assessment of how nutrients may interact in immune function is complex and more difficult. Investigators often seek to strengthen inferences by inclusion of *in vivo* tests. For example, *in vivo* methods of immune function assessment are based on two main approaches: antibody response to vaccine or delayed-type hypersensitivity (DTH) reaction. In the first method immunisation with appropriate antigens (viral or bacterial) can elicit serum antibodies. Sheep red blood cells (SRBC) are often used as antigens. Haemaglutination (HA) assay measures serum antibody concentration (titer) against antigens. This assay provides information about humoral immunity (B cell responsiveness) and its association with cell-mediated immunity (T cell cooperation). In the second, DTH reaction method is used to assess cell-mediated immune function. It is measured by skin testing.

## General Strategies to Assess the Impact of a Nutrient on Immune Function

**What are the best predictors of immune status?** This is a challenge for research workers with interest in interface between nutrition and immunity because 'Immunity' is an extremely broad concept. Chew and Park (2004) proposed some general strategies to assess the impact of a nutrient on immune function. These include immunoglobulin production (total IgM and IgG) in blood as indexes of immunity, cytokine concentrations in biological samples, immune cell (T and B cells) proliferation by the addition of specific chemicals (mitogens), index for humoral immune system and delayed-type hypersensitivity (DTH) assay.

The development of cytokine biology has provided a critical means of clarifying the fundamental impact of nutrients on immune response. **Cytokines are produced in response to microbial threat and aid in the recruitment and activation of immune cells to protect the host.** Naturally nutrients appear to affect the immune system deeply through regulatory mechanisms affecting the expression and production of cytokines. The type of cytokine pattern produced is crucial for the response to infectious pathogens. Hence, serious nutrient imbalance will ultimately compromise the development of the future immune response. Malnutrition promotes susceptibility to pathogens. Even subclinical infections directly affect nutrient intake and metabolism. Severe, acute infection will have a very strong impact.

Immune deficiency and susceptibility to infection are often directly linked with malnutrition. Many of the infections observed in human protein-energy malnutrition (PEM), such as tuberculosis, herpes, *Pneumocystis carinii* pneumonia and measles, are caused by intracellular pathogens, indicating that the cellular immune system is particularly affected (Keusch, 1993).

It is well known that cytokine production during the acute-phase response (APR) to generalised sepsis can lead to loss of lean tissue and body fat (Lin et al, 1998). Interestingly, this cascade of events can be altered by nutritional intervention.

## Nutritional Immunology

The emerging field of nutritional immunology has benefitted from the evolution of cellular and molecular immunology (Cunningham-Rundles, 2001). In order to evaluate the effects of nutrients on immune function, Cunningham-Rundles (2002) suggested that the presence of nutrients in the local environment have important regulatory effects on the immune system. Over the last decade, there has been a renewed interest in the analysis of the metabolic basis of immune function; new physiological links and potential immunoregulatory pathways have been discovered.

## Nutritional Support of Immunity

The immune system is functioning at all times. However, specific immunity becomes activated when the host is challenged by pathogens. Immune system activation is associated with a marked increase in the demand for substrates (nutrients) that can be supplied from exogenous sources (i.e. from the diet) and/or from endogenous pools. The cells of the immune system are metabolically active and are able to utilise glucose, amino acids and fatty acids as fuels.

Energy generation involves electron carriers, which are nucleotide derivatives [e.g. nicotinamide adenine dinucleotide (NAD), flavin adenine dinucleotide (FAD)] and a range of coenzymes. The electron carriers and coenzymes are usually derivatives of vitamins: thiamine pyrophosphate is derived from thiamine (vitamin $B_1$), FAD and flavin mononucleotide (FMN) from riboflavin (vitamin $B_2$), NAD from nicotinate (niacin), pyridoxal phosphate from pyridoxine (vitamin B$_6$), coenzyme A from pantothenate, tetrahydrofolate from folate and cobamide from cobalamin (vitamin B$_{12}$). In addition, biotin is required by some enzymes for activity. The final component of the pathway for energy generation (the mitochondrial electron transfer chain) includes electron carriers that have iron or copper at their active site. Several other micronutrients (e.g. selenium, zinc) are also needed by the cells.

## Respiratory Burst/Oxidative Burst

An important component of the immune response is oxidative burst. When exposed to pathogens, phagocytes (including neutrophils, macrophages and eosinophils) undergo marked changes in the way they handle oxygen to generate reactive oxygen species (ROS). Firstly, their rate of oxygen uptake increases greatly. This is accompanied by (i) the production of large amounts of superoxide (powerful microbiocidal agents to kill pathogens) and hydrogen peroxide and (ii) the metabolism of large quantities of glucose through the hexose monophosphate shunt. The phagocyte respiratory burst is essential for host defence to pathogens. Here oxygen is used not for respiration but to kill pathogens. Concomitantly, glucose is oxidised through the hexose monophosphate shunt to regenerate the NADPH that has been consumed through the reduction of molecular oxygen to generate superoxide. The phagocyte respiratory burst is driven by both membrane-bound and cytosolic subunits of the phagocyte NADPH oxidase. See Fig. 3.3.

## Cellular Proliferation is a Key Component of the Immune Response Providing Amplification and Memory

Immune defences are dependent upon cell replication and production of proteins with biological activity. Prior to the cell division, there must be replication of DNA and then of all cellular components (proteins, membranes, intracellular organelles, etc.). In addition to energy, this clearly needs a supply of nucleotides (for DNA and RNA synthesis), amino acids (for protein synthesis), fatty acids, bases and phosphate (for phospholipid synthesis), and other lipids (e.g. cholesterol) and cellular components. Although nucleotides are synthesised mainly from amino acids, some of the cellular building blocks cannot be synthesised in mammalian cells and must come from the diet (e.g. essential fatty acids, essential amino acids, minerals). Amino acids (e.g. arginine) are precursors for synthesis of polyamines, which have roles in the regulation of DNA replication and cell division. Various micronutrients (e.g. iron, folic acid, zinc, magnesium) are also involved in nucleotide and nucleic acid synthesis.

In recent years, more specific molecular mechanisms by which the nutrients support immunity have been elucidated. For example, vitamin B$_6$ is required for the formation of lymphocyte receptor that is involved in lymphocyte trafficking between blood, lymphoid tissues and peripheral tissues.

Thus, **the roles for nutrients in immune function are many and varied.** Hence, an adequate and balanced supply of these nutrients is essential, if an appropriate immune response is to be mounted. Our understanding of the molecular basis for nutrient action on immune function is incomplete, although there is evidence to suggest that it involves effects on surface receptor/protein regulation, production of mediators and redox status.

## Immune Cells and Antioxidants

Immune cells rely heavily on cell-cell communication, particularly via membrane-bound receptors, to work effectively. Cell membranes are rich in PUFA. If peroxidised, the modified-PUFA can lead to a loss of membrane integrity, altered membrane fluidity (Baker and Meydani, 1994) and alterations in intracellular signalling and cell function. It has been shown that exposure to ROS can lead to a reduction in cell-membrane-receptor expression (Gruner et al, 1986). Hence, the immune system is particularly vulnerable to oxidative damage. But immune cell integrity is essential in order to mount a response to overcome the stress. Hence, antioxidant nutrients help to maintain this integrity.

As mentioned earlier, phagocytic granulocytes also undergo respiratory bursts to produce oxygen radicals to destroy intracellular pathogens. However, these oxidative products can, in turn, damage healthy cells, if they are not eliminated. Antioxidants serve to stabilise these highly reactive oxygen species (ROS), thereby maintaining the structural and functional integrity of cells. Therefore, antioxidants are very important to the immune defence and health of humans and animals.

**Antioxidant vitamins and metalloenzymes:** Tissue defence mechanisms against free radical damage generally include vitamin C, vitamin E (alpha and gamma tocopherol) and β-carotene as the major vitamin antioxidant sources. In addition, several metalloenzymes that include glutathione peroxidase (selenium), catalase (iron) and superoxide dismutase (copper, zinc and manganese) are also critical in protecting the internal cellular constituents from oxidative damage. The dietary and tissue balance of all these nutrients are important in protecting tissues against free radical damage. Nitrogen oxides can only be destroyed by a second form of vitamin E, gamma tocopherol.

Both *in vitro* and *in vivo* studies show that the antioxidant vitamins generally enhance different aspects of cellular and non-cellular immunity. The antioxidant function of these vitamins could, at least in part, enhance immunity by maintaining the functional and structural integrity of important immune cells. A compromised immune system will result in reduced animal production efficiency through increased susceptibility to diseases, leading to increased morbidity and mortality.

## Effect of Protein Energy Malnutrition (PEM) on Immune Function

Protein energy malnutrition often considered a problem solely of developing countries, is being reported now even in the most of the affluent countries. Moderate malnutrition in the developed world is encountered amongst the elderly, premature babies, hospitalised patients and patients with various diseases (e.g. cystic fibrosis, acquired immunodeficiency syndrome, some cancers). The interaction between malnutrition and impaired immunity was explored nearly 100 years ago, but it was not until late 1950s that malnutrition was firmly established as one of the causes of increased susceptibility to infection. It is now recognised that both malnourishment and over-nutrition adversely impact immunity.

Practically all forms of immunity may be affected by protein energy malnutrition. But non-specific defences and cell-mediated immunity are more severely affected than humoral (antibody) responses. Protein energy malnutrition causes atrophy of the lymphoid organs (thymus, spleen, lymph nodes, tonsils) in laboratory animals and humans.

A large number of studies in animals have demonstrated the adverse effects of protein deficiency on immunity. Saho et al (2009) reported that protein calorie malnutrition (PCM), essential lipid deficiency and vitamin and mineral deficits resulted in some aspects of impaired immunity. In view of the nutrients' need for the immune system, it is not surprising that protein deficiency diminishes immune responses and increases susceptibility to infection. Immune defences are dependent upon cell replication and the production of proteins with biological activities (e.g. antibodies, cytokines, acute phase proteins).

- The circulating white blood cell count can be increased, but this is due to increased numbers of **neutrophils;** the absolute and relative numbers of monocytes, lymphocytes, CD4+T cells and CD8+T cells are decreased.
- The decline in the number of circulating **T lymphocytes** is proportional to the extent of malnutrition. The proliferative response of T lymphocytes to mitogens and antigens is decreased by malnutrition, as is the synthesis of the cytokines IL-2 and

interferon- $\gamma$ (IFN-$\gamma$) and the activity of NK cells.

- Production of cytokines by monocytes, including TNF-$\alpha$, IL-1 and IL-6, is also decreased by malnutrition.

- The *in vivo* delayed-type hypersensitivity (DTH) response to challenge with specific recall antigens is reduced by malnutrition. Bactericidal activity and respiratory burst of neutrophils are decreased by malnutrition, but the phagocytic capacity of neutrophils and monocytes appears to be unaffected.

Hence, it is important to recognise that **appropriate supplementation of macro- and micronutrients are taken care for nourishment of the immune system**.

## Metabolic Requirements for Neutrophil Extracellular Traps (NETs) Formation

Neutrophils are the first cells to be attracted to infected or sterile wounded tissues. They not only provide immune protection but also contribute to healing and recovery. They kill bacteria by engulfment and formation of phagosomes, which fuse with lysosomes to create phagolysosomes. Microbes are killed by oxidative and non-oxidative mechanisms, such as enzymes that catalyse the formation of reactive oxygen and nitrogen species (ROS and RNS), and the release of proteases, iron-binding proteins and defensins.

In 2004, a new functional capacity of neutrophils was identified with the release of neutrophil extracellular traps (NETs). They composed of DNA, histones and microbicidal peptides, with the ability to kill some bacterial species. Several studies have addressed the possible mechanisms that account for NETs formation. Among several others, hyper-citrullination of histones and the formation of reactive oxygen species are required for this process to take place. From the metabolic point of view, it is known that neutrophils contain fewer and less active mitochondria than other immune cells such as lymphocytes and macrophages and that they derive their energy mainly from glycolysis.

Studies conducted by Rodriguez-Espinosa et al. (2015) showed that the formation of NETs is dependent primarily on glucose and, to a lesser extent, on glutamine. This would be expected because glucose is one of the main metabolic substrates and the principal energy source of neutrophils, whereas glutamine accounts for > 20% of the free amino acid pool in plasma, and both have metabolically overlapping functions such as NADPH production and redox homeostasis. In addition, glutamine supports glutathione biosynthesis, whose absence favours oxidative damage in some cell types. The results provide evidence on the strict dependence on glucose and glycolysis for NETs formation.

## IMMUNOMETABOLISM—METABOLIC REGULATION OF T LYMPHOCYTES

One of the most fundamental cellular requirements is the ability to access sufficient and appropriate nutrients to support essential cellular functions. As cells are stimulated to grow, proliferate, or die, their metabolic requirements change and it is important that cellular metabolism matches these demands. Although immune cells spend a significant amount of time in blood, where nutrients are generally abundant, the manner in which these cells uptake and utilise nutrients remains of fundamental importance. Now, it is understood that the regulation of nutrient uptake and utilisation is critically important for the control of immune cell number and function.

## Cellular Metabolism in Resting and Activated Immune Cells—Aerobic Glycolysis

Cellular metabolism is distinct between a resting cell and an activated cell. Cancer cells are proliferative that is they are highly activated. In a seminal finding nearly a century ago, Otto Warburg first observed that rather than relying on mitochondrial oxidative pathways for maximal energy generation, cancer cells use the less efficient process of glycolysis, producing lactic acid even in the presence of sufficient oxygen. Interestingly,

Warburg was also one of the first to study leukocyte metabolism and found the same to be true of activated leukocytes: resting leukocytes use primarily an aerobic oxidative metabolism, whereas stimulation leads to a shift toward glycolysis as the primary metabolic programme. These findings were contrary to classical biochemistry of the time for mammalian cells, as it was believed that cells would rely on the conversion of pyruvate to lactate only when mitochondria were damaged or if oxygen was not present. As activated cells used glycolysis even in the presence of oxygen and this metabolic programme was termed **aerobic glycolysis.**

## Why Activated Lymphocytes Choose Aerobic Glycolysis Over More Energy-Efficient Mitochondrial Oxidative Pathways?

Metabolism must match cell functional demands. Both cancer cells and stimulated lymphocytes are signalled to grow and rapidly proliferate. They share, therefore, a metabolic demand to prioritise efficient and rapid biosynthesis over efficient energy/ATP production. The shift from oxidative metabolism to glycolysis is perfectly suited to match this shift in metabolic demand because oxidative metabolism funnels glucose-derived pyruvate to the mitochondria for oxidation potentially down to carbon dioxide, while glycolysis produces many intermediates that can be used for biosynthesis. In addition to increased glycolysis, some glucose transitions through the mitochondria and a portion of the tricarboxylic acid (TCA) cycle to generate citrate for lipid synthesis. To allow continued TCA flux as citrate molecules are removed to produce lipid membranes, glutamine oxidation increases in a process of anapleurosis that can provide $\alpha$-ketoglutarate for the TCA cycle and metabolic intermediates for biosynthesis of a variety of macromolecules. Thus, although aerobic glycolysis is best characterised by increased rates of glycolysis, coordinated action of glycolysis and mitochondrial metabolism is essential.

## Immunometabolism

Metabolism and immunology have been recently merged to form the rapidly advancing field of immunometabolism. Metabolism generates energy for organisms to sustain all kinds of biological functions. The immune system requires an adequate energy supply for its optimal function. Immunometabolism field explores the interaction between metabolic activities and immune responses.

Metabolic and immune pathways are intimately linked in that key metabolic enzymes and energy metabolites have a direct influence on pro- and anti-inflammatory responses of macrophages. In response to danger signals, activated macrophages reprogram nutrient metabolic pathways (e.g. enhancing aerobic glycolysis) to meet heightened energy requirements and generate sufficient biomolecules to mount an effective innate immune response. Lysine deacetylases are dual regulators of both metabolic pathways and inflammatory responses of macrophages. Lysine acetylation regulates the activity, stability and/or localisation of metabolic enzymes, as well as inflammatory responses in macrophages (Shakespear, M.R. et al, 2018, Trends in Immunology, 39: 473–488).

## Metabolic Control of Regulatory T Cell Development and Function

During the activation and differentiation of T cells, the balance between glycolysis and lipid oxidation shifts in order to cater for the cell's energy requirements. There is increasing evidence that shows how metabolism has an important role in regulating immunity and a series of molecules have been described to play a functional role in both metabolism and the regulation of immune responses. Upon cognate antigen stimulation, naive CD4+T cells are activated and differentiated into Th1, Th2, Th17 or follicular helper (Tfh) effector lineages dependent on instructive cytokine mileu, while some of the effector T cells eventually become memory T cells.

## Regulatory T Cells and Immune Function

Foxp3$^+$ regulatory T cells (Tregs) are a specialised T cell population that provides dominant suppression over effector T cells as well as other immune cells. (1) The majority of Tregs develop in the thymus (tTregs), where they are selected by strong or intermediate T cell receptor (TCR) signals, while escaping negative selection. (2) Tregs can also be converted from naive T cells in the periphery (pTregs), generally at mucosal surfaces that interface with the environment, or in *in vitro* assays (iTregs), particularly in the presence of the anti-inflammatory cytokine transforming growth factor-β (TGF-β).

Expression of the **transcription factor Foxp3** is essential for Treg development and function and it is regulated by genomic regulatory elements termed 'conserved noncoding DNA sequences (CNS) 1–3'. The Treg lineage development is governed by both genetic and epigenetic programmes.

Host-derived nutrients (e.g. short chain fatty acids derived from commensal microbiota) and hormones play an important role in the generation, proliferation and survival of Tregs. Such nutrients control Treg homeostasis and function in the gut associated lymphoid tissue (GALT). Compared to naive T cells, Tregs exhibit unique metabolic activities characterised by low to modest glycolysis and elevated mechanistic target of rapomycin (mTOR) activity and nutrient metabolism.

These exciting new studies indicate that **Tregs could serve as a "liaison" between immunity and metabolism**, that is, immune function is affected by metabolic fitness through modulation of Tregs at three levels of regulation: host nutritional status, commensal microbes and the cellular metabolism of Tregs themselves (Zeng and Chi, 2015).

## Host Metabolism and Regulatory T Cells

It has been reported that host metabolic status and multiple nutrient metabolites impact Treg homeostasis and this may in turn have bearing in metabolic disorders and associated inflammation (Zeng and Chi, 2015). Various vitamins and their metabolites control Treg trafficking and survival.

**Vitamins and their metabolites that control Treg trafficking, generation and survival:** A variety of immunological disorders can result from deficiency of various vitamins. Among these, vitamins A, D, B$_3$ (niacin and nicotinic acid) and B$_9$ (folic acid) have been linked to Treg biology.

### Vitamin A in the form of Retinoic Acid

Dietary sources of vitamin A include all-trans-retinol, retinyl esters and β-carotene. These are first converted to all-transretinal by alcohol dehydrogenases or short chain dehydrogenases/reductases, which are ubiquitously expressed. All-transretinal is then oxidised to all-transretinoic acid (RA) by retinal dehydrogenases, which are selectively expressed by dendritic cells (DCs) in GALT.

Retinoic acid has pleiotropic effects on the host immune system. Specifically, it promotes the effector functions of CD4+T cells, supports the generation of immunoglobulin A (IgA) secreting B cells in GALT, mediates the balance between innate lymphoid cell (ILC) 3 and ILC2, and controls secondary lymphoid organ development.

Retinoic acid also imprints gut-homing specificity on T cells and B cells by inducing the expression of α4β7 integrin and CCR9, two receptors critical for trafficking to the small intestine, and this process is dependent on the activity of the p38 signalling pathway in mucosal DCs.

Retinoic acid has an important role in shaping Treg development and function in the gut. Of note, different T cell lineages do not represent irreversibly differentiated endpoints. In particular, iTregs and Th17 subsets exhibit considerable plasticity, in that they can be reciprocally regulated by cytokines and cellular metabolism. Retinoic acid synthesis from vitamin A in the intestine is dependent upon CD103$^+$ DCs in the mesenteric lymph nodes (MLN) and the small intestine lamina propria (LP).

CD103+ DC-derived RA, in combination with TGF-β, induces Foxp3 expression in naive T cells and these pTregs preferentially home to MLN and the small intestine. This mechanism has significant physiological implications because it underlies tolerance induced by oral or food-derived antigens, known as oral tolerance, which is critically dependent on pTreg generation. Thus, retinoic acid promotes TGF-β-mediated pTreg generation and homing in GALT and maintains mucosa immune tolerance.

## Vitamin D

Vitamin $D_3$ is synthesised in the skin from 7-dehydrochelesterol under sunlight, or acquired from the diet. Vitamin $D_3$ is further metabolised into $25(OH)D_3$ and $1,25(OH)_2D_3$, the most biologically active form, in the liver, kidney and many immune cells. The cellular action of $1,25(OH)_2D_3$ is mediated by the vitamin D receptor (VDR), a ligand-dependent transcription factor. The VDR is expressed by most cells of the immune system, including regulatory T cells and antigen-presenting cells, such as dendritic cells and macrophages. Because of this, 1,25 $(OH)_2D_3$ is produced and acts locally to regulate the immune response. $1,25(OH)_2D_3$ inhibits T cell proliferation and cytokine production, as well as inducing Foxp3 expression and enhancing the suppressive activity of Tregs. Moreover, it can induce tolerogenic DCs that enhance Treg generation and mediate transplantation tolerance.

Vitamin D response elements (VDRE) have been identified in the 'conserved noncoding sequence region' of the human Foxp3 gene and these could underlie how vitamin $D_3$ induces Foxp3 expression. However, vitamin $D_3$ has been shown to be required for human T cell activation. Additionally, mice lacking VDR contain normal numbers of functional Tregs in spleen and thymus and do not develop overt systemic autoimmune disorders. Nonetheless, they do have low-grade

inflammation (LGI) in the colon manifested by increased expression of IL-1β and TNF-α. Therefore, the physiological relevance of vitamin $D_3$ metabolites on Treg induction remains to be ascertained (Zeng and Chi, 2015).

## Folic Acid (Vitamin B₉)

Tetrahydrofolate (folic acid) is required for DNA synthesis, repair and methylation. It is particularly involved in cell proliferation and survival. Folate plays a critical role in nucleic acid and prolactin synthesis by supplying one-carbon units needed for DNA and histone methylation. A deficiency of folate significantly alters the immune response. tTregs (Foxp3+ regulatory T cells [Tregs] developed in thymus) constitutively express high level of folate receptor4 (FR4), which binds folic acid and delivers its derivatives into cells. The importance of dietary folic acid to Tregs is revealed by the selective reduction of intestinal Tregs in mice fed with folic acid-deficient diet or treated with an inhibitor that disrupts folic acid metabolism. It promotes Treg cellularity by inhibiting apoptosis. Further, its deficiency leads to increased colonic inflammation, which can be ameliorated by transfer of FR4+ tTregs. Tregs purified from human peripheral blood mononuclear cells (PBMC) also preferentially express FR4 relative to other lymphocytes. Thus, vitamin $B_9$ metabolism maintains gut Treg survival and restricts intestinal inflammation.

## Niacin (Vitamin B₃)

Vitamin $B_3$ (niacin and nicotinic acid) is an essential nutrient. Deficiency of vitamin $B_3$ in humans leads to pellagra, a disease characterised by intestinal inflammation, diarrhoea, dermatitis and dementia. Vitamin $B_3$ signals through the G-protein-coupled receptor (GPR) 109a. This interaction induces anti-inflammatory properties, including the expression of retinal dehydrogenases in colon macrophages and DCs, which in turn induce Treg differentiation. GPR109a-deficient mice contain reduced colonic Tregs and show increased susceptibility to colonic inflammation. Thus, vitamin $B_3$ promotes colonic Treg generation and maintains colon homeostasis (Zeng and Chi, 2015).

## METABOLIC PATHWAYS THAT SUPPORT T CELL DEVELOPMENT AND IMMUNITY

### Mobilising T Cells out of Quiescence in Times of Pathogen Invasion

Simply stated, we are what we eat. Our genetics, coupled with environmental influences, dictate how we metabolise the nutrients that we consume and how this shapes our growth, function and overall health (M.D. Buck et al, 2015). The same principles hold true at the cellular level. Just as a track runner quickly engages his/her muscles to propel himself/ herself from rest to sprint in response to a starting gun, pathogen-derived or inflammatory signals drive T cells out of quiescence, resulting in rapid modulation of gene expression and the acquisition of new functions. These changes range from increased production of cytokines and cytolytic molecules to the ability to undergo cell division and migration. Intimately integrated into this programme of activation is the regulation of cellular metabolism.

The engagement of specific metabolic pathways profoundly affects cell differentiation and function. **Metabolic reprogramming** is controlled by key receptor signalling events and growth factor cytokines, as well as availability of nutrients. In addition, metabolic products provide substrates that can alter the functional fate of a cell through posttranslational modifications (PTMs) or epigenetic remodelling. Several recent articles have covered these and other emerging topics in T cell metabolism (Lochner et al, 2015; Palmer et al, 2015).

### Lymphocyte Metabolism

Lymphocytes must adapt to a wide array of environmental stressors as part of their normal development, during which they undergo a dramatic metabolic remodelling process. Diverse metabolic pathways and metabolites have been found to regulate lymphocyte signalling and influence differentiation, function and fate.

T cells engage specific metabolic pathways during development that underpin their differentiation and function. T cells cycle through states of metabolic quiescence and activation. Naive T cells mature and exit from the thymus into the periphery. As quiescent cells, they primarily oxidise glucose-derived pyruvate in their mitochondria via oxidative phosphorylation, or they use fatty acid oxidation to generate ATP for their metabolic needs. Once in the periphery, a mature naive T cell is triggered to activate to effector T cells. Activated effector T cells follow aerobic glycolysis. See page 42 for details on aerobic glycolysis.

Although aerobic glycolysis is less efficient than oxidative phosphorylation at yielding great amount of ATP per molecule of glucose, aerobic glycolysis can generate metabolic intermediates important for cell growth and proliferation and provides a way to maintain redox balance (NAD+/NADH) in the cell (Fig. 2.5). For example, glucose-6-phosphate and 3-phosphoglycerate (3PG) produced during glycolysis can be metabolised in the pentose phosphate and serine biosynthesis pathways, respectively, donating important precursors for nucleotide and amino acid synthesis.

### Metabolic Pathways that Support T Cells

Glucose can also enter the mitochondria as pyruvate, where it is converted to acetyl-CoA and joins the TCA cycle by condensing with oxaloacetate to form citrate. Breakdown of substrates in the TCA cycle not only provides reducing equivalents for oxidative phosphorylation, but also precursors for biosynthesis. Glucose-derived citrate can be exported into the cytosol to generate acetyl-CoA by ATP citrate lyase (ACL) for use in lipid synthesis. Similarly, oxaloacetate can be used to produce aspartate, an additional precursor for generating nucleotides (Fig. 2.5).

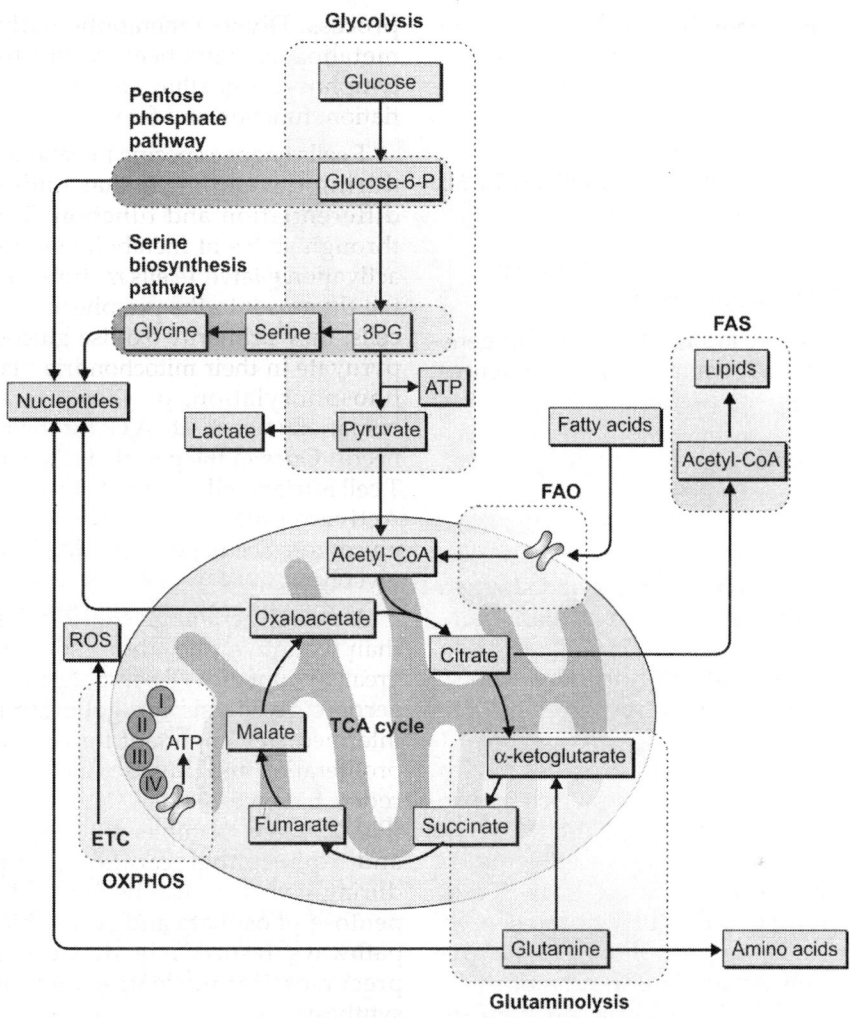

**Fig. 2.5:** Metabolic pathways that support T cells (*Source*: M.D.Buck et al, 2015)

ATP is the molecular currency of energy in the cell. It can be derived from glucose through two integrated pathways. (1) glycolysis, the enzymatic breakdown of glucose to pyruvate in the cytoplasm. (2) The TCA cycle, where pyruvate is converted to acetyl-CoA in the mitochondria and shuttled through several enzymatic reactions to generate reducing equivalents to fuel oxidative phosphorylation. Other substrates can also be metabolised in the TCA cycle, such as glutamine via glutaminolysis or fatty acids via fatty acid oxidation (FAO). These connected biochemical pathways can also provide metabolic precursors for biosynthesis.

Intermediates from glucose catabolism during glycolysis can shuttle through the pentose phosphate and serine biosynthesis pathways to fuel nucleotide and amino acid production. Oxaloacetate from the TCA cycle can similarly be used to generate aspartate for use in nucleotide synthesis. Precursors for amino acid and nucleotide biosynthesis can be obtained from glutamine. Citrate from the TCA cycle can be exported from the mitochondria and converted to acetyl-CoA for fatty acid synthesis (FAS). Reactive oxygen species (ROS) generated from the electron transport chain (ETC) during oxidative phosphorylation (OXPHOS) can also act as secondary signalling molecules (Fig. 2.5).

## Importance of Transcription Factors and Signalling Pathways in T Cell Development

Several transcription factors and signalling pathways coordinately support and regulate this change in T cell metabolic programmes after activation. (1) Growth factor cytokines such as IL-2 and ligation of costimulatory molecules promote the switch to glycolysis through the enhancement of nutrient transporter expression and activation of the key metabolic regulator mTOR. mTOR exists as two complexes, mTORC1 and mTORC2; these integrate extrinsic and intrinsic signals related to nutrient levels, energy status and stress to induce changes in cellular metabolism, growth and proliferation. (2) CD28 ligation enhances phosphatidylinositol 3-kinase (PI3K) activity, which recruits 3-phosphoinositide-dependent protein kinase-1 (PDPK1) and Akt. PDPK1, together with mTORC2, phosphorylates Akt, which in turn activates mTORC1. (3) Both Akt and mTOR promote aerobic glycolysis and support effector T cell differentiation, growth and function. Akt regulates nutrient transporter expression and can phosphorylate the glycolytic enzyme hexokinase II, promoting its localisation to the mitochondria and augmenting its enzymatic activity. (4) mTORC1 activation increases protein translation via phosphorylation of 4E-BP1 and p70S6 kinase and promotes lipid synthesis by activating SREBP2 (sterol regulatory element-binding protein 2).

## Transcription Factors

The up-regulation of transcription factors c-Myc, estrogen-related receptor $\alpha$ (ERR$\alpha$) and hypoxia inducible factor-1$\alpha$ (HIF-1$\alpha$) coordinately drives the expression of genes involved in intermediary metabolism that fuel the rapid proliferation of effector T cells during clonal expansion. c-Myc has been shown to be a critical regulator of metabolic reprogramming after T cell activation. c-Myc drives the expression of enzymes that promote aerobic glycolysis and glutaminolysis and coordinates these metabolic pathways with lipid, amino acid and nucleic acid synthesis. HIF-1$\alpha$, a transcription factor that responds to oxygen levels, also increases glucose uptake and catabolism through glycolysis.

## Metabolite Succinate

ROS is produced as a general byproduct of mitochondrial metabolism. But recent studies have specifically linked the metabolite succinate to both the generation of ROS and activation of HIF-1$\alpha$ in settings of inflammation or injury (Tannahill et al, 2013; Chouchani et al, 2014). Innate immune receptor activation increases intracellular succinate from glutamine via glutamine-dependent anerplerosis and the $\gamma$-amino-butyric acid shunt pathway and this leads to HIF-1$\alpha$ stabilisation and activation (Tannahill et al, 2013). Given that mitochondrial ROS and HIF-1$\alpha$ activity are important for the metabolic reprogramming of naive T cells after activation, **it is interesting to speculate that the metabolite succinate may also support the transition from a naive to an activated effector T cell.**

## Metabolic Programming of T Helper Cell Differentiation

Activation of T cells is intimately tied to the engagement of specific metabolic pathways, so it is no surprise that distinct-metabolic programmes also support the differentiation of CD4 T helper (Th) cells into their separate lineages. The results of Delgoffe et al (2009) are consistent with the metabolic profiles of these cells: Th1, Th2, and Th17 cells strongly engage glycolysis via mTOR signalling, whereas FoxP3+ regulatory T (Treg) cells depend more on the oxidation of lipids. Th17 cells in particular have been found to heavily rely on glycolysis for their development and maintenance, stimulated by HIF-1α activity downstream of mTOR.

## Substrate Utilisation in Activated T Cells

**Carbohydrates:** Glucose is a key metabolic substrate for T cells. Upon T cell activation, glucose transporter Glut1 traffics to the cell surface from intracellular vesicles. Overexpression of Glut1 in mice results in larger naive T cells and an increased number of CD44[hi] T cells. It suggests that glucose acquisition mediates early steps in T cell activation, such as promoting the expression of activation markers and increasing cell size. Consistent with these observations, T cell specific deletion of Glut1 impairs CD4 T cell activation, clonal expansion and survival (Macintyre et al, 2014).

When deprived of glucose, CD8 T cells display defects in functional capacity with reduced IFN-γ, granzyme and perforin production. More recently it was shown that T cells can become activated and proliferate when glucose catabolism through aerobic glycolysis is limited, as they can rely on oxidative phosphorylation. However, in this case, effector function is compromised, with impaired cytokine production caused by posttranscriptional regulation by the glycolytic enzyme GAPDH. When disengaged from glycolysis, GAPDH can function as a RNA-binding protein (RBP) and prevent the translation of cytokine messenger RNAs containing AU-rich elements in their 3-UTRs. Therefore, in addition to providing precursors for biomass, augmenting aerobic glycolysis in activated T cells allows for the acquisition of full effector function.

## Amino Acids

i. Glucose is a critical substrate for T cells. But glutamine is also essential during T cell activation. T cells increase the expression of glutamine transporters and their deletion impairs the transition to an effector T cell. Clear differences in concentrations of other amino acids also exist in quiescent compared with activated T cells, corresponding to their distinct metabolic requirements. Recent research has begun to uncover the vast array of additional amino acid transporters and catabolising enzymes that regulate amino acid levels, revealing important roles for amino acids in T cell metabolism and function.

ii. Deficiency in the neutral amino acid transporter S1c7a5 (LAT1), which transports leucine, prevents the metabolic reprogramming, clonal expansion and/or effector function of both CD4 and CD8 T cells (Hayashi et al, 2013; Sinclair et al, 2013). These cells had impaired mTORC1 activation and were unable to induce key metabolic processes, such as enhancing glutamine and glucose uptake (Sinclair et al, 2013). This deficiency, however, did not impair the ability of CD4 T cells to differentiate into Treg cells. Additionally, protein expression of the key metabolic transcription factor, c-Myc, was diminished, despite its increased mRNA expression upon activation (Sinclair et al, 2013). This raises the intriguing question of whether leucine deficiency results in posttranslational regulation of c-Myc expression.

Results from another study suggest that modulation of intracellular leucine concentrations can be used to regulate metabolic reprogramming. It was found that the expression of the cytosolic branched chain aminotransferase (BCATc), which can reduce intracellular leucine concentrations through a transamination reaction, limited the mTORC1 activation (Ananieva et al, 2014). BCATc expression was upregulated upon CD4 T cell activation, and T cells that lacked BCATc had increased intracellular leucine, which correlated with enhanced activation of mTORC1 and glycolytic phenotype. Increased BCATc expression has been observed in anergic T cells, which have impaired metabolic function (Zheng et al, 2009; Ananieva et al, 2014). These data could suggest that leucine depletion by BCATc contributes to T cell anergy through suppression of mTOR activity.

iii. The alanine serine and cysteine transporter system (ASCT2/S1c1a5), which also transports glutamine, is another solute carrier whose expression increases after T cell activation. It was recently found that loss of ASCT2 decreased glutamine import and impaired oxidative phosphorylation and glucose metabolism in activated CD4T cells (Nakaya et al, 2014). Surprisingly, the loss of ASCT2 did not inhibit proliferation or IL-2 production. However, ASCT2-deficient cells cultured *in vitro* had a decreased ability to differentiate into Th1 and Th17 cells, but not Th2 or Treg cells. Interestingly, glutamine transport into cells can substantially enhance leucine transport via S1c7a5, as increased intracellular glutamine levels result in glutamine export and concomitant import of leucine by this transporter (Nicklin et al, 2009). Supporting this additional role for glutamine in T cell activation, addition of leucine to T cells lacking ASCT2 helps rescue their polarisation defects (Nakaya et al, 2014).

iv. Depletion of extracellular arginine has been found to impair T cell proliferation and aerobic glycolysis, but not mitochondrial oxidative phosphorylation (Fletcher et al, 2015). However, T cells can partially compensate by synthesising arginine *de novo* via an argininosuccinate 1 (ASS 1)–dependent process, provided extracellular concentrations of citrulline are sufficient.

v. A recent study suggests that intracellular recycling of amino acids also contributes to T cell amino acid homeostasis. Cytosolic protease tripeptidyl peptidase II (TPPII) digests proteins for the recycling of amino acids. Hence deficiency of TPPII leads to increased sensitivity to perturbations in intracellular amino acids concentrations, which reflected in impaired IFN-γ production and a susceptibility to viral infections (Lu et al, 2014). Lack of TPPII activity in both human and murine T cells resulted in impaired glycolysis caused by enhanced degradation of the key glycolytic enzyme hexokinase II, an effect that likely contributed to their impaired cytokine production (Lu et al, 2014).

vi. Many products of amino acid catabolism also have important nonanaplerotic roles that can alter cell signalling and function. (a) The metabolic byproduct of tryptophan catabolism, kynurenine, can ligate the aryl hydrocarbon receptor and enhance polarisation of CD4 T cells to a Treg phenotype (Mezrich et al, 2010). (b) Another example is catabolism of phenylalanine by IL-4-induced gene 1 protein (IL4I1). When highly expressed by tumours or APCs, IL4I1 can inhibit T cell proliferation (Boulland et al, 2007). This effect appears to be caused by the production of $H_2O_2$, a product of phenylalanine catabolism. IL4I1 is also expressed in Th17 and Treg cells (Santarlasci et al, 2012). However given that low concentrations of $H_2O_2$ can act as a signalling molecule (Veal et al, 2007), IL4I1 might also play a role in cell signalling pathways independent of mechanisms that inhibit proliferation.

vii. Fluctuations in environmental amino acid concentrations, as well as metabolic products from amino acid catabolism, can dramatically alter T cell activity and polarisation. A well-documented example of this is indoleamine-2,3-dioxygenase (IDO)-mediated tryptophan catabolism. IDO, which is often expressed at high levels by APCs or tumour cells, can deplete tryptophan within a tissue microenvironment and this in turn can lead to inhibition of effector T cell proliferation and induction of anergy. Depletion of tryptophan causes activation of the 'integrated stress response inducer' general control nonderepressible 2 (GCN2) kinase. This results in the inhibition of translation, initiation and metabolic remodelling. See chapter 'Amino acids and Immunity'.

viii. Studies into the interactions of APCs or tumour cells with T cells have highlighted multiple pathways through which APCs modulate extracellular concentrations of amino acids, or their catabolic products, to regulate T cell responses. In a tumour, TGF-β-producing DCs can enhance expression of transporters for histidine, leucine, valine and tryptophan, depleting these amino acids from the extracellular micro environment and directly impairing T cell proliferation.

Treg cells can also enhance expression of particular amino acid catabolising enzymes, including arginase 1, histidine decarboxylase, threonine dehydrogenase and IL4I1, in skin grafts and bone marrow–derived DCs. Limitations in these amino acids, singularly or in combination, enhanced Treg cell polarisation when T cells were activated *in vitro*.

Although depletion of amino acids from the microenvironment appears to be a way in which APCs can negatively regulate T cell activity, the opposite also occurs, whereby APCs can support T cell activation through supplementing a microenvironment (with amino acid). For example, DCs and monocytes can release cysteine, which is thought to support T cell activation and function. Cysteine supply is a limiting factor in T cell proliferation and is used extensively for protein and glutathione synthesis, as well as providing beneficial catabolic products, such as taurine, which may support T cell function through regulating osmolality.

**Lipid metabolism:** Lipids or fatty acids encompass another critical substrate group for T cells. They are a vital component of cell membranes, provide a high yielding energy source, and can also supply substrates for cell signalling and PTMs (Lochner et al, 2015;

Thurnher and Gruenbacher, 2015). After T cell activation, the demand for lipids rapidly increases. Within 24 hours, *in vitro*-activated T cells augment fatty acid synthesis (FAS), while concomitantly decreasing FAO, thus enhancing the accumulation of fatty acid metabolites needed for membrane synthesis. c-Myc and mTOR have important roles in coordinating these metabolic changes. SREBP transcription factors are critical for reprogramming lipid metabolism. SREBPs (Sterol response element binding proteins) induce expression of genes involved in FAS and mevalonate pathways, which supply *de novo* synthesised fatty acids and cholesterol, respectively (Thurnher and Gruenbacher, 2015). CD4 T cells deficient in Raptor, and thus mTORC1 signalling, have impaired *de novo* FAS, most likely caused by reduced expression of SREBP1 and SREBP2 protein.

## Exogenous Cholesterol Supplementation

Loss of SREBP function in CD8 T cells results in a failure to induce metabolic pathways needed for clonal expansion during a viral infection. **Exogenous cholesterol** rescues the defects in SREBP-deficient T cells, suggesting a lack of cholesterol is the main limiting factor. This requirement for cholesterol synthesis is consistent with results showing that perturbing sterol homeostasis in activated T cells impairs T cell proliferation. Liver X Receptor (LXR) targets genes that are involved in cholesterol cellular transport. The inhibitory effect of LXR activation can be overcome through the addition of mevalonate (Fig. 2.6), a cholesterol precursor (Bensinger et al, 2008).

Inhibition of 3-hydroxy-3-methylglutaryl-coenzymeA (HMG-CoA) reductase, an enzyme in the mevalonate pathway (See cholesterol biosynthesis, Fig. 2.6), results in a Th2 cell bias in the experimental autoimmune encephalomyelitis (EAE) disease model, due to impaired biosynthesis of isoprenoids and a subsequent reduction in prenylation of Ras and RhoA GTPases (Youssef et al, 2002). These data suggest that in addition to cholesterol homeostasis, other products of the mevalonate pathway can also influence T cell differentiation. The impact of commonly used drugs that lower cholesterol by inhibiting

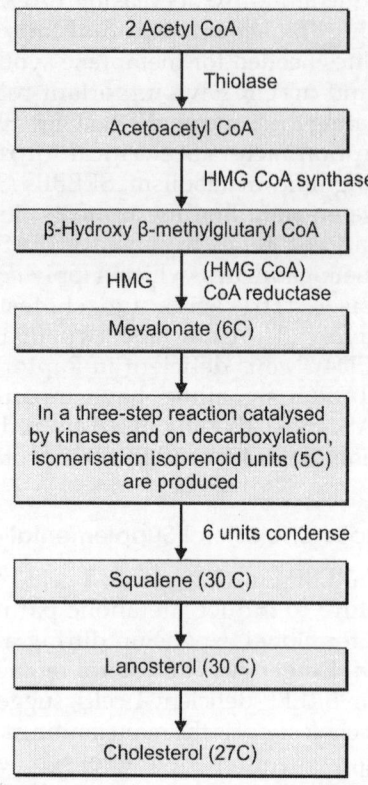

**Fig. 2.6:** Outline of cholesterol biosynthesis

HMG-CoA reductase can affect both prenylation and cholesterol synthesis, and thus it is plausible these drugs have multiple effects on activated T cells.

**The synthesis of fatty acids is also important for effector T cell function.** Although activated T cells readily acquire and use extracellular fatty acids, it appears that there may also be cell-intrinsic requirements for *de* novo-synthesised fatty acids (Berod et al, 2014; O'Sullivan and Pearce, 2014; O'Sullivan et al, 2014).

- Inhibition of acetyl-CoA carboxylase 1 (ACC1, an enzyme in FAS), was shown to limit Th17 cell differentiation and promote the development of Treg cells.

- Inhibition of ACC1 impaired phospholipid synthesis in Th17 cells, while also impairing glycolytic flux, both through aerobic glycolysis and the TCA cycle. In contrast, Treg cells were able to sustain their requirements for fatty acids through acquisition from extracellular sources (Berod et al, 2014).

- ACC1 deficiency also impairs Th1 and Th2 development, suggesting that CD4 effector T cells have a common requirement for FAS (Berod et al, 2014). In contrast, T cell-specific deletion of ACC1 does not impair CD8 effector T cell development after infection, although effector T cell expansion is diminished due to increased cell death, indicating that FAS is required for the persistence of CD8 effector T cells.

- Collectively, these findings suggest that there are varying requirements for *de novo*-synthesised fatty acids between different T cell subsets.

- Interestingly, defects after ACC1 inhibition in either Th17 cells or CD8 effector T cells can be rescued through the addition of excess free fatty acids to the media (Berod et al, 2014), indicating that these cells can compensate for the lack of FAS if the extracellular fatty acid supply is plentiful.

- Addition of extracellular fatty acids can also enhance T cell proliferation. It suggests that lipid released from adipose tissue may enhance T cell proliferation *in vivo*.

## Utilisation of FAO in Effector T Cells

Although in general the balance of FAS to FAO within effector T cell populations is weighted heavily toward FAS, effector T cells can use FAO (Byersdorfer et al, 2013; O'Sullivan et al, 2014). Given that the demand for energy is high in these cells, it is likely that they need some metabolic flexibility in their fuel sources, an idea that is consistent with recent work highlighting the importance of adenosine monophosphate-activated protein kinase (AMPK) in effector T cell function (Blagih et al, 2015). The extent to which FAO occurs in effector T cells is likely to be highly context dependent, in part due to the heterogeneity of this population of cells during an immune response. Results of several studies suggest that the utilisation of FAO in effector T cells may be influenced by several factors, such as activation state, exposure to antigen, inflammatory signals, and microenvironmental nutrient availability.

## Memory T Cell Metabolism

Effector T cell populations contract after pathogen clearance and undergo apoptosis, leaving behind a small population of long-lived memory T cells that can respond vigorously upon antigen rechallenge (Williams and Bevan, 2007). Although both naive and memory T cells acquire effector functions upon activation, memory T cells have an accelerated response to antigen, proliferate faster and produce more cytokines than their naive counterparts. Work of Buck et al (2015) and others have shown that changes in metabolism also drive memory T cell development.

**AMPK and mTOR:** AMPK is important for the development of memory T cells. Increases in intracellular AMP-to-ATP concentrations activate the 'energy stress sensor' AMPK, a signal that also promotes FAO (Jones and Thompson, 2007). Administration of **metformin** (the metabolic stressor and AMPK activator) enhances the generation of memory T cells after infection. In addition, AMPK allows for effector T cells to metabolically adapt during nutrient stress and modulates T cell effector function through suppression of mTOR. **Rapamycin** inhibits mTOR and this boosts memory T cell development *in vivo*. Loss of the mTORC1-negative regulator TSC1 compromises formation of memory T cell precursors that are present during the primary effector response. Similarly, suppressing mTORC2 fosters memory T cell generation (Pollizzi et al, 2015).

Inhibition of mTOR and activation of AMPK also strongly stimulate the catabolic process of autophagy. Autophagy has been shown to support T cell viability and bioenergetics after activation (Hubbard et al,

2010). Consistent with the idea that activation of catabolic pathways promotes the development of memory T cells, a recent study found that deletion of the autophagy molecules Atg5 or Atg7 compromised the formation of CD8 memory T cells after viral infection (Xu et al, 2014).

**FAO and Memory T cells:** Work of Buck and coworkers has shown that CD8 memory T cells are dependent on FAO for their development, long-term persistence and ability to robustly respond to antigen stimulation. Enhancing FAO in memory T cells through increased expression of carnitine palmitoyl-transferase 1a (CPT1a) (a critical mitochondrial transporter of long-chain fatty acids and rate limiting step to β-oxidation) increases CD8 memory T cell numbers after infection. During an immune response, common γ chain cytokines like IL-15 and IL-7 have an essential role in supporting catabolic metabolism by promoting mitochondrial biogenesis, CPT1a expression, and FAO. As a result, memory T cells have increased mitochondrial mass and greater spare respiratory capacity (SRC) compared with naive and effector T cells, which endows them with a bioenergetic advantage for survival and recall after antigen rechallenge.

The specific role of FAO in promoting memory T cell development and survival remains to be elucidated, but it appears that metabolic reprogramming associated with FAO enhances mitochondria-associated processes. Induction of FAO in memory T cells enhances spare respiratory capacity (SRC), which is the reserve capacity of mitochondria to produce energy over and above normal energy outputs. This parameter is probably important for the longevity of memory T cells, especially in times of stress or nutrient restriction, conditions that may present themselves when infection is resolved and growth factor signals are scarce. Surprisingly, endothelial cells, unlike most other cell types, use carbon derived from FAO for nucleotide synthesis and proliferation (Schoors et al, 2015), providing another way in which FAO supports cell function.

O'Sullivan et al (2014) reported that memory T cells preferentially use *de novo* FAS to fuel FAO. Specifically, CD8 memory T cells use glucose to produce triglycerides (TAGs) that are subsequently hydrolysed by lysosomal acid lipase (LAL) to support mitochondrial FAO. It was also recently shown that glucose metabolism is critical for CD4 memory T cell survival, and this is controlled by Notch signalling (Maekawa et al, 2015). The requirement for FAS in CD8 memory T cells is supported by a recent study showing that glycerol import into the cell via IL-7-induced aquaporin-mediated transport is required for memory T cell longevity (Cui et al, 2015). Glycerol is the molecular backbone for TAGs. Aquaporin 9 (AQP9)-deficient T cells had reduced glycerol import and TAG synthesis and impaired memory T cell survival after viral infection (Cui et al, 2015).

The reasons why CD8 memory T cells synthesise and then catabolise fatty acids in an apparently futile cycle rather than simply acquire extracellular fatty acids are not understood. However, this synthesis/catabolism cycle has also been shown to occur in muscle and adipose tissues (Dulloo et al, 2004). If viewed on a purely energetic level, this process appears counter-productive, as there would be no net gain in ATP. It is possible that building and burning fatty acids allows memory T cells to sustain their glycolytic and lipogenic machinery while maintaining mitochondrial health during times of quiescence, allowing for the rapid recall ability that is characteristic of memory T cells after antigen recognition and activation (Buck et al, 2015).

## T Cell Metabolic Reprogramming During its Activation

It is an exciting time for the field of immunometabolism. We are just beginning to understand the many connections between metabolism and gene regulation in T cells (Buck et al, 2015). Protein acetylation is a reversible post-translational modification (PTM) that influences epigenetic changes mediated by histone acetyltransferases (HATs) and histone deacetylases (HDACs) and also controls the actions of transcription factors and molecular chaperones. Acetyl-CoA and NAD+ generated from oxidative metabolism are used for HAT and HDAC activity. T cell metabolic reprogramming during activation increases cytosolic NAD+ and citrate (the precursor of acetyl-CoA), which may direct cell-fate decisions through protein acetylation.

## Circadian Rhythm and Lymphocyte Metabolism

Acetylation also affects the activity of circadian clock proteins. Organisms rely on the cell autonomous transcription-translation oscillator loop managed by solar time to accommodate physiological changes brought about by the daily pattern of rest, activity and feeding (Curtis et al, 2014). The circadian clock also in part regulates Th17 cell development (Yu et al, 2013). Circadian rhythm controls nutrient acquisition and metabolic flux, and it will be interesting to see how the body's internal clock may connect to lymphocyte metabolism, regulation, and function (Rey and Reddy, 2013).

## Intermediates from Glucose, One-carbon and Serine and Glycine Metabolism Support T cell Growth and Proliferation

Intermediates from glucose catabolism can be converted into substrates that are needed to support cell growth and proliferation. Many common features are shared between 'activated T cells' and 'proliferating cancer cells'. Hence, the leads from one-carbon metabolism in cancer research involving the serine and glycine biosynthetic pathways may have implications for T cell metabolism. Role of one-carbon metabolism in generating units for nucleic acid synthesis from folate has long been known. Now it is recognised that this pathway is an important source of NADPH to maintain redox balance and methyl groups for methylation (Locasale,

2013; Fan et al, 2014). Serine and glycine metabolism also have a vital role in cell survival under harsh environmental conditions of nutrient scarcity and hypoxia. T cells also migrate and travel to sites of infection and must adapt to these hypoxic or nutrient-depleted environments (Pearce et al, 2013).

## METABOLIC REQUIREMENTS FOR PLASMA CELL FORMATION AND ANTIBODY PRODUCTION

### Nutrient Needs of Plasma Cell Secretion

Humoral immunity (B lymphocytes) is generated and maintained by antigen-specific antibodies that counter infectious pathogens. Plasma cells are the major producers of antibodies during and after infections, and each plasma cell produces some thousands of antibody molecules per second. This magni-

tude of secretion requires enormous quantities of amino acids and glycosylation sugars (see Appendix) to properly build and fold antibodies, biosynthetic substrates to fuel endoplasmic reticulum (ER) biogenesis and additional carbon sources to generate energy. Lam and Bhattacharya (2018) has reviewed these aspects of plasma cell biology.

### Intermediary Metabolism in Plasma Cell Formation and Maintenance

Naive resting B cells have scant cytoplasm and endoplasmic reticulum. They appear to have relatively few energy or biosynthetic requirements (Fig. 2.7). However, activation of naive B cells [in vitro with mitogens such as bacterial lipopolysaccharide (LPS)] leads to increased glucose transporter expression, glucose uptake, glycolysis and oxidative phosphorylation (Fig. 2.7). Germinal center

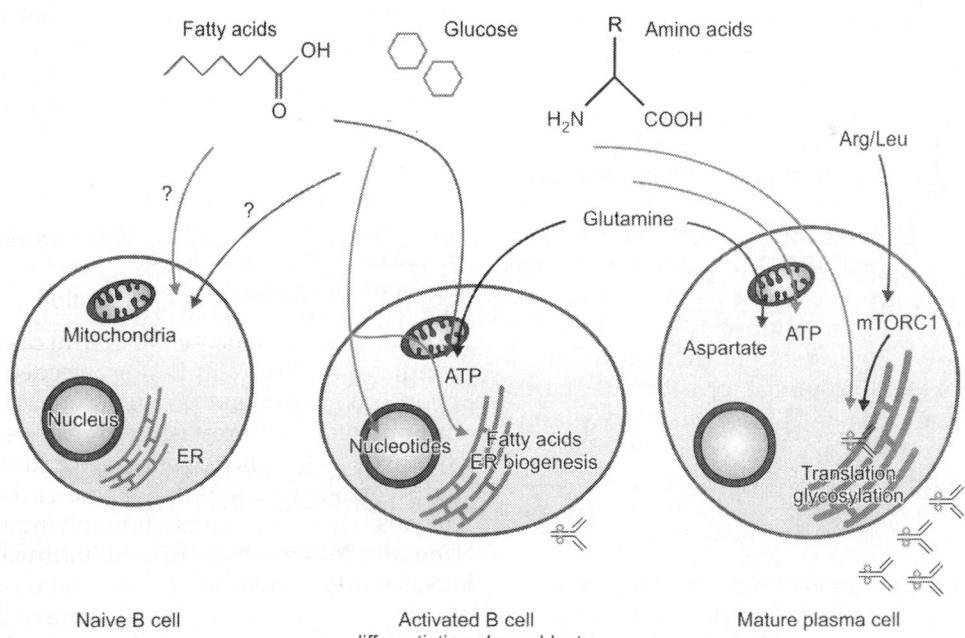

**Fig. 2.7:** Major metabolic fates of nutrients during B cell differentiation into plasma cells. *Source:* Lam and Bhattacharya (2018). The known metabolic fates of glucose, amino acids and fatty acids are shown as B cells (left) differentiate into plasma cells (right). Arrows passing through mitochondria indicate a metabolic process that takes place in that organelle, while the endoplasmic reticulum (ER) and nucleus indicate sites where the end-products of nutrients are used

B cells *(in vivo)* also rely on glycolysis, although these cells import relatively little glucose. After activation, glucose-derived carbons can be found not only in glycolytic and tricarboxylic acid cycle intermediates but also in cataplerotic biosynthetic pathways that generate fatty acids including phosphatidylethanolamine, phosphatidylcholine, ceramide and cholesterol (Dufort, F.J. et al, 2014).

These *de novo* synthesised fatty acids are crucial for the initial expansion of the endoplasmic reticulum that occurs during plasma cell differentiation as well as for the expression of hallmark transcription factors such as Prdml(Dufort et al, 2014). With marked endoplasmic reticulum (ER) expansion coupled with increased translation of ER-associated proteins and the production of copious amounts of antibodies, nearly 70% of the transcriptome is devoted to immunoglobulin synthesis. Fatty acids also undergo β-oxidation to generate ATP.

Once plasma cells are formed, the metabolic requirements switch to support antibody production and organelle maintenance rather than biogenesis (Fig. 2.7). Some of these changes are mediated by the aforementioned transcription factor Prdml, which promotes the expression of amino acid transporters. Amino acids such as leucine and arginine activate the mechanistic target of rapamycin complex 1 (mTORC1) in plasma cells that enhances protein synthesis. B cell-intrinsic genetic manipulation of the mTORC1 pathway suggests that this pathway is essential for the optimal formation of plasma cells from activated precursors. Once plasma cells are fully differentiated, mTORC1 is predominantly used to enhance antibody production.

### Distinct Change in Metabolic Pathways during B Cell Differentiation into Plasma Cells

Within intestinal B cells, diet-derived vitamin $B_1$ is essential for promoting oxidative phosphorylation and plasma cell formation, but is dispensable once plasma cells are already formed (Kunisawa et al, 2015). Intestinal IgA+ plasma cells instead utilise diet- and gut microbiota-derived short-chain fatty acids as at least a small portion of the required carbon sources for the electron transport chain and to maintain cellular fatty acid content.

Glucose continues to be utilised by plasma cells once they are fully mature, but is preferentially shunted into metabolic pathways distinct from those employed during B cell activation (Fig. 2.7). Moreover, glucose is potentially imported by unique cell-surface transporters in mature plasma cells.

During initial B cell activation and differentiation, glucose is used primarily for glycolysis, oxidative phosphorylation, lipid synthesis and the pentose phosphate pathway (PPP), whereas glucose taken up by mature plasma cells is primarily diverted into the hexosamine pathway (HSP) to glycosylate antibodies. However, upon depletion of energy reserves, glucose can be diverted from the hexosamine pathway back to glycolysis, and the resultant pyruvate can be used for respiration.

This glucose, when catabolised, also stabilises expression of anti-apoptotic Mcl1, a factor that is essential for plasma cell survival. Glucose thereby maintains energy reserves and survival pathways that promote long-term maintenance of antibody-secreting cells. This is another example of how a nutrient (glucose) that is involved in antibody assembly (glycosylation sugars) is also used to promote plasma cell survival (Lam and Bhattacharya, 2018).

### THE MULTIFACETED ROLE OF NRF2 IN MITOCHONDRIAL FUNCTION

#### Nrf2 is the Master Regulator of the Cellular Redox Homeostasis

- The transcription factor nuclear factor erythroid 2 p45-related factor 2 (Nrf2) is the master regulator of the cellular redox homeostasis.
- Nrf2 is well-equipped to counterbalance the mitochondrial ROS production and is

critical for maintaining the redox balance in the cell (Hayes and Dinkova-Kostova, 2014).

- Following exposure to oxidants or electrophiles, Nrf2 accumulates in the nucleus.
- There, it binds to antioxidant response elements (ARE) in the upstream regulatory regions of genes encoding detoxification and antioxidant enzymes, leading to their enhanced transcription.

## Nrf2 and the Cellular Redox Homeostasis

- Nrf2 has been associated with cytoprotective functions in animal models of a range of human disease conditions and has been implicated in the regulation of over 600 target genes.
- Nrf2 targets include antioxidant enzymes, proteins involved in xenobiotic metabolism and clearance, protection against heavy metal toxicity, inhibition of inflammation, repair and removal of damaged proteins, as well as other transcription and growth factors.
- Nrf2 regulates the expression of γ-glutamyl cysteine ligase catalytic (GCLC) and modulatory (GCLM) subunits, glutathione reductase (GR), as well as the four enzymes [i.e. malic enzyme 1 (ME1), isocitrate dehydrogenase 1 (IDH1); glucose-6-phosphate dehydrogenase (G6PD) and 6-phosphogluconate dehydrogenase (6PGD), that are responsible for the generation of NADPH, all of which are involved in the biosynthesis and maintenance of reduced glutathione (GSH).
- In turn, GSH, the principal small molecule antioxidant in the mammalian cell, counterbalances the production of ROS.
- Now, it has emerged that one of the important functions of Nrf2 is to modulate mitochondrial function, as part of its role as a **master regulator of cytoprotective gene expression** and the cellular redox homeostasis (Fig. 2.8).

## Nrf2 affects Mitochondrial Function at Multiple Levels

- Nrf2 activation increases the mitochondrial membrane potential, the availability of substrates for respiration and ATP production.
- Nrf2 positively regulates the levels of NADPH by enhancing the expression of genes encoding the enzymes of the pentose phosphate pathway [(PPP) i.e. G6PD and 6PGD] and malic enzyme 1 (ME1) and isocitrate dehydrogenase 1 (IDH1). In addition to NADPH, ME1 regenerates pyruvate, which can cycle back to the mitochondria.
- Nrf2 also regulates the levels of GSH by enhancing the expression of genes encoding enzymes involved in its biosynthesis and regeneration from its oxidised form, GSSG, including glutathione reductase (GR).
- Nrf2 negatively regulates the four critical enzymes involved in fatty acid synthesis (FAS), i.e. ATP-citrate lyase (ACL), acetyl-CoA carboxylase, fatty acid synthase and stearoyl CoA desaturase.
- A decrease in the levels of malonyl-CoA may increase mitochondrial fatty acid oxidation (FAO) by relieving its inhibitory function on carnitine palmitoyltransferase 1 (CPT1), which mediates the transport of long-chain fatty acids into the mitochondria.

## MITOCHONDRIAL DYNAMICS AT THE INTERFACE OF IMMUNE CELL METABOLISM AND FUNCTION

Immune cell differentiation and function are crucially dependent on specific metabolic programmes dictated by mitochondria, including the generation of ATP from the oxidation of nutrients and supplying precursors for the synthesis of macromolecules and post-translational modifications (PTMs). The many processes that occur in mitochondria are intimately linked to their morphology that is shaped by opposing fusion and fission events (Rambold and Pearce, 2018).

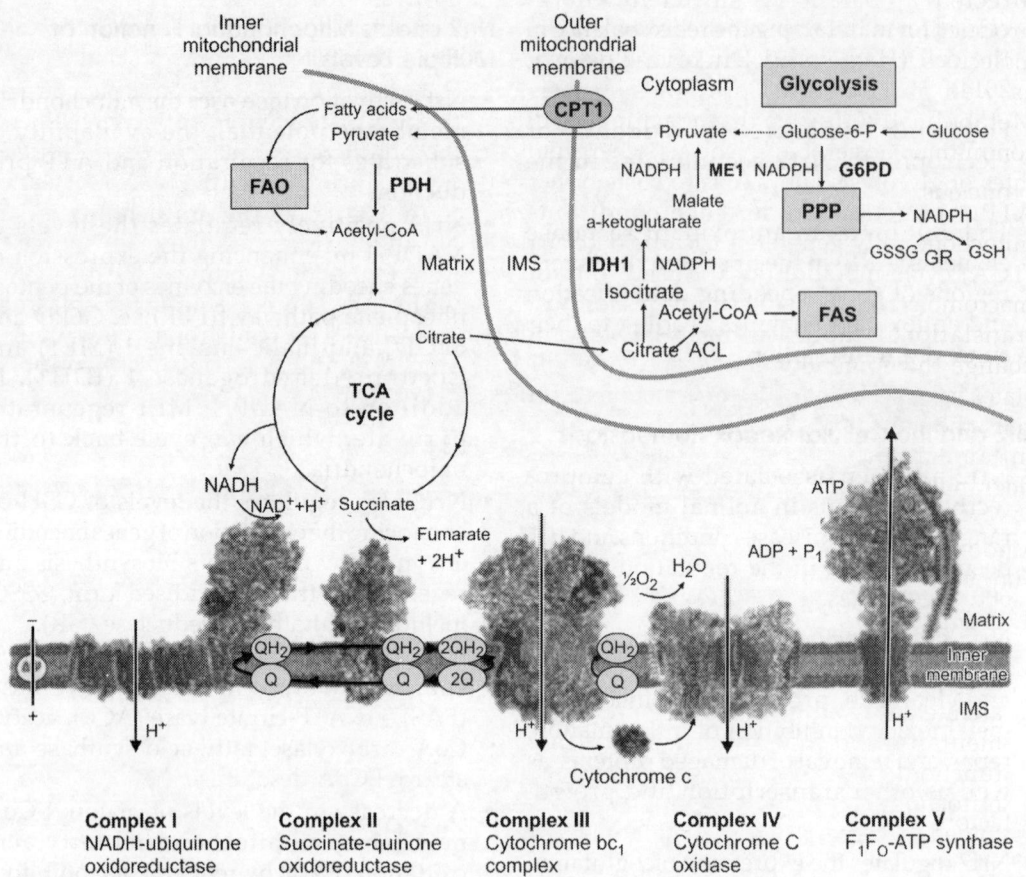

**Fig. 2.8:** Nrf2 affects mitochondrial function at multiple levels. Source: Holstrom et al, (2016); Sazanov, (2015). IMS, mitochondrial intermembrane space; for other abbreviations see the text

## Metabolic Shifts during Immune Responses

For an immune response to proceed, specialised cells of the immune system morph from a state of relative quiescence to one of high activity. A prime example of a cell type that undergoes this transformation is the T lymphocyte. Initially patrolling our body as quiescent naive T cells, these cells become rapidly activated upon antigen detection to T effector (Teff) cells that proliferate, secrete cytokines and migrate to the sites of infection. Once the antigen load is reduced and supportive signals wane, the vast majority of Teff cells die, while a small number of long-lived memory T (Tmem) cells persist over time, maintaining a state of relative quiescence.

It is now well-established that T cells, as well as several other immune cell types such as B cells, macrophages and dendritic cells, must reprogramme their cellular metabolism to acquire their different phenotypic and functional states.

**Catabolic metabolism:** Cells such as Tmem cells, regulatory T cells and alternatively activated (M2) macrophages rely on catabolic metabolism where nutrients are fully degraded and shuttled toward energy-generating pathways. As such, they rely on mitochondrial activity driven, e.g. by pyruvate- or fatty acid-driven oxidative phosphorylation.

**Anabolic metabolism:** By contrast, the anabolic metabolism of activated cells is directed at balancing sufficient energy production with the synthesis of macro-molecules that are necessary for cell division as well as DNA and protein synthesis. Metabolically this is often achieved by commitment to aerobic glycolysis, where high rates of glycolysis allow cells to sustain their ATP production. Under such conditions, mitochondrially generated tricarboxylic acid (TCA) cycle metabolites are used to build macromolecules, provide substrates for post-translational modifications (PTMs) and change the epigenetic landscape. Anabolic states have been linked to the function of Teff cells, the activation of dendritic cells and pro-inflammatory (M1) macrophages and the degranulation of mast cells.

## Mitochondrial Metabolism and Its Cellular Functions

1. **Production of ATP:** The mitochondria are known as the powerhouse of the cell. Mito-chondria are characterised by a complex architecture and high degree of compart-mentalisation that are crucial for their function. They are composed of an outer mitochondrial membrane and a heavily folded inner mitochondrial membrane, the site of the electron transport chain. Histori-cally, the major role of mitochondria was thought to be to the efficient coupling of substrate oxidation through the TCA cycle to ATP production by the electron trans-port chain. In fact, mitochondria produce up to 36 ATP from one molecule of glucose, compared to two ATP from glycolysis, and are thus a more efficient source of cellular ATP. In addition to pyruvate derived from glucose, mitochondria can utilise fatty acids or amino acids and oxidise them in the TCA cycle. The substrate-driven fueling of the TCA cycle generates the reducing equivalents NADH and $FADH_2$ that provide electrons to the electron transport chain. By transferring electrons to mole-cular oxygen, the electron transport chain pumps protons across the inner mito-chondrial membrane, resulting in the generation of the proton-motive force that

is utilised to produce ATP by the ATP synthase. The ATP production is the major role of the electron transport chain.

The process of providing the cell with the bulk of its energy is intimately linked to the production of reactive oxygen species (ROS) during oxidative phosphorylation. In most cells, the mitochondria and NADPH oxidase are the main sources of ROS. Our understanding of the role of ROS within the cell is becoming increasingly complex. The traditional view of ROS simply being a harmful byproduct of respiration is giving way to a more intricate picture where the role of ROS as an important signalling molecule is emerging (Nickel et al, 2014; Mehta, M.M. et al, 2017). It is, however, becoming evident that an imbalance in the generation of ROS is a common feature in several disease states, ranging from neurodegeneration and diabetes to cardiovascular disease and cancer (Pham-Huy et al, 2008).

2. **Utilisation of TCA cycle intermediates:** In addition to the production of ATP, an equally important function of mitochond-ria is the utilisation of TCA cycle intermediates in anabolic or regulatory reactions. For example, citrate can be transported into the cytosol where acetyl-CoA is generated to drive fatty acid synthesis and protein acetylation. Simi-larly, the TCA cycle intermediate α-ketoglutarate is required for function of the α-ketoglutarate-dependent dioxygenase family of proteins, while fumarate and succinate are inhibitors of these proteins. Thus mitochondria regulates widespread functions through its metabolic modes.

## IMMUNE MICROENVIRONMENT— RELATIONSHIP BETWEEN NUTRIENTS AND IMMUNE RESPONSES

### "You are What you Eat"

The phrase "you are what you eat" has been used to convey the idea that one's diet, healthy or otherwise, has a big influence on one's well-being. This works through the immune cells. The identity of an immune cell, the pro- and anti-inflammatory charac- teristics of immune cells, can be significantly influenced by the nutrients that are available to it in the local microenvironment. That is the nutrients available to the immune cell in its local microenvironment matters most and this reflects on one's well-being or otherwise.

At the same time there is an increasing appreciation that there is an inflammatory component to the majority of diseases. A detailed understanding of the relationship between nutrients and immune responses is likely to reveal exciting opportunities for developing new approaches to promote health and well-being and to treat inflam- matory diseases (Wall et al, 2016).

## Basics of T Cell Metabolism

The primary duty of naive T cells is immune surveillance. T cells stay in close proximity to B cells and antigen presenting cells (APCs) in secondary lymphoid tissues and are poised to respond to presentation of specific antigen.

**Metabolic switching:** Upon stimulation, T cells undergo a dramatic shift in metabolism that is marked by increased nutrient uptake and glycolysis. Activated T cells switch from oxidative to glycolytic metabolism. This shift is somewhat counterintuitive, as glycolysis is less efficient than oxidative phosphorylation when considered as a source of ATP. Known as the Warburg Effect or aerobic glycolysis (see page 42), ATP is generated primarily from glycolysis even in the presence of oxygen. T lymphocytes also induce aerobic glycolysis during effector responses (Wang et al, 1976). Aerobic glycolysis can be highly efficient at promoting biosynthesis essential for effector function and rapid proliferation, but also relies on high levels of nutrient uptake, which may change with tissue location, inflammation, or even time of day.

Activated T cells are considered pre- dominantly glycolytic with increased gly- colysis and lactate production and large changes in uptake of anabolic precursors such as glucose and amino acids (Buck et al, 2015;

Can et al, 2010; Sinclair et al, 2013). Metabolic switching is likely due to increased metabolic demand for energy, reducing equivalents and precursors for cell components (Wang et al, 2011). Cells that fail to meet this metabolic demand undergo programmed cell death.

**Metabolic reprogramming:** Carbon tracing for glucose and glutamine has recently shown that a majority of carbon cell mass in rapidly proliferating cells, including T cells, is derived from amino acids and not glucose (Hosios et al, 2016). However, a high flux of both glucose and glutamine is required for effector T cell (Teff) function (Carr et al, 2010). After successful T cell proliferation and immunological clearance of pathogens, Teff responses are diminished and memory T cells emerge with naive-like oxidative phos- phorylation metabolism (Sukumar et al, 2016). This metabolic reprogramming event is paramount to transition of effector cells to memory, as memory T cells (Tmem) require oxidative metabolism.

## T Cell Subsets and Metabolic Specification

Depending on the extrinsic cell signals, T cells can differentiate into effector T cells (Teff) and regulatory T cells (Treg) functionally distinct subsets that utilise and require diverse metabolic programmes. The balance between inflammatory effector T cells (Teff) and suppressive regulatory T cells (Treg) is tightly regulated during immune responses. But dysregulation occurs as nutrients change in obesity, chronic inflammation and cancer. These observations supported the potential for distinct metabolic programmes for different T cell subsets.

CD4 subsets or CD8 effector or memory populations have clearly distinct metabolic programmes (Buck et al, 2015; MacIver et al, 2013). Teff activate and generally utilise aerobic glycolysis (reminiscent of cancer cells), while Treg show to predominantly rely on mitochondrial oxidative pathways. Similarly, activated CD8T cells utilise glycolysis, while memory CD8T cells utilise lipid oxidation.

Increased effector Th1 cells and macrophage infiltration and decreased Treg in obese subjects have been found based on histological analysis of visceral adipose tissue. Hyperglycemia itself has been shown to enhance cell survival in general by increasing glycolysis and inhibiting caspases via NFκB expression (Ramakrishnan et al, 2011). These shifts in T cell subsets may have significant implications for immunity.

Further, T cell subsets are not fixed but have a great deal of plasticity. It is now clear that CD4 subsets can switch from one functional subset to another. Th17 cells can become Th1 cells and regulatory T cells can become effector cells based on microenvironmental cues and epigenetic programming.

## Metabolic Regulators of T cells

### i. mTOR and AMPK

- The mTOR and AMPK pathways have significant and opposing roles in T cell metabolic programming and differentiation.
- AMPK is an AMP-sensitive signalling kinase gets activated to boost catabolic metabolism and inhibit anabolic growth in times of stress, when nutrient availability is low or ATP synthesis decreased. AMPK can also phosphorylate TSC2 and RAPTOR to inhibit mTOR signalling (Inoki et al, 2003).
- When biosynthetic nutrients are abundant, mTOR integrates extracellular signalling and sensing of essential amino acids. This promotes anabolic metabolism through transcriptional activity and direct action to promote glycolysis and lipogenesis (Porstmann et al, 2008).
- The mTOR and AMPK pathways can be generalised as a rheostat, where AMPK induces catabolic metabolism and oxidative phosphorylation that slow proliferation, whereas the mTOR pathway promotes anabolic growth pathways to drive proliferation during

activation. However, the role of mTOR in T cell metabolism is quite complicated.

### ii. Myc

- The transcription factor Myc is also an important modulator of T cell metabolism.
- Myc is growth factor-induced and commonly mutated or overexpressed in cancer cells to promote glycolytic programming and glutamine uptake and catabolism.
- Myc interacts with a variety of signalling and transcriptional networks that regulate cell growth, cell death and metabolism. Indeed, there are few anabolic pathways untouched by Myc.
- T cell activation leads to Myc upregulation and Myc is essential for appropriate Teff activation (Wang et al, 2011).
- Consistent with the role of Myc in cancer to promote aerobic glycolysis, Myc-deficient T cells fail to upregulate glycolysis and glutaminolysis following activation (Wang and Green, 2012).
- Myc-high cells become effectors and Myc-low daughter cells become memory T cells (Verbist et al, 2016) with reduced glycolysis and mTOR signalling.

### iii. HIF-1 α

- Hypoxia Inducible Factor1α (HIF-1α) is an important transcriptional regulator of T cell metabolism in response to environmental stress.
- HIF-1α can strongly promote glycolysis in conditions of hypoxia and is regulated by oxygen sensing mechanisms and mTORC1 signalling, which promotes HIF-1α protein translation.
- While mTORC1-mediated regulation provides a link to other nutrient sensing mechanisms, HIF-1α was initially discovered because it is

upregulated in low-oxygen environments.

- When lymphocytes move into environments with low oxygen tension, HIF-1α becomes important to promote adaptation.

- Upon T cell activation, however, HIF-1α is selectively required for generation of Th17 cells. This may act through interaction with the Th17 transcription factor RORγT.

- It may also specifically regulate the degradation of Foxp3 (Treg-associated transcription factor), thus preventing Treg generation.

## Metabolites as Signalling Molecules: Glyceraldehyde-3-phosphate and Phosphoenolpyruvate

In addition to signalling pathways that directly regulate T cell metabolism, it is also now apparent that metabolites and metabolic pathways in turn regulate signalling and differentiation events. This bidirectional connection ensures that cells only proceed to activate or differentiate if nutrient conditions are appropriate. In response to limiting glucose, it was recently shown that reduced glycolysis allows glyceraldehyde-3-phosphate dehydrogenase (GAPDH), the enzyme responsible for catalysing glyceraldehyde-3-phosphate to glycerate 1,3-bisphosphate in the glycolysis pathway, to translocate to the nucleus and modify IFNγ translation in T cells (Chang et al, 2013). While a role for GAPDH in translation has been previously shown, the modification of transcript for IFNγ specifically correlated with induction of glycolytic metabolism to provide a new link between this metabolic enzyme and inflammation (Chang et al, 2013).

Similarly, the glycolytic metabolite phosphoenolpyruvate may directly modify calcium signalling and T cell activation, to link glucose availability and T cell receptor induced signalling.

It is likely that other metabolic enzymes and metabolites will have additional moon-lighting jobs but have yet to be discovered. Our incomplete understanding of the metabolic regulation of T cells is slowly being filled in, opening new targets of potential treatment for diseases of autoimmunity, immune-deficiency and cancer (Johnson et al, 2016).

## Metabolic and Nutrient Requirements of T Cells

### Nutrient Availability—Glucose

Beyond the changes in signalling pathways that directly modify metabolic pathways intrinsic to T cells, access to extracellular nutrients and the regulation of nutrient uptake are also essential for T cell function. In some cases, nutrient levels are altered or may not be present, such as in tumour environment. Even if adequate nutrients are available, however, appropriate transporters must be present on the cell surface. Indeed, T cell activation leads to a sharp upregulation of nutrient transporter expression and cell surface trafficking to increase metabolic substrate availability and remove waste products.

The glucose transporter Glut 1 and the amino acid transporters SLC1a5 and SLC7a5 are upregulated and traffic to the cell surface in response to PI3K/Ak1/mTORC1 signalling to allow T cells to uptake glucose and amino acids, including large neutral amino acids and glutamine (Sinclair et al, 2013; Macintyre et al, 2014; Nakaya et al, 2014). Likewise, Mct 1 and Mct4 transport lactate out of cells to maintain glycolysis and redox balance and are also upregulated upon activation. These changes can have significant impact on T cell activation and fate. T cells rely strongly on high rates of glucose uptake and elevated Glut 1 expression can enhance activation and glycolysis of effector T cells, leading to a Systemic Lupus Erythematosus (SLE) like-disease (Michalek et al, 2011). Conversely, Glut 1-deficient T cells have decreased glucose uptake and reduced Teff proliferation, activation and function.

## Nutrient Availability—Glutamine and Amino Acids

Besides glucose, availability and metabolism of amino acids have significant impacts on T cell metabolism. Glutamine in particular is an important substrate for highly proliferative cells (MacIver et al, 2013). Glutamine is the most abundant amino acid in circulation (Newsholme et al, 2003) and is a critical fuel for anabolic metabolism. As proliferative cells remove citrate from the TCA cycle to generate fatty acids for various structures such as cell membrane, glutamine is internalised and converted to glutamate, then the TCA intermediate, $\alpha$-ketoglutarate ($\alpha$-KG). In addition, glutamine is essential for nucleotide synthesis, generation of glutathione and provides glutamate that is used to facilitate transport of additional amino acids. Because proliferative T cells closely resemble the metabolic state of cancer cells, glutamine metabolism also likely contributes to T cell metabolism and function.

In addition to providing metabolic substrates, amino acids have direct activating effects on mTORC1. Low amino acid levels inhibit mTOR association with lysosome and thus prevent downstream signalling for cell growth and proliferation (Verbist et al, 2016). While the essential amino acid leucine is likely the key substrate for mTORC1 amino acid sensing, T cells deficient in the large neutral amino acid transporter (SLc7a5), also fail to maintain mTORC1 activity and support anabolic metabolism (Poncet et al, 2014). S1c7a5 deficient T cells failed to properly activate and maintain mTORC1 signalling and, as a consequence, failed to upregulate Glut1 and induce glycolysis necessary for effector T cell activation.

## Metabolism and Epigenetic Modifications in T Cells

Another mechanism by which nutrient status and metabolic pathways may influence T cell signalling and differentiation is through epigenetic modification of DNA and histones. The two primary epigenetic modifications,

methylation and acetylation, each use metabolites as substrates.

## Methylation and Demethylation

DNA methylation is controlled by DNA methyltransferase and requires methyl groups donated by S-adenosylmethionine derived from the one carbon metabolism pathway. This pathway integrates nutrients from glycolysis, amino acids and choline or folate. Associated with reduced gene transcription, methylation of DNA is heritable and stable, but responds to dietary influences. Indeed, reduced dietary methionine was found to lower DNA methylation. Conversely, the dioxygenase enzymes that demethylate DNA, such as TET2, require $\alpha$-KG as a substrate. Thus both methylation and demethylation events are metabolically sensitive.

## Acetylation and Deacetylation

Acetylation and deacetylation of histones and other proteins also play significant roles in gene transcription and cell function, affecting growth and proliferation. Increased availability of acetyl-CoA enhanced global acetylation of histones, even when nutrients were limited (Joyce et al, 2016). Lysine acetylation can also affect enzymatic activity and protein interactions (Choudhary et al, 2014). The Treg-associated transcription factor, Foxp3, e.g. is stabilised by hyperacetylation, leading to increased Foxp3 expression and higher Treg numbers. This increased acetyl-CoA allowed for the acetylation of GAPDH, enhancing glycolysis and boosting CD8+ function. Because T cells rely so strongly on glycolytic reprogramming, epigenetic and protein modifications could be a significant contributor to T cell function and inflammatory responses by linking substrate availability, diet and metabolism.

Modification of epigenetic marks can have major functional consequences. Myc expression is required for T cell activation but methylation of the enhancer regions usually bound by Myc prevents Myc association and reduces gene expression. A study of CD8+ T lymphocytes from geriatric and young patients showed methylation status of T cells was significantly more variable in geriatric CD8+ T cells and this correlated with decreased immune function.

## Tumour Infiltrating Lymphocytes and Metabolic Adaptation

Tumour cells can be highly glycolytic and poorly vascularised, causing the tumour microenvironment to have reduced glucose and amino acid levels (Ye et al, 2010), while simultaneously accumulating lactate, increased acidity and other waste products. Tumour infiltrating lymphocytes (TILs) thus face the challenge of engaging in active cell metabolism necessary for effector function when substrates are limited by nutrient availability. High lactate levels inhibited proliferation and cytokine production in human cytotoxic lymphocytes (CTL), which was attributed to disruption of a required lactate gradient, prevention of lactate export and metabolic perturbation (Fischer et al, 2007). Additionally, in squamous tumours, highly glycolytic tumours had reduced CD8+ T cell infiltration (Ottensmier et al, 2016).

## Circadian Rhythm Regulation of Cell Metabolism

It has been appreciated for some time that immune responses are influenced by time of day and circadian rhythms that are closely linked to metabolic status. Entrainment of the circadian rhythm is generally provided by sunlight, sleep cycles and feeding. The daily cycles of feeding and sleeping connect energy homeostasis with metabolic substrate availability, as feeding schedules correlate with availability of glucose and amino acids in the blood (Scheiermann et al, 2013) and loss of the normal circadian cycle can effect body weight and metabolic disorder. A key function, therefore, of circadian rhythms is to coordinate metabolism with nutrient availability. The transcription factors Clock and BMAL1 constitute the original basis for circadian

cycling and these form dimers to induce transcription of oscillatory inhibitory proteins PER (PER1-3), Cry (Cry 1 and 2) and REV-ERB (Dibner et al, 2010). The rise and fall of these transcription factors Clock and BMAL1 and their downstream protein targets establish the cell-intrinsic circadian rhythm.

Lymphocytes show the same 24 hours circadian cycling as most other mammalian cells. Because the expression of Clock and BMAL1 is under control of retinoic acid receptor-related orphan nuclear receptors (RORs), it is possible that transcriptional regulation of Clock genes is partially under control of RORyt, the regulator of Th17 development.

## Immune Microenvironments are Nutrient Restrictive

Most cells in the body have a constant supply of nutrients, which are required to sustain cellular metabolism and functions. However, in certain microenvironments this is not always the case. For example, at inflamed sites the influx of inflammatory cells such as neutrophils and monocytes increases nutrient consumption and can lead to low glucose availability and tissue hypoxia (Taylor and Colgan, 2007). Neutrophils have low levels of mitochondrial respiration and few functional mitochondria and as a result have a high demand for glucose to fuel glycolytic energy production as well as to support other cellular processes and effector functions (Rodriguez-Espinosa et al, 2015). At sites of infection there is additional demand for nutrients caused by the infecting pathogen.

Glucose levels can drop during infection. Tumour cells consume large amounts of glucose and other nutrients such as glutamine and as a result the tumour microenvironment can become depleted of nutrients. Additionally, tumour cells and tumour promoting immune cells such as myeloid derived suppressor cells express enzymes such as arginase and indoleamine-2, 3-dioxygenase (IDO) that consume arginine and tryptophan, respectively. Solid tumours can also become hypoxic due to insufficient vascularisation.

## Immune Microenvironments have Altered Nutrients that can Shape Immune Responses

It is known that metabolic syndrome is a clustering of conditions including central obesity, dyslipidaemia and hypertension that increases the risks of morbidities such as cancer and cardiovascular disease. Another feature of metabolic syndrome is altered immune function (Andersen et al, 2016). Fatty acids, cholesterol and cholesterol derivatives have all been proposed to have roles in controlling immune function and the dysregulated systemic levels of these molecules in patients with metabolic syndrome is likely to underpin the observed alterations in immune function (Spann and Glass, 2013). The levels of molecules like oxysterols can also be altered in discrete immune microenvironments. For instance, tumour cells release oxysterols into the tumour microenvironment and activated macrophages make large amounts of the oxysterol 25-hydroxycholestrerol (25HC). It is also clear that dietary and microbiome derived molecules such as short chain fatty acids have a role to play in the control of immune responses.

Therefore, many of the environments in which immune cells operate can have variable levels of important nutrients, including glucose, amino acids, fatty acids and cholesterol/oxysterols. These molecules are all important for cellular metabolism or as structural components of the cell, but importantly, these molecules can also directly impact upon immune signalling pathways to influence immune activation, differentiation and function. Indeed, there is a growing appreciation that nutrients are important cues that can shape immune responses. Let us discuss them.

## Various Nutrient Sensing Signalling Pathways and the Roles they Play in Regulating the Function of Immune Cells

### Glucose and Glutamine Sensing

Glucose and glutamine are important fuels that feed into different parts of the ATP generating pathways of the cell, glycolysis and oxidative phosphorylation, but can also supply various biosynthetic pathways. The levels of these fuels can impact upon multiple signalling pathways that are integral to the control of immune responses.

a. **AMPK/mTORC1 signalling:** AMPK is a complex multi-subunit kinase that is an acute sensor of cellular energy homeostasis becoming activated, when energy levels are decreased. Activated AMPK functions to restore energy homeostasis by turning off anabolic processes that consume ATP (such as fatty acid synthesis) and up-regulating catabolic processes that generate ATP (such as glycolysis). In activated T cells AMPK can be activated within an hour of being placed in limiting concentrations of glucose. Similarly, hypoxia or glutamine deprivation will activate AMPK in immune cells that rely on mitochondrial ATP production. Indeed, glutamine deprivation also results in AMPK activation in antigen stimulated T cells. This highlight the importance of both glucose and glutamine for ATP production in activated T cells.

Some recent studies in T cells demonstrate that AMPK is a key metabolic regulator that provides T cells with the metabolic plasticity to adapt to energy stress that will occur in nutrient restrictive conditions, such as those found in inflammatory microenvironments. T cells lacking AMPK have a striking defect in their ability to generate memory CD8 T cell responses.

AMPK also controls the function of mammalian Target of Rapamycin complex 1 (mTORC1) as activation of AMPK results in the inhibition of mTORC1 (Rolf et al, 2013; Blagih et al, 2015). mTORC1 is also an important metabolic regulator and has widespread roles in controlling immune cell functions (Powell et al, 2011). Therefore, glucose or glutamine levels can impact upon an AMPK/mTORC1 signalling axis that is important in the control of immune responses.

b. **O-linked β-N-acetylglucosamine transferase (OGT):** In addition to supplying glycolysis and oxidative phosphorylation, glucose and glutamine are also (approximately 2–5% of total glucose) used for generation of uridine diphosphate N-acetylglucosamine (UDP-GlcNAc) through the hexosamine biosynthetic pathway (HBP; Benhamed et al, 2014). UDP-GlcNAc is utilised by glycosyltransferases for various cellular processes including O-GlcNAcylation, the reversible addition of N-acetylglucosamine (GlcNAc; see appendix) to proteins on serine or threonine residues. O-linked GlcNAc transferase (OGT) adds GlcNAc to proteins, while O-linked GlcNAc hydrolase (OGA) removes the GlcNAc from serine/threonine residues.

O-GlcNAcylation has emerged as one of the most abundant post-translational modifications (PTMs) that can control many aspects of protein function including stability, localisation and transcriptional activity (Bond et al, 2015). O-GlcNAcylation can compete with protein phosphorylation as both types of modification target serine and threonine residues on a protein. As a result, there can be extensive crosstalk between these two protein modification pathways (Hart et al, 2011).

Levels of UDP-GlcNAc and protein O-GlcNAcylation are dependent on the supply of both glucose and glutamine in T cells arguing that OGT and O-GlcNAcylation are important nutrient sensing mechanisms (Swamy et al, 2016). OGT is essential for normal T cell development, activation and clonal expansion (Swamy et al, 2016; Golks et al, 2007).

A number of signalling molecules that are important for T cell function are found to be O-GlcNAcylated including c-Myc, nuclear factor of activated T cells (NFAT) and NFκB (Swamy et al, 2016; Golks et al, 2007; Ramakrishnan et al, 2013). Indeed, OGT and O-GlcNAcylation are essential for sustaining c-Myc protein expression in CD8 cytotoxic T cells. There is evidence to suggest that glucose/glutamine dependent O-GlcNAcylation has an important role for other aspects of immune function.

c. **Glycolytic flux links glucose to immune signalling; *Phosphoenolpyruvate*:** The glycolytic metabolite phosphoenolpyruvate (PEP) can affect $Ca^{2+}$ signalling and activation of NFAT transcription factor in antigen stimulated T cells. PEP represses sarco/ER $Ca^{2+}$-ATPase (SERCA) activity, which is responsible for $Ca^{2+}$ reuptake into the ER. PEP, therefore, enhances cytosolic $Ca^{2+}$ signalling and promotes NFAT nuclear activity.

T cells activated in low glucose have reduced PEP levels, reduced cytosolic $Ca^{2+}$ signalling and reduced nuclear NFAT, leading to defective T cell activation (Ho et al, 2015).

**GAPDH functions:** The function of the glycolytic enzyme glyceraldehyde-3-phosphate dehydrogenase (GAPDH) is also sensitive to glycolytic flux in T cells. GAPDH has additional roles outside its function as a glycolytic enzyme including acting an RNA binding protein to inhibit the translation of certain proteins including IFNγ and IL2 in T cells.

The rate of glycolytic flux in activated T cells controls the balance of these different GAPDH functions; high rates of glycolysis prevent GAPDH binding to IL2 and IFNγ mRNA and thereby maximise the production of these cytokines. On the other hand, if glucose is limiting, reduced glycolytic flux allows GAPDH to inhibit IFNγ and IL2 production.

*Amino Acid Sensing*

Amino acids are important for biosynthetic pathways in immune cells, including protein and nucleotide synthesis. Furthermore, they can also be directly metabolised to generate immunomodulatory molecules such as nitric oxide; arginine is a substrate for inducible nitric oxide synthase (iNOS). Thus, it is not surprising that immune cells, in particular lymphocytes, greatly increase amino acid uptake in response to immune stimulation.

**Amino acids are critically important in the generation of effector cells:** Amino acids of particular importance to lymphocytes include glutamine, methionine, tryptophan, arginine and leucine. Depletion of any of these amino acids results in impaired responses to immune activation (Van Baren and Van den Eynde, 2015; Rodriguez et al, 2007; Ananieva et al, 2016). T lymphocytes increase nutrient uptake in response to antigen stimulation through up-regulating the expression of nutrient transporters. This is critically important in the generation of effector cells. Indeed T cells lacking the glucose transporter Glut 1, the large neutral amino acid transporter Slc7a5, or the glutamine transporter ASCT2 fail to differentiate into effector cells (Macintyre et al, 2014; Sinclair et al, 2013).

**Amino acids can be signalling molecules:** In addition to the role for amino acids as cellular fuels, certain amino acids can also be considered important signalling molecules. A number of signalling pathways important for immune responses are acutely sensitive to changes in the levels of certain amino acids and these are discussed below.

i. **Amino acids and mTORC1:** In recent years the serine threonine kinase mTORC1 has emerged as a central regulator of immune cell function. mTORC1 has diverse roles in controlling the function of immune cells in both the adaptive and innate arms of the immune system (Powell et al, 2011; Weichhart et al, 2015). For instance, in T cells mTOR signalling is essential for lineage commitment of Th1 and Th17 effector cells, whilst in macrophages Rheb-dependent activation of mTORC1 has been implicated in monocyte-macrophage differentiation and mature macrophage phagocytosis.

*The regulation of this kinase complex is complicated:* mTORC1 activity is turned on by growth factor or antigen signalling and switched off by other signalling pathways including AMPK, as described earlier. However, mTORC1 activity is also acutely sensitive to the availability of certain amino acids and this arm of mTORC1 regulation overrides other signalling pathways; in the absence of amino acids mTORC1 is turned off even in the presence of strong growth factor signalling.

The mTORC1 activity is controlled by amino acid availability in mammalian cells. Amino acids act through various amino acid sensors that promote the activity of the Rag GTPases to facilitate mTORC1 activation (Bar-Peled and Sabatini, 2014). Cytosolic sensors for leucine and arginine have been identified as Sestrin2 and Castor, respectively (Wolfson et al, 2016; Chantranupong et al, 2016) and the solute transporter Slc38a9 has been identified as a lysosomal arginine sensor (Wang et al, 2015).

In activated lymphocytes, mTORC1 activity is exquisitely sensitive to leucine availability (Sinclair et al, 2013). Leucine is essential for mTORC1 activity in immune cells, while the evidence for a similar sensitivity to arginine is lacking. Interestingly, effector T cells up-regulate Slc7a5-mediated leucine transport in response to arginine deprivation. More work is required to elucidate the respective roles for arginine and leucine sensing in immune cells (Walls et al, 2016).

Glutamine availability is also essential for mTORC1 activity in activated lymphocytes. This is because glutamine is required for efficient leucine uptake into these cells through the Slc7a5 amino acid transporter (Sinclair et al, 2013). Slc7a5 is an obligate antiporter: one amino acid in, one amino acid out. Slc7a5 has high import affinities for large neutral amino acids including leucine, valine, tryptophan and methionine and a high export affinity for glutamine. Thus, in the context of amino acid sensing and the impact on mTORC1, Slc7a5 will transport glutamine out of the cell whilst importing leucine into the cell.

ii. **Amino acids and c-Myc:** The transcription factor c-Myc (myelocytomatosis oncogene) is a key controller of the metabolic reprogramming seen in T cells in response to antigen stimulation (Wang et al, 2011) as well as macrophages responding to M-CSF (Liu et al, 2016). One role for c-Myc is to promote or sustain the expression of a cohort of nutrient transporters, including glucose transporters, amino acid transporters and the transferrin receptor (CD71). The importance of iron transport for lymphocyte function is evident in patients that have a missense mutation in their transferrin receptor. These patients have severe immunodeficiency characterised by impaired T and B cell function.

c-Myc levels are dependent on glutamine fuelled O-GlcNAcylation in effector T cells (Swamy et al, 2016). c-Myc protein expression is effectively "fine-tuned" by amino acid availability, which is dependent on amino acid levels in the local microenvironment and levels of amino acid transporter expression. This mechanism for regulating c-Myc expression is important for immune responses.

*General control non-derepressible 2 kinase (GCN2):* This is a serine/threonine protein kinase. GCN2 senses low cellular amino acid levels through binding to uncharged transfer RNA (tRNA) leading to kinase activation and subsequent phosphorylation of eukaryotic initiation factor 2a (eIF2a) (Grallert and Boye, 2013).

In dendritic cells, GCN2 activiation in response to virus (or live virus vaccination) enhances antigen presentation to CD8 cells (Ravindran et al, 2014). Conversely, GCN2 activity in gut APC restrains excessive Th17 responses. Thus, amino acid levels and GCN2 signalling acts to balance the immune response by inducing autophagy and cross-presentation of viral antigens in APCs and limiting excessive ROS accumulation and inflammasome activity during cellular stress.

Amino acid sensing by GCN2 is also important for lymphocytes. The enzyme Indoleamine 2,3-dioxygenase (IDO) suppresses T cell responses, at least in part, by depleting tryptophan levels leading to the activation of GCN2 within the T cell. Activation of GCN2 in CD8 T cells results in proliferative arrest and anergy, while in CD4 T cells GCN2 activation can lead to the generation of regulatory T cells.

## *Fatty Acid Sensing and Immune Function: G Protein Coupled Receptors (GPCR)*

Free fatty acids (FFA) can be obtained from three sources: (1) exogenously through diet, (2) produced by the gut microbiome and (3) can also be produced from breakdown of triglycerides in the liver and adipose tissue. While FFA can be used as a cellular fuel for generating ATP, they also act as ligands for several G protein coupled linked receptors (GPCR) (Talukdar et al, 2011).

Many immune cell types have been demonstrated to express GPCR receptors for FFA including macrophages, neutrophils, T cells and dendritic cells (Alvarez-Curto and Milligan, 2016). These receptors can be classified based on the carbon number of their fatty acid ligands. GPR40 and GPR120 (also called Fatty acid receptor (FFAR) 1 and FFAR4, respectively) are responsive to long-chain fatty acid (LCFA, >C12), while GPR43, GPR41 (also called FFAR2 and FFAR3, respectively) are activated by short-chain fatty acids (SCFA, C2-C6) (Ichimura et al, 2009). GPR109a (also called hydroxycarboxylic acid receptor 2) is ligated specifically by the 4 carbon SCFA butyrate. Medium-chain fatty acids (MCFA C9-14) appear to signal through GPR84 and also GPR40 (Wang et al, 2006).

i. **SCFA sensing:** SCFA, such as acetate, propionate and butyrate, can be produced by a number of tissues, notably the liver, but the major source of SCFA is the gut microbiome. SCFA are metabolic byproducts of intestinal microbiota fermentation that can be taken up by the gut and reach the circulation via the portal vein and the liver (Tremaroli and Backhed, 2012).

*SCFA produced in the gut are used*

1. As a fuel source for certain cells including colonic epithelial cells.

2. Microbiome derived SCFA are also important fuels for B cell responses (Kim et al, 2016). Mice with low SCFA production due to microbial insufficiency were defective for pathogen-specific antibody responses, while a SCFA-supplemented diet restored normal B cell responses (Kim et al, 2016).

3. SCFA can also function as potent signalling molecules that have an anti-inflammatory effect on the function of immune cells. **SCFA signalling occurs through the GPCRs:** GPR43, GPR41 and GPCR109a; GPR41 is expressed primarily on adipocytes, GPR43 is highly expressed on polymorphonuclear leukocytes (PMNs) and lymphocytes and GPR109a is expressed on various immune cells including neutrophils and macrophages but not lymphocytes (Smith et al, 2013).

4. SCFA can impact upon the differentiation of both CD4 and CD8 T subsets, promoting CD4 regulatory T cell (Treg) formation and optimal CD8 memory T cell responses (Balmer et al, 2016; Zeng and Chi, 2015). Tregs are important in maintaining immune homeostasis and Tregs numbers in the colon lamina propria are dependent on the gut microbiome; germ-free mice have dramatically reduced Treg numbers in the colon (Zeng and Chi, 2015). SCFA also suppress the production of pro-inflammatory mediators from neutrophils, such as TNFα and nitric oxide (Vinolo et al, 2011).

5. Additionally, SCFA can have direct actions in the cells independent of

GPRs, notably SCFA can impact upon the levels of protein acetylation.

6. Acetate can directly impact upon cell signalling as it can be converted to acetyl-CoA, the substrate for protein acetylation reactions. Butyrate and propionate also promote protein acetylation as they are inhibitors of histone deacetylases (HDAC). Elevated levels of acetate promote the acetylation of the glycolytic enzyme GAPDH facilitating elevated glycolytic flux and robust CD8 memory T cell responses (Balmer et al, 2016). HDACs deacetylate histones as well as non-histone substrates including NFκB. Butyrate- or propionate-mediated inhibition of HDACs promotes FoxP3 expression in T cells. SCFA-mediated inhibition of HDACs also potentiates the ability of DCs to promote Treg differentiation and inhibits pro-inflammatory macrophage and neutrophil function (Vinolo et al, 2011).

ii. **LCFA sensing:** GPR120 is strongly activated by omega 3 fatty acids including the essential fatty acid, α-linolenic acid that is not endogenously synthesised. Therefore, GPR120 is important in responding to diet obtained fatty acids. GPR120 is highly expressed in CD11c+ macrophages and adipocytes (Oh et al, 2010). Exogenously derived omega 3 fatty acids, including docosahexaenoic acid (C22, DHA) and eicosapentaenoic acid (C20, EPA) have clear anti-inflammatory effects on macrophages. Ligation of GPR120 by DHA results in decreased TLR2/3/4 and TNFα mediated signal transduction leading to reduced pro-inflammatory cytokine production (TNFα, IL6, IL1β) (Oh et al, 2010; Yan et al, 2013).

The anti-inflammatory function of GPR120 involves the sequestration of TAB2 to bind to β-Arrestin-2 rather than TAK1, leading to decreased TAK1 signalling and decreased NF κB and JNK activation (Oh et al, 2010). There is also evidence that LCFA inhibit the activation of the NLRP3 inflammasome. DHA acting through GPR120, and also GPR40, suppresses caspase 1 cleavage and IL1-β secretion in macrophages by increasing β-arrestin-2 binding to NLRP3 (Yan et al, 2013).

iii. **MCFA sensing:** There is evidence that MCFAs such as capric acid, lauric acid can impact upon the function of certain immune cells. The MCFA receptor GPR84 is highly expressed on macrophages and neutrophils. The data suggests that MCFA, acting through GPR84, can enhance LPS-induced IL-12 and TNFα expression in macrophages (Wang et al, 2006). Ligation of GPR84 also induces the production of IL8 and chemotactic responses in human polymorphonuclear leukocytes. Therefore, the data available suggests that, in contrast to SCFA and LCFA, MCFA have pro-inflammatory effects on immune cell function (Walls et al, 2016).

**CD36 scavenging receptor:** CD36 is a well-characterised receptor for triacylglycerol substrates and is highly expressed in scavenging immune cells such as macrophages (Feng et al, 2000). CD36 is responsible for receptor mediated endocytosis of triacylglycerol-rich lipoprotein particles, such as low density lipoproteins (LDL) and very low density lipoproteins (VLDL) and also has a high affinity for oxidised LDL (oxLDL). Triglycerides can be used to generate intracellular FFA to fuel oxidative phosphorylation following fatty acid oxidation in the mitochondria. Macrophage polarisation to M1 or M2 phenotypes is closely linked to cellular metabolism; M1 macrophages rely on glycolysis while M2 are fuelled by fatty acid oxidation and oxidative phosphorylation. IL-4 induced CD36 is crucial for generating M2 macrophages; CD36 deficiency disrupts M2 macrophage metabolism and polarisation. Therefore, CD36 expression can affect immune function by supplying cellular metabolic pathways, but additionally CD36-

mediated scavenging can also directly impact upon immune signalling pathways.

In macrophages, CD36 mediates the internalisation of various molecules, such as oxLDL, and the subsequent lysosomal conversion of these molecules into crystals, such as cholesterol crystals, that then activate the NLRP3 inflammasome to promote IL1β production (Sheedy et al, 2013). Further, CD36 also augments TLR4–6 signalling to prime the inflammasome, inducing the expression of inflammatory genes including IL1β and NLRP3 (Sheedy et al, 2013). In macrophages, ligation of CD36 with oxLDL also leads to the recruitment of the plasma membrane ion transporter Na+/K+ATPase and the subsequent activation of the Src family kinase Lyn. Therefore, CD36 is important in controlling macrophage function through supporting the oxidative metabolism of fatty acids and also through promoting inflammatory signalling.

*Cholesterol and Oxysterol Sensing*

Cholesterol is an important component of the plasma membrane that is involved in maintaining membrane integrity and fluidity, but cholesterol also has roles in signal transduction. There are multiple branches off the cholesterol biosynthesis pathway that generate intermediates important for steroid hormone production and protein prenylation and in the regulation of immune responses (Bah et al, 2016). Cholesterol can also be oxidised into various oxysterol molecules, such as 25-hydroxycholesterol (25HC), that are important in the control of various aspects of the immune cell function.

Cholesterol, oxysterols or indeed flux through the cholesterol biosynthesis pathway can directly regulate signal transduction pathways including those involved in the type 1 interferon response. While oxysterols have a substantially shorter half-life compared to cholesterol, there is evidence that the levels of these molecules can accumulate in discrete immune microenvironments. In particular, activated macrophages and tumour cells have been shown to produce and secrete oxysterols. Activated macrophages also upregulate the expression of cholesterol 25-hydroxylase (CH25H) and produce large amounts of 25HC.

**Macrophage-derived 25HC can have direct immunoregulatory effects:** 25HC affects the plasma membranes of host cells to suppress viral fusion. But many of the immunoregulatory effects of 25HC on the immune response are through changes in signalling pathways. Under certain conditions, systemic levels of oxysterols can also be elevated. Patients (human beings) with aspects of metabolic syndrome (e.g. hypercholesteremia, type II diabetes or hyperlipidemia) have elevated plasma levels of oxidised cholesterol species. Healthy individuals injected with LPS showed increased plasma levels of 25HC, arguing that inflammatory processes can also promote elevated levels of systemic oxysterols (Diczfalusy et al, 2009).

**Signal transduction pathways that are sensitive to levels of cholesterol:** Now let us know about the signal transduction pathways that are sensitive to levels of cholesterol and oxysterols and the role they play in controlling immune responses.

**Sterol response element binding proteins (SREBP) signalling:** SREBP are transcription factors. These are the master regulators of fatty acid and cholesterol synthesis as they promote the expression of most of the enzymes in these biosynthetic pathways. SREBP transcription factors are activated through a complex mechanism that involves the transport of a precursor SREBP protein from the endoplasmic reticulum to the Golgi apparatus, multiple protease cleavage events and the subsequent translocation of the cleaved active transcription factor to the nucleus.

Further, SREBP has been described to have a number of direct immunoregulatory roles. The intermediates in the cholesterol biosynthetic pathway can act as agonists for RORγt transcription factors and so impact upon the differentiation of Th17 CD4 T cells (Hu et al, 2015). The oxysterol, 7β,26-dihydroxycholesterol (7β,26-HC), has been identified as a potent RORγt agonist and enhances the differentiation of Th17 CD4 T cells in mice and humans.

## Cholesterol Crystals can Potentially Affect Immunological Signalling Pathways

Free cholesterol has very low solubility in aqueous environments and for this reason cholesterol is complexed to apoproteins for transport in the bloodstream. However, in pathologies such as atherosclerosis, elevated levels of free cholesterol result in the formation of cholesterol crystals within arterial plaques and within the macrophages at these sites. These cholesterol crystals stimulate inflammatory signalling pathways through activation of the NLRP3 inflammasome (Grebe and Latz, 2013). As mentioned earlier, CD36 is important for inflammatory signalling in macrophages due to its function as a lipid transporter but also due to its interaction with inflammatory signalling pathways. Indeed, CD 36 seems to be particularly important for the formation of cholesterol crystals in macrophages in the context of atherosclerosis (Grebe and Latz, 2013).

## Oxysterols as Ligands for Nuclear Receptors

A number of different oxysterol species, including 22(R)-hydroxycholesterol, 24(S)-hydroxycholesterol, 27-hydroxycholesterol and 70,26-dihydroxycholesterol (70,26-HC) are ligands for Liver X receptors (LXRs). LXRs form a permissive heterodimer with retinoid X receptor (RXR) and regulate transcription through binding to LXR response elements. In the absence of ligand, LXRs act as transcriptional repressors but switch into transcriptional activators when ligand in bound.

LXRs are best characterised as important regulators of systemic sterol homeostasis and control the expression of a panel of genes involved in sterol transport between cells and tissues. LXRs are also described to have important immunoregulatory roles. LXRs facilitate the phagocytosis and clearance of apoptotic cells, LXRs promote cholesterol efflux to prevent lipotoxicity and LXRs inhibit the expression pro-inflammatory genes by suppressing NFκB and AP1 activities (Gonzalez et al, 2009). LXRs are also important for maintaining neutrophil homeostasis and in lymphocytes LXR agonists inhibit mitogen driven proliferation. Additionally, LXRs have a role in the differentiation of different CD4 T cells subsets.

## Reference

Silvestre-Roig C, Fridlender ZG, Glogauer M, Scapini P. Neutrophil Diversity in Health and Disease. Trends in Immunology, 2019; 40(7):565.

# 3

# Prooxidants and Antioxidants

## FREE RADICALS, ANTIOXIDANT ENZYMES AND ANTIOXIDANT NUTRIENTS

### Introduction

Oxygen is a vital component for living beings and constitutes about one-fifth of the atmospheric gases. This is a paramagnetic gas that is consumed continuously during respiration and also regenerated by plants during photosynthesis. Oxygen in the atmosphere exists in the diatomic state. One atom of oxygen is bonded to another to make a molecule of oxygen (Fig. 3.2). In this state, oxygen is at its lowest energy level. Each atom of oxygen molecule contains four pairs of electrons (six electrons being in the outer shell) and the two unpaired electrons present in the outer shell are shared by both the atoms.

Most of the molecular oxygen consumed by aerobic cells is reduced to water at the expense of electrons flowing down the respiratory chain of mitochondria. Respiratory process involves the transport of electrons via cytochromes to molecular oxygen. The cytochromes in the electron transport chain or respiratory chain are arranged in a sequence of $b \rightarrow c_1 \rightarrow c \rightarrow aa_3$. However, small amounts of oxygen are used (by oxygenases or oxidases) in enzymatic reactions in which one (monooxygenase) or both atoms (dioxygenase) of the oxygen molecule are directly inserted into the organic substrate molecule to yield hydroxyl groups. Monooxygenases are also called hydroxylases or mixed-function oxygenases, while dioxygenases are also called oxygen transferases.

Oxygen is one of the essential elements mandatory for oxidative metabolic reaction involved in energy production for living organisms. Besides, it also participates in various reactions generating toxic compounds such as reactive oxygen species (ROS) considered harmful for physiological system (Zorov et al, 2014). These will be studied later in this section.

### Free Radicals

The outermost orbital in an atom or molecule contains two electrons, each spinning in opposite directions. The chemical covalent bond consists of a pair of electrons, each component of the bond donating one electron each. A free radical may be defined as a molecule or molecular fragment that contains one or more unpaired electrons in its outer orbital (Fig. 3.1). It is generally represented by a superscript dot (R). Note the difference between oxygen and superoxide anion radical in the Fig. 3.2.

So this loss of electron produces a free 'radical' or 'oxidant', which is highly reactive. Free radicals have an unpaired electron and are very electrophilic (i.e. they react to gain another electron). Free radicals are formed by

73

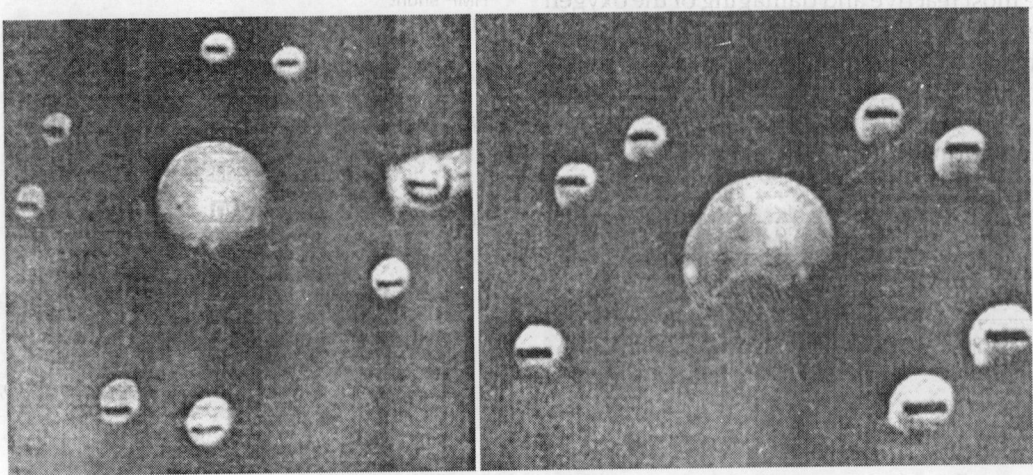

**Fig. 3.1:** Left side = normal oxygen atom with all paired electrons; one electron is in the process of jumping out. Right side = free radical, with an unpaired electron

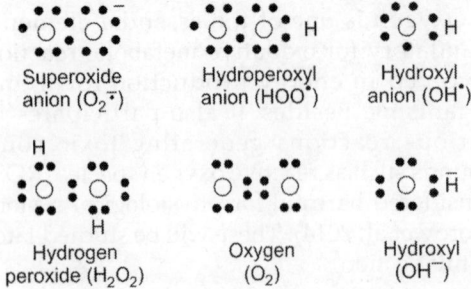

Superoxide
anion ($O_2^{\cdot-}$)

Hydroperoxyl
anion (HOO$^{\cdot}$)

Hydroxyl
anion (OH$^{\cdot}$)

Hydrogen
peroxide ($H_2O_2$)

Oxygen
($O_2$)

Hydroxyl
(OH$^-$)

**Fig. 3.2: Some free radicals.** Please compare hydroxyl onion (free radical) with hydroxyl, which is not a free radical. Also compare oxygen with superoxide anion

$$O_2 \xrightarrow{(+)\,e^-,\,2H^+} O_2^- \xrightarrow[(-)\,H_2O]{(+)\,e^-,\,H^+} H_2O_2 \xrightarrow{(+)\,e^-,\,H^+} OH^{\cdot} \xrightarrow{(+)\,e^-,\,H^+} H_2O$$

*Oxygen; superoxide anion; hydrogen peroxide; hydroxyl radical; water*

But excess production (of free radicals) can cause several health hazards. The slowest form of oxidation is rusting and since we live in an oxygen atmosphere, everything is subject to oxidation.

### Reactive Oxygen Species

Free radicals are highly reactive molecules containing one or more unpaired electrons. The term 'reactive oxygen species (ROS)' is a collective one that includes not only oxygen-centred radicals but also some non-radical derivatives of oxygen, such as hydrogen peroxide ($H_2O_2$), singlet oxygen and hypochlorous acid (HOCl) (Table 3.1). Important characteristics of the ROS are extreme reactivity, short lifespan, generation of new ROS by chain reaction and damage to various tissues. Hydrogen peroxide can get very easily breakdown, particularly in the presence of transition-metal ions [e.g. ferrous ($Fe^{2+}$) iron], to produce the hydroxyl radical,

the body as a consequence of normal breathing and metabolism. Indeed, various calculations of electron escape from electron-transport chain in mitochondria gave an estimation of about 200 billion of free radicals in every cell everyday to be produced in physiological conditions (Surai, F., 2006). They are potentially damaging to biological system. However, body's antioxidant nutrients neutralise them, as depicted below, to save the system.

**The sequential univalent reduction steps of oxygen may be represented as follows:**

the most reactive and damaging of the oxygen free radicals. The cytochrome oxidase and other proteins that reduce oxygen (to water) have been designed not to release superoxide anion. However, a small amount is unavoidably formed.

**Table 3.1:** Radicals and non-radical reactive oxygen and nitrogen species

| Radicals | Non-radicals |
|---|---|
| **Reactive Oxygen Species** | **Reactive Oxygen Species** |
| Superoxide ($O_2^{\bullet-}$) | Hydrogen peroxide ($H_2O_2$) |
| Hydroxyl ($OH^\bullet$) | Singlet oxygen ($^1O_2$) |
| Hydroperoxyl ($HO_2^\bullet$) | Hypochlorous acid (HOCl) |
| **Reactive Nitrogen Species** | |
| Nitric dioxide ($NO_2^\bullet$) | |
| Nitric oxide ($NO^\bullet$) | |

**Nitric oxide ($NO^\bullet$):** It is a free radical gas produced endogenously from arginine in a complex reaction (see below) that is catalysed by nitric oxide synthase (NOS). Nitric oxide diffuses freely across membranes but has a short life, less than a few seconds, because it is highly reactive. The other reactive nitrogen species (RNS) is nitric dioxide ($NO_2^\bullet$).

$$\text{Arginine} \xrightarrow[\text{NOS}]{\text{NADPH}} \xrightarrow[\text{NOS}]{O_2} \text{Citrulline} + NO^\bullet$$

### Generation of Free Radicals

1. Free radicals are constantly produced during the normal oxidation of foodstuffs, due to leaks in electron transport chain in mitochondria.
2. Some enzymes such as xanthine oxidase and aldehyde oxidase form superoxide anion radical, hydrogen peroxide.
3. NADPH oxidase in the inflammatory cells (neurtrophils, eosinophils, monocytes and macrophages) produces superoxide anion by a process of respiratory burst during phagocytosis (Fig. 3.3). Along with the

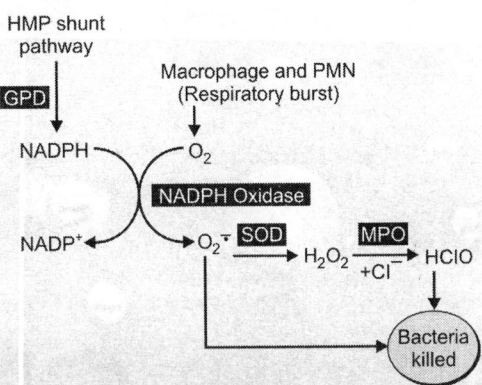

**Fig. 3.3.** Generation of ROS in macrophages (GPD, glucose-6-phosphate dehydrogenase, SOD, superoxide dismutase; MPO, myeloperoxidase; HClO, hypochlorous acid; PMN, polymorphonuclear leukocytes)

activation of macrophages, the consumption of oxygen by the cell is increased drastically, hence this is called respiratory burst.

4. Macrophages also produce nitric oxide (NO) from arginine by the enzyme nitric oxide synthase. NO is part of reactive nitrogen species (RNS) Table 3.1.
5. Peroxidation is also catalysed by lipooxygenase in platelets and leukocytes.
6. Free radicals are generated by ionising radiation, cigarette smoke and inhalation of air pollutants. Light of appropriate wavelength can cause photolysis of oxygen to produce singlet oxygen. Singlet oxygen is not a free radical but extremely reactive. All these are illustrated in Fig. 3.4.
7. Hydrogen peroxide in the presence of free iron can generate hydroxyl radical ($OH^\bullet$), which is highly reactive (compared to hydrogen peroxide) (Fig. 3. 5).

**Free radicals are produced from both endogenous and exogenous sources.**

### Endogenous Free Radicals

Free radicals are generated endogenously mainly from two sources. The first is by leakage from the mitochondrial electron-transfer chain, as part of normal cellular

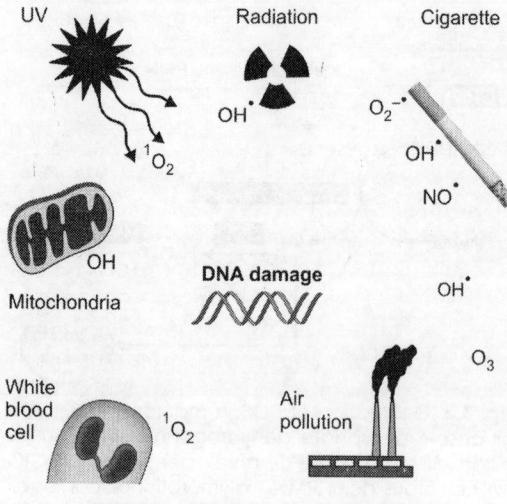

**Fig. 3.4:** Formation of free radicals

$$Fe^{++} + H_2O_2 \longrightarrow Fe^{+++} + OH^{\bullet} + OH^{-} \text{ (Fenton reaction)}$$

$$O_2 + H_2O_2 \xrightarrow{\text{Iron}} O_2 + OH^{\bullet} + OH^{-} \text{ (Haber-Weiss reaction)}$$

**Fig. 3.5:** Iron produces free radicals exogenous free radicals

metabolism. The second is as part of the respiratory-burst activity of leukocytes, which is involved in microbial killing.

**Intracellular free radicals** arise from autooxidation and inactivation of thiols, flavins and other small molecules, and from the activity of certain cyclooxygenases, lipooxygenases, dehydrogenases, oxidases and peroxidases as well as electron transport systems. Reactive oxygenated free radicals are continuously generated within the cell predominantly by oxidases and electron transport systems.

**Intracellular sites cf free radical generation** include all organelles and subcellular structures, especially mitochondria, peroxisomes, lysosomes and major cellular membranes like endoplasmic reticulum, plasma and nuclear membranes.

Common types of free radicals generated within the cell are peroxy, alkoxy, hydroxyl, hydroperoxyl and superoxide radicals. In addition, hydrogen peroxide and singlet

oxygen are also generated. These are not free radicals but molecules that are very reactive and capable of causing damage to tissues. Superoxide radical is explained later.

*Exogenous Free Radicals*

Exogenous sources of free radicals include ozone, tobacco smoke, environmental pollution, UV radiation, anaesthetics and some organic solvents, e.g. chloroform. The formation of free radicals is catalysed by ultraviolet light and certain ions (copper, iron) and the presence of either increases the rate of oxidation dramatically (Figs 3.4 and 3.5).

It is reported that more free radicals are found in smokers than in non-smokers. Free radicals are believed to be associated with cancer, atherosclerosis, high blood pressure, osteoarthritis and immune deficiency.

## Superoxide Anion ($O_2^{\bullet}$) and its Biological Effects

*Superoxide anion*

Superoxide anion is a byproduct of normal metabolism. The pathway for production of superoxide anion in biological system includes both enzyme-catalysed reactions and non-enzymatic reactions. The examples of enzymatic reactions are NADPH oxidase, xanthine oxidase, etc. Phagocytic oxidative bursts and mitochondrial electron chain leakage are other sources of generation. The non-enzymatic reactions that lead to the generation of this oxidant molecule are the transfer of electrons from quinine/semi-quinone to oxygen and certain photochemical reactions where electron is transferred from excited state photoactive molecule to the oxygen. The major events associated with the release of superoxide anion in biological system are chemotaxis, oxidation of proteins, inactivation and degradation of proteins and lipids.

Superoxide anions are involved in inflammatory disorders, carcinogenesis and various other genetic disorders. They are also involved in photosensitisation reactions such as those observed following administration of hematoporphyrins, a mixture of porphyrins used for the detection and management of neoplasm in the photodynamic therapy of cancer patients.

## Biological Effects of Superoxide Anion

The $O_2^{\bullet-}$ released from activated neutrophils also produce chemotactic substances by reacting with certain components of blood plasma. This allows neutrophiles to recruit others and thereby producing a local inflammatory reaction. Superoxide anions are toxic and need to be removed before other intermediates of dioxygen reduction are formed from it.

Superoxide anion can attack deoxyribonucleic acid (DNA) at either the sugar or the base which results into fragmentation, base loss and strand breaks with a terminally fragmented sugar residue. This has been observed during the exposure of bacteria and mammalian cells to $H_2O_2$, $O_2^{\bullet-}$, gamma radiation or ozone. Superoxide anion is relatively less reactive with short lifespan to the tune of milliseconds at neutral pH. It is relatively a weak oxidant which can oxidise compounds like ascorbate, sulfite and certain catecholamines. But this has been shown to be a potent reductant.

## Oxidative Stress

Free radicals play an important role in various physiological functions such as cell to cell interaction and cell signalling. When there is an increased ROS/RNS production that goes undefended by antioxidants, there occurs an oxidative stress (OS).

Oxidative stress may result from cumulative damage caused by reactive oxygen species (ROS). This kind of oxidative stress is present throughout life and is thought to be a major contributor to the ageing process. The immune system is particularly vulnerable to oxidative damage, since many immune cells produce these reactive compounds as part of the body's defence mechanisms.

Ageing, cancer, ischemic heart disease, hypertension, arthritis and cataract are currently thought to be a result of oxidative stress, i.e. the generation of excess free radicals and peroxides in the tissues. These oxidants oxidise several blood constituents including the lipids. Oxidised blood lipids are more atherogenic.

These oxidant stressors may precipitate a deficiency of several trace and ultratrace elements such as copper, selenium, manganese, boron, zinc, since they are involved in oxidative metabolism and antioxidant action.

## Damage to Macromolecules

ROS can cause damage to all of the major classes of macromolecules. They cause strand breaks in DNA (Halliwell and Aruoma, 1991), which can potentially lead to subsequent mutation and tumour-cell formation. Free-radical-mediated damage to proteins of the lens (of the eye) leads to formation of cataract. Lipids with several double bonds are probably most susceptible to free radical attack. This oxidative destruction of PUFA (lipid peroxidation) can be extremely damaging, since it proceeds as a self-perpetuating chain reaction.

Generation of ROS in excess of the amounts that can be dealt with by the body's antioxidant protective mechanisms seems to be a major contributor to several degenerative disorders in humans such as cancer, cardiovascular disease, stroke, cataract, degeneration of the macula region of the retina, immunosenescence and to the ageing process. Indeed, it is probably crucial to try to balance the production of ROS and the antioxidant defence system from as early an age as possible to prevent many age-related disorders.

Strong associations between diets rich in antioxidant nutrients and a reduced incidence of cancer have been observed in several epidemiological studies (Block et al, 1992; Giovannucci, 1999). That is why it has been suggested that antioxidants boost the body's immune system (Bendich and Olson, 1989).

## Mechanism of action of Reactive Oxygen Species

A mild oxidative stress is not harmful, but it acts positively. It results in a physiological response and upregulating the antioxidant defences as well as redistribution of antioxidants. But in case of severe uncontrolled oxidative stress, there may occur cell death, organ and/system failure. The possible reasons for oxidative stress injury are alterations of cell membranes caused by free radicals. These are due to lipid peroxidation, protein oxidation, nucleic acid modification, increase in intracellular $Ca^{+2}$ concentrations and signal transductions.

Oxygen radicals and other ROS cause modifications of proteins leading to changes in protein function, chemical fragmentation, or increased susceptibility to proteolytic attack as well as an altered enzyme activity.

## What are Antioxidants?

Antioxidants give an electron to a free radical without themselves becoming harmful, thus stop the chain reaction of free radicals or oxidants that damage cellular components and membranes. Antioxidants are considered important nutraceuticals on account of many health benefits.

## Natural and Synthetic Antioxidants

Naturally occurring antioxidants such as vitamins C, A and E, carotenoids, polyphenols and other micronutrients can remove peroxides and free radicals and thereby reduce the oxidative stress in tissues. Selenium has antioxidant activity due to its role in glutathione peroxidase. Polyphenols from plant sources also have antioxidant activity.

A number of synthetic antioxidants are used as preservatives to prevent autooxidation of lipids in foods and feeds. Synthetic antioxidants available are propyl-, octyl- or dodecyl-gallate, butylated hydroxyanisole (BHA), butylated hydroxytoluene (BHT), ethoxyquin, nordihydroguaiaretic acid (NDGA), diphenyl-P-phenylenediamine (DPPD). NDGA and DPPD have been banned by FDA. BHA and BHT are phenolic compounds and ethoxyquin is not a phenolic but quinoline compound. Very much disturbing information is available on these chemicals. Now, it appears beyond a shadow of a doubt, at some level of ingestion, synthetic antioxidants are inducers or promoters of neoplasia, i.e. cancer.

Consumer has become informed of that ready to eat convenience products could be laced with carcinogens in the form of preservatives. Vitamin E - based preservatives are good for this purpose.

## End products of Metabolic Pathways as Antioxidants

Some end products of degradative metabolic pathways play important roles as protective agents, e.g. urate, bilirubin. Bilirubin, urate and ascorbate are the three principal antioxidants in plasma.

### Urate

It is very efficient scavenger of highly reactive and harmful oxygen species-namely, hydroxyl radicals, superoxide anions, singlet oxygen and oxygenated haeme intermediates in high Fe valence states (+4 and +5). Indeed, urate is about as effective as ascorbate as an antioxidant.

The increased level of urate in humans compared with prosimians and other lower primates may contribute significantly to the longer lifespan of humans and to the lower incidence of human cancer. Urate, the ionized form of uric acid, is the end product of purine metabolism in humans.

### Bilirubin

It is the end product of haeme metabolism in mammals, while biliverdin is the end product in reptiles and birds. Bilirubin is a very effective antioxidant. It scavenges two hydroperoxy radicals. On a molar basis, bilirubin bound to albumin is about a tenth as effective as ascorbate in affording protection against water-soluble peroxides. Bilirubin is an especially potent antioxidant in membranes, where it rivals vitamin E.

## Antioxidant Enzymes that Ameliorate the toxicity of dioxygen

The antioxidant enzymes are located intracellularly. As a result, they act only on free radicals produced and retained within the cell.

## Superoxide Dismutases (SOD)

Superoxide anion is unstable in aqueous medium and gets dismutated either spontaneously or through an enzyme-catalysed reaction. The enzyme responsible for its fast dismutation is known as superoxide dismutase (SOD). Hence, it is one of the principal chain-breaking antioxidants, the other being vitamin E that traps peroxide free radicals.

The rate of autodismutation is at least four times less in magnitude compared to enzyme-catalysed reaction. Three isozymes of SOD have been reported to exist which perform dismutation reaction with comparable efficiency. These are manganese containing isozyme (Mn-SOD), iron-containing isozyme (Fe-SOD) and copper and zinc-containing isozyme (Cu, Zn-SOD). Mn-SOD and Cu, Zn-SOD differ in their cellular locations. The former is located in the mitochondrial matrix, while Cu, Zn-SOD is cytoplasmic. Cu, Zn-SOD is found in the red blood cells and other tissue cells. The activity of cytoplasmic Cu, Zn-SOD and that of mitochondrial Mn-SOD are reduced in individuals deficient in copper and manganese, respectively. Cu, Zn-SOD activity is not affected by zinc deficiency.

Superoxide dismutase is absent from anaerobic organisms. Since the production of $O_2^{\bullet-}$ occurs in the presence of oxygen, the respiring cells face a great threat of $O_2^{\bullet-}$-mediated injury and need enough amount of superoxide dismutase, which catalytically scavenges these anion radicals with great efficiency. SOD provides protection against oxygen toxicity and against the oxygen-mediated enhancement of the lethal effect of antibiotics, such as streptonigrin, etc. SOD imparts resistance towards hyperoxia.

**Exogenous supplemented SOD**: There is ordinarily very little SOD present in extracellular fluids. In certain $O_2^{\bullet-}$-mediated health disorders, levels of this enzyme are depleted and are not sufficient to combat the situation of excessive generation of these radicals. Therefore, the exogenous supplemented enzyme may afford protection against $O_2^{\bullet-}$-mediated tissue injury.

## Other Antioxidant Enzymes

In addition to SOD, catalase and glutathione peroxidase protect the system against hyperoxia. Copper-containing plasma protein, ceruloplasmin has some antioxidant property. Glutathione peroxidase and catalase catalyse the decomposition of hydrogen peroxide resulting from dismutase and other metabolic activities.

**Peroxisomes contain oxidases:** Peroxisomes are small membrane-bound compartments that are present in the cells of most eukaryotes. These organelles contain oxidases that generate hydrogen peroxide and catalase which degrade $H_2O_2$ to water and oxygen. Peroxisomes are devoid of DNA. Peroxide forming and destroying reactions are confined mainly to peroxisomes, a biological adaptation which minimises damages to cellular constituents by peroxides.

## Reduced Glutathione and Oxidised Glutathione

Glutathione ($\gamma$-L-glutamyl-L-cysteinylglycine) is ubiquitous in nature. It protects red blood cells (erythrocytes) from oxidative damage. It is present at high levels in animal cells ($\sim 5$ mM) and serves as a sulfhydral buffer. Glutathione plays a key role in detoxification by reacting with hydrogen peroxide and organic peroxides, the harmful products of aerobic life. It is thus indispensable for all aerobic life forms. It is also essential for the normal function of mitochondria. **Glutathione has been labelled as the largest nonenzymatic antioxidant defence of the body.**

Glutathione peroxidase destroys peroxides at the expense of reduced glutathione (GSH). In the process, GSH is converted into oxidised glutathione (GSSG).

Peroxide + GSH → GSH Peroxide
GSH Peroxide → GSSG + Hydroxyacids

The resultant GSSG is subsequently reduced back to GSH at the expense of NADPH in a reaction catalysed by glutathione reductase (a flavoprotein).

GSSG + NADPH → GSH + NADP$^+$

Thus, it cycles between a reduced thiol form (GSH) and an oxidised form (GSSG), in which two tripeptides are linked by a disulphide bond. The ratio of GSH to GSSG in most cells is greater than 500. Peroxidases catalyse an analogous reaction in which alkyl peroxide is reduced to water and an alcohol by a reductant. For example, the reductant could be cytochrome C or ascorbate.

### Antioxidant System—Selenium has been Considered as the "Chief Executive of The Antioxidant System"

There are three major levels of antioxidant defence and selenium (Se) participates in all of them. The first level is based on the activity of antioxidant enzymes with SOD as chief to detoxify superoxide radical. Se-dependent GSH-Px, catalase and metal-binding proteins are also integral part of the first level of antioxidant defence. The GSH-Px also belongs to the second level of antioxidant defence, since it is responsible for detoxification of lipid hydroperoxides formed as a result of reaction of lipid peroxides with such antioxidants as vitamin E. Indeed, an optimal interaction between vitamin E and GSH-Px provides an important mechanism of antioxidant defence. Recently, it has been shown that SeMet could affect activity of DNA repairing enzymes. This means that Se also belongs to the third level of antioxidant defence. Taking into account the possible role of all 25 known selenoproteins, selenium has been considered as the "Chief executive of the antioxidant system".

The understanding that all antioxidants in the body are working as a team, called the antioxidant system, creates an additional interest in antioxidant interactions. Indeed, **vitamin E recycling** is shown to be the most important mechanism of the antioxidant defences. This means that, if the recycling is effective, even low levels of vitamin E could provide a substantial antioxidant protection. If recycling is broken, probably even high levels would not provide the antioxidant protection.

### Free Radical Scavenger Systems

The superoxide anion gets dismutated to hydrogen peroxide by superoxide dismutase (SOD). Hydrogen peroxide is also a potent oxidant. It is detoxified by the reaction with reduced glutathione (GSH) catalysed by glutathione peroxidase (Fig. 3.6). The oxidised glutathione (GSSG), in turn, is reduced by glutathione reductase (GR) in the presence of NADPH (Fig. 3.6). [This NADPH is generated with the help of glucose-6-phosphate dehydrogenase (GPD) in HMP shunt pathway (Fig. 3.3). Therefore, in GPD deficiency, the RBCs are liable to lysis Fig. 3.6a]. When $H_2O_2$ is generated in large quantities, the enzyme catalase is also used for its removal.

### Dietary Antioxidants and their Mechanism of Action

Higher organisms have evolved a variety of antioxidant defence systems either to prevent

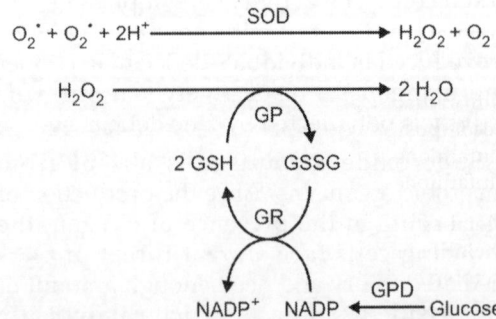

**Fig. 3.6:** Free radical scavenging enzymes (SOD, superoxide dismutase; GP, glutathione peroxidase; GSH, reduced glutathione; GSSG, oxidised glutathione; GR, glutathione reductase; GPD, glucose-6-phosphate dehydrogenase; $O_2^{•}$, superoxide anion radical

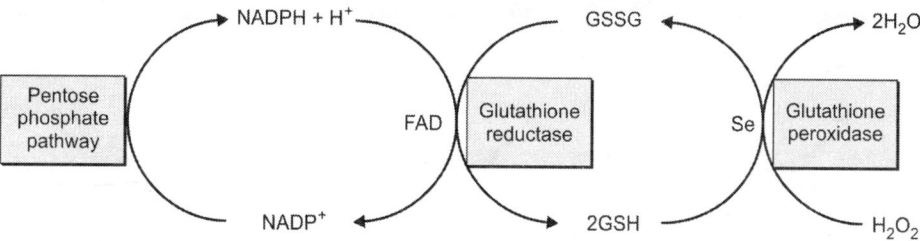

**Fig. 3.6a:** Role of the pentose phosphate pathway in the glutathione peroxidase reaction of erythrocytes. GSSG, oxidised glutathione; GSH, reduced glutathione; Se, selenium cofactor

the generation of ROS or to intercept any of these ROS that are produced. These defence systems exist in both the aqueous and membrane compartments of cells and can be enzymic or non-enzymic in nature. The enzymes contain metal ions at their active sites and these metal ions must be obtained from the diet, while the diet is the source of many non-enzymic components of the body's antioxidant defence system (e.g. antioxidant vitamins).

While the endogenous antioxidants (superoxide dismutase, glutathione peroxidase [GSH-Px], catalase, etc.) are controlled via cell to cell interaction and cell signalling, the exogenous antioxidants (vitamins C and E, beta-carotene and various plant pigments and free amino acids, peptides and proteins) depend solely on the diet of an individual (Table 3.2).

**Principal chain-breaking antioxidants** include superoxide dismutase, which traps superoxide free radicals and vitamin E, which traps peroxide free radicals. The tocopheroxyl free radical product is reduced back to tocopherol by ascorbic acid (vitamin C). The ascorbate free radical is converted to ascorbate and dehydroascorbate, which are not free radicals.

## Antioxidant Nutrients

### Vitamin C

Vitamin C (ascorbate and dehydroascorbate; Fig. 3.7) has a broad-spectrum of antioxidant activities due to its ability to react with numerous aqueous free radicals (water-soluble free radical scavenger) and reactive oxygen species. It is a simple molecule, derived from glucose and can readily undergo oxidation

| Table 3.2: Types of antioxidants depending on their action | | |
|---|---|---|
| *Preventive* | *Scavenging* | *Repair Enzymes* |
| Suppress formation of free radicals | Inhibit chain initiation, break chain propagation | Repair the damaged biomolecules |
| **Non-radical decomposition:** Catalase, glutathione peroxidase, glutathione-S-transferase | **Hydrophilic:** Vitamin C, uric acid, bilirubin, albumin | Lipases<br>Proteases<br>DNA repair enzymes |
| **Metal sequestration by chelation:** Transferrin, lactoferrin, ceruloplasmin, haptoglobin, ferritin | **Lipophilic:** Vitamin E, carotenoids, flavonoids | |
| **Quenchers:** Superoxide dismutase, vitamin E, carotenoids, flavonols and phenolics | | |

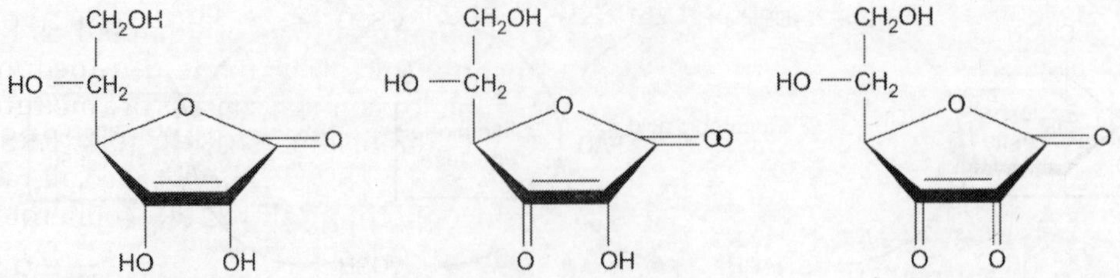

Ascorbate                    Monodehydroascorbate           Dehydroascorbate
                             (semidehydroascorbate)

**Fig. 3.7:** Ascorbic acid or vitamin C. Dehydroascorbate is the oxidised form; monodehydroascorbate has one oxygen reduced; and ascorbic acid has both oxygens reduced

and reduction. Its synthesis involves formation of L-gulonolactone from glucose, which is converted to ascorbic acid by the enzyme L-gulonolactone oxidase (Fig. 3.8).

Vitamin C is found in high concentrations in circulating phagocytic cells (leukocytes) and it appears to be utilised during infections. Ascorbic acid helps to protect these cells from oxidative damage. Unlike deficiencies of $B_6$, E and $B_2$, deficiency of vitamin C does not cause atrophy of lymphoid tissue. In guinea pigs, vitamin C was shown to be important in maintaining normal primary and secondary antibody responses and was important for neutrophil function (Anderson and Lukey, 1987). Ascorbic acid is reported to have a stimulating effect on the phagocytic activity of leukocytes, the function of the reticuloendothelial system and the formation of antibodies. Vitamin C can stimulate the production of interferons, the proteins that protect cells against viral attack (Siegel, 1974).

It forms the first line of defence in plasma exposed to a variety of oxidant insults, including aqueous free radicals, activated polymorphonuclear leukocytes and cigarette smoke. When compared with other water-soluble antioxidants, vitamin C offers the most effective protection against plasma lipid peroxidation. Since it is water-soluble, it protects other antioxidants such as vitamins A and E and essential fatty acids.

Vitamin C is an electron donor and therefore a reducing agent. All known physiological and biochemical actions of vitamin C are due to its action as an electron donor; by donating its electrons, it prevents other compounds from being oxidised. In the process of sparing fatty acid oxidation, tocopherol is oxidised to the tocopheryl free radical. Ascorbic acid can donate an electron to the tocopheryl free radical, regenerating the reduced antioxidant form of tocopherol. Thus, it does vitamin E recycling.

One of the protective effects of vitamin C may partly be mediated through its ability to reduce circulating glucocorticoids (Degkwitz, 1987). The suppressive effect of corticoids on neutrophil function in cattle was alleviated with vitamin C supplementation (Roth and Kaeberle, 1985).

Vitamin C is the most important antioxidant in extracellular fluids and can protect biomembranes against lipid peroxidation damage by eliminating peroxyl radicals in the aqueous phase before the latter can initiate peroxidation (Frei et al, 1989). Vitamins C and E supplementation resulted in a 78% decrease in the susceptibility of lipoproteins to mononuclear cell-mediated oxidation (Rifici and Khachadurian, 1993).

*Tocopherols and Tocotrienols*

Vitamin E is a generic name for two classes of isoprenoid compounds, tocopherols and tocotrienols (Fig. 3.9). There are total 8 compounds that exhibit vitamin E activity, i.e. 4 tocopherols ($\alpha$, $\beta$, $\gamma$, and $\delta$) and similarly 4 tocotrienols ($\alpha$, $\beta$, $\gamma$, and $\delta$). The most popular is $\alpha$-tocopherol, commonly called vitamin E. The only metabolic function of vitamin E as a cellular antioxidant, it is

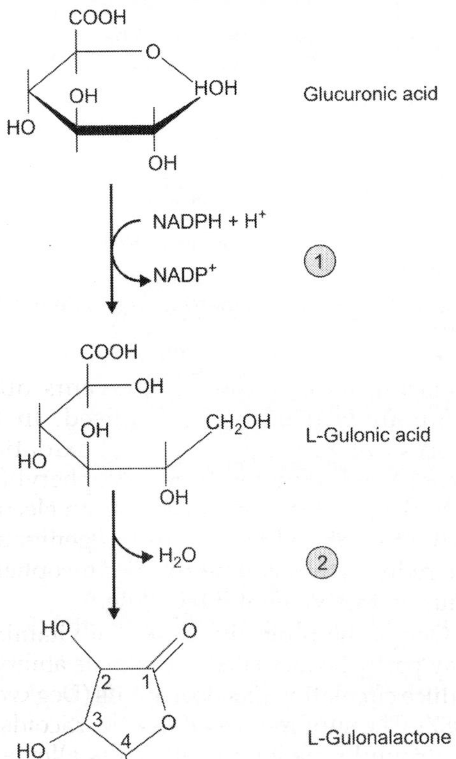

COOH

OH    HOH    Glucuronic acid

HO

OH

$\curvearrowright$ NADPH + H$^+$

$\curvearrowright$ NADP$^+$    ①

COOH

OH

OH    CH$_2$OH    L-Gulonic acid

HO

OH

$\rightarrow$ H$_2$O    ②

HO    O

2  1

3  4  O    L-Gulonalactone

HO

5

HO — CH

6

CH$_2$OH

$\curvearrowright$ O$_2$    ③

$\rightarrow$ H$_2$O$_2$

HO    O

O

HO    Ascorbic acid

HO — CH

CH$_2$OH

**Fig. 3.8:** Synthesis of vitamin C from glucose

responsible for stabilising cell membranes. Cell membranes contain PUFA, which are stabilised against free radical damage by the presence of vitamin E as an integral part of membranes.

The natural form of vitamin E is RRR-α-tocopherol (older name d-α-tocopherol). Synthetic vitamin E consists of a mixture of all eight stereoisomers (RRR, RSR, RRS, RSS, SRR, SSR, SRS, SSS) and is called all-racemic-α-tocopherol or all-rac-α-tocopherol (older name dl-α-tocopherol).

**Vitamin E molecules are recycled:** It is the major lipid-soluble biological antioxidant in the body and is required for protection of membrane lipids from peroxidation. Since free radicals and lipid peroxidation are immuno-suppressive, it is considered that vitamin E should act to optimise and even enhance the immune response. This molecule acts as a **chain-breaking antioxidant,** intercepting lipid peroxyl radicals and so terminating lipid-peroxidation chain reactions. Similarly vitamin E protects the animal from the detrimental effects of protein oxidation.

In functioning as an antioxidant, the phenolic hydroxyl group on the chromanol ring of tocopherol reacts with free radicals, causing termination of the auto-oxidation chain reaction, particularly within the membranes where vitamin E resides. This action is called **free-radical scavenging** and involves donation of the phenolic hydrogen to a fatty acid free radical. This action is also called **free-radical quenching.** In this process, an inactive tocopheroxyl free radical is formed, which is converted to tocophery-lquinone. The quinone form is reduced back to the tocopherol form by ascorbic acid; thus **vitamin E molecules are recycled** and can repeatedly function as antioxidants.

In laboratory animals, vitamin E deficiency decreases spleen lymphocyte proliferation, NK cell activity, specific antibody production following vaccination and phagocytosis by neutrophils and increases the susceptibility of animals to infectious pathogens (Bendich, 1993; Meydani and Beharka, 1998; Han and Meydani, 1999).

Considerable attention is presently being directed to the role vitamin E and selenium play in protecting leukocytes and macrophages during phagocytosis, the mechanism

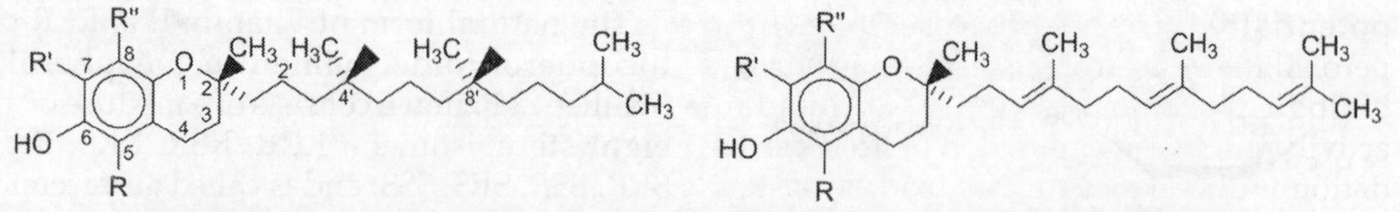

| Compound | R | R' | R" | Compound |
|----------|-----|-----|-----|-----------|
| α-Tocopherol | $CH_3$ | $CH_3$ | $CH_3$ | α-Tocotrienol |
| β-Tocopherol | $CH_3$ | H | $CH_3$ | β-Tocotrienol |
| γ-Tocopherol | H | $CH_3$ | $CH_3$ | γ-Tocotrienol |
| δ-Tocopherol | H | H | $CH_3$ | δ-Tocotrienol |

**Fig. 3.9:** The structures of various forms of vitamin E

whereby animals immunologically kill invading bacteria. Both vitamin E and selenium may help these cells to survive the toxic products that are produced in order to effectively kill ingested bacteria.

Macrophages and neutrophils from vitamin E-deficient animals have decreased phagocytic activity. Large doses of vitamin E protected chicks and poults against *Escherichia coli* with increased phagocytosis and antibody production. Since vitamin E acts as a tissue antioxidant and aids in quenching free radicals produced in the body, any infection or other stress factors may exacerbate depletion of the limited vitamin E stores from various tissues.

During stress and disease, there is an increase in production of glucocorticoids, epinephrine, eicosanoids and phagocytic activity. Eicosanoid and corticoid synthesis and phagocytic respiratory bursts are prominent producers of free radicals that challenge the animal antioxidant systems. Vitamin E has been implicated in the stimulation of serum antibody synthesis, particularly IgG antibodies (Tengerdy, 1980).

The protective effects of vitamin E on animal health may be involved with its role in reduction of glucocorticoids, which are known to be immunosuppressive. Daily vitamin E (as *dl*-α-tocopheryl acetate) supplementation at 450 IU per head in newly received feedlot cattle, stressed by long distance shipment and changes from green forage to high grain feedlot diets, improved early performance (Lee et al, 1985). Higher levels have been shown to positively influence both cellular and humoral immune status of ruminant species and thus vitamin E has an important role in improving health (Rizvi et al, 2014).

Antioxidants, including vitamin E, play a role in resistance to viral infection. Vitamin E deficiency allows a normally benign virus to cause disease (Beck et al, 1994). In mice, enhanced virulence of a virus resulted in myocardial injury that was prevented with vitamin E adequacy. Selenium or vitamin E deficiency leads to a change in viral phenotype, such that a virulent strain of a virus becomes virulent and a virulent strain becomes more virulent (Beck, 1997).

## Carotenoids and Vitamin A

**Carotenoids:** Carotenoids are an abundant group of plant pigments; over 600 individual carotenoids are known. They contain a long chain of conjugated double bonds and this chain has antioxidant activity. Among carotenoids some have a β-ionone ring (e.g. β-carotene), while others do not have (e.g. lycopene). β-ionone ring is necessary for vitamin A activity.

Beta carotene can function as a **chain-breaking antioxidant.** It deactivates reactive chemical species such as singlet oxygen, triplet photochemical sensitisers and free radicals which would otherwise induce potentially harmful processes (e.g. lipid peroxidation). β-carotene displays an efficient biological radical-trapping antioxidant activity through its inhibition of lipid peroxidation induced by xanthine oxidase system. The carotene deficiency is associated with a higher incidence of cancer and increased carcinogenesis.

Carotenoids have been shown to have biological actions independent of vitamin A. They can enhance many aspects of immune functions, act directly as antimutagens and anticarcinogens, protect against radiation damage and block the damaging effects of photosensitisers. Carotenoids are also suggested to induce phase II detoxification system as well as enhance T cell mediated immune responses.

In animal models, β-carotene and canthaxanthin have protected against UV-induced skin cancer as well as some chemically induced tumours. In some of these models, an enhancement of tumour immunity has been suggested as a possible mechanism of action of these carotenoids (Bendich, 1989).

The vitamin A is formed in the body after absorption of β–carotene (provitamin A). The provitamin A is absorbed via esterification with cholesterol and/or fatty acid. Compared with α–tocopherol, β–carotene is a relatively weak antioxidant. Vitamin A acts as a radical scavenger.

**Vitamin A:** Vitamin A plays a role in the maintenance of mucosal surfaces (i.e. essential for maintaining epidermal and mucosal integrity), in the generation of antibody responses to T cell-dependent and independent antigens, in haematopoiesis and in the function of T and B lymphocytes, natural killer (NK) cells and neutrophils. Vitamin A regulates keratinocyte differentiation. It is now recognised that vitamin A modulates many different aspects of immune function, including components of both nonspecific immunity (e.g. phagocytosis, maintenance of mucosal surfaces) and specific immunity (e.g. generation of antibody responses). The influence of vitamin A on different aspects of immune function is attributed to the action of vitamin A and related metabolites as modulators of gene transcription.

**Effects of vitamin A deficiency on host defence:** Much of our knowledge of vitamin A and immune function is derived from experimental animal studies involving mice, rats and chickens. Role of vitamin A deficiency has been assessed on immune responses in the experimental animals. Vitamin A deficiency affected the metabolism and functions of lymphoid organs. Vitamin A deficient animals showed a marked atrophy of spleen, thymus and the weights of these organs were reduced. Such animals are more susceptible to parasitic infections as compared to controls. Vitamin A deficiency also leads to increased incidence of lung cancer, bronchial carcinoma and cancer of oral cavity and severity of infectious diseases, and this has been linked to an impaired immune response.

**Vitamin A deficiency impairs mucosal immunity:** There is a close relationship between vitamin A status and the expression of mucins and keratins. Mucins are large glycoconjugates that are found on cell surfaces and secreted into the lumens of the gastrointestinal, respiratory and genitourinary tracts. Mucins are also secreted on the bulbar and palpebral conjunctivae of the eye. Vitamin A deficiency impairs mucosal function through several mechanisms: (i) loss of cilia in the respiratory tract; (ii) loss of microvilli in the gastrointestinal tract; (iii) loss of mucin and goblet cells in the respiratory, gastrointestinal and genitourinary tracts; (iv) squamous metaplasia with abnormal keratinisation in the respiratory and genitourinary tracts; (v) alterations in antigen-specific secretory immunoglobulin A (IgA) concentrations; (vi) impairment of mucosal-associated immune-cell function (vii) decreased integrity of the gut.

Loss of mucin and goblet cells and sqamous metaplasia of the conjunctiva and cornea are also well known. The loss of mucin that occurs in vitamin A deficiency constitutes a serious impairment of mucosal immunity. Breakdown in gut barrier integrity and impaired mucus secretion facilitate entry of pathogens.

**Vitamin A deficiency alters immune cell activity :** Vitamin A deficiency appears to impair **haematopoiesis** of some lineages, such as CD4+ lymphocytes, NK cells and erythrocytes. Retinoids have been implicated in the maturation of pluripotent stem cells to cell lineages that produce different haematopoietic cell lines, such as lymphocytes, granulocytes and megakaryocytes.

**Natural killer (NK) cells:** Vitamin A deficiency reduces the number of circulating NK cells and impairs NK cell cytolytic activity. NK cells play a role in anti-viral and anti-tumour immunity that is not major histocompatibility complex (MHC)-restricted and they are involved in the regulation of immune responses. The cytolytic activity of NK cells was reduced by vitamin A deficiency (Zhao et al, 1994).

**Neutrophils** play an important role in non-specific immunity because they phagocytose and kill bacteria, parasites, virus-infected cells and tumour cells. Retinoic acid plays an important role in the normal maturation of neutrophils.

**T and B lymphocytes and antibody response:** Vitamin A appears to modulate the balance between T-helper type 1- and T-helper type 2-like responses. Retinoids appear to play a role in the differentiation and activity of cells of the monocyte/macrophage lineage.

Vitamin A deficiency impairs the growth, activation and function of B lymphocytes. B lymphocytes have been shown to utilise a metabolite of retinol, 14-hydroxy-4, 14-retro-retinol, instead of retinoic acid, as a mediator for growth.

The hallmark of vitamin A deficiency is an impaired capacity to generate an antibody response to T cell-dependent antigens (Semba et al, 1992, 1994) and T cell-independent type 2 antigens, such as pneumococcal polysaccharide (Pasatiempo et al, 1989).

Both low and high vitamin A intakes resulted in impaired immune responses. Low dietary vitamin A level caused reduced antibody production, defective T cell responses and reduced phagocytosis and decreased resistance to infection by bacteria, virus and protozoa. Optimum immune responses in growing chicks and poults were observed at 3–10 times higher dietary vitamin A levels than specified by NRC.

**Vitamin D:** Vitamin D receptors (VDR) have been identified in most cells of the immune system, suggesting that it has immunoregulatory properties. According to the classic genomic action of vitamin D,1,25 $(OH)_2D_3$ is released from its serum-binding protein, diffuses through the cell membrane and binds to a classic zinc finger-containing receptor (the vitamin D receptor; VDR) in the nucleus (Macdonald et al, 1994). There is some interaction between the nuclear co-receptors of vitamins A (retinoid X receptor; RXR) and D, as well as thyroxin; the receptors form heterodimers in different combinations, which can affect target gene transcription (Haag, 1999). Over the last decade, it has become clear that in addition to the slow genomic mode of action, vitamin D can also act via rapid non-genomic actions, which involve a number of second messenger pathways. See Chapter 9 on vitamin D for more information.

## Folic Acid and B-group Vitamins

**Folic acid** deficiency in laboratory animals causes thymus and spleen atrophy and decreases circulating T cell numbers, the activity of cytotoxic T lymphocytes and spleen lymphocyte proliferation, but does not alter phagocytosis or bactericidal capacity of neutrophils. In contrast, **vitamin $B_{12}$** deficiency decreases phagocytosis and the bactericidal capacity of neutrophils. **Vitamin $B_6$** deficiency in laboratory animals causes thymus and spleen atrophy, decreases lymphocyte proliferation and the DTH response and increases allograft survival.

## Cysteine

In mammals, cysteine is made from two other amino acids, methionine and serine.

Methionine furnishes the sulphur atom and serine furnishes the carbon skeleton in the synthesis of cysteine. Cysteine is required for synthesis of glutathione.

*Selenium*

Vitamin E and the trace element selenium share the property of preventing peroxidation of unsaturated fatty acids in cell membranes. They are uniquely suited as **cellular antioxidants.** Virtually all of the disorders and deficiency signs associated with these two nutrients can be explained by their antioxidant properties (an exception is the role of selenium in the thyroid gland). See Chapter 8 on Selenium for details.

**Vitamin E and selenium have complementary roles as antioxidants:** Vitamin E is incorporated into the structure of cell membranes and thus is first line of defence against oxidant and free radical damage. It is situated so as to immediately neutralise oxidants before they can initiate chain reactions. If any oxidants escape the protective action of vitamin E, selenium (as a component of glutathione peroxidase) is a second line of defence. There is considerable variation among species and tissues in their reliance to either vitamin E or selenium as antioxidants. For example, ruminant muscle tissue is highly dependent on selenium to prevent nutritional muscular dystrophy (white muscle disease) whereas in chickens, vitamin E is more effective. Some species, such as rabbits, have **non-selenium dependent glutathione peroxidase and, therefore, are not susceptible to selenium deficiency.**

*Zinc*

The essential requirement of zinc (Zn) was first documented in animal studies in the 1930s for the growth and survival of animals. Zinc is a cofactor for many enzymes, including Cu-Zn superoxide dismutase, the **cytoplasmic antioxidant** and is therefore involved in protecting host cells from the cytotoxic effects of free radical species produced during immune responses. High zinc can also result in copper depletion and copper deficiency impairs immune function. Thus, zinc has a key role in supporting **DNA, RNA and protein synthesis and progress through the cell cycle.**

**Zinc is very important for cell replication.** Zn influences the activity of multiple enzymes, which act at the very basic levels of replication and transcription. These include DNA polymerase, thymidine kinase, DNA-dependent RNA polymerase, terminal deoxyribonucleotidyl transferase and aminoacyl tRNA synthetase and the family of transcriptional regulators known as Zn-finger DNA-binding proteins. In addition, Zn forms the active enzymatic sites of many metalloproteases. DNA polymerase regulates DNA replication and its activity is zinc-dependent. Thymidine kinase is crucial for the synthesis of phosphorylated pyrimidines and it is also very sensitive to dietary zinc depletion.

In fact, zinc is required for expression of multiple genes regulating mitosis, including thymidine kinase, ornithine decarboxylase and *c-myc*. Several transcription factors, such as nuclear factor kappa B (NFκB), metallothionein transcription factor 1 (MTF-1) and 'really interesting new gene' (RING) contain Zn-finger-like domains, which may be influenced by changes in intracellular pools of Zn. In addition, Zn deprivation affects also the activity of RNA polymerase, which is needed for transcription.

**Zinc plays a role in multiple aspects of T lymphocyte activation and signal transduction:** Zinc has a number of key roles relating to cell signalling, cell activation, gene expression, protein synthesis and apoptosis. Zinc is crucial for the normal development of immune cells. It plays an important role in maintaining the activity of a range of immune cells, including neutrophils, monocytes, NK cells, B cells and T cells, and Zn-deficient individuals have increased susceptibility to a variety of pathogens.

Zinc deficiency in animals is associated with a wide range of immune impairments. Zinc deficiency has a marked impact on bone marrow, decreasing the number of nucleated cells and the number and proportion of cells that are lymphoid precursors. Providing optimum level of zinc for deficient individuals improves the immune function and host defence leading to significant decreases in the incidence and severity of infectious diseases.

**Zinc and apoptosis:** The major mechanism of cell death in the body and in cell culture is apoptosis, a form of cell suicide characterised by a decrease in cell volume, dramatic condensation of the chromatin and cytoplasm and fragmentation of nuclear DNA. Apoptosis is a normal physiological process, enabling a variety of important processes, from epithelial turnover to T and B cell development. The dysregulation of such a basic process would, therefore, have important health consequences.

Zinc-deficient animals exhibit enhanced spontaneous and toxin-induced apoptosis in multiple cell types. Thymic atrophy is a central feature of zinc deficiency. It is now known that this atrophy is accompanied by apoptotic cell death of thymocytes. Several studies have demonstrated that zinc is a regulator of lymphocyte apoptosis *in vivo* and *in vitro*.

**Zinc plays a role in antioxidant defence,** protecting cells from the damaging effects of oxygen radicals that are generated during immune activation. Zinc is a component of the cytosolic superoxide dismutase enzyme. It also regulates the expression of metallothionein and metallothionein-like proteins in lymphocytes. Metallothionein is the primary zinc-binding and transport protein in the body. Superoxide dismutase and metallothionein have antioxidant activity (Prasad, 1993). Membrane zinc levels are strongly influenced by dietary zinc levels. Its concentration in cell membranes appear to be important in preserving their integrity through poorly defined mechanisms involving binding to thiolate groups. Zinc release from thiolate bonds can prevent lipid peroxidation. In addition, nitric oxide induces zinc release from metallothionein, which may limit free-radical membrane damage during inflammation.

**Zinc and Thymulin:** Thymulin is a nine-peptide hormone (Glu-Ala-Lys-Ser-Gln-Gly-Gly-Ser-Asn) secreted by thymic epithelial cells. Zinc is bound to thymulin in a 1:1 stoichiometry via the side-chain of asparagine and the hydroxyl groups of the two serines. The binding of zinc results in a conformational change, which produces the active form of thymulin. Thymulin binds to high-affinity receptors on T cells and promotes T cell maturation, cytotoxicity and interleukin (IL)-2 production. Thymulin activity *in vitro* and *in vivo* in both animals and humans is dependent on plasma zinc levels, such that marginal changes in its intake or availability affect thymulin activity. Thymulin may be used to know the status of zinc similar to transferrin that provides useful information regarding iron status.

## Copper

Zinc and iron impair copper uptake so that taking high doses of these might induce mild copper deficiency. Copper deficiency has been described in premature infants and in patients receiving total parenteral nutrition.

Copper deficiency in experimental animals and farm animals impairs a range of immune functions and increases susceptibility to bacterial and parasitic challenges. Human studies show that subjects on a low-copper diet have decreased lymphoctye proliferation and IL-2 production, while copper administration reverses these effects. As with many other micronutrients, excess copper can be immunosuppressive.

## Iron

Iron is the fourth most common element on earth and is one of the most studied nutrients in human health. Iron exists in two main forms: ferric ($Fe^{3+}$) and ferrous ($Fe^{2+}$). The ease of oxidation and reduction of iron makes it a unique trace element for many cellular redox reactions. Iron is required by virtually all living cells for many biochemical reactions, especially for aerobic and anaerobic energy metabolism and cell proliferation. The importance of iron in immunity was first recognised only in the late 1960s and early 1970s. Majority (67 to 75%) of body iron circulates in blood in the form of haemoglobin. Iron status is evaluated by the concentration of serum ferritin, blood haemoglobin and serum transferring receptor and transferrin saturation.

**Iron absorption and transport:** Iron is predominantly absorbed in the duodenum. In its free form, iron is a potent prooxidant known to induce peroxidation of lipids, proteins and nucleic acids. Extracellular iron circulates in blood bound to transferrin. One transferrin molecule has two iron-binding sites. Under physiological conditions, cells take up iron from plasma by enclocytosis, whereby one transferrin molecule binds to one transferrin receptor molecule, and the complex is transferred to the cytoplasm by invagination. As a result of low pH in the endosome, iron is released to the cytoplasm, where it is either used for various cellular functions or incorporated into ferritin.

Upon loss of iron, the apotransferrin-transferrin-receptor complex is transported back to the cell membrane, where apotransferrin is released into the bloodstream and the transferrin receptor is available for a new round of transferrin binding. The mechanism by which the apotransferrin-transferrin-receptor complex is transported to the cell membrane remains unclear. However, Sainte-Marie et al (1997) suggests that changes in free cytoplasmic calcium concentrations might be involved in the recycling of transferrin receptor.

**Effects of iron deficiency on immunity:** Iron deficiency has multiple effects on immune function in laboratory animals and humans. Iron-deficient individuals have normal phagocytic function but there is impaired ability to kill bacteria by neutrophils, probably as a result of an alteration in respiratory burst. Iron deficiency is associated with gastrointestinal and respiratory infections.

**T cells: Iron metabolism by immune cells and the effects of its deficiency on their functions:** Resting T cells do not express the transferrin receptor on their cell surface and therefore either do not take up iron from their environment or take up very little. Upon T cell activation, T cells express surface transferrin receptors in the G0/G1 phase of the cell cycle before the initiation of DNA synthesis, but after induction of interleukin (IL)-2 secretion. The increase in transferrin receptor concentrations is believed to be to ensure sufficient iron uptake to support the activity of ribonucleotide reductase for the biosynthesis of deoxyribonucleotides.

In mice, iron deficiency reduces the proportion of total T cells, helper T cells and cytotoxic/suppressor T cells in the spleen (Kuvibidila et al, 1990). Recent data suggest that iron deficiency decreases thymocyte proliferation and thus induces atrophy.

**Natural killer (NK) cells:** Similar to T lymphocytes, resting NK cells do not express surface transferrin receptor and they probably take up very little iron from the environment (Kemp, 1993). However, upon activation, they express the transferrin receptor on their surface. There is no information on the effects of iron deficiency on NK cell activity in human subjects. In rats, iron deficiency markedly reduces NK cytotoxicity against the YAC-1 target cell line (Spear and Sherman, 1992).

**B cells:** In contrast to T cells, resting B cells express low levels of the transferrin receptor, which implies that they continuously take up small quantities of iron (Neckers et al, 1984). Upon activation with a mitogen, up to 80% of B cells express surface transferrin receptor, and hence exhibit increased iron uptake. This suggests that iron deprivation may also affect certain B cell functions.

**Monocytes and macrophages:** Although monocytes do not express transferrin receptor, macrophages do (Testa et al, 1991). Macrophages differ from lymphocytes or other cell types because they upregulate the expression of surface transferrin receptor when cultured in an iron-rich medium. This makes sense because macrophages are involved in iron storage and require iron for cytotoxic activity (Jiang and Baldwin, 1993).

Although the production of 'macrophage migration inhibitory factor' is reduced in iron-deficient adults, production of IL-1 is not, and macrophage cytotoxicity is only slightly reduced.

**Neutrophils:** Iron concentrations in neutrophils are affected by the iron status of the host. Iron level can be low in iron deficiency and it is elevated in iron overload. Neutrophils can take up iron from iron-saturated transferrin (Brieland and Fantone, 1991), although transferrin receptors have never been demonstrated on the neutrophil surface (Parmley et al, 1983).

Several neutrophil responses have been assessed in both iron-deficient humans and laboratory animals. Although neutrophil phagocytosis remains normal in iron deficiency, intracellular killing of bacteria is significantly impaired in both humans and laboratory animals. In parallel with this reduced bactericidal killing, the activity of myeloperoxidase (Myeloperoxidase [MPO] is an iron-dependent enzyme involved in neutrophil killing of bacteria) is impaired.

**Mechanisms of impaired immunity in iron deficiency and iron overload:** The mechanisms by which iron deficiency impairs cell-mediated and non-specific immunity are not fully understood, but they are multi-factorial. They include reduced activity of iron-dependent enzymes (specifically ribonucleotide reductase), reduced cytokine secretion, a reduced number of immunocompetent T cells and, very probably, altered **signal transduction.** Specific steps of signal-transduction pathways that are potentially regulated by iron remain to be identified.

However, **protein kinase C** activity and its translocation to the plasma membrane in murine spleen lymphocytes and human T cell lines are impaired by iron deficiency. Furthermore, iron chelation reduces production of mRNA for protein kinase C. One early event in T cell activation pathways (that is also reduced by iron deprivation) is the hydrolysis of cell-membrane phosphatidylinosito 1-,4-,5-bisphosphate by phospholipase C (a zinc-dependent enzyme) (Kuvibidila et al, 1998). The end-products of this enzymatic reaction, inositol 1,3,5-triphosphate and diacylglycerol, regulate protein kinase C activity.

Both protein kinase C activation and the hydrolysis of cell-membrane phospholipids are crucial for signal transduction that leads to T cell proliferation and many functions. But both are reduced by iron deficiency. The altered protein kinase C activation and hydrolysis of cell-membrane phospholipids may lead to impaired immune responses in iron-deficient humans and laboratory animals.

Similarly, iron overload has detrimental effects on cell-mediated and non-specific immunity. Therefore, iron deficiency and iron overload affect susceptibility to certain types of infections.

### Isoflavones and Flavonoids

Isoflavones are structural isomers of the flavonoids. Isoflavones are primarily present as glycosides, genistin, daidzin and glycetin. Isoflavones exhibit antioxidant property both *in vivo* and *in vitro*. Isoflavones are found in soybeans.

### Phenolics

Phenolic compounds contain aromatic rings with hydroxyl groups; polyphenolics have more than one hydroxyl group. These phenolic groups function as antioxidants by providing hydrogen to reduce oxidants. Vitamin E functions via its labile phenolic group on position 6 (Fig. 3.9), as an anti-oxidant. An example of a phenolic antioxidant is resveratrol (Fig. 3.10). It occurs in grape skins and is the substance responsible for the healthful effects of red wine.

Many fruits and berries are good sources of antioxidants due to their flavonoid and polyphenol contents. Plums are a good

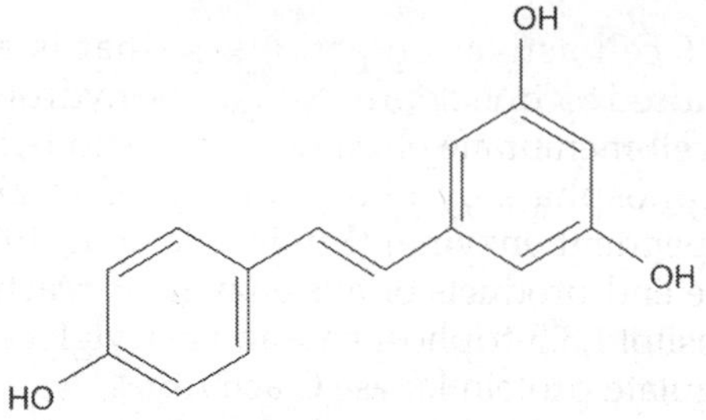

**Fig. 3.10:** Resveratrol

source. The addition of plum juice concentrates to meat products aids in their preservation by reducing lipid peroxidation and off-flavour.

The extensive conjugated P electron systems of phenolics allow ready donation of electron or H atoms from hydroxyl moieties to free radicals. In particular, polyphenols (mainly flavanols such as catechin, epigallocatechin, etc.) in tea may have important functions as nutritional antioxidant. Epidemiological studies in humans have shown that tea consumption is inversely related to the risk of strokes, chronic heart diseases, certain cancers and liver disorders. **Green tea polyphenols** have also been suggested to have protective role in cardiovascular diseases. Many herbs also possess antioxidant activity because of a high phenolic content. Polyphenols are widespread constituents of fruits, vegetables, cereals, dry legumes, chocolate, and beverages, such as tea, coffee or wine.

*Alpha Lipoic Acid (ALA)*

Alpha lipoic acid is a naturally occurring potent antioxidant. A major property of ALA is that it can serve as a pro-glutathione agent and enhance the cellular glutathione level. Both lipoate and dihydrolipoate have remarkable ROS detoxifying properties and scavenge hydroxyl radical, hydrogen peroxide and singlet oxygen. Also it can chelate metal ions. Lipoate also suppresses TNF-$\alpha$, induced activation of NFкB. It is also reported to protect vitamin E. Lipoic acid has been suggested to be beneficial in diabetes and heart diseases. See page 94 for more information on ALA.

*Curcumin*

*Curcuma longa* is a polyphenol derived from dietary spice turmeric. It possesses diverse anti-inflammatory and anticancer properties following oral or topical administration. Curcumin has potent antioxidant and free radical-removing properties which prevent DNA damage. Also see later page 112 for details on curcumin. **Garlic** and **onion** have also been used in research and suggested to be protective in gastrointestinal cancers.

**Antioxidant Foods**

Vitamins E and C, carotenoids and polyphenols from plant sources are examples of naturally occurring antioxidants. The phenolic group has antioxidant property. Plant parts rich in antioxidants are usually bright coloured. Fruit-eating birds, humans and other primates have well-developed colour vision, which aids in selection of an antioxidant-rich diet. Carnivores, which do not rely directly on plants for antioxidants, have poor colour vision (Benzie, 2003).

Yellow or orange vegetables and fruits, green leafy vegetables, eggs, cereals and pulses are the principal sources of antioxidants and micronutrients (Table 3.3). These should form good part of the diet to diminish the effects of oxidative damage caused by the free radicals that are formed inside the cells during the course of normal metabolism as well as those formed due to the polluting environment.

A high intake of fresh fruit, root vegetables and fruiting vegetables has been shown to be associated with reduced mortality, probably as a result of their high content of vitamin C, provitamin A carotenoids and lycopene.

**RANCIDITY OF DIETARY FAT –LIPID PEROXIDATION**

The unpleasant odour and taste that fats may develop on ageing are due to hydrolysis of the glycerides into free fatty acids and glycerol or to oxidation of unsaturated fatty acids in oils. Unsaturated bonds in lipid molecules are the prime targets of free radicals. Rancid fats

| Table 3.3: Dietary sources of antioxidant vitamins | |
| --- | --- |
| Vitamin C | Citrus fruits, blackcurrants, kiwi fruit, strawberries<br>Red peppers, broccoli, Brussels sprouts |
| Vitamin E | Whole grains, vegetable oils, wheat germ, eggs |
| Carotenoids | |
| β-carotene | Carrots, broccoli, watercress, spinach, apricots |
| Lycopene | Tomatoes and processed tomato products (sauce and paste) |
| Lutein | Peas, spinach, broccoli and dark green leafty vegetables |
| β-cryptoxanthin | Mandarins, apricots, orange peppers |

deplete the body's vitamin E, vitamin C and beta-carotene, the antioxidants.

## Rancidity is of Three Types

1. **Hydrolytic rancidity:** Hydrolytic rancidity occurs when fats containing short-chain fatty acids, such as butyric or caproic, are hydrolysed, releasing these malodourous fatty acids. The edible fat may frequently be rendered completely unacceptable to the consumer. The enzymes, lipases are mostly derived from bacteria and moulds.

2. **Oxidative rancidity:** Oxidative rancidity is the more important form of rancidity. The unsaturated fatty acids readily undergo oxidation. The products of oxidation include shorter chain fatty acids, fatty acid polymers, aldehydes, ketones, epoxides and hydrocarbons. The acids and aldehydes are major contributors to the smells and flavours associated with oxidised fat and significantly reduce its palatability. This autocatalytic reaction process is explained under lipid peroxidation.

3. **Oxidation of saturated fatty acids:** Oxidation of saturated fatty acids results in the development of sweet, heavy taste and smell due to the formation of methyl-ketones, as in the production of various cheeses. This is known as **ketonic rancidity.**

Highly refined fats begin to absorb oxygen immediately upon exposure to it. Natural fats, however, may vary considerably in this induction period before oxidation begins. Certain unsaturated fats are quite resistant. This resistance is due to the presence of antioxidants such as phenols, quinones, tocopherols, gallic acid and gallates. Many vegetable oils have these natural antioxidants, whereas, ordinarily animal fats do not.

## Lipid Peroxidation

Peroxidation (auto-oxidation) of lipids exposed to oxygen is an important factor in the deterioration of fat-containing feeds and also for damage to tissues *in vivo*. This damage to tissues may be important as a cause of cancer, inflammatory diseases, athero-sclerosis and ageing. Lipophillic molecules, like polyunsaturated fatty acids (PUFA), are very liable to oxidation by superoxide radicals to form the corresponding peroxides in a process called lipid peroxidation. The deleterious effects of lipid peroxidation are due to free radicals generated during peroxide formation from PUFAs. Prolonged or repeated heating of PUFAs also produce peroxides, free radicals, etc. **Lipid peroxidation occurs in three phases: initiation, propagation and termination.**

• Initiation begins with a fatty acid reacting with a metal (e.g. iron) or an existing free radical. Hydroperoxide (ROO•), RO• and OH• are the free radicals formed, R being the hydrocarbon portion of a fatty acid.

• Propagation involves reaction of the free radicals with oxygen to produce more free radicals.

• Termination is through antioxidants. Antioxidants either reduce the rate of initiation (e.g. catalase, peroxidases) or interfere with chain propagation. Hence, now it is clear that lipid peroxidation is prevented by natural or synthetic antioxidants.

Peroxidation is a non-enzymatic process initiated by free radicals, which are formed in the course of normal metabolism in the presence of trace metals (e.g. iron, copper) or by ionising radiation. That is why they are prooxidants.

Once initiated by free radicals, lipid peroxidation is autocatalytic. These prooxidants are produced during the processing of a fat and the presence of optimum heat, light and moisture greatly accelerate the oxidative process. PUFA are of the methylene-interrupted type, i.e. a $CH_2$ group exists between the two double bonds. Any of the free radicals like the peroxy, alkoxy or hydroxyl radical can propagate the reaction either by abstracting H from methylene carbon or by reacting with oxygen to produce more radicals. The double bond shifts to the conjugated form and the free radical can then unite with oxygen to a form a peroxide and then with hydrogen to form a hydroperoxide. The hydroperoxides can polymerise with other hydroperoxides to form a film as in the drying of linseed oil paint. It can also breakdown into aldehydes and ketones which are odourous.

$-CH_2-CH=CH-CH2-CH=CH$  Methylene-interrupted double bond

$\downarrow$ H• Free radical

$-CH_2-CH=CH-C•H-CH=CH$

$\downarrow$

$-C•-CH=CH-CH=CH$  Conjugated form of double bond

$\downarrow$ O + H•

$-CH-CH=CH-CH=CH$

|

OOH (Hydroperoxide)

**Autoooxidation of methylene-interrupted unsaturated fatty acid**

Fatty acid peroxides are very unstable. They disintegrate rapidly into fragments, leading to loss of fatty acids from membrane lipids and damage the biological membrane. Free radical damage may denature the proteins. In addition, certain degradation products of PUFA peroxides can react with biomolecules.

**Lipid peroxidation is prevented by antioxidants:** Lipid peroxidation causes extensive damage to biomembranes. Lipid peroxidation in mitochondria would lead to uncoupling of oxidative phosphorylation since enzymes involved in the energy production are associated with mitochondrial membrane. The lipid peroxidation reaction can be stopped if antioxidants are present which promptly replace the H once it has been abstracted.

## ANTIOXIDANT FEED SUPPLEMENTS

### Dietary Supplementation of Oregano in Broiler Chickens

Intensive farming of broilers involves stressful conditions that reduce animal welfare, quality of chicken meat and performance. Dietary supplementation of plant extracts improves performance and meat quality. Oregano *(Origanum vulgare L.)* is known for its antimicrobial, antifungal, insecticidal and antioxidant properties.

Sabino et al (2018) studied the effect of oregano aqueous extract-supplemented diet on gene expression in broiler chickens. Whole liver transcriptome of 10 birds fed with a supplemented diet versus 10 control birds was analysed using the RNASeq technique. One hundred and twenty-nine genes were differentially expressed with an absolute log fold change > 1. RNA-Seq analysis revealed that oregano modulated liver transcriptome expression. The analysis revealed a massive downregulation of genes involved in fatty acid metabolism and insulin signalling pathways in broilers fed with the oregano aqueous extract supplementation.

Down-regulated genes could be associated to chicken lean line, suggesting the potential beneficial effect of oregano supplementation in reducing both abdominal and visceral fat deposition. Downregulation of insulin signalling pathway related genes suggest that dietary oregano supplementation might be adoption in obesity and diabetes conditions.

## Dietary Supplementation of Bamboo Vinegar in Pigs

Bamboo vinegar is a natural liquid manufactured from bamboo. Bamboo vinegar powder (BVP) has been regarded as a potential alternative to antibiotic growth promoter in animal production. Yu et al. (2017) evaluated the effects and mechanism of bamboo vinegar powder (BVP) supplementation at 0.5 to 1.5% level on the antioxidant ability of pigs.

Bamboo vinegar powder supplementation improved the antioxidant ability of the liver in finishing pigs by increasing the activity of some antioxidant enzymes and decreasing the activity of oxidative stress enzymes. BVP supplementation could change the gene expression of antioxidant and oxidative stress enzymes. The improved antioxidant ability of both liver and blood may be due to the activation of the Nuclear related factor 2 (Nrf2)-Are pathway.

With the BVP-supplemented diets, the activities of glutathione peroxidase (GSH-Px) and superoxide dismutase (SOD) in the blood increased, the activities of GSH-Px and catalase in the liver also increased, the activity of total antioxidant capacity (T-AOC) increased both in the liver and blood, but the activity of iNOS in the liver and blood decreased ($P$ <0.05). Moreover, the gene expressions of nuclear related factor 2 (Nrf2), catalytic subunit of glutamate-cysteine ligase (GCLC), NAD(P)H quinone dehydrogenase 1(NQO1), haeme oxygenase 1(HO1), Glutathione peroxidase (GSH-Px) and catalase in the liver were also increased due to the addition of BVP ($P$ < 0.05).

## Alpha-lipoic Acid: An Invaluable Feed Supplement

Alpha-lipoic acid (1,2-dithiolane-3-pentanoic acid; ALA) is an integral component of mitochondria that can regulate energy metabolism. It has been reported that α-lipoic acid (Fig. 3.11) can scavenge free radicals, replenish endogenous antioxidants as well as act as a coenzyme in carbohydrate

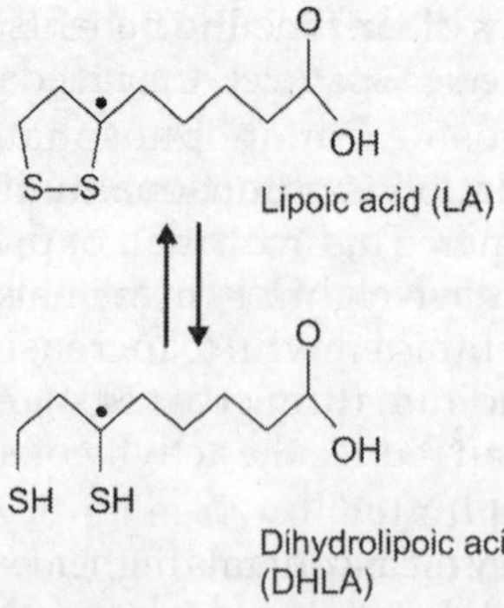

Fig. 3.11: Structure of alpha-lipoic acid and dihydrolipoic acid

metabolism in the chicken birds (Packer et al, 2001). Alpha-lipoic acid is both fat and water soluble and therefore, can easily be absorbed and transported across cell membranes resulting in optimal nutrient availability (Kofuji et al, 2008).

## Alpha Lipoic Acid is an Inimitable Feed Supplement

1. Alpha-lipoic acid can exist in both oxidised as well as reduced form. Between the two, the reduced form, dihydrolipoic acid (DHLA) is a potent antioxidant and its dietary supplementation under normal glucose level facilitates mobilisation of fatty acid as per β-adrenergic response to isoproterenol (Moini et al, 2002).

2. Alpha-lipoic acid is naturally occurring dithiol synthesised from octanoic acid in mitochondria and involved as cofactor using α-keto acid dehydrogenases in mitochondrial reactions.

3. Alpha-lipoic acid and DHLA quench reactive oxidative species as well as other radicals generated through the oxidation of different substrates mainly lipids and proteins in lipophilic and hydrophilic domains.

4. Alpha-lipoic acid has the capability to be absorbed in intestine and can also cross the blood–brain barrier. It can also impart hypotriglyceridemic and hypoglycemic properties in chicken birds along with

variety of therapeutic benefits (Gonzalez-Perez and Gonzalez-Castaneda, 2006).

5. Adenosine 5-monophosphate activates protein kinase functionality in the hypothalamus. This activation of protein kinase results in weight loss in animals by limiting feed intake, while increasing energy expenditure (Kim et al, 2004). Alpha-lipoic acid can reduce the activity of adenosine 5-monophosphate.

6. Poultry meat contains higher level of PUFA in relation to other meats thereby making it more prone for oxidation. Dietary supplementation of ALA is a pragmatic strategy to enhance the oxidative stability of poultry meat and meat-based products (Shen and Du 2005). Its supplementation has a protective role as a feed supplement in poultry nutrition. It has been reported in humans that ALA administration increased serum superoxide dismutase activity and diminished malonaldehydes generation with age-related macular degeneration (Sun et al, 2012).

## Mechanism of Action of Alpha-lipoic Acid

Alpha-lipoic acid is considered as a metabolic antioxidant in two ways:

1. It is involved in oxidative metabolism as lipoamide and as an essential cofactor for mitochondrial $\alpha$-keto acid dehydrogenase complexes. It is considered essential for normal oxidative metabolism. However, exogenous $\alpha$-lipoic acid is rapidly taken up by cells and is converted to dihydrolipoate (Mackenzie et al, 2006) as shown in Fig. 3.12. The reducing power of ALA comes from NADH that also modulates NADH/NAD, and NADPH/NADP ratios thereby affecting cell metabolism. It is involved in cell metabolism by acting as antioxidant to retard mitochondrial dysfunction.

2. It is a crucial mitochondrial cofactor for neurodegeneration carried out by changing calcium homeostasis (Diaz-cruz et al, 2003). The mechanism of action revealed that alpha-lipoic acid is exogenously provided and is readily uptaken by a variety of cells and tissues that ALA is rapidly reduced by NADH- or NADPH-dependent enzymes to DHLA. Additionally, as an antioxidant, it is a potent scavenger of ROS like hydroxy radicals, hypochlorous acid and singlet oxygen, but not superoxide or peroxyl radicals (Packer et al, 1997). Moreover, this antioxidant can

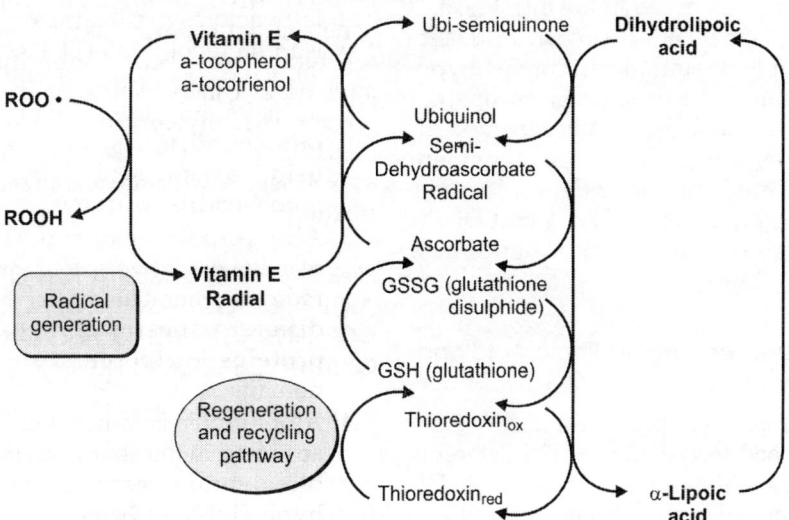

**Dihydrolipoate reduces (recycles) the major cell antioxidants-vitamins C & E, glutathione thioredoxin and ubiquinol**

**Fig. 3.12:** Pathways by which dihydrolipoate recycles vitamin E and other antioxidants

effectively clear the hydroxyl, peroxyl and superoxide radicals as well as enhance the antioxidant enzymes like glutathione peroxidase, catalase and superoxide dismutase, etc. concentrations by providing reducing substrate and regenerating them to reduce free radicals to promote the lipid stability in birds and meat products (Srilatha et al, 2010).

In mitochondria, the reduction of α-lipoic acid to DHLA takes place with the help of α-keto acid dehydrogenase complexes. However, DHLA is mainly found at oxidant production site. Moreover, mitochondria are considered vital for neurodegeneration mechanism because of its involvement in calcium homeostasis. Gonzalez-Perez (2011) also documented that during indo-1-loaded T cells in a flow-cytometric system, the provision of α-lipoic acid partially protected against oxidant-induced perturbation of intracellular calcium homeostasis that also imparts beneficial effects in neurodegenerative disorders.

Moreover, DHLA can also reduce glutathione disulphide, dehydroascorbate and semidehydroascorbyl radical and ubiquinone resulting in the regeneration of vitamin E from its radical oxidised form and to reduce thioredoxin (Fig. 3.12). Alpha-lipoic acid has the ability to be absorbed in the intestine and also can cross the blood–brain barrier. Therefore, its supplementation can impart hypotriglyceridemic and hypoglycemic properties in chicken birds along with other therapeutic benefits including stress management (Gonzalez-Perez and Gonzalez-Castaneda, 2006). However, the *in vivo* ALA and DHLA concentration remain indecisive until now (Sohaib et al, 2018).

## Synergism between Alpha-lipoic Acid and Alpha-tocopherol

The provision of α-lipoic acid and α-tocopherol enriched feed enhances lipid stability of broiler microsomal fraction of meat. The correlation between antioxidant activity and total phenolics indicated the antioxidant potential of these antioxidants. The α-lipoic acid and vitamin E are considered as potent nutritional antioxidants for poultry birds because α-lipoic acid helps to recycle vitamin E (Fig. 3.12).

The decline in lipid peroxidation and oxidative storability in meat can be achieved through providing dietary antioxidants to birds. The supplementation of α-lipoic acid to birds also increased total phenolics as well as α-lipoic acid content of the thigh and breast meat without affecting the protein level. It is also revealed from thiobarbituric acid reactive substances (TBARS) and DPPH analysis that provision of α-lipoic acid and α-tocopherol to birds also increased antioxidant potential of meat (Yasin et al, 2012).

Alpha-lipoic acid is a multifunction antioxidant that is produced in small amount by the cells along with its dietary supplementation facilitates fatty acid mobilisation, energy expenditure and can scavenge free radicals in poultry birds. It exists in oxidised as well as reduced form.

Alpha-lipoic acid has growth promoting, anti-inflammatory, antioxidative, immunostimulatory, and hypocholesterolemic properties when fed as dietary supplement to farm animals particularly chicken birds.

It can be concluded that α-lipoic acid as a feed additive/supplement imparts some beneficial antioxidative as well as hypocholesterolemic prospects. Alpha-lipoic acid as antioxidant can be accumulated in tissues and organs thereby, protect fresh meat from oxidation and increases antioxidant potential as well as oxidative stability of meat and meat fractions.

## EFFECT OF SUPPLEMENTATION OF ANTIOXIDANTS INDIVIDUALLY OR IN COMBINATION WITH OTHERS ON THE OXIDATIVE STATUS IN BROILERS

### Supplementation of n-3 PUFA: Pros and cons

Broiler chickens demand a high-energy concentration in their feed (3200 kcal/kg ME in finisher feed; ICAR, 2013), which is achieved through supplementation of feeds with various fats and oils. Moreover, there is an increasing demand for 'functional foods', in which supplementation with n-3 polyunsaturated fatty acids (PUFA)-rich plant oils is becoming an accepted practice to ensure a favourable fatty acid composition of meat. However, it is often overlooked that n-3 PUFA are very susceptible to oxidation.

Studies have shown that a high dietary n-3 PUFA inclusion affects the oxidative status of broilers and can cause a pronounced oxidative stress (Estevez, 2015). The oxidative stress is also due to an enlarged production of reactive oxygen species (ROS) *in vivo* (Gladine et al, 2007). Supplementation with n-3 PUFA oils can cause an imbalance between reductants and oxidants *in vivo* and consequently induce damage to different macromolecules such as DNA, proteins and lipids, which can lead to impaired activity, apoptosis and necrosis of different cells. Additionally, a high dietary intake of n-3 PUFA led to enhanced levels of them in meat and tissues, thereby increasing the susceptibility of the animal products to oxidative deterioration because of higher malondialdehyde (MDA) (Estevez, 2015).

## Exposure to High Temperature

High environmental temperatures also have been reported as one of the most important causes of oxidative stress for a long-time (Gursu et al, 2004; Akbarian et al, 2016).

## Dire need of Antioxidant Supplementation

Broilers exposed to a stressful environment, e.g. high temperatures or increased dietary n-3 PUFA, have higher demands for dietary antioxidants as protection from oxidative stress. Creating n-3 PUFA-enriched products requires additional antioxidants in the feed due to oxidative stress (Leeson and Summers, 2001). Even though poultry can endogenously synthesize vitamin C, it was shown that under heat stress, dietary supplementation with vitamin C could alleviate the oxidative stress (Leeson and Summers, 2001). This suggested that the endogenous synthesis of vitamin C may not be sufficient in all stress conditions.

## Synergism Among Vitamins C and E and Selenium

As it has been known for a long-time, vitamins E and C and selenium have important roles in the antioxidative defence network and can work efficiently only in synergism. Vitamin E inhibits free radical-mediated lipid peroxidation, but is oxidised and depleted fast, if not regenerated by vitamin C. The antioxidant activity of vitamin C is restored by selenium-containing enzymes.

## Individual Versus Combination of Antioxidants Supplementation

1. Cinar et al (2014) showed that dietary supplementation with a combination of vitamins E and C resulted in better protection in copper-induced oxidative stress than the individual supplementation at the same level.
2. Sahin et al (2002) obtained similar results in hens reared at a high ambient temperature, as a combination of vitamins E and C lowered serum MDA to a greater extent than supplementing these vitamins separately.
3. Lower concentrations of MDA in the serum, liver, heart and kidney were also found in Japanese quails under heat stress when fed a combination of vitamin C and folic acid than when supplementing them individually (Sahin et al, 2003b).
4. Harsini et al. (2012) showed that the combination of selenium and vitamin E was more effective in antioxidative protection in broilers under heat stress than their individual use.
5. Similarly, Skrivan et al (2012) showed that a combination of vitamin C and selenium lowered TBARS in broilers fed a PUFA diet more than the supplementation of only selenium.

Leskovec et al (2018) conducted a trial to investigate whether the combined supplementation of vitamin E, vitamin C and selenium was superior to their sole supplementation concerning the oxidative stress induced by a high n-3 dietary PUFA intake in broiler chickens. Analyses of malondial-dehyde (MDA), vitamin C, and $\alpha$- and $\gamma$-tocopherols in plasma, antioxidant capacity of water (ACW) and lipid (ACL) soluble compounds in serum and glutathione peroxidase (GSH-Px) and superoxide dismutase (SOD) activities in whole blood were performed.

The inclusion of high amounts of $\alpha$-tocopherol in diets led to high concentration of $\alpha$-tocopherol in plasma and breast muscle. Lower plasma and breast muscle MDA concentrations were detected in comparison to the control group, since $\alpha$-tocopherol protects lipids from oxidation.

The results indicated that vitamin E is the most effective antioxidant to alleviate oxidative stress caused by high dietary PUFA and that the supplementation with additional vitamin C and selenium did not have clear synergistic effect. However, further studies are warranted to get clarity on the issue (Leskovec et al, 2018).

## PROOXIDANTS AND ANTIOXIDANTS—THEIR BALANCE IN THE INTESTINE: A HEALTHY GUT IS A PREREQUISITE TO A SOUND GENERAL HEALTH

In commercial animal production a range of various stresses are responsible for economical losses due to decreased productive and reproductive performance of animals. It has been proven that at the molecular level nutritional, technological, environmental and internal/biological stresses are associated with overproduction of free radicals (prooxidants), disturbances of redox balance and oxidative stress (Surai and Fisinin, 2016a; b).

A delicate balance between antioxidants (antioxidant enzymes, glutathione, synthetic antioxidants and dietary antioxidant nutrients) and prooxidants in body cells is an important determinant of various physiological processes. An integrated antioxidant system is built in the animal body with the sole purpose of maintenance of this balance. This system was developed during evolution to provide an antioxidant defence and give a chance for animals to survive in the oxygenated atmosphere. Recent data suggest

that the antioxidant-prooxidant balance starts in the intestine. Relationship between food and human health has attracted attention of scientists for many years. Various antioxidants of fruits and vegetables are widely accepted to be responsible for prevention of oxidative damage in the gastrointestinal tract (GIT). Indeed, antioxidant-prooxidant balance in the digestive tract is considered to be a major determinant of human and animal health (Surai et al, 2003; 2004).

### Antioxidant—Prooxidant Balance

Antioxidant enzymes and glutathione can be synthesised in the body and diet is the major provider of antioxidant nutrients that possess antioxidant properties or facilitate synthesis of antioxidant enzymes. When food is consumed and reaches the stomach and then the small intestine, it contains a range of antioxidants but may also contain a range of potentially dangerous substances (prooxidants) (Fig. 3.13). Thus diet plays a crucial role in the very important task of maintaining a fine balance between antioxidants and prooxidants in the intestine (Surai et al, 2003).

### Prooxidants in the GIT

*Generation of Oxidised Lipids*

It is known that free radicals are produced as a natural consequence of the normal metabolic activity and as part of the immune system's strategy for destroying invading microorganisms. Surai (2006) reported the impact of free radicals on cellular metabolism due to their participation in lipid peroxidation reactions. It is clear from the published data that lipid peroxidation in food is an important source of toxic products and a potential source of free radicals in the digestive tract.

It is generally accepted that low-level oxidation of lipids in meat and milk during storage and processing is practically unavoidable. In fact, lipid stability in meat and meat products depends on many factors. They include species, muscle type, the amount and type of fat in the diet, the nutritional status of

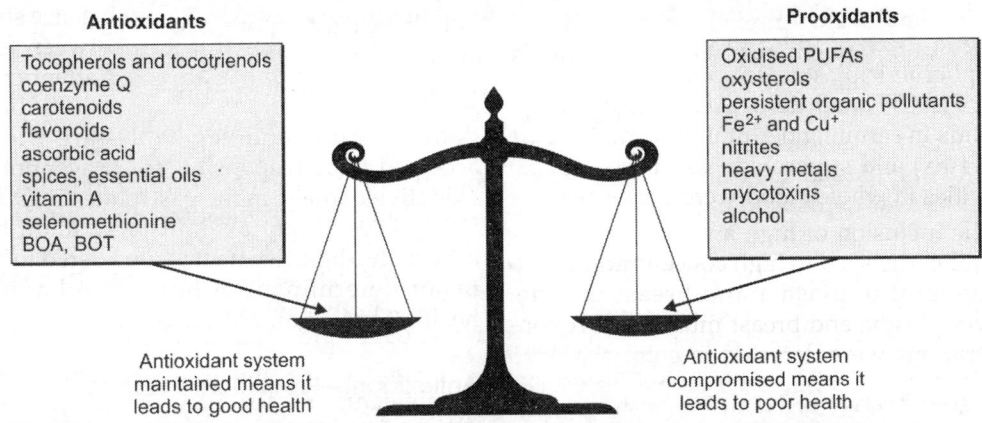

**Fig. 3.13:** Antioxidant-prooxidant balance in the intestine (*Adapted from* Surai et al, *2003*)

the animal at slaughter, the presence or absence of disease or infection and the type of processing to which the meat is subjected. Fish and fish oil are especially susceptible to peroxidation due to presence of highly unsaturated docosahexaenoic (DHA, 22:6n-3), docosapentaenoic (DPA, 22:5n-3) and eicosapentaenoic (EPA, 20:5n-3) fatty acids.

The primary products of lipid peroxidation are lipid hydroperoxides (LOOH). LOOH are not stable and can decompose (in the presence of transition metal ions) to produce new free radicals and cytotoxic aldehydes that contribute to the flavour deterioration of foods and biological oxidation and can cause oxidative stress. Lipid peroxidation is associated with the formation of a wide range of secondary aldehyde products such as n-alkenals, trans-2-alkenals, 4-hydroxy-trans-2-alkenals, 4-hydroxy nonenal (4-HNE) and melondialdehyde (MDA). Among them, MDA appears to be the most mutagenic product of lipid peroxidation, whereas 4-HNE is the most toxic one (Ayala et al, 2014). In fact most of the oxidised lipids in foods come from fats and oils heated at high temperature in particular from frying fats (Dobarganes and Marquez Ruiz, 2003).

**Effect of oxidised lipids:** Oxidised lipids are partly absorbed in the digestive tract and incorporated into membrane phospholipids altering their structure and properties (Hayam et al, 1994). The consumption of oxidised fats is associated with diarrhoea, liver enlargement, growth depression and histological changes in tissues of experimental animals.

In animal models, it has been shown that oxidised lipids in the diet can suppress growth (Lin et al, 1989), reduce vitamin E level in tissues increasing their susceptibility to lipid peroxidation (Sheehy et al, 1994), increase tissue protein oxidation (Hayam et al, 1997) and increase the number of aberrant crypts in the intestine (Yang et al, 1998). The gastrointestinal epithelium of swine and chickens responded to this oxidant stress by increased enterocyte turnover and the gut associated immune system is compromised (Dibner et al, 1996).

Toxic and mutagenic 4-HNE and MDA can damage the proteins and phospholipids by covalent bonding and cross-linking. Indeed, 4-HNE is highly reactive toward nucleophilic thiol and amino groups and could form covalent adducts with various cellular macromolecules, including lipids, proteins and nucleic acids. This leads to various detrimental consequences of cellular structure and metabolism, including inhibition of protein and DNA synthesis, dysregulation of enzyme activities, alteration in mitochondrial coupling (Hu et al, 2017). Therefore, major systems of the animal body are affected due to lipid peroxidation.

Acrylamides are formed in food products - chiefly in potato chips, potato fries, cereals and bread. It has been reported that acrylamide caused an increase in lipid peroxidation and decrease in glutathione contents and activity of glutathione S-transferase in the rat liver in a dose dependent manner.

## Cholesterol Oxidation Products

Cholesterol oxidation products (oxysterols) are commonly found in foods of animal origin and they are formed during food processing, storage and cooking. Examples: fresh egg yolk contains negligible levels of cholesterol oxide, while spray-dried egg yolk powder is a rich source of cholesterol oxides. Similarly, fresh meat is almost free of cholesterol oxides but cooked meat products are considered to be a substantial source of cholesterol oxides in the diet. Therefore, cholesterol oxides can be found in the diet and they are cytotoxic and potentially can be involved in lipid peroxidation in the intestine.

Recent findings suggest that oxysterols may modulate cytotoxicity by inducing apoptosis with consequential oxidative stress. Oxysterols can also replace cholesterol in membranes, perturbing permeability, stability and other membrane properties (Guardiola et al, 1996), which are extremely important in relation to enterocyte membranes in the intestine.

## Iron Ions are Involved in Free Radical Generation

Muscle tissue is rich source of iron bound to proteins in the form of myoglobin. Meat can also contain some haemoglobin residues from residual blood and iron-containing cytochromes. The main problem with iron nutrition is its reactivity and possible involvement in free radical generation. Iron ions are considered to catalyse the formation of the hydroxyl radical and accelerate the decomposition of lipid hydroperoxides (Davies and Slater, 1987) and to stimulate lipid peroxidation (Minotti and Aust, 1987). Numerous compounds, including haeme and nonhaeme

iron, have been reported to act as catalysts of lipid oxidation in food system.

The iron content of plant foods is dismally low. Milk is a poor source of iron. Anaemia is rampant in the vulnerable group of human population. Hence food fortification has been advocated. Iron fortification of various foods could represent another source of potentially dangerous free iron in the digestive tract. Therefore, iron supplements could also be involved in lipid peroxidation in the intestine.

It is necessary to mention that other mineral supplements can also be involved in stimulation of lipid peroxidation in the intestine. Surai (2002) reported that selenite can generate free radicals when present in combination with reduced glutathione. Iron can also interact with other nutrients stimulating free radical production. For example, it has been shown that iron in combination with the secondary bile acids (lithocholic and deoxycholic acids) and the vitamin K group can generate free radicals.

Clearly meats and meat-containing products are an important source of free iron which can be involved in generation of free radicals and lipid peroxidation in the digestive tract. These are additional to iron fortified-foods and iron supplements, which represent another possible source of iron in the GIT.

## Nitrate, Nitrite and Peroxynitrite

Nitrate and nitrite are added to the food as preservatives. Vegetables (e.g. lettuce, potato, etc.) and drinking water comprise a major source of nitrates. Therefore, humans and animals are subjected to significant nitrate and nitrite levels in foods and water, as well as those formed *in vivo*.

Nitrites and nitrates are formed from nitrogenous sources by microorganisms in saliva and intestine. These are considered to be the major source of human exposure under physiological conditions. It is generally accepted that nitrate is concentrated in the saliva and rapidly converted to nitrite by facultative anaerobic bacteria. It was shown that nitrite could be converted to nitric oxide (NO) under the highly acidic conditions (pH 3) that occur in the lumen of the stomach. This NO can be a source of another reactive free radical peroxynitrite (ONOO⁻), which is 1000 times more oxidising than $H_2O_2$ and has half-life in solution about 1–2 seconds (Van Dyke, 1997). It is well-accepted that peroxynitrite is a potent cytotoxic agent (Squadrito and Pryor, 1998).

Peroxynitrite can also affect antioxidant system by changing activities of antioxidant enzymes. In fact peroxynitrite has been shown to inhibit the activities of catalase, GSH-Px and promote lipid peroxidation. Moreover, it appears that ONOO⁻ can oxidise a variety of essential molecules (e.g. sulfhydryls, thiols, ascorbate, proteins, DNA) and trigger injurious processes, including lipid peroxidation. On the other hand, peroxynitrite may be decomposed forming highly reactive hydroxyl radical and nitrogen dioxide. The amount of nitrates and nitrites in the diet in combination with other prooxidants in the digesta can be involved in free radical formation and lipid peroxidation.

**Cadmium** depletes reduced glutathione (GSH) and protein-bound sulfhydryl groups, resulting in enhanced production of reactive oxygen species such as superoxide, hydroxyl radicals, and hydrogen peroxide (Stohs et al, 2001). The ROS production is associated with lipid peroxidation, enhanced excretion of urinary lipid metabolites, modulation of intracellular oxidised states, DNA damage, membrane damage, altered gene expression, and apoptosis. On the other hand, GSH and α-tocopherol offer significant protection against cadmium toxicity in rats by diminishing oxidative stress via raising GSH concentration and reducing lipid peroxidation.

It is believed that **lead** can alter certain membrane bound enzymes and may cause oxidative stress. **Mercury** is also a strong prooxidant able to increase lipid peroxidation and decrease GSH content in liver of Swiss albino mice. Heavy metal concentrations in major food sources are quite low, but data from nutritional supplements is disturbing. In combination with other prooxidants, heavy metals can potentially be involved in generation of free radicals and cause oxidative stress in the GIT.

### Persistent Organic Pollutants

Persistent organic pollutants (POPs) comprise a class of chemicals that are among the most insidiously dangerous compounds and it includes many organochlorine pesticides. Examples of persistent organic pollutants found in foods include dioxins, polychlorinated biphenyls (PCBs), polybrominated diphenyl ethers and some pesticide chemicals. Six seasonal vegetables (60 samples) were monitored during 1996–1997 in India to determine the magnitude of pesticidal contamination by insecticide residues representing four major chemical groups, i.e. organochlorine, organophosphorus, synthetic pyrethroid and carbamate. The tested samples showed 100% contamination with low but measurable amounts of residues (Kumari et al, 2002). Organochlorines can cause oxidative stress.

*Dieldrin* exposure caused depolarisation of mitochondrial membrane in a dose-dependent manner, stimulated generation of ROS and significantly increased lipid peroxidation. Unlike oxidised glutathione, the content of total glutathione declined significantly after exposure to cyclodiene insecticides. Membrane leakage and peroxide production were significantly enhanced by the pesticides. Furthermore, this dieldrin-induced oxidative stress could be associated with modulation of gene expression.

The results of Hassoun et al. (1993) demonstrated that the four structurally dissimilar polyhalogenated hydrocarbons (lindane, DDT, chlordane and endrin) could produce oxidative stress in rats with significant increases in hepatic lipid peroxidation and DNA damage. Therefore persistent organic pollutants represent an important health hazard for humans and animals and they also can be involved in promotion of lipid peroxidation in the GIT.

## Mycotoxins

In general, main mycotoxin contaminants of the food including aflatoxin $B_1$, fumonisins, $T_2$ toxin, DON, zearalenone and ochratoxin are shown to compromise antioxidant system and stimulate lipid peroxidation *in vivo* and *in vitro* (Surai, 2002). Mycotoxins are considered to be unavoidable contaminants of the most food and feed ingredients and they are potent prooxidants. Therefore even in comparatively low concentrations (lower than officially allowed limits) they still represent an important source of free radical generation in the GIT.

## Alcohol

Exposure of the intestinal mucosa to ethanol leads to morphological injuries and impairs the absorptive capacity creating an oxidative stress in the small intestine. During ethanol metabolism the antioxidant system is compromised, with reduced levels of vitamin E, selenium and GSH. Therefore, it has been suggested that the underlying mechanism of 'intestinal epithelial barrier dysfunction' induced by alcohol is due to oxidative injury to the cytoskeleton. Therefore, alcohol can be involved directly or indirectly in the free radical production and lipid peroxidation in the intestine. It seems likely that alcohol in combination with other prooxidants can be a source of free radicals in the GIT (Surai, 2006).

## Immune System of the Gut Could also be a Source of Free Radical Production in the Intestine

The gastrointestinal tract is considered to represent the largest immune organ of the animal body responding to the challenge of bacteria or food antigens by production of ROS (Halliwell et al, 2000). Intestinal epithelial cells secrete macrophage inflammatory protein 2 (MIP-2). It is a chemokine that attracts neutrophils and its secretion from intestinal epithelial cells is enhanced by inflammatory stimuli such as IL-1 and the production of MIP-2 by epithelial cells is responsible for increases leukocyte migration into the intestine. In particular, increased neutrophil migration into the intestine and activation of myeloperoxidase (MPO) are shown to be a result of induced inflammatory bowel disease-like colitis in transgenic mice. MPO is a haeme protein secreted by activated neutrophils, monocytes and some macrophages. Non-pathogenic, resident bacteria have a specific role in releasing butyrate, a normal bacterial metabolite. Thus, intestinal epithelial cells are directly involved in immune processes apart from their routine functions.

Further, in specific pathological conditions enterocytes could become a target of mucosal immune factors. The intestinal immune response to enteric antigens includes production of T helper-1-type cytokines that affects the gut epithelium in several ways. T cells produce macrophage migration inhibitory factor (MIF) that inhibits macrophage migration and has pleitropic activities on immune and inflammatory responses, cell growth and glucose metabolism. MIF is also produced by macrophages and endothelial cells. Human intestinal epithelial cells are reported to be a major source of MIF.

It has been also suggested that paracrine factors of intestinal epithelium increased the phagocytic capacity of intestinal monocytes/macrophages to be ready for immune and inflammatory responses. A characteristic feature of inflammation is the concomitant peroxidation of lipids and formation of bioactive lipid peroxidation products. It has been demonstrated that principal role for myeloperoxidase (MPO) is promotion of oxidant stress at sites of inflammation. It has been shown that this enzyme serves as a major enzymatic catalyst of lipid peroxidation by formation of NO-derived oxidants (Zhang et al, 2002). Thus intestinal immune system can generate free radicals in response to various antigens including microbes and some food allergens.

## The Gastrointestinal Tract (GIT) as a Major Site of Antioxidant Action

**Mucosal surfaces covered by the layer of epithelial cells** of GIT represent the most critical interface between the organism and its environment, since the mucosal interstitia of the intestine is continuously exposed to large amounts of dietary and microbial antigens. Therefore, epithelial cells engage in cross talk with luminal bacteria and their products and produce mediators and signals that are key components of host innate and acquired mucosal immunity (Maaser and Kagnoff, 2002).

The mucosal immune system is a first line of defence against foreign antigens, including microbial and dietary antigens. Under normal circumstances, it employs tightly regulated dynamic mucosal intra- and internets consisting of inductive (e.g. Peyer's patch) and effector (e.g. intestinal lamina propria) tissues and maintains an appropriate immunological homeostasis between the host and mucosal environments (Kiyono et al, 2001). Therefore, the mucosal immune system has evolved efficient mechanisms to distinguish potentially pathogenic from nonpathological antigens. However, loss of these mucosal defence mechanisms may alter immunological homeostasis in the gastrointestinal tract and induce pathological changes including chronic active inflammation, mucosal atrophy and tissue injuries (Nagura et al, 2001). It is important to stress that under inflammatory conditions in the intestine the maintenance of the epithelial barrier could be broken.

Diet is a potent mechanism for altering the environment of cells of most organs, particularly the gastrointestinal tract. Nutrient metabolism provides an essential stimulus for the induction, differentiation and maintenance of the mucosal immune system (Cunningham-Rundles, 2001). Therefore changes in diet, through the composition of the lumen environment, alter the expression of genes encoding for proteins that signal to the mucosal immune system (Sanderson and Naik, 2000). In fact **enterocytes act as immune cells** having receptors for bacterial products and expressing a variety of molecules on their surface responsible for interaction with immunocytes within the intestine (Sanderson, 2001).

It is necessary to stress that the nutrient requirements to maintain this kind of highly active immune system in the digestive tract could be quite high. In fact different sources of injury, such as nutritional, infectious or allergic, to the intestinal mucosa act via a common mechanism of cell-mediated immune damage. Nutrient repletion is required for restoration of immune function (Cunningham-Rundles, 2001). In particular, the immunomodulating properties of natural antioxidants (Surai, 2002) could be of great advantage for the intestinal immunity.

## Antioxidant Defences in the GIT

Diet provides a range of antioxidants necessary to balance the prooxidants in the intestine and to maintain a healthy gut. An effective antioxidant protection in the gastrointestinal tract is needed to maintain gut health and this protection is based on food derived antioxidants (Surai et al, 2004).

### Coenzyme Q (CoQ)

Coenzyme Q is the only fat-soluble antioxidant synthesised in the body. Coenzyme Q, also known as ubiquinone, has one quinone group and 10 isoprenyl units. Coenzyme $Q_{10}$ exists both in an oxidised and a reduced form, ubiquinone and ubiquinole, respectively. Therefore the ubiquinole/ubiquinone ratio is considered to be a sensitive marker of oxidative stress and an altered ubiquinole/ubiquinone ratio is the first sign of lipoprotein exposure to oxidative stress. Tissue CoQ originates from endogenous synthesis and from food. Meat and fish are the major sources of this compound. $CoQ_{10}$ is characterised by comparatively slow absorption in humans with blood values reaching a maximum after 6 h and this potentially slow absorption of CoQ could be an advantage for antioxidant protection in the GIT.

It is believed that exogenous CoQ, protects cells from oxidative stress by conversion into its reduced antioxidant form by cellular reductases. In particular cytosolic NADPH-CoQ reductase is responsible for cellular CoQ redox cycle as an endogenous antioxidant. Further, the selenoenzyme thioredoxin reductase is an important ubiquinone reductase and can explain how selenium and coenzyme Q, by combined action, may protect the cell from oxidative damage.

Since CoQ is an essential part of oxidative phosphorylation complex in mitochondria, the majority of endogenous CoQ is found in these organelles. However, exogenous CoQ is usually found in the extramitochondrial fractions including lysosomes and Golgi vesicles. $CoQ_{10}$ protects efficiently not only membrane phospholipids from peroxidation but also mitochondrial DNA and membrane proteins from free-radical-induced oxidative damage.

## L-Ascorbic Acid or Vitamin C

Vitamin C is a hydrophilic antioxidant functioning in an aqueous environment and possessing high free-radical-scavenging activity. It can participate in vitamin E recycling thus maintaining efficient antioxidant defence. Due to its high reducing potential, in combination with iron ions, vitamin C can be a prooxidant. However, it is believed that in physiological conditions and in the GIT, vitamin C performs mainly its antioxidant functions.

## Selenium

The main food sources of selenium are cereals, meat and fish. Selenomethionine represents the major natural form of selenium in feed and food ingredients. This compound itself is considered as an antioxidant apart from it being an important source of selenium for selenoprotein synthesis. Hence selenium has a special place in antioxidant defences in the GIT, it being an integral part of a range of selenoproteins expressed in the intestine.

Selenium and/or vitamin E pre-treatments ameliorated the disturbances in prooxidant-antioxidant balance in the GIT. This amelioration has been confirmed with histopathological findings.

## Selenium-dependent enzymes in antioxidant defence of GIT

*Glutathione:* Glutathione (GSH) is the most abundant non-protein thiol in mammalian cells. GSH is abundantly distributed in the mucosal cells of GIT in man and its highest concentration is found in the duodenum. It is considered to be an active antioxidant in biological systems providing cells with their reducing milieu. GSH thiolic group can react directly with $H_2O_2$, superoxide anion, hydroxyl radicals, alkoxyl radicals, hydroperoxides (Meister and Anderson, 1983). Therefore, a crucial role for GSH is as free radical scavenger, particularly effective against the hydroxyl radical, since there are no enzymatic defences against this species of radical. Usually decreased GSH concentration in tissues is associated with increased lipid peroxidation. Furthermore in stress conditions, GSH prevents the loss of protein thiols and vitamin E. It plays an important role as a key modulator of cell signalling. Animals and human are able to synthesise glutathione. Further, foods also provide GSH.

Food-derived antioxidant enzymes would be inactivated during thermal food processing. However, GIT contains internally-originated antioxidant enzymes SOD, GSH-Px and catalase and they represent an important mechanism of the enterocyte defence from oxidative damage. A specific gastrointestinal GSH-Px (GI-GSH-Px) has been described in 1993, which could be considered to be a barrier against hydroperoxide resorption (Brigelius-Flohe, 1999) and this enzyme should be considered as a major antioxidant defence in the intestine. Furthermore, in the gastrointestinal tract there are at least three more selenoproteins including plasma GSH-Px, selenoprotein P and thioredoxin reductase. In fact many other antioxidant compounds could improve antioxidant defence by up-regulating the expression of various GSH-Px in the gut.

Glutathione and glutathione-dependent enzymes contribute significantly towards intestinal antioxidant defences. Peroxide detoxification pathway in the intestine is based on the GSH redox system, where GSH-Px reduces peroxides at the expense of GSH oxidation. Oxidised glutathione is reduced back to the active form by glutathione reductase utilising reducing potential of NADPH which is produced in the pentose phosphate pathway. It is known that exogenous GSH provided rat small-intestinal epithelial cells with significant protection against injury induced by t-butyl hydroperoxide or menadione. Thus, rat small-intestinal epithelial cells can utilise plasma GSH to support intracellular detoxification systems that function in protection against chemically induced injury. On the other hand, decreased intestinal GSH concentration was associated with an increased susceptibility to oxidative injury, metal intoxication and various intestinal pathologies.

**Glutathione S-transferase** (GST) may be important to protect the intestinal cells and tissues against toxic electrolytes and ROS. The level of this antioxidant enzyme is increased as a result of the elevated oxidative stress in the intestine.

## Carotenoids

Carotenoids comprise a family of more than 600 compounds responsible for a variety of bright colours in the leaves, flowers, fruits (pineapple, citrus fruits), vegetables (carrots, tomatoes), insects, bird plumage and marine animals (Pfander, 1992). These pigments provide different colours from light yellow to dark red and when complexed with proteins they can produce green and blue colourations.

Yellow, orange and green fruits and vegetables provide a range of carotenoids. β-carotene, α-carotene and β-cryptoxanthin are the major provitamin A carotenoids, while lutein, zeaxanthin and lycopene are major carotenoids that are not converted to vitamin A.

In general carotenoids are not toxic for humans. There is no evidence that conversion of β-carotene to vitamin A contributes to vitamin A toxicity. However, extremely high consumption of carotenoids for a long-time could cause hypercarotenemia. It can lead to yellowing of the skin which eventually returns to normal after carotenoid exclusion from the diet.

Carotenoid assimilation from the diet varies significantly depending on many diverse conditions and a substantial proportion of ingested carotenoids could be found in all segments of the digestive tract. Therefore, in combination with other dietary antioxidants, carotenoids could promote antioxidant defence in the GIT.

## Flavonoids and other Polyphenols

Flavonoids are low molecular weight polyphenolic substances based on the flavan nucleus. They are widespread in nature, occurring in all plant families and are found in considerable quantities in fruits, vegetables, grains, tea, coffee, cocoa, beer and red wine. The major flavonoid classes include flavonols, flavones, flavanones, flavanols (catechins), anthocyanidins, isoflavones, dihidroflavonols and chalcones (Cook and samman, 1996). Dietary intake of flavonoids is the highest in vegetables.

In general flavonoids can prevent LDL oxidative modification by scavenging ROS, chelating transition metal ions or inhibiting lipoxygenase and this leads to the prevention of atherosclerosis. For example, a number of studies have shown that consumption of soy is antiatherogenic and the isoflavones (genistein, diadzein and biochanin) of soy are most likely responsible for this effect.

Flavonoids and other polyphenols could provide efficient antioxidant protection in the lower gut due to their comparatively low efficiency of absorption in the small intestine (Halliwell et al, 2000). Dietary polyphenols can also modulate *in vivo* oxidative damage in the gastrointestinal tract of rodents supporting the hypothesis that dietary polyphenols might have both a protective and a therapeutic potential in oxidative damage-related pathologies.

**Naringin,** a citrus bioflavonoid, plays an important role in regulating antioxidative capacities by increasing the SOD and catalase activities, up-regulating the gene expressions of SOD, catalase and GSH-Px and protecting the plasma vitamin E in high cholesterol-fed rabbits.

Since flavonoids are consumed in concentrations usually much higher than other antioxidant compounds, their protective effect during digestion is of great importance. For example, flavonoids not only prevented an accumulation of peroxidised lipids but also could switch prooxidant properties of haeme-proteins to antioxidant ones.

**Cereal brans contain significant quantities of the phenolic** ferulic acid and diferulic acid. Their potential health benefits include protection of LDL from oxidative modification, reduction in atherogenesis, inhibitory effects on tumour promotion and chemopreventive properties and have been related mostly to their antioxidant activity.

*Spices and Essential Oils*

Addition of **spices** to food is a common procedure in most cultures. The seasonings contribute a pleasant flavour. It has been shown that they contain a range of antioxidant compounds. Spices are effective in preventing food deterioration during storage and this explains why traditional diets in countries with high temperature (India, Thailand, Mexico, etc.) are usually rich in spices. **Essential oils** from aromatic and medicinal plants have been shown to have antibacterial, antimycotic and antioxidant properties.

*Other Antioxidant Mechanisms*

The gastrointestinal mucosa has a variety of defence mechanisms consisting of functional (mucus-alkaline secretion, mucosal microcirculation), humoral (prostaglandins and nitric oxide) and neuronal (capsaicin sensitive sensory neurones) factors to deal with various aggressive factors including free radicals and toxic products of their metabolism. Furthermore, **oxidative stress at the cellular level is reduced by enzymatic and nonenzymatic antioxidant mechanisms.**

## Adaptation to Stress

To adapt to environmental changes and survive different types of injuries, eukaryotic cells have evolved networks of different responses that detect and control diverse forms of stress. A new mechanism of such adaptive defence of the gastrointestinal mucosa at the intracellular level has been characterised and this is known as the **heat shock response** that is considered to be a universal fundamental mechanism necessary for cell survival under a variety of unfavourable conditions (Santoro, 2000).

Recently 'vitagene concept' of animal adaptation to stress has been developed (Surai and Fisinin, 2016c). In fact, the term 'vitagene' was introduced by Rattan (1998) who suggested that adaptation to stress is mediated by a complex network of several genes called 'vitagenes'. Later this 'vitagene concept' has been developed and adapted to human health by Calbrese and colleagues (Calabrese et al, 2007). The vitagene family includes heat shock proteins, thioredoxin/thioredoxin reductase system, superoxide dismutase and sirtuins. The cytoprotective heat shock proteins (HSP) function as molecular chaperones in regulating cellular homeostasis and promoting survival. HSPs (HSP 60, HSP 70 and HSP 32 or haeme oxygenase-1 [HO-1]) play an important role in gastric and mucosal defence under conditions of stress.

Surai et al. (2017a) reported that the vitagene net work can be modulated by nutritional means. In particular, vitamins A, D, E, C as well as selenium, carnitine, taurine and silymarin are shown to affect vitagenes and improve adaptive ability of birds to various stresses.

## Antioxidant-Prooxidant Balance in the Intestine: Synergistic Effect of Different Antioxidants

Synergistic effect of different antioxidants is of great importance. For example, lycopene acts synergistically, as an effective antioxidant against LDL oxidation, with several natural antioxidants such as vitamin E, the flavonoid glabridin, the phenolics rosmarinic acid and carnosic acid and garlic. Similarly synergistic interactions between isoflavones and ascorbic acid have been shown.

It was shown that antioxidant enzymes play a key role in rendering the intestinal mucosal cells resistant to iron-induced oxidative damage in rats (Srigiridhar and Nair, 1997). It was also shown that supplementation of vitamin E alone or in combination with ascorbic acid protects the GIT of Fe-deficient rats against Fe-mediated oxidative damage during Fe repletion (Srigiridhar and Nair, 2000).

## Linoleic Acid and Vitamin E

The dietary concentration of linoleic acid significantly affected oxidation of pig jejunal mucosa and vitamin E has a protective effect. Pigs supplemented with $\alpha$-tocopheryl acetate showed lower cell desquamation in their jejunal mucosa, while a higher cell desquamation was found in the groups fed diets containing the higher concentration of linoleic acid. Vitamin E also protects the rat colon from oxidative stress associated with inflammation. In fact, vitamin E supplementation increased the colonic vitamin E levels, reduced colonic weight and damage score, prevented lipid peroxidation and diarrhoea, reduced interleukin-1$\beta$ levels and preserved glutathione reductase activity and total glutathione levels.

## Antioxidant-Prooxidant Balance in Various Parts of the Intestine

Presence of antioxidants in the GIT is an essential factor preventing lipid peroxidation in the stomach, small intestine and colon. In fact, total antioxidant activity and activities of SOD and catalase were higher in the rat mucosa/submucosa of the small intestine than in the colon.

Indeed, the antioxidant-prooxidant balance in various parts of the intestine would ultimately depend on the level of antioxidants and prooxidants provided with the diet and released by cells themselves as well as on the level of absorption of both antioxidants and prooxidants. The conditions are favourable for lipid peroxidation in the stomach, since major antioxidants and prooxidants are there before absorption or major metabolism and the pH is also favourable.

In the small intestine this balance will be more variable since many antioxidants, mainly vitamins E, A, C and carotenoids will be effectively absorbed. However, efficiency of absorption of iron is quite low and is available for stimulation of peroxidation. On the other hand, after lipid absorption, concentrations of substrates of peroxidation will be substantially decreased. Furthermore, various flavonoids will also be available for antioxidant defence. Finally, in the colon/rectum, levels of vitamins E, A, C are low, although various flavonoids and some carotenoids are present (Halliwell et al, 2000) as well as iron, but the lipid concentration would be low. Therefore, in each part of the digestive tract there is a possibility of oxidative stress and damage to various biological molecules.

## Antioxidant—Prooxidant Balance in the Intestine and Animal Health

1. Published data clearly indicate that antioxidant-prooxidant balance in human intestine is an important determinant of the intestinal integrity and efficiency of nutrient absorption and assimilation. From the one hand, it was suggested that a compromised antioxidant-prooxidant balance in the intestine could lead to the development of various diseases. On the other hand, consumption of dietary antioxidants, including those, which are not well-absorbed in the small intestine, could improve intestinal health and help in maintaining general health.

   The prooxidants listed here also applies to animals. Thus animals obtain feed with oxidised PUFAs, iron supplements, nitrites and nitrates, heavy metals, persistent organic pollutants, mycotoxins and some other compounds possessing prooxidant properties. Animal diets may have rather higher level of prooxidants.

2. **A compromised antioxidant-prooxidant balance in the intestine can trigger apoptosis of enterocytes:** Taking into account recent information on the effect of redox status of the cell on the apoptosis, it is possible to suggest, that apoptosis of enterocytes could be triggered by a compromised antioxidant-prooxidant balance in the intestine. This could lead to inflammatory reactions, decreased efficiency of absorption of various nutrients and decreased productive and reproductive performances of farm animals and poultry. Therefore, development of various animal diseases where intestinal inflammation and necrosis/apoptosis are involved could be affected by antioxidant-prooxidant balance in the intestine (Surai, 2006).

## What 'to do' to have a Healthy Diet?

It is clear that in most cases food-producers and consumers themselves are responsible for increased levels of prooxidants in the diet and ultimately in the GIT. Therefore, there is a need 'for changes in ways the food is produced, prepared, stored and eaten'. It is possible to improve the situation both at the producer and consumer levels.

## What Should be Done at the Producer Level?

1. To enrich meats and meat-related food with vitamin E: This technological solution can substantially decrease lipid peroxidation in meat during processing, storage and cooking. It seems likely that enrichment of fish with vitamin E also be beneficial in terms of prevention of lipid peroxidation. Similarly enrichment of eggs with vitamin E can also substantially decrease lipid peroxidation and cholesterol oxide formation. In addition, vitamin E in the egg yolk is in highly available free-tocopherol form that could be a major benefit at the level of digestion.

2. To enrich meat, milk and eggs with organic selenium: Selenium is absolutely essential for expression of GI-GSH-Px, the main defence against lipid peroxide absorption in GIT. This is responsible for decomposition of lipid peroxides. If activity of this enzyme is optimal, the lipid peroxides found in the GIT will not be able to be absorbed and hence, peroxides will not be found in the blood. Hence, selenium enrichment could be beneficial in terms of preventing lipid peroxidation in meat or eggs. Selenium is also important for expression of other selenoproteins (e.g. thioredoxin reductase, etc.), which play an important role in antioxidant defence in the intestine and in other tissues.

3. To enrich eggs with carotenoids: These natural antioxidants will be a part of the complex antioxidant defence system interacting with other antioxidants in the GIT and they *per se* can also provide antioxidant protection.

4. **To improve product storage by decreasing oxygen availability and lipid peroxidation.**

5. **To minimise storage of cooked products, which are especially susceptible to peroxidation.**

6. To change the methodology in the fast food restaurants: To change frying oils more often and use olive oil which is less sensitive to peroxidation (Quiles et al, 2002) and to enrich frying oils with natural antioxidants (e.g. tocopherol mixture). It would be advantageous to serve fast food with bigger portions of salads and use more sauces providing additional antioxidants. Some other oils (e.g. rapeseed oil) enriched with tocopherols can also be considered to be useful.

7. **To produce antioxidant-enriched sources, especially for fast food restaurants.**

## What Should be Done at the Consumer Level?

• To choose olive oil (or other antioxidant-enriched oils keeping the economics in mind) for frying food: This will decrease accumulation of oxidation products. Rapeseed oil enriched with tocopherols is also an important medium for frying. Consuming less oil may be a better option.

- To use more spices and herbs during cooking: This will decrease oxidation and prevent accumulation of the lipid peroxides.

- To encourage daily consumption of vegetables and fruits and antioxidant-enriched food products, choose boiled eggs rather than fried eggs, decrease usage of cooked food after storage, decrease consumption of fryed, fast food.

The protective effects of vegetables and fruits against development of various cancers, especially cancers related to the digestive tract, are based on provision of a variety of antioxidants which are not always well-absorbed. Thus, they provide antioxidant protection in the large intestine and prevent oxidative damage and possible mutagenic effect. There is a reason for some antioxidants to be absorbed partially and in that way they provide antioxidant protection in lower parts of the intestine. For example, tocotrienols possess high antioxidant activity. They are not well-absorbed from the food and feed and would be found in the digesta in colon providing antioxidant protection in the lower intestine (Surai, 2006).

## We are what we Eat—We are what our food-animals have Eaten?

Recent achievements in biochemistry and molecular biology, together with epidemiological data have changed our thinking about food. It became increasingly clear that our diet plays a pivotal role in maintenance of our health and a disbalanced diet can cause serious health-related problems. It seems likely that antioxidants are among the major regulators of many physiological processes and therefore a balance between antioxidants and prooxidants in the diet, GIT, plasma and tissues is an important determinant of the state of our health.

Plants contain thousands of phenolic compounds. Dietary polyphenols are of great interest due to their higher consumption (in comparison to other antioxidants such as vitamin E), because of their antioxidant and possible anticarcinogenic activities.

Some dietary constituents which are not well absorbed could have health-promoting properties by maintaining antioxidant-prooxidant balance in the large intestine, where concentration of other antioxidants (vitamin E, carotenoids, ascorbate) could be low, but prooxidants (iron) and substrates of oxidation are still present. This protective effect in the large intestine could be responsible for bowl cancer prevention. Therefore, there could be a biological reason for some nutrients (examples: tocotrienols, flavonoids, carotenoids) not to be absorbed, but be involved in antioxidant protection in the lower gut (Surai, 2006).

## DIRECT AND INDIRECT ANTIOXIDANTS AND THEIR CYTOPROTECTION ABILITIES

### Inherent Oxidant and Antioxidant System

Oxygen is indispensable to aerobic organisms. However, its metabolism can lead to the generation of reactive oxygen species (ROS). For example, in the liver, ROS are produced in the mitochondria and endoplasmic reticulum of hepatocytes through the action of cytochrome p450 enzymes. These generated ROS affect major cellular components such as lipids, DNA and proteins (Cichoz-Lach and Michalak, 2014). Hepatocytes are equipped with molecular strategies that maintain balance between the oxidant and antioxidant system.

Intracellular damage is detectable even in healthy young animals, indicating that the intrinsic antioxidant system is not sufficient to completely eliminate ROS (Sohal et al, 2002). Therefore, a diet with high quality antioxidants is critical for maintaining a high-level of protection against ROS. Cellular protection against ROS can be mediated by direct and indirect antioxidants (Dinkova-Kostova and Talalay, 2008). Antioxidant group that do not activate KEAP1- Nrf2 pathway is considered as direct antioxidants, while the group that activate the KEAP1- Nrf2 pathway as indirect antioxidants.

## Nrf2 Transcription Factor

The nuclear factor related erythroid factor 2 (Nrf2) transcription factor is a master regulator of several antioxidant response genes. Nrf2 is bound to Kelch-Like-ECH Associated Protein 1 (KEAP-1) protein by interacting with cysteine residue and is normally present in cytoplasm of cell. However, during oxidative stress Nrf2 get dissociated from KEAP-1 and translocated to the nucleus. Under normal conditions, Nrf2 is constantly degraded in a KEAP-1-dependent manner via the ubiquitin–proteasome pathway (Kobayashi et al, 2004). In the presence of electrophiles or ROS, Nrf2 accumulates in nuclei, forms a hetero-dimer with small Maf proteins, and finally activates cytoprotective genes through antioxidant response element (ARE)/electrophile response element (EpRE) (Itoh et al, 1997).

## Direct Antioxidants

Direct antioxidants are generally small molecules, such as polyphenols and sulphur-containing amino acids (Silvia et al, 2012) that undergo redox reactions and scavenge ROS. Examples are chlorogenic acid, gallic acid, rosmarinic acid, cyanidin-3-O-glucoside.

## Indirect Antioxidants

Indirect antioxidants activate the KEAP1-Nrf2 pathway and thereby induce the expression of cytoprotective proteins such as phase II enzymes, xenobiotic transporters and drug metabolizing enzymes against xenobiotics and ROS (Suzuki and Yamamoto, 2015). Indirect antioxidants may or may not be redox active (or ROS absorptive). However, these compounds activate the KEAP1- Nrf2 pathway and induce a series of phase II enzymes that are active in antioxidant action and detoxification. Examples are curcumin,

sulforaphane, quercetin, isoriquirigenin, lycopene.

## Utilities of the Direct Antioxidants

1. Chlorogenic acid is one of the most abundant phenolic acids in the human diet, with coffee, fruits, nuts and vegetables being major sources (Shahidi and Ambigaipalan, 2015). It reportedly has antioxidant, anti-carcinogenic and hypotensive effects.

2. Gallic acid is also a phenolic acid found in various teas, nuts and fruits (Shahidi and Ambigaipalan, 2015). It has strong antioxidant, anti-inflammatory, anti-mutagenic and anticarcinogenic actions.

3. Rosmarinic acid, a polyphenol, is found in a variety of plants. It has antioxidant, antibacterial, anti-inflammatory and antiviral actions (Petersen, 2013).

4. Cyanidin-3-O-glucoside is an anthocyanidin and is found in several plants, flowers and fruits (Serraino et al, 2003). It has anti-inflammatory, neuroprotective, antimicrobial, antiviral, antithrombotic and epigenetic actions.

## Utilities of the Indirect Antioxidants

1. Curcumin, a polyphenol, is found in the rhizome of turmeric *(Curcuma longa)*. Curcumin induces the expression of human glutathione S-transferase P1 via activation of the KEAP-1- Nrf2 pathway in HepG2 cells. Curcumin has anti-inflammatory, antimicrobial, anticancer and anti-Alzheimer activities.

2. Sulforaphane is an isothiocyanate derived from broccoli and other cruciferous vegetables (Kensler et al, 2013). Sulforaphane activates the KEAP-1-Nrf2 pathway and protects cells from oxidative stress, inflammation and DNA damage due to radiation, neurodegeneration and cancer.

3. Quercetin is a polyphenol that activates the KEAP-1-Nrf2 pathway and widely exists in caper, black chokeberry, onion, tomato, and lettuce (Wang et al, 2016). Quercetin has attracted increasing attention due to its antioxidant, anti-obesity, anti-carcinogenic, antiviral, antibacterial and anti-inflammatory actions.

4. Isoriquiritigenin, a chalcone compound, is found in licorice *(Glycyrrhiza uralensis)* (Asl and Hosseinzadeh, 2008). Isoriquiritigenin activates the KEAP-1-Nrf2 pathway. It has antiviral, antimicrobial, antioxidative and anti-cancer actions, as well as immunomodulatory, hepatoprotective and cardioprotective actions.

5. Lycopene, a carotenoid, is found in red fruit and vegetables (e.g. papayas, tomatoes, and red peppers) (Petyaev, 2016). Lycopene modulates various cellular redox signalling, including the KEAP-1-Nrf2 pathway and may act beneficially against cancer and cardiovascular diseases.

## Cytoprotection abilities between direct and indirect antioxidants

Study conducted by Joko et al (2017) suggests that indirect antioxidants might be more cytoprotective against oxidation (and more cytotoxic also) than direct antioxidants. Thus indirect antioxidants might be more useful in cytoprotection than direct antioxidants. The strong cytoprotective abilities of the indirect antioxidants can be explained, at least partly, by the expression of multiple antioxidant proteins induced through activation of the KEAP-1-Nrf2 pathway (Joko et al, 2017).

However, indirect antioxidants, especially those with high n-octanol/water partition coefficient (logP), can exhibit cytotoxicity. Hence, caution should be exercised regarding their use in humans. In this regard, indirect antioxidants like 3,5-dihydroxy-4-methoxybenzyl alcohol (DHMBA) and sulforaphane might serve as safe ingredients in antioxidant/functional foods. Joko et al (2017) suggested the need to conduct larger scale studies to address this issue.

3,5-dihydroxy-4-methoxybenzyl alcohol (DHMBA)

## CURCUMIN—A NATURAL PHENOLIC COMPOUND WITH ANTIBACTERIAL, ANTIVIRAL, ANTI-INFLAMMATORY AND ANTIOXIDATIVE EFFECTS

Curcumin is a natural phenolic compound extracted from the root of turmeric, a member of the *Zingiberaceae* family. It has been extensively studied because of its anti-proliferative and anti-inflammatory activities and it is thought to be a promising agent with potential applications such as in cancer prevention, cardiovascular, gastrointestinal disorders and diabetes (Hajavi et al, 2017; Khajehdehi, 2012; Ravindran et al, 2007). Curcumin is designated by the United States Food and Drug Administration as a food additive that is generally recognized as safe (GRAS). It is used as a supplement and sold in several forms as capsules, tablets and energy drinks (Gupta et al, 2013).

## Bioavailability of Curcumin

Curcumin is responsible for the bright yellow colour of the turmeric root and its chemical name is 1,7-bis (4-hydroxy 3-methoxy-pheny1)-1,6-heptadiene-3,5-dione (1E-6E) (Ravindran et al, 2007). Turmeric is usually used as a spice, giving flavour and natural colouring to food and its average intake by Asians varies from 0.5 to 1.5 g/day/person, which does not produce toxic symptoms. Its bioavailability is low and the levels in plasma and target tissues are low because of slow intestinal absorption, rapid metabolism and conjugation to hydrophilic molecules in the liver with biliary excretion, poor solubility in water and clearance of the body.

## Anti-inflammatory Effect of Curcumin

There are several hypotheses that can explain the anti-inflammatory effect of curcumin as down regulation of transcription factors like cyclooxygenase-2 (COX-2), signal transducer and activator of transcription 3 (STAT3) and IκB kinase β (IκKβ) (inhibitor of nuclear factor kappa-B; NFκB). Curcumin seems able to decrease cytokines synthesis, improve nitric oxide (NO) bioavailability and scavenging of reactive oxygen species (ROS) [that promote inflammation and oxidative stress, which are common complications in several chronic diseases including chronic kidney disease (Alvarenga et al, 2018)].

## Curcumin is a Bifunctional Antioxidant

Curcumin has broad biological functions. It has been reported that curcumin is a bifunctional antioxidant because of its ability to react directly with reactive species and to induce an upregulation of various cytoprotective and antioxidant proteins. It has been established that curcumin exerts antioxidant activity directly by reducing the scavenging ROS such as superoxide anion ($O_2^{\bullet-}$), hydroxyl radicals ($^{\bullet}OH$), hydrogen peroxide ($H_2O_2$), singlet oxygen ($^1O_2$), peroxynitrite and peroxyl radicals ($ROO^{\bullet}$). Therefore, these mechanisms might explain some of the cytoprotective effects of this compound (Trujillo et al, 2013). It promotes intestinal alkaline phosphatase (IAP) activity.

Moreover, in the mitochondria, due to the high flow of electrons during the process of oxidative phosphorylation, ROS are produced and usually are partially removed by antioxidant enzymes located in the mitochondrial matrix, such as manganese-dependent superoxide dismutase (SOD) and/or released into the cytosol and detoxified by endogenous antioxidant systems.

Excess ROS production (associated with deficiency of the endogenous antioxidant system) may lead to the oxidation of specific mitochondrial biomolecules, resulting in mitochondrial dysfunction. A large body of evidence has shown that mitochondrial dysfunction is the main culprit of different diseases, especially in non-communicable diseases such as cancer, neurodegenerative diseases and cardiovascular disease (CVD) (Oliveira et al, 2016).

Curcumin also exerts antioxidant effects upon mitochondria through decreased production of ROS and upregulation of antioxidant enzymes, thus, inhibiting mitochondrial damage and contributing to the preservation of the important functions of this organelle (Aparicio-Trejo et al, 2017). Further, it has been demonstrated that curcumin may trigger mitochondrial biogenesis (Oliveira et al, 2016).

Curcumin is an indirect antioxidant, since it activates the KEAP1-Nrf2 pathway. Curcumin is able to induce the master regulator of antioxidant response, the Nrf2 (Tapia et al, 2012). Treatment with curcumin significantly increased Nrf2 and hemo-oxygenase-1 (HO-1) expression in the neonatal rats with hypoxic-ischemic brain injury (Cui et al,

2017). Nrf2 is bound to its cytosolic repressor protein, KEAP1. Curcumin may modulate Nrf2 by modification of KEAP1, thereby releasing Nrf2. Then Nrf2 is translocated into the nucleus, where it binds as a heterodimer to the antioxidant responsive element (ARE) in DNA to initiate target gene expression including: quinone oxidoreductase 1 (NQO1), glutathione S-transferase (GST), HO-1, glutathione peroxidase (GSH-Px), glutamate cysteine ligase (GCL), catalase, superoxide dismutase (Cardozo et al, 2013).

Thus, curcumin upregulates the activity of Nrf2, which is crucial for cytoprotection against various forms of stress due to the ability of the Nrf2 to antagonise the transcription factor NFκB. NFκB is an important regulator of genes encoding pro-inflammatory cytokines during inflammatory responses (Cardozo et al, 2013).

In addition, curcumin has been found to attenuate NFκB activity by inhibiting IκB (inhibitor of kinases) degradation, thus preventing NFκB translocation to the nucleus, suppressing pro-inflammatory gene expression and downregulating pro-inflammatory cytokines, such as tumour necrosis factor alpha (TNF-α), interleukin (IL-)1 and IL-6 (Liu et al, 2014).

## Curcumin is a Natural Agonist of PPAR-γ

Curcumin is also a natural agonist of peroxisome proliferator-activated receptor-γ (PPAR-γ). This PPAR-γ is a member of the nuclear receptor superfamily of ligand-activated transcription factors that has been found to be involved in anti-inflammatory signalling pathways. PPAR-γ binds to PPAR-responsive elements (PPRE) in the regulatory region to initiate target gene expression.

Inhibitory effects of PPAR-γ on NFκB activation have been demonstrated in multiple cell systems (Liu et al, 2014). Thus, PPAR-γ pathway may be a critical mediator of the protective anti-inflammatory effects of curcumin (Liu et al, 2014). Curcumin mediated anti-inflammatory and antioxidant effects involving Nrf2, NFκB, PPAR-γ and mitochondria are depicted in Fig. 3.14.

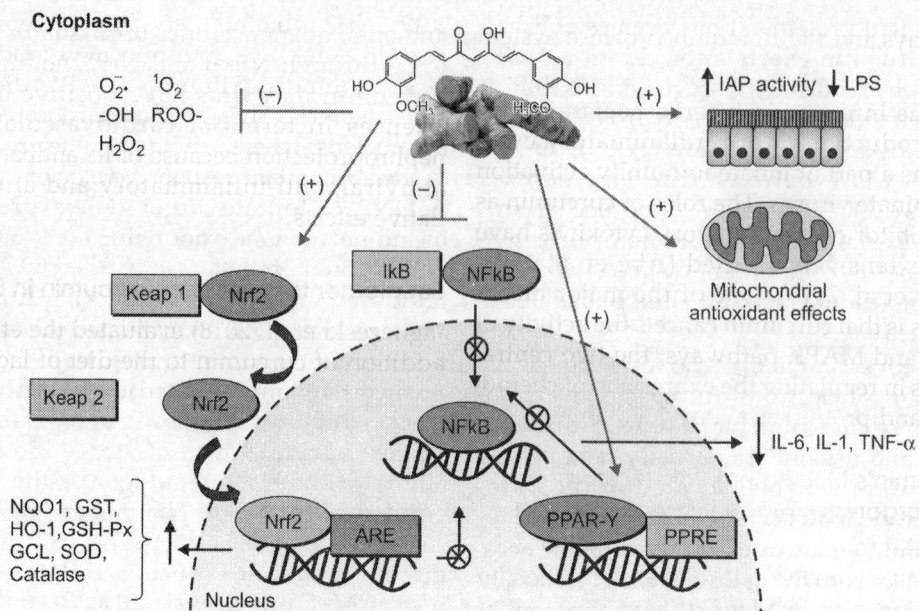

**Fig. 3.14:** Curcumin mediated anti-inflammatory and antioxidant effects in CKD. *Source:* Alvarenga et al, 2018

## Curcumin as an Antiviral Drug

Curcumin has been studied extensively for its pleiotropic activity, including anti-inflammatory, anti-oxidant and anti-tumour activity. Curcumin's pleiotropic activities against viruses emanate from its ability to modulate numerous molecular targets that contribute to various cellular events, such as transcription regulation and the activation of cellular signalling pathways such as inflammation and apoptosis likely via intermolecular interactions.

Accumulated evidence indicated curcumin plays an inhibitory role against infection of numerous viruses. These mechanisms involve:

1. Either a direct interference of viral replication machinery, or
2. Suppression of cellular signalling pathways essential for viral replication.

### Curcumin Targets Critical Steps of Virus Replication Cycle

As a single unit, a virus cannot equip all the enzymes required for their replication. They commandeer cellular machinery for their efficient reproduction and metabolic processes. However, an antiviral agent must stop the viral growth in infected cells, without affecting surrounding normal cells. Hence, specific processes of the virus replicative cycle, which include attachment/penetration, uncoating, genome replication, gene expression, assembly and release, have been attractive targets for chemotherapeutic intervention.

One of the bio-functions of curcumin is revoking the infection of viruses, by targeting the viral entry, or solely attacking the viral components essential for viral replication.

### Curcumin Suppresses Intercellular Signalling Cascades Prerequisite for Efficient Virus Replication

Viral infection damages the cell as they compete with the host cell for their cellular apparatus. Viruses for their advantage, survival and replication could hijack various intracellular signalling cascades such as NFκB, PI3K/Akt, MAPK signalling pathways and the ubiquitin protease system (UPS).

Virus infection is often associated with overproduction of pro-inflammatory cytokines as a part of innate immunity activation to eliminate viruses. The roles of curcumin as an inhibitor of inflammatory cytokines have been extensively studied (Abe et al, 1999; Yadav et al, 2015). One of the major mechanisms is that curcumin cancels the activity of NFκB and MAPK pathways, the two central signals in regulating the expression of chemokines and pro-inflammatory cytokines.

## Curcumin's Multipotent Role Against Microorganisms Made it a Wonder Drug

Curcumin's multipotent role against organisms like bacteria, fungi, virus as well as its synergistic effects like antioxidant potential, anti-inflammatory and anti-tumoral activities has made it a wonder drug. However, one of the drawbacks of curcumin is its poor bioavailability. The advances of nanotechnology has helped to circumvent the challenges faced with curcumin drug delivery by using various nano-carriers such as nanoparticles, curcumin nanocrystals, polymeric micelles, dendrimers, nano-liposome-encapsulated curcumin, polymeric micelles and solid-lipid nanoparticles. Thus, the various nano-carriers provide better permeability, resistance to metabolic processes and increased blood circulation (Mathew and Hsu, 2018).

Several signalling pathways could be a potential target of curcumin and this broad mechanism of action of curcumin may make this spice a promising adjuvant therapy for chronic kidney (CKD) patients (Alvarenga et al, 2018). This is because CKD is characterised by profound metabolic and nutritional alterations resulting in increased systemic inflammation and oxidative stress that are thought to be due to factors such as downregulation of Nrf2 and upregulation of NFκB that directly or indirectly could be affected by curcumin. Thus, some of the more important pathways for the anti-inflammatory anti-proliferative and antioxidant activities of curcumin seems to be through NFκB and Nrf2 modulation. Curcumin may thus have positive consequences in terms of cardiovascular and nephroprotection because of its antibacterial, antiviral, anti-inflammatory and anti-oxidative effects.

## Supplementary Effect of Curcumin in Sheep

Jaguezeski et al (2018) evaluated the effect of addition of curcumin to the diet of lactating ewes (at 100 mg/kg feed) on their health, productive performance and milk quality. Levels of ROS were lower, but the activities of antioxidant enzymes increased significantly in the blood of the ewes. Milk yields were increased and there was a reduction in somatic cell count (SCC) and protein oxidation in milk; unsaturated fatty acid oleic acid increased, while saturated fatty acid hexadecanoic acid decreased in the milk. The authors concluded that the addition of curcumin in sheep diet had antioxidant and anti-inflammatory effects and it improved productive performance and milk quality; sheep receiving 80 mg/animal/day has higher digestibility of neutral detergent fibre and consequently increased milk production.

Molosse et al (2019) evaluated the addition of curcumin in concentrate feed of nursing lambs (15 day-old) at concentrations of 100 (the group T100) and 200 (the group T200) mg/kg for 30 days on their growth and health, as well as on the prevention of coccidiosis. Nursing lambs fed with concentrate containing curcumin showed higher body weight and weight gain. Rahmani et al (2018) demonstrated that a diet containing 200 mg/kg of curcumin increased intestinal villous surface area and enhanced the uptake of nutrients in broilers and prevented intestinal histopathological lesions also contributing to improved animal performance. The addition of curcumin in the diet increased total antioxidant levels and exerted anti-inflammatory action, as well as altered the activity of enzymes (serum creatine kinase activity was higher and pyruvate kinase was lower) involved on adenosine triphosphate (ATP) metabolism, which may have contributed to weight gain.

Curcumin has been used as an additive due to its nutritional, medical and pharmacological properties (Wang et al, 2018). Earlier, Yarru et al (2009) demonstrated that curcumin exerts positive effects in the expression of genes linked to immunological and antioxidant systems, as well as improves some parameters related to animal performance. Also, it is known that curcumin acts as a potent eliminator of reactive oxygen species (ROS), protecting the haemoglobin against nitrite and lipid peroxidation-induced oxidation (Srinivasan and Sambaiah 1991), and consequently, minimising the oxidative stress of lambs in periods of higher sanitary challenges, such as nursing (Molosse et al, 2019).

## ROLE OF OXIDANT-ANTIOXIDANT BALANCE IN ENHANCING REPRODUCTIVE EFFICIENCY OF DAIRY ANIMALS

**Free radicals and antioxidants** remain in equilibrium

Normally reactive oxygen species (ROS) and antioxidants remain in equilibrium. When this equilibrium can be interrupted as a consequence of overproduction of ROS or over-depletion of antioxidants, oxidative stress (OS) occurs (Celi, 2011). Numerous studies have reported the physiological as well as pathological involvement of oxidants and antioxidants in mammals. Reproductive processes lead to dynamic changes in metabolism and energy consumption, which may be responsible for the excessive production of byproducts.

There are two major types of free radical species, namely ROS and reactive nitrogen species (RNS) (Chauhan et al, 2014). ROS are formed by the partial reduction of molecular oxygen occurring usually within the cells under an aerobic condition (Rizzo et al, 2012). ROS have been implicated in the adjustment of the reproductive events such as oocyte maturation, steroidogenesis, the regulation of

follicular fluid environment, folliculogenesis, corpus luteal function and luteolysis.

## Enzymatic Antioxidants and Non-Enzymatic Antioxidants

Antioxidants can be divided into enzymatic antioxidants and non-enzymatic antioxidants (Chauhan et al, 2014). Superoxide dismutase (SOD), catalase, glutathione peroxidase (GSH-Px), glutathione reductase (GRx), thioredoxin reductase, peroxiredoxin, haeme oxygenase (HO) are the enzymatic antioxidants against ROS.

The non-enzymatic antioxidants can be categorised into metabolic antioxidants (endogenous antioxidants) and nutrient antioxidants (exogenous antioxidants).

Metabolic antioxidants such as lipoic acid, glutathione, L-ariginine, melatonin, uric acid, bilirubin, metal-chelating proteins, ceruloplasmin and transferrin are known as endogenous antioxidants as they can be synthetised in the body. Nutrient antioxidants such as vitamins A, C, D and E, beta-carotene and other carotenoids, trace metals (selenium, manganese, zinc), polyphenols, flavonoids, omega-3 and omega-6 fatty acids are known as exogenous antioxidants as they cannot be produced in the body and must be provided through foods or supplements (Pham-Huy et al, 2008).

Enzymatic and non-enzymatic antioxidants work in concert to protect against ROS-induced cellular damage (Sordillo and Aitken, 2009). For example, SOD enzymes are dependent on trace minerals, copper and manganese, in the dismutation of $O_2^-$ to $H_2O_2$. Subsequently, the reduction of $H_2O_2$ to water and oxygen is mediated by catalases or the selenium-dependent enzymes. The reduction of $H_2O_2$ and other hydroperoxides is coupled to the oxidation of reduced glutathione (GSH) to the oxidised state (GSSG). The GSSG is converted by the glutathione reductase system to GSH, which becomes available for further glutathione peroxidases- or thioredoxin reductases-mediated metabolism. Reduced GSH can scavenge preformed reactive metabolites and also participate in regenerating and maintaining the functional forms of other antioxidant enzymes such as vitamins. For example, vitamin E radicals formed during the neutralisation of lipid free radicals in the cell membranes are recycled back to reduced vitamin E by peroxidase enzymes using GSH as a cofactor. Dietary micronutrients such as vitamin E and selenium are recognised as important tools to enhance antioxidant defence mechanisms and reduce health disorders of dairy cattle during periods of increased metabolic demands.

## Elevated Foetal and Maternal Metabolism During the Final Stages of Pregnancy

It is well-established that reproduction increases energy expenditure by augmenting the metabolic rate (Nilsson, 2002). Elevated metabolism results in increased production of ROS and, therefore, unless the antioxidant defences are also enhanced, it might expose the organism to the negative effects of oxidative stress (OS). The ovary is a metabolically active organ and, hence, it produces ROS.

An increase in both foetal and maternal metabolism can be observed during the final stages of pregnancy as a consequence of rapid foetal growth and at the start of the lactation, as a result of colostrum and milk production. The resulting enhanced mitochondrial activity in both foetal and maternal tissues results in an over-production of ROS (Aurousseau et al, 2006) as observed in dairy cows during the last trimester of pregnancy (Castillo et al, 2005) and the beginning of the lactation (Pedernera et al, 2010).

It is important to consider that excessive consumption of reducing equivalents, provided by reduced nicotinamide adenine dinucleotide phosphate (NADPH), by both antioxidant defence and metabolic reactions, can result in NADPH depletion. The OS-induced depletion of reducing equivalents can reduce the amount of NADPH required by other important physiological processes (several reductive processes in addition to biosynthesis) and the consequent upregulation of the pentose monophosphate shunt

would redirect glucose from other pathways such as milk production, resulting in decreased productivity (Lean et al, 2014). Therefore, ROS accumulation may lead to a disruption of the oxidant–antioxidant balance, resulting in oxidative stress (Celi and Gabai, 2015).

## Disorders of Oxidant-antioxidant Balance During Reproduction

A growing body of evidence indicate that the antioxidant-prooxidant (redox) balance is an important regulator of mammalian reproductive functions including ovarian follicular development, ovulation, fertilisation, luteal steroidogenesis, endometrium receptivity and shedding, embryonic development, implantation and early placental growth and development.

The characterisation of the oxidant-antioxidant balance is attracting a high level of interest in ruminant physiology (Celi, 2011) as it may have a pivotal role in the regulation of several physiological functions including reproduction. In dairy cows, disorders of the oxidant-antioxidant balance have been observed during several reproductive pathologies, such as retained placenta, mastitis, embryonic mortality, follicular cysts and repeat breeder syndrome. Moreover, one of the main constraints on conception rate is the elevated rate of early embryonic death that occurs before Day 21 post-insemination, causing 30–50% losses (Cook, 2009).

## Role of Free Radicals and Antioxidants in Female Reproduction

The presence of ROS in the female reproductive tract has been established through several veterinary and medical studies. ROS exert both physiological and pathological effects in the female reproductive events. Their involvement in reproductive functions has been depicted in the Fig. 3.15. Superoxide ($O_2^{\cdot-}$) is generated during normal metabolism by the activity of the NADPH oxidase. Dietary imbalances and high metabolic load also stimulate the activity of the NADPH oxidase,

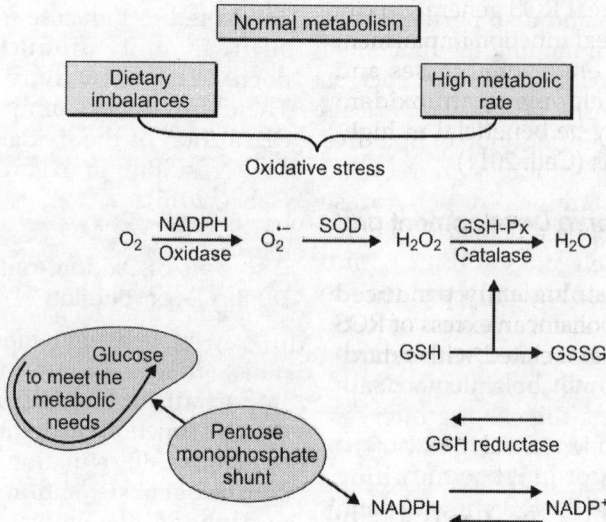

**Fig. 3.15:** Role of oxidative stress in the animal

leading to oxidative stress if not removed by the antioxidant system. In normal conditions, $O_2^{\bullet-}$ converted to hydrogen peroxide ($H_2O_2$) by superoxide dismutase (SOD); $H_2O_2$ is then converted to water ($H_2O$) by the activity of glutathione peroxidase (GSH-Px) and catalase. Reduction of peroxides is accompanied by oxidation of reduced glutathione (GSH), which can be regenerated from glutathione disulfide (GSSG) by reducing equivalents from NADPH, which is generated by the pentose monophosphate shunt.

During folliculogenesis, superoxide radicals are produced by normal cellular metabolism and steroidogenesis (Sugino, 2005). The mechanism of action of SOD involves the dismutation of superoxide anion to $H_2O_2$. SOD plays a central role in antioxidative reactions. Three isozymes are generated by mammalians: SOD1 encodes Cu, Zn-SOD and is mainly cytosolic, while SOD2 encodes Mn-SOD and is located in the mitochondria of ovarian follicular cells. SOD3, which encodes the extracellular form, is similar to Cu, Zn-SOD in structure. Growing follicles, granulose cells of Graffian follicles and ovulated follicles all produce both enzymatic and non-enzymatic antioxidants to preserve themselves

from the oxidative damage of ROS (Rizzo et al, 2012).

## Similarities Between Ovulation and Inflammation

The ovulatory event has several similarities to a controlled inflammatory reaction. Inflammation is accompanied by an increase in prostaglandin synthesis, cytokine production, activity of proteolytic enzymes such as matrix metalloproteinases and increased vascular permeability. These inflammatory reactions seem to be modulated by ROS ultimately leading to the rupture of the follicle wall, resulting in ovulation (Sugino, 2005).

Within the ovary, leukocytes and endothelial cells located near pre-ovulatory follicles are deemed to be the main sources of ROS (Sugino, 2005). Lower plasma biological antioxidant potential, glutathione levels and higher milk superoxide dismutase level, but lower milk glutathione peroxidase and glutathione concentrations, have been reported in ovulated cows than in anovulated herd mates (Talukder et al, 2015). These findings support the notion that the decrease in antioxidant status before ovulation may be a crucial event preceding the ovulatory response.

As the excess of luteal ROS generation can be a cause of early luteal function impairment in early pregnancy, embryonic losses and early conceptus development, antioxidant supplementation may be beneficial in high-yielding dairy animals (Celi, 2011).

## Oxidative Stress, Embryo Development and Embryo Mortality

While ROS are physiologically produced during embryo metabolism, an excess of ROS production has been associated with retardation of embryo growth or embryo death (Celi, 2010), extending the calving interval and increasing days open in dairy cows. The increase in cytokine production resulting from the stimulation of the inflammatory and immune response enhances the secretion of molecules such as $PGF_2\alpha$ or nitric oxide that are harmful for embryo survival and development. In the normal situations, embryos are protected by a complex antioxidant network, such as enzymes (SOD and GSH-Px) and other molecules (transferrin, ascorbic acid) that are present in the oviduct (Celi, 2010). The antioxidant network seems to be upregulated during key physiological events. Indeed, soon after fertilisation, an increase in luteal SOD and catalase activities has been observed (Rizzo et al, 2012), while Miszkiel et al (1999) reported the presence of β-carotene and ascorbic acid in the corpora lutea (CL) of pregnant cows and sows.

In oxidative stress due to ROS accumulation, ROS can damage several biological targets such as DNA, RNA, cholesterol, lipids, carbohydrates and proteins (Celi and Gabai, 2015). Indeed, during oxidative stress, DNA mutations are more common in mitochondria than in the nucleus. When damaged, embryo mitochondrial DNA may lead to alteration of embryonic metabolism and development. Oxidation of proteins and lipids can lead to an increase in advanced oxidative protein products (AOPP) and malondialdehyde (MDA). Dairy cows diagnosed with embryo mortality after Day 25 of artificial insemination have shown higher AOPP and MDA levels (Celi et al, 2011, 2012).

In dairy cows, high nutrient demands during early lactation often result in a negative nutrient balance, which is typically associated with increased non-esterified fatty acid (NEFA) concentrations. These elevated NEFA concentrations have also been reported in the microenvironment of the growing oocyte, jeopardising oocyte development and embryo quality (Van Hoeck et al, 2011). High concentrations of β-carotene have been observed in the plasma of cows that ovulated during the first follicular wave, compared with the low concentrations in anovulatory cows (Kawashima et al, 2009).

In agreement with this observation, precalving dietary supplementation with β-carotene resulted in a higher number of cows ovulating postpartum (Kawashima et al, 2010). The positive effect of dietary β-carotene supplementation on dairy-cow fertility might be related to its conversion to vitamin A in the ovary (Schweigert, 2003). These observations bring further evidence to the importance of a correct oxidant-antioxidant balance for optimal reproductive function.

## Maintenance of a Correct Oxidant-Antioxidant Balance is Imperative During Pregnancy

The rapid foetal growth that can be observed during the final stages of pregnancy is accompanied by an increase in placental and maternal metabolism that, in turn, make the dam and the foetus susceptible to oxidative stress (Rizzo et al, 2012). The development of an adequate antioxidant system in the uterus, embryo and placenta is deemed to be a crucial event for the establishment and maintenance of pregnancy. When an excessive production of ROS occurs during the initial stages of placenta development, several adverse pregnancy outcomes such as embryo resorption, miscarriage, intrauterine growth restriction and pre-eclampsia can be observed in domestic animals (Rizzo et al, 2012).

**Oxidative status may also affect key transcription factors** (hypoxia-inducible factor, nuclear factor κB, activator protein-1 and apoptotic factor) and, hence, alter gene expression during development of the embryo (Celi, 2010). Overexpression of these transcription factors affects vascular development, decreases apoptosis and increases the pro-inflammatory state, further modifying the cellular redox status and arresting the growth of the embryo (Cell, 2010). An increase in the activity of Mn-SOD and GSH-Px has been observed in sheep placentomes during early placental development, indicating that these changes could be considered as a physiological response of the placentomes to ROS-induced oxidative stress (Garrel et al, 2010). Therefore, the maintenance of a correct oxidant—antioxidant balance is imperative during embryonic development (Rizzo et al, 2012).

**Dietary supplementation of β-carotene improves fertility:** Climatic stress can result from an over-abundant production of ROS, which can impair health, welfare and reproduction especially in grazing ruminants, either as a direct consequence of the increased ROS production, or indirectly through the reduced quality of fresh or preserved forages (Chauhan et al, 2014). Most of the β-carotene is found in vegetative plants and its concentrations decline as plants mature and the majority of grains and fermented feeds are characterised by very low concentrations of β-carotene as a consequence of heat damage and breakdown during storage (Johansson et al, 2014).

Hence, dietary supplementation of antioxidants might represent a useful strategy to improve fertility (Celi, 2011). Pregnancy rate at 120 days postpartum can be increased by 14% in heat stressed-cows upon supplementation with β−carotene for at least 3 months. Also, prepartum supplementation with β-carotene is associated with a lower incidence of retained placenta in multiparous cows. Other studies have also demonstrated the beneficial effects of dietary supplementation of β−carotene on fertility, with improved conception rates, uterine involution, ovulation and reduced incidence of cystic ovaries and early embryonic death.

**Measuring oxidants and antioxidants in milk samples helps in monitoring oxidative stress:** Measurement of biomarkers of oxidative stress in milk is less invasive. Milk can have antioxidant, antimicrobial and immunomodulatory properties. Several enzymes can be found in milk, with some of them, such as xanthine oxidase (XO) and lactoperoxidase (LP), being sources of ROS. To balance the prooxidant effect of these enzymes, several non-enzymatic antioxidants can also be identified both in the lipid (vitamin E, carotenoids and ubiquinol) and water (vitamin C) phase of milk. The endogenous milk enzymes are secreted and arise through blood plasma, secretory cell cytoplasm, the apical membrane of the mammary cell and somatic cell as leukocytes. Among the antioxidant enzymes, SOD, GSH-Px and catalase have been quantified in milk (Przybylska et al, 2007). It seems that measuring oxidants and antioxidants in milk samples may be a convenient way for monitoring oxidative stress status in dairy species. Further, assessment of biomarkers of oxidative stress in biological samples (plasma and milk) may pave the way for prediction of ovulation.

## ROLE OF OXYLIPIDS IN THE REGULATION OF OXIDATIVE STRESS IN DAIRY CATTLE

A considerable amount of research was conducted in order to find out the factors that contribute to compromised immunity and health disorders in periparturient dairy animals. Uncontrolled or impaired inflammatory responses that contribute oxidative stress are linked directly to increased health disorders during this critical period in the production cycle of cow/buffalo. Increased incidence of diseases such as mastitis, metritis and retained placenta has been attributed to the underlying oxidative stress.

### Reactive Metabolites

The oxidants 'reactive oxygen species (ROS) and reactive nitrogen species (RNS)' are referred to as **reactive metabolites.** They are produced both in physiological and pathological states. Reactive metabolites are normal products of metabolism and are essential for signalling functions. They are necessary for cellular processes including proliferation, differentiation and metabolic adaptations. For example, reactive oxygen species $O_2^-$ and $H_2O_2$ participate in phosphorylation of various proteins that are part of signalling networks such as mitogen-activated protein kinase (MAPK) phosphatases, by oxidising thiol-containing cysteine residues (Sordillo and Mavangira, 2014).

Excessive production of reactive metabolites leads to oxidative stress.

The level of production of reactive metabolites is increased during pregnancy and the onset of lactation in dairy cows because of increased metabolic demands. Reactive metabolites also increase during regulated inflammatory processes to levels necessary for effective innate and adaptive immune functions (Sordillo and Aitken, 2009). In contrast to the physiological production of reactive metabolites, uncontrolled inflammation is characterised by excessive levels of reactive metabolites that contribute to the pathology of diseases.

During the inflammatory conditions mitochondria and peroxisomes are major source of excessive reactive metabolite production, while significant contributions also come from upregulated enzyme pathways. Inducible nitric oxide synthase (iNOS), xanthine oxidase (XO) and the nicotinamide adenine dinucleotide phosphate oxidase (NOX) enzymes are all upregulated by inflammatory stimuli. Inducible NOS (iNOS) is upregulated and generates excess nitric oxide, which induces widespread vasodilation and generation of peroxynitrite in acute inflammation (Sorokin, 2016).

## Nrf2 Activates Antioxidant Response Elements in the Promoter Regions of Antioxidant Response Genes

i. Cells have an elaborate system of antioxidants that neutralise, metabolise and delay the production of oxidants. Antioxidants include endogenous enzymes and non-enzymatic pool of dietary antioxidants. Enzymatic and non-enzymatic components collectively contribute to the overall cellular antioxidant potential, which is crucial for defence against oxidative cellular damage during inflammatory-based diseases (Mavangira and Sordillo, 2018).

ii. Activation of antioxidant response genes is another important mechanism essential for limiting the excessive reactive metabolite accumulation. For example, during oxidative stress Nrf2 acts as a master regulator of several antioxidant response genes.

In normal (unstimulated) condition, Nrf2 is bound to Kelch-Like-ECH Associated Protein 1 (KEAP-1) protein and is present in the cytoplasm. During oxidative stress (or in the presence of Nrf2 agonist), oxidation of the cysteine residues dissociates Nrf2 from KEAP-1 and translocates to the nucleus. After forming dimers with other transcription factors, **Nrf2 activates antioxidant response elements in the promoter regions of antioxidant response genes** (Ruiz et al, 2013). Several Nrf2 target genes showed increased expression in peripartal dairy cows (Gessner et al, 2013). Nrf2 target genes include the enzymes catalase, glutathione peroxidase, thioredoxin reductase, haeme oxygenase, superoxide dismutase and acute phase proteins such as haptoglobin and serum amyloid A.

## Oxylipids

During oxidative stress, ROS can modify polyunsaturated fatty acids (PUFA) associated with cellular membranes, resulting in the biosynthesis of oxidised products called oxylipids. These oxylipids depending on their precursor fatty acid have the capacity of either enhancing or resolving inflammation. Oxylipids can directly or indirectly target sites of ROS production and thus control the degree of oxidative stress. Oxylipids are of two types: ROS oxylipids (non-enzymatic) and non-ROS oxylipids (enzymatic) (Fig. 3.16). Non-ROS oxylipids are cyclooxygenase (COX)-,

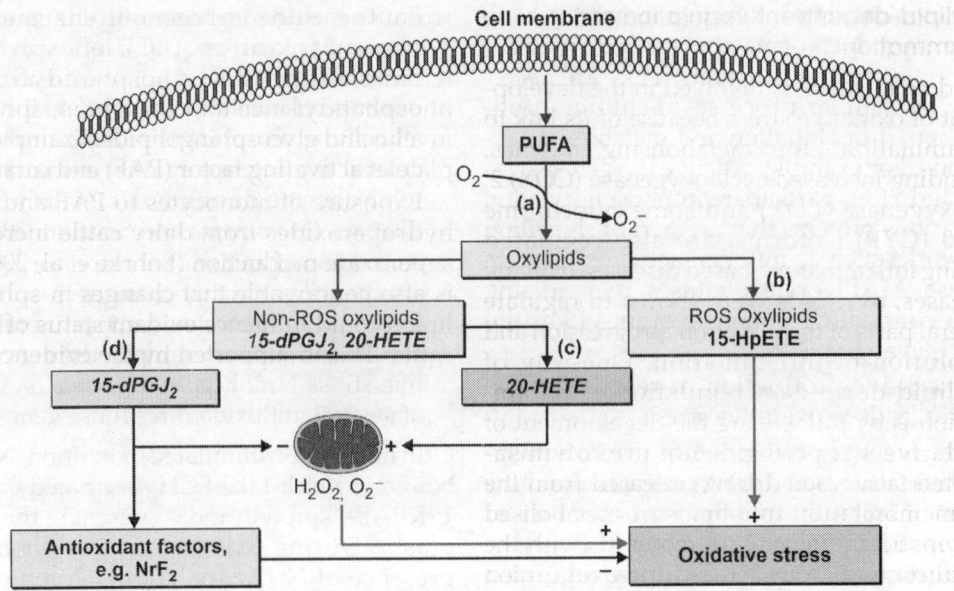

**Fig. 3.16:** Oxylipid-dependent regulation of inflammation. + induce production; – decrease production

lipooxygenase (LOX)- and cytochrome p450 (CYP)-derived oxylipids.

## Role of Oxylipids in Oxidative Stress

Omega 6 (n-6) PUFA such as arachidonic acid (AA) and linoleic acid (LA) and omega 3 (n-3) PUFA including α-linolenic (ALA), eicosapentaenoic acid (EPA) and docosahexaenoic acid (DHA) are the common substrates for oxylipid synthesis. Metabolism of the PUFA substrates occurs after their hydrolysis from cell membrane phospholipids catalysed by members of the phospholipase (PL) enzyme family, predominantly by PLA2. Alternatively, PUFA are metabolised while still esterified in cell membranes. This explains their ability to modify cell function by altering the properties of the cell membrane lipid bilayer (Milne et al, 2015).

The enzymatic pathways of COX LOX and CYP are involved in metabolising PUFA with evidence of substrate preferences. For example, CYP enzymes will readily oxygenate EPA and DHA over linoleic acid and arachidonic acid when incubated with equimolar concentrations of these PUFA (Arnold et al, 2010). Nonenzymatic pathways

are also involved in the oxygenation of PUFA mediated by free radicals such as $O_2^-$.

The general mechanism of oxylipid biosynthesis follows the removal of susceptible hydrogen atoms from PUFA structure and the concurrent or subsequent insertion of one or more oxygen molecules. The oxygenation of PUFA generates lipid hydroperoxides that add to the pool of ROS during oxidative stress (Sordillo and Mavangira, 2014). The LOX enzymes exist as several isoforms including 5-, 8-, 12- and 15-LOX based on the site of oxygen insertion in the PUFA substrate.

The hydroperoxides are potent ROS metabolites that were shown to participate in the development of pathological conditions, e.g. the LA derived-13- hydroxyl-octadecadienoic acid (13-HODE), 13-hydroperoxyoctadecadienoic acid (13-HpODE) and the arachidonic acid-derived 15-hydroxyperoxyeicosatetraenoic acid (15-HpETE). Since, the effects of 15-HpETE and 13-HpODE are similar to the direct effects of $H_2O_2$, these primary oxygenation metabolites serve as inherent reactive electrophiles that can exacerbate oxidative stress during acute inflammation.

## Oxylipid-dependent Regulation of Inflammation

Lipid metabolism is involved in the development of oxidative stress because of its link to inflammation. Lipid metabolising enzymes, including increased cyclooxygenase (COX) 2, lipoxygenase (LOX) and some cytochrome p450 (CYP) isoforms, are also regulated during inflammatory-based diseases. In many diseases, oxylipids were shown to regulate several parts of the initiation, progression and resolution of inflammation. One-way of oxylipid-dependent regulation of inflammation is by influencing the development of oxidative stress (Fig. 3.16). (a) Polyunsaturated fatty acids (PUFA) released from the cell membrane phospholipids are metabolised enzymatically to produce oxylipids with the production of ROS such as superoxide anion in the process. (b) Some of the primary oxylipids (hydroperoxides from the LOX pathway) are potent ROS such as the arachidonic acid-derived 15-hydroperoxyeicosatetraenoic acid (15-HpETE) that can directly damage cellular macromolecules.

Other oxylipid metabolites target sites of reactive metabolite production like the mitochondria (NOX enzyme pathway) to induce production (c) such as is the case of the cytochrome p450-derived 20-hydroxyeicosatetraenoic acid (20-HETE). (d) Other oxylipids such as the dehydration product of prostaglandin D2 (15-dPGJ$_2$) (exerts antioxidant effects) decrease reactive metabolite production by directly decreasing production or by stimulating antioxidant factors such as Nrf$_2$. The link between oxylipids and oxidative stress, therefore, offers opportunities for modulating inflammatory processes by directly targeting the metabolic pathways of these metabolites.

## Other Lipid Mediators and Oxidative Stress

In addition to the oxylipid products of lipid metabolism, other lipid mediators can also induce oxidative stress and may be relevant in inflammatory conditions of the dairy cow. These other lipid mediators can be derived from the major phospholipids such as phosphatidylcholine (PC), phosphatidylethanolamine (PE), phosphatidylserine, phosphatidyl-inositol, cardiolipin, sphingomyelin and glycosphingolipids. Examples are platelet activating factor (PAF) and ceramide.

Exposure of monocytes to PAF and lipid hydroperoxides from dairy cattle increased superoxide production (Lohrke et al, 2005). It is also conceivable that changes in sphingolipids could influence oxidant status of dairy cattle. This is supported by the evidence that 'higher body condition dairy cows' suffered greater oxidative stress compared to those with lower body condition (Bernabucci et al, 2005). Greater plasma concentrations of sphingolipids, especially, ceramide were reported in 'overconditioned (obese) dairy cows' (Rico et al, 2015). Ceramide is an intracellular mediator that links NOX stimulation and the resulting increased mitochondrial ROS production.

## Oxylipids are useful Biomarkers of Oxidative Stress

The challenges experienced in the accurate diagnosis of oxidative stress may be addressed by further evaluating effectiveness of macromolecular (DNA, protein and lipids) damage products (Mavangira and Sordillo, 2018). Because PUFAs are highly susceptible to peroxidation during oxidative stress, specific peroxidation metabolites offer a better opportunity for accurate oxidative stress diagnosis in dairy cattle. The metabolism of PUFA occurring non-enzymatically with free radical-mediated hydrogen abstraction, followed by addition of oxygen and intramolecular rearrangement generates **stable oxylipid products**. The metabolism of arachidonic acid, e.g. generates isomers of prostaglandins known as isoprostanes (IsoPs) (Milne et al, 2015).

## Stable Oxylipid Products: Isoprostanes

Both mastitis and metritis are examples of dairy cow diseases whose incidence increases with declining antioxidant capacity (Miller et al, 1993). The demonstration of $15\text{-}F_{2t}\text{-}IsoP$ in these diseases suggests a utility of this oxylipid in assessing the role of oxidative stress in inflammatory conditions of dairy cattle.

i. Isoprostanes are currently considered as gold standard markers of oxidative stress and are utilised in human patients with oxidative stress (e.g. sepsis, atherosclerosis, coronary heart disease; Milne et al, 2015). In dairy cattle specifically, $15\text{-}F_{2t}\text{-}IsoP$ concentrations were elevated during coliform mastitis (Mavangira et al, 2016) and with retained foetal membranes. Retained foetal membranes frequently predispose dairy cattle to the development of metritis.

ii. Hydroxyl metabolites derived from arachidonic acid and linoleic acid have been utilised as oxidative stress markers; examples are 9-HETE and 9-HODE.

### Regulation of Oxylipid Metabolising Systems –Antioxidant Supplementation

Supplementation of antioxidants including selenium and vitamin E in the periparturient period has been associated with decreased postpartum disorders (Miller et al, 1993). However, antioxidant supplementation does not always result in beneficial outcomes. Bouwstra et al (2010a,b) showed an increased occurrence of mastitis following supplementation of vitamin E at low or high doses in animals starting with plasma vitamin E concentration of $>14.5$ µg/mL. Such a discrepancy may be explained by the possibility of vitamin E participating in the sequential free radical formation as a consequence of a deficient vitamin E regeneration system (VERS).

Oxylipid biosynthesis can be influenced by targeting pathways through modifying cellular redox status. Selenium is essential for maintaining the glutathione peroxidase system vital for cellular redox balance. Dairy cows consuming insufficient dietary selenium had increased pro-inflammatory oxylipid production.

### Modification of Oxylipids Through Supplementation of PUFA to have more Antioxidative Oxylipids

Modification of dietary PUFA substrate may be the obvious approach to modifying oxylipid biosynthesis. In humans and in pigs, the supplementation of PUFA altered the oxylipid profiles in peripheral blood leukocytes and plasma, respectively. In ruminants, however, this is not possible because of the happenings of rumen degradation and synthesis.

Recent studies in dairy cattle found that supplementation with n-3 PUFA through direct infusion into the abomasum could effectively modify both plasma and peripheral blood leukocyte PUFA content (Ryman et al, 2017). Evidence suggestive of the potential for n-3 PUFA supplementation in reducing inflammatory gene expression including IL-6, and IL-8 was accompanied by decreased ROS production in bovine endothelial cells (Contreras et al, 2012). Much remains to be determined on how PUFA substrate supplementation can be fine-tuned to balance the antioxidative oxylipids and those with prooxidative effects during disease in dairy cattle (Mavangira and Sordillo, 2018).

### OXIDATIVE STRESS—ROLE OF PROTEIN OXIDATION ON ANIMAL NUTRITION AND HEALTH OF FARM ANIMALS

### Introduction

Dairy cows undergo several physiological changes during the onset of lactation that can impact the magnitude and duration of the inflammatory responses. Higher nutrient demands necessary for (1) parturition and (2) onset of lactation come through coordinated shifts in nutrient partitioning. During the first month of lactation, 75% of disease incidence occurs due to the oxidative stress. Compromised immunity is the consequence.

### Oxidative Stress

Oxidative stress refers to the damage occurring to cellular macromolecules as a consequence of an imbalance between oxidants and antioxidants (Halliwell, 2007).

## Important Causes of Oxidative Stress (OS)

Uncontrolled or impaired inflammatory responses have been linked directly to increased health disorders such as mastitis and metritis (Sordillo and Mavangira, 2014). The metabolic (nutrient partitioning) and inflammatory events and environmental factors (heat stress) are the most important causes of oxidative stress. Uncontrolled inflammation is characterised by excessive levels of reactive metabolites (reactive oxygen species and reactive nitrogen species). In dairy cows conditions such as high milk yield, negative energy balance, diet, etc. contribute to increase the oxidative stress.

Several observations suggest that excessive lipid mobilisation plays a pivotal role as a link between altered energy metabolism, oxidative stress and decreased immune system efficiency (Sordillo and Mavangira, 2014; Sordillo and Raphael, 2013). Indeed, the adipose tissue secretes a great number of substances involved in the modulation of the immune response (Sodillo and Aitken, 2009; Contreras and Sordillo, 2011). Further, during excessive adipose tissue mobilisation, adipose tissue produces pro-inflammatory cytokines, while the production of adiponectin is reduced. In addition, changes in bovine nonesterified fatty acid (NEFA) concentrations and composition may alter the response of monocyte and neutrophil (Raphael and Sordillo, 2013).

Activated phagocytes and neutrophils represent another source of oxidative stress, which contribute by generating hydrogen peroxide and superoxide via a respiratory burst, and the release of the enzyme myeloperoxidase (MPO). The enzyme MPO gives rise to the potent oxidant hypochlorous acid, which plays an important role in killing invading pathogens. However, excessive generation of this oxidant can cause tissue damage and it is believed to be involved in a number of human and animal diseases.

## Effects of Oxidative Stress

Oxidative stress can virtually damage all biological molecules (DNA, RNA, cholesterol, lipids, carbohydrates and proteins).

## Oxidant-induced Damage to Macromolecules

Increased production of ROS in peripartum dairy cattle, the decrease in the total antioxidant capacity and the accumulation of lipid peroxidation products negatively impact normal functions of plasma membranes.

Lipids are the major macromolecules present in plasma membranes of cells and their internal organelles and their oxidation can impact the function and viability of cells. Lipid peroxidation products and secondary by-products also may induce toxic modification of proteins and DNA resulting in cell death. The damage to DNA may be a direct oxidation of bases or adduct formation with either lipid or protein oxidation products affecting cellular structure, function, or viability (Celi, 2011). DNA damage is thought to contribute to carcinogenesis, ageing and neurodegenerative diseases through mutations, genome instability and perturbed signalling. Furthermore, lipid peroxidation-derived aldehydes and their exocyclic adducts could be implicated in mutations (Kawai and Nuka, 2018).

Proteins are the molecules most susceptible to oxidative damage in cells because of oxidisable functional groups of the amino acids. Proteins have various and unique biological functions. Their oxidation can result in structural changes. Consequently, protein oxidation can affect cellular function because of altered protein structure. Altered protein structure occurs when thiol groups in amino acid residues such as cysteine and lysine are covalently modified resulting in alteration or loss of function. Celi and Gabai (2015) reviewed various aspects of oxidative damage to proteins, with emphasis on using oxidised proteins as markers of oxidative stress in veterinary medicine. Further the involvement of protein oxidation in pathological conditions relevant to farm animals had also been discussed.

## Protein Oxidation

It has been estimated that proteins can scavenge up to 75% of free radicals, such as hydroxyl. Protein oxidation is defined as the covalent modification of a protein induced either directly by ROS or indirectly by reaction with secondary by-products of oxidative stress. Indeed, proteins exposure to ROS causes modification of amino acid side chains and alteration of the protein structure leading to functional changes disturbing cellular metabolism associated with several pathological states (Ahmed et al, 2017).

In fact, increased side-chain hydrophilicity, side-chain and backbone fragmentation, aggregation via covalent crosslinking or hydrophobic interactions, protein unfolding and altered conformation, altered interactions with biological partners and modified turnover are observed due to protein oxidation (Davies, 2016). Oxidative damage to proteins can affect their functions as receptors, enzymes, transport, or structural proteins, etc. Oxidised proteins can also generate new antigens and provoke immune response.

Reactions of ROS with proteins and peptides can induce alterations to both the backbone and side chains. Circulating polymorphonuclear neutrophils (PMNs) are attracted to the site of infection and release oxidants and proteases to destroy the invading pathogens. Enzymes and oxidants secreted by both bacteria and PMNs result in the damage of the mammary cells and milk components, milk proteins in particular.

## Protein Carbonylation

Products of protein side chain oxidation are relatively stable and there are several assays available for their detection. The most frequently used biomarker of protein oxidation is the carbonyl assay, which measures protein carbonyl groups. Protein carbonylation occurs when ROS attack the amino acid side chains of proline, arginine, lysine and threonine in presence of transition metals ($Fe^{2+}$, $Cu^+$, etc.).

Protein carbonylation is the most frequent irreversible transformation and accumulation of protein carbonyls that have been observed in several human diseases. In general, the accumulation of oxidised proteins depends on the rate of their clearance. Degradation of oxidised proteins is influenced by the presence and the activity of specific proteases and the extent of their chemical modification: mildly oxidised proteins are highly prone to degradation, while extremely oxidised proteins (i.e. carbonylated) can form cross-links and aggregates and these are poor substrates for proteolysis.

Advanced oxidation protein products (AOPP) can be defined as synthetic markers of protein oxidation. AOPP contain abundant dityrosine and disulfide bridges, which allow cross-linking and carbonyl groups. In humans, fibrinogen and serum albumin modifications and dityrosine cross-links are the major contributors to AOPP formation.

## Oxidation of Cysteine and Methionine

Proteins rich in cysteine and methionine residues are particularly prone to oxidative stress (OS) damage. In the case of cysteine, oxidation leads to the formation of disulphide bonds, mixed disulphides and thiyl radicals, while methionine sulphoxide is the major product of methionine oxidation. The oxidation of cysteine and methionine is reversible as cells are equipped with systems, such as methonine sulphoxide reductase, glutathione, and thioredoxin redox system, capable of reversing the oxidation. It seems that the reversible oxidation/reduction of methionine may prevent the formation of more damaging forms of protein oxidative modification, namely protein carbonyl formation. Oxidation of cysteine and methionine can also result in the reversible formation of disulphides bonds between thiol groups.

## Protein Oxidation in Farm Animals

*Female Reproduction*

It is apparent that oxidative stress plays a crucial role in the cause and progression of a number of reproductive events, such as fertilisation and early embryo development and it seems that OS is involved in the regulation of the female reproductive system at different levels. Published works of P. Celi et al and A. Rizzo et al have shown that oxidative stress is associated with embryonic losses in dairy cows and that OS is involved in the pathogenesis of follicular cysts and repeat breeder syndrome in dairy cows.

It has been observed that the development of subclinical endometritis seems to be a common event in dairy cows after artificial insemination. That means pathogens are often introduced in the uterus during the artificial insemination procedure. When uterine physical defences are breached, the next line of defence is represented by neutrophils and macrophages triggering an inflammation process subsequently. The activated leukocyte and vasoactive substances released during inflammation can increase blood vessel permeability. This results in plasma protein leaking into the endometrial surface (Singh et al, 2008). Therefore, the increase in plasma advanced oxidation protein products (AOPP) in cows/buffaloes that experience embryonic mortality might be indicative of subclinical uterine infection. Hence, the assessment of oxidative stress and protein oxidation in particular, might improve our understanding of the role of OS and protein oxidation in the pathophysiology of reproductive wastage.

**Is pregnancy characterised by a pro-inflammatory state?** Gestation is considered to be associated with oxidative stress arising from increased placental mitochondrial activity and production of ROS. Interestingly, the placenta also produces ROS affecting placental function including trophoblast proliferation and differentiation and vascular reactivity (Myatt and Cui, 2004).

As consequence of the rapid foetal growth during the last trimester of pregnancy and the production of large amounts of colostrum and milk at the beginning of lactation, both maternal and foetal metabolism are increased in consequence of augmented mitochondrial activity in maternal tissues and the conceptus (Pedernera et al, 2010). This results in an increase in the production of ROS, particularly in dairy cows during late gestation (Castillo et al, 2005) and early lactation.

Considering that the activity of monocytes and macrophages is increased during pregnancy and that the concentration of several markers of oxidative stress is concomitantly increased, it could be argued that pregnancy is characterised by a pro-inflammatory state. The observation of a positive correlation between AOPP and C-reactive protein during pregnancy brings further support to the association between inflammation and OS during pregnancy.

Wen et al (2009) suggested that the important reproductive tasks such as oestrus, gestation, birth and lactation cause reproductive stress. In particular gestation is considered as constant oxidative stress for the gilt/sow. The reproductive performance of sows was shown to be related to their oxidative stress status during gestation and lactation (Zhao et al, 2013) with a risk of compromised growth and health of foetuses as well as postpartum growth of piglets. Mahan et al (2007) reported that pregnant sows were characterised by low antioxidant defences; they had low serum vitamins E and C, serum selenium and GSH-Px activity.

**Antioxidant supplementation helps to overcome the negative effects on reproductive performance:** Antioxidant supplementation is one possible approach to reduce oxidative stress during late gestation. Supplementation of gilts' diets with plant extract silymarin decreased liver and circulating protein carbonyls (Farmer et al, 2014). Conversely, the administration of polyphenol-rich foods (dried tomatoes, dried apples, dried green tea leaves and raw soy grains) in pregnant ewes resulted in an increase in protein carbonyls and a decrease in lipid peroxidation and non-protein thiols (Bubols et al, 2014). Hence, a thorough analysis of antioxidants–animal interactions is necessary to achieve a deeper understanding of the effects of antioxidant supplementation in animal diets. The use of 'plant products' rich in antioxidants is a new goal in animal nutrition (Makker et al, 2007; Celi, 2013), which needs to be explored (Celi and Gabai, 2015).

## Neonatal Physiology

Mammalian neonates are exposed (to environmental oxygen) abruptly from the hypoxic intrauterine environment to the relatively hyperoxic external environment at birth. In response to the changes in extracellular environmental conditions, the cells of newborn animals generate large amount of ROS leading to neonatal oxidative stress. Important predisposing factors include reduced antioxidant defences and presence of free iron, which enhances the Fenton reaction leading to production of highly toxic hydroxyl radicals. A compromised redox balance (an imbalance between antioxidant- and oxidant-generating systems) leads to oxidative damages. In a study designed to evaluate the oxidant/antioxidant balance in dairy calves from birth to weaning, it has been reported that antioxidative defences increased with time in newborn calves.

Newborn piglets are shown to suffer seriously from birth oxidative stress due to the immature antioxidative system (Yin et al, 2013). The activities of two major antioxidant enzymes (SOD and GSH-Px) in the piglet plasma and ileal Nrf2 significantly increased during the first week after birth preventing lipid and protein oxidation in piglet plasma (Yin et al, 2013).

## Feeds and Method of Feeding

In dairy cattle prolonged concentrate feeding increased lipid peroxidation and decreased α-tocopherol and ferric reducing ability of plasma (Wullepit et al, 2009). An increase in oxidative stress has also been observed when high levels of starch have been fed to dairy cows (Gabai et al, 2004). It has been demonstrated that an increase in dietary concentrate content and a reduction in dietary NDF content are associated with an increase in ruminal endotoxin (Zabeli and Metzler-Zabeli, 2012), which may stimulate the production of pro-inflammatory cytokines, ROS, and bioactive lipids.

Studies of P.Celi, Raadsma, Robinson show an increase in AOPP concentration in dairy cows and in growing dairy calves when they are fed on maize silage. Silage is characterised by low antioxidant content and when its level in the diet is increased, it could lead to oxidative stress. Further, as the antioxidant capacity of rumen bacteria is less developed than that of aerobe microbes, the lower antioxidant content of the silage might also expose ruminal bacteria to oxidative stress, impairing their activity, growth and finally decreasing ruminant production. Indeed, a negative correlation between AOPP concentration and milk yield has been observed in dairy cows.

In horses, the ingestion of excessive amount of **rapidly fermentable carbohydrates** (e.g. starch from cereal grains or sugar and fructans from pasture) can induce laminitis (a condition that has been associated with oxidative stress). Rapidly fermented carbohydrates induce lactic acid production and increase hindgut mucosal permeability. Therefore, endotoxins [lipopolysaccharides (LPS)], exotoxins (protease) and amines are released by the disturbed gut microflora leading to the activation of neutrophils, release of cytokines and other inflammatory and OS mediators, which ultimately lead to the activation of matrix metalloproteinase that results in laminitis (Harris et al, 2006).

Interestingly, an increase in AOPP concentration has been observed in obese ponies subjected to high level of energy restriction. This observation may be attributed to the high level of lipomobilisation as reflected by the increase in triglycerides and NEFA concentrations, which are then prone to oxidation. This observation further supports the link between energy balance, metabolism and oxidant - antioxidant balance (Pedernera et al, 2010).

Supplementing pigs' diet with *L-methionine* resulted in a reduction of melondialdehyde (MDA) and protein carbonyl levels in duodenal mucosal samples, indicating a decrease in oxidative stress in the mucosa of the duodenum (Shen et al, 2014). It may be due to the greater efficiency of L-methionine, compared to DL-methionine, in enhancing GSH synthesis in the intestinal mucosa. L-methionine is also known to be a potent ROS scavenger. In duodenal mucosal cells, free L-methionine and L-methionine residues in protein act as endogenous antioxidants (Shen et al, 2014).

Oxidised feeds can induce protein oxidation in birds. In poultry, feeding diets with oxidised oil or animal-vegetable fat increased plasma protein carbonyl content. Dietary antioxidant supplementation with organic selenium and minerals or with saponins is able to reduce oxidative stress in poultry by eliminating or decreasing the production of protein carbonyls. Therefore, Celi and Gabai (2015) proposed inclusion of AOPP and protein carbonyl in the panel of biomarkers to study the relationships between OS, nutrition, metabolism and gut health in veterinary medicine.

## Respiratory Diseases

The respiratory system is a major site of oxidative stress insult and it appears that pulmonary oxidative stress is crucial for the progression of respiratory disease especially in horses. Lungs are quite susceptible to LPS, a major component of the outer membrane of gram-negative bacteria.

Studies in piglets have shown that ampelopsin (a flavonoid with known antioxidant activity) is able to reduce the lung protein carbonyl content in LPS-challenged piglets.

Recently in a study designed to evaluate oxidative stress responses in foetal lambs exposed to intra-amniotic endotoxin, a significant increase in protein carbonyls was observed in their bronchoalveolar lavage fluid (BALF) and in their plasma. Therefore, the investigation of proteins oxidation could represent a novel tool to study the role of oxidative stress in the etiopathogenesis of respiratory diseases in veterinary medicine (Celi and Gabai, 2015).

## Animal Management Practices

Marco-Ramell, A. et al (2011 and 2012) observed an increase in plasma protein oxidation in pigs housed at high densities and in cattle living in hard conditions. While these observations could be due to several factors (nutrition, environmental conditions), they also suggest that animals might adopt different behavioural strategies in order to cope with stress. That is why oxidative stress biomarkers have been proposed as new and reliable indicators of animal welfare, since stress of any origin can deplete the body's antioxidant resources.

## Protein Oxidation in Heat/Cold Stress— Need for Higher Levels of Antioxidants

Heat stress has been implicated in the generation of oxidative stress either through excessive ROS production or decreased antioxidant defences (Chauhan et al, 2014b). Heat stress increases AOPP concentration in sheep and pigs, while supra-physiological doses of vitamin E and selenium are able to reduce the oxidation of plasma protein (Liu et al, 2015). The lower AOPP concentration in heat stressed lambs fed supra-physiological doses of vitamin E and selenium is indicative of protective role of these two antioxidants against the oxidative stress damage of proteins induced by heat stress. These findings reinforce the need for higher levels of antioxidants than the current recommended levels under stressful conditions.

Studies in broiler chickens have also demonstrated that high temperatures induce both lipid and protein oxidation. It seems that acute heat stress might induce oxidative stress by disrupting the respiratory chain complex. Interestingly, low ambient temperature conditions increase the amount of protein carbonyls in liver and lung of broiler chickens. Cold can be considered as a stressor and therefore lower temperature can induce oxidative stress.

The increase in AOPP during heat stress was accompanied by an increased expression of TNF-α (Chauhan et al, 2014b). This suggests a strong association between protein oxidation and mediators of pro-inflammatory responses (Celi, 2010) indicating that heat stress leads to undesired pro-inflammatory responses that may compromise animal performance (Chauhan et al, 2014a). Therefore, the manipulation of dietary micronutrients and antioxidants has the potential to prevent the effects of oxidative damage (Chauhan et al, 2014a) thereby enhancing animal resilience to heat stress.

**Oxidised protein products in milk can be noninvasive tools that reflects oxidative status of the animal:** A state of oxidative stress can be observed in the periparturient cow in response to the copious milk yield and mammary gland remodelling. At least three sources of OS can be identified: the shift in cellular metabolism during the transition period, the contribution of immune cells (PMN and phagocytes) and the intensive mammary epithelial cell replacement occurring after termination of milking. In a preliminary study,

Celi and Gabai, (2015) observed that plasmatic AOPP significantly decreased, while plasmatic carbonyl groups significantly increased in cows around parturition.

Between two consecutive milking bouts most of milk produced resides within mammary alveoli and ducts for a significant time, exposing milk proteins to the action of oxidising enzymes, such as MPO, lactoperoxidase and xanthine oxidase present in the surrounding mammary and immune cells. Thus, oxidative stress biomarkers in colostrum and milk may reflect the oxidative status within the mammary gland. Hence, oxidised protein products in milk and whey can be noninvasive tools for investigating the oxidative status of the dairy cow (Celi and Gabai, 2015).

**Conclusion:** Animal health and welfare are crucial for a sustainable production system. How, the inevitable oxidative stress during the animal's life stages influence metabolism and health is of great interest. The study of oxidant/antioxidant balance is contributing to the understanding of important pathways involved in regulation of cellular functions and metabolism. When ROS accumulates because of high metabolic rates, this may result in an impairment of the redox balance leading to oxidative stress. Stress can negatively impact immune function and health of the animals. Hence, future research should investigate the strategies needed in the maintenance of redox homeostasis in all the life stages.

# Oxidative Stress Combating Potential of Plant Phenols

## IMPACT OF NATURAL PLANT PRODUCTS ON IMMUNOMODULATION IN ANIMALS

### Primary and Secondary Plant Products

Plants provide herbivore animals an array of chemicals with the potential to improve their health and well-being. Plant products may be categorised into primary and secondary: Primary products are meant for primary roles of photosynthesis, respiration, growth and development of the plants, while the secondary category phytochemicals protect plants from consumers and pests by adversely affecting their cellular and metabolic processes (Cozier et al, 2006). But at low doses and in appropriate mixtures, they can have beneficial effects on animal nutrition and health (Provenza, 2008). That is the silverline for animal nutritionists to use the secondary products profitably. These phytochemicals are variously called: plant secondary compounds or plant secondary metabolites (PSC or PSM) or secondary plant metabolites (SPM).

### Beneficial Effects of Primary and Secondary Compounds

#### Primary Compounds

Certain 'primary' compounds have the potential to function as medicines. For instance, certain polysaccharides, polymers of glucose (glucans), mannose (mannans), xylose (hemicellulose) and fructose (levans) provide immune-stimulating and antineoplasic activity (Tizard et al, 1989). The importance of amino acids and proteins has long been recognised in immune function. Nutritional immunology is emerging as a new discipline exploring the role of nutrients in the metabolism and function of cells of the immune system (Li et al, 2007).

#### Secondary Compounds

Eating plants high in tannins is a way for herbivore animals to reduce internal parasites and alleviate bloat by binding those tannins to proteins in the rumen. By this process tannins also enhance nutrition through provision of high-quality 'bypass' protein to the small intestines, since plant protein is unavailable for digestion and absorption until it reaches the more acidic abomasum (Barry et al, 2001). Plant-derived alkaloids such as terpenes and phenolics also have antiparasitic properties (Kayser et al, 2003), while sesquiterpene lactones have anti-tumourigenic, anti-amoebic, anti-bacterial, anti-fungal and cardiotonic properties (Huffman et al, 1998).

### Plant-derived Immunomodulators for the Grazing Animals

Natural landscapes are diverse mixtures of plant species. They may be considered as

131

nutrition centres and pharmacies with vast arrays of primary (nutrient) and secondary (pharmaceutical) compounds vital in the nutrition and health of plants, herbivores and people (Provenza, 2008). Consumers increasingly demand products that are "clean" and "green". These emerging trends reflect increasing appreciation of the health benefits of natural plant products and provide a spur for seeking novel/alternative approaches to control disease with secondary plant compounds. The use of natural plant products as immunomodulators has the potential to enhance animal health.

Plant-derived immunomodulatory compounds have been used in traditional remedies for both humans and animals. Provenza and Villalba (2010) reviewed how the natural plant products can benefit the animals by way of preventing and combating the diseases through immunomodulatory effects with an aim to provoke discussion and spur readers into new ways of studying the relationships among foraging behaviour, natural plant products and immune responses in the herbivores.

## Can Natural Plant Products "Modulate" Immune Responses?

Mammalian immunomodulators such as signalling compounds from the immune system include interferon gamma (IFN-γ), granulocyte colony-stimulating factor and granulocyte-macrophage colony-stimulating factor (GMCSF) (Schepetkin and Quinn, 2006). In addition, some carbohydrates isolated and purified from microorganisms have immune-stimulating properties.

Phagocytic cells of the innate immune system do not recognise every possible antigen, unlike T and B cells. Instead, they recognise a few highly conserved structures called "pathogen-associated molecular patterns" (PAMP), present in many different microorganisms and interact with receptors on the surface of immune cells (Janeway et al, 2005).

Lipopolysaccharides (LPS) from the gram-negative bacteria cell wall, peptidoglycan from the gram-positive bacteria cell wall, the sugar mannose from some viruses and glucans from fungal cell walls are recognised by innate immune cells (Carroll, 2008). Collectins bind to these carbohydrates on various microorganisms and to specific receptors on phagocytic cells, thus facilitate enhanced phagocytosis by the innate immune system. For example, cows fed a mannan oligosaccharide (MOS) has enhanced immune response to rotavirus, which tended to enhance the subsequent transfer of rotavirus antibodies to calves (Franklin et al, 2005).

These complex carbohydrates (LPS, peptidoglycan, mannans, glucans), common in fungi and yeasts, are also present in vascular plants. Galactomannans (copolymers of galactose and mannose) are found in seeds of soya beans, glucans in oats and arabinogalactans in Juniper (Tizard et al, 1989). All these compounds stimulate macrophage function, from phagositosis to nitric oxide and cytokine production. Likewise, plants from the genus *Echinacea* contain arabinogalactans, fructofuranosides and heteroxylans that increase mouse, rat and human macrophage activity. Thus natural plant products modulate immune response.

Supplementing oligosaccharides may promote the formation of antioligosaccharide antibodies in the gut (Srinivasan et al, 1999), which in turn may enter the bloodstream and enhance the immune response to oligosaccharides in some virus-containing vaccines. Epithelial cells lining the respiratory, gastrointestinal and urogenital mucous membranes function not only as terminal effector sites but also as inducers of mucosal humoral immunity.

## Is Ingesting Immunomodulators that Act as Adjuvants Beneficial?

The immunomodulatory carbohydrates may also act as adjuvants, improving phagositosis and enhancing the immune response (Franklin et al, 2005). Stimulation of the innate immune system is essential for activating the adaptive immune response. For instance, macrophages and dendritic cells initiate the adaptive immune response by presenting an antigen to CD4+ T cells via the class II MHC antigen (Beutler, 2004).

The release of pro-inflammatory cytokines (PIC; interleukin-1, interleukin-6, tumour necrosis factor-$\alpha$ and interferon) by cells of the innate immune system during infection initiates the acute phase response (APR) and the adaptive immune response. These responses alter protein and lipid metabolism and thus influence growth and efficiency of gain (Johnson, 1997).

The production of these **signalling compounds** from macrophages and monocytes at the site of infection is characterised by fever, increased synthesis of the acute phase proteins (APP) by the liver, increased circulating white blood cells, as well as increased sleep, decreased feed and water intake, decreased social and sexual behaviour, decreased aggressive behaviour, increased pain reactivity and increased activity of the stress axis (Carroll, 2008). Thus, the ingestion/administration of compounds that "stimulate" the immune system through an adjuvant-like mechanism for preventive/protective purposes **affects the production and well-being of animals.**

The direct anti-parasitic, anti-fungal and anti-bacterial positive characteristics of plant secondary compounds/metabolites (PSC/PSM) are accompanied with negative impacts as cellular and physiological processes of the disease-inducing agents can also adversely affect the host. Thus, the potential benefits associated with consuming certain immunostimulants by animals must be traded-off against their potentially negative consequences on the host (Provenza and Villalba, 2010). However, it is beneficial to treat endoparasites in humid areas. This is an option to be of use in situations of demand.

## Some Oligosaccharides Stimulate Immune Responses without Inflammation

Some oligosaccharides seem to stimulate immune responses without causing inflammation thereby providing modulatory instead of stimulatory effects (non-inflammatory activation). Example the cell walls of yeasts such as *Saccharomyces cerevisiae*, mannan oligosaccharides (MOS). Pigs supplemented with MOS have a greater proportion of blood lymphocytes/neutrophils (without an increase in acute-phase proteins) and they also have higher weight gains and better feed efficiencies. These effects suggest mannan supplementation alleviates alterations in immune function that result in an inflammatory response (Davis et al, 2004). Pigs supplemented with MOS produced less pro-inflammatory (TNF-$\alpha$) and more anti-inflammatory (IL-10) cytokines than unsupplemented pigs (Che et al, 2008), which also suggests an immunomodulatory effect without the negative impacts of inflammation.

## Mucosal Immunity and Natural Plant Products

The mucosal immune system is different in many ways from its systemic counterpart. The mucosa is directly exposed to the external environment and continuously stimulated by antigens from commensal bacteria, dietary antigens and pathogens in far greater quantities each day than the systemic immune system has to endure in a lifetime (Mayer, 2003). Thus normal mucosal immune responses are generally associated with suppression and regulation rather than stimulation of the immune system.

Different components of the mucosal immune system respond specifically to exogenous antigens. The first line in this defence is the secretory IgA system, which produces abundant mucosal antibodies (SIgA) that mainly inhibit bacterial/viral attachment to the underlying epithelium and the inflammatory effects of other immunoglobulins. The commensal bacteria release immunomodulatory factors such as polysaccharides that regulate the balance between inflammatory/anti-inflammatory cytokines. These immunomodulatory factors in turn enable tolerance of these bacteria in the gastrointestinal tract. Thus, mucosal immunity can be modulated by administering exogenous polysaccharides or by modifying the commensal microflora.

For instance, polysaccharides present in the cell walls of some plants, yeast and fungi are potent inductors of macrophages and some favour the production of anti-inflammatory cytokines (Schepetkin and Quinn, 2006). These cytokines initiate the recruitment of antigen-presenting cells such as dendritic cells and macrophages that bind to the bioactive polysaccharide through mannose receptors causing non-inflammatory activation (Porporatto et al, 2003). The polysaccharide chitosan favours immunosuppressory responses rich in anti-inflammatory cytokines that stimulate the production and differentiation of regulatory myeloid cells at local and systemic levels (Porporatto et al, 2007).

## Natural Plant Products have Potential to Regulate Local and Systemic Immune Responses

Interactions occur between gut-associated myeloid tissues and commensal bacteria or their structural components that lead to modulation of T- or B cell mediated immune responses, either locally or systemically. For instance, the immune system favours some microbes allowing commensal microbes to persist on mucosal surfaces, while eliminating disease causing pathogens.

- Early colonisation of intestines of 1-day-old chicks by a probiotic containing *Lactobacillus acidophilus, Bifidobacterium bifidum* and *Streptococcus faecalis* enhanced the systemic antibody responses to sheep red blood cells (SRBC) in chickens.

- Administering probiotics also enhances serum and intestinal natural antibodies to several foreign antigens.

This suggests that the effect of probiotic bacteria in reducing colonisation of intestinal pathogens may be due in part to stimulation of natural antibodies. Thus, the **bacteriostatic/ bactericidal** effects of some natural plant products on the gastrointestinal microflora have the potential to regulate local and systemic immune responses through a **probiotic** effect, besides the effects of polysaccharides on mucosal immunity.

## Effects of Specific PSC or PSM or SPM on immune function

Phenolic compounds are widely distributed throughout the plant kingdom. They can be classified into two groups: the flavonoids and the nonflavonoids. See page 142.

### Flavonoids

Flavonoids are a large group of SPM and possess numerous potentially health-beneficial biological activities. The main effects of flavonoids on immune responses may derive from their different mechanisms of action such as protein binding, active site interference, or antioxidant effects. Several flavonoids specifically affect the function of enzymes involved in generating inflammatory responses. Dietary flavonoids seem to modulate the inflammatory response and have primarily inhibitory effects on T lymphocytes (Middleton et al, 2000). Many of the structurally diverse flavonoids stimulate natural killer (NK) cell activity and have thus great potential as diet-derived immuno-modulatory chemoprotective agents (Burkard et al, 2017; The Journal of Nutritional Biochemistry, 46: 1–12). Some flavonoids also alter immune responses which could be involved in immunosurveillance of tumours, e.g. quercetin.

Cocoa flavonoids modulate the cellular immune response *in vitro*, inhibiting the production of ROS (hydrogen peroxide and superoxide anion) by lymphocytes and granulocytes. Cocoa liquor phenols inhibit the proliferation of lymphocytes and the production of immunoglobins. They also modulate the secretion of PIC by myeloid cells (Lamuela-Raventos et al, 2005).

## Condensed Tannins

By making the protein unavailable for digestion and absorption until it reaches the more acidic abomasum, tannins enhance nutrition by providing high-quality protein to the small intestines (Barry et al, 2001) in ruminants. This high-quality 'bypass' protein has the potential to enhance the immune response and increase resistance to gastrointestinal nematodes (Min et al, 2004). 'Bypass' amino acids like arginine, glutamine and cysteine can enhance immune responses as these amino acids regulate activation of T and B lymphocytes, natural killer cells and macrophages, gene expression and lymphocyte proliferation and the production of antibodies, cytokines and other cytotoxic substances (Li et al, 2007).

Condensed tannins have bactericidal effects (Min et al, 2002), which may impact intestinal bacteria. Hence, changes in populations of commensal bacteria in the gastrointestinal tract may stimulate gut-associated myeloid tissues and consequently modulate T- or B-cell-mediated immune responses. Calves treated with **green tea polyphenols** had more beneficial commensal species of *Bifidobacterium* and *Lactobacillus* and fewer harmful *Clostridium perfringens*. Thus, through their effects on intestinal bacteria, **tannins may have probiotic effects** that indirectly impact the immune system.

## Alkaloids

Alkaloids are a diverse group of nitrogen-containing compounds, present in about 20% of plant species, mostly derived from amino acids. Many of the alkaloids have been used as pharmaceuticals, stimulants, narcotics and poisons.

**Some alkaloids have been tested for their impacts on immune function.** Punarnavine, an alkaloid from *Boerhaavia diffusa*, enhanced natural killer (NK) cell activity, antibody-dependent cellular cytotoxicity and antibody-dependent complement mediated cytotoxicity in tumour-bearing mice. In contrast, PIC were significantly reduced by punarnavine. The

extract (cepharanthin) of *Stephania cepharantha* Hayata contains biscoclaurine alkaloids. These are widely used in Japan to treat many acute and chronic diseases because directly or indirectly they activate macrophages through T cell-associated effects. Supplementing cattle consuming endophyte-infected tall fescue with Tasco-Forage, an extract of the seaweed *Ascophyllum nodosum,* enhanced monocyte cell function, thus improving innate immunity, likely due to its antioxidant activity.

**Some alkaloids may have immunosuppressant effects.** Ergot alkaloids in endophyte-infected tall fescue impair immune function. This may be due to altered antioxidant status, including vitamin E, in both the plant and the animal.

## Terpenes

Terpenes are a large and varied class of hydrocarbons derived biosynthetically from units of isoprene. They represent one of the most diverse classes of plant secondary metabolites (PSM). They were identified from fragrances, etc.

Terpenes extracted from *Zanthoxylum rhoifolium* significantly improved NK cell cytotoxicity *in vitro* and *in vivo* in tumours. Terpenes in *Ginkgo biloba* (e.g. ginkgolides and bilobalide) reduce the production of some pro-inflammatory cytokines. Some terpenes also are immunosuppressive agents.

Terpenes have bacteriostatic and bactericidal properties and they have selective effects on ruminal bacteria (Villalba et al, 2006a). As with tannins, the selective effects of terpenes on the gastrointestinal tract could have indirect effects on immunomodulation.

### *Antrodia Cinnamomea* Powder Supplementation

*Antrodia cinnamomea* (a precious and unique medical fungus) exhibits antioxidant and immunomodulatory properties. *Antrodia cinnamomea* powder (ACP) was supplemented at 0.1, 0.2 and 0.4% in broiler chickens diets for 35 days. Its phenolics include triterpenoids. The experimental findings revealed that ACP could induce the Nrf2-dependent pathway and decrease the NFκB-dominated inflammatory signalling pathway. Antioxidant genes dominated by Nrf2 genes, such as HO-1 and GCLC, were up-regulated, while inflammatory-related genes, such as IL-1β and IL-6, ruled mainly by NFκB were down-regulated. Body weight enhancement with ACP supplementation further implied the promising effects exerted by ACP (Lee et al, 2018; Poultry Science, 97: 2419–2434).

## Learning about Foods and Animal Self-medication: Dynamic Interplay between Flavour and Postingestive Feedback

The biochemical diversity present in the nature provides animals with the opportunity to enhance their health and well-being. Provenza et al (2003) have recommended providing the animals with a variety of biochemically diverse plant species, allowing them to learn to consume so that the immunomodulatory effects of specific bioactive compounds are enhanced without negatively impacting their health, welfare and production.

Food preference in herbivore animals develops due to the dynamic interplay between flavour and postingestive feedback, which are determined by an animal's physiological condition and a plant's chemical characteristics (Provenza, 1995; Provenza and Villalba, 2006). Animals use flavours (taste, smell, texture) to discriminate among the feeds. Postingestive feedback calibrates a food's flavour with its homeostatic utility. If a particular food provides chemicals that are required by an animal at a certain point in space and time, then the animal will associate the flavour of that food with a benefit to the body and preference will increase. In contrast, if a food supplies chemicals that provide negative effects to the body or compounds not needed in that particular point in time, postingestive feedback will cause a decline in food preference and intake. Thus, **food selection in animals is the constant quest for substances in the external environment that provide a homeostatic benefit to the internal environment.**

Nutrients, toxins and medicines are the labels scientists use to better comprehend foraging complexity. But for the animal that grazes/browses/ingests all these nutrients, toxins and medicines are the means to survive and produce (Villalba and Provenza, 2007).

**Preference for PEG, bentonite or dicalcium phosphate:** Sheep increase intake of medicinal substances such as polyethylene glycol (PEG) (a polymer that attenuates the aversive effects of tannins) as tannin concentrations in their diet increase. They discriminate the medicinal effects of PEG from "nonmedicinal" substances by selectively increasing intake of PEG after eating a meal high in tannins. They also forage in locations where PEG is present, rather than where it is absent, when offered nutritious feeds high in tannins in different locations.

Similarly, sheep select an anti-acid (sodium bentonite) after ingesting a meal that causes ruminal acidosis. They prefer substances that neutralise the effects of tannins (e.g. PEG) and oxalic acid (e.g. dicalcium phosphate) after ingesting meals with these PSM.

Sheep also increase preference for tannin-containing foods when they are infected with endoparasites relative to when parasitic loads are not present. From these findings, it can be inferred that **animals have capacity to learn to ingest immunomodulatory substances that restore health**.

**Beneficial effects of offering diverse feeds:** Herbivores exposed to varied diets may ingest PSC or PSM under normal situations, simply as a consequence of consuming multiple foods. Consuming diverse feeds likely play (1) a significant role in preventing disease and maintaining health. (2) Sheep eat more when offered choices of feeds with various toxins that affect different detoxification mechanisms (Lyman et al, 2008). (3) Animals may minimise the negative effects of SPC through the effect of self-medication (Villalba and Provenza, 2007).

Huffman et al (1998) reported that African great ape routinely consumed 192 recognised plant food species thereby reaping the nutrition and health benefits of the diverse array of compounds found in foods. Eating diverse diets thus undoubtedly provides all the advantages of bioactive compounds such as immunomodulators with health-maintenance effects (Provenza and Villalba, 2010).

## Interactions Among PSC/PSM

When animals graze chemically diverse pastures the secondary compounds (PSC or PSM) may interact with each other, thus reducing the potential immunomodulatory properties of any (or) all of the bioactive compounds available. For instance, condensed tannins evidently form stable complexes with proteins, saponins, alkaloids and terpenes. Tannins, terpenes and alkaloids can co-occur in the digesta of animals consuming diverse diets and thus the biological activity of plant secondary metabolites (PSM) may be reduced significantly after the formation of such complexes.

Natural plant products may provide herbivore animals with plant secondary compounds/metabolites (PSC/PSM), which modulate the immune system at local and systemic levels. These secondary compounds may not only have a **direct effect** on pathogens due to their negative impacts on cells and metabolic processes, they may also provide the consumers with **indirect effects** on health through their probiotic and immunomodulatory properties that may lead to prevention instead of treatment of disease. Plant secondary compounds or metabolites are 'no longer just toxins' but valuable nutrients when administered appropriately as per the physiological state of the animal (Provenza and Villalba, 2010).

## BIOLOGICAL ACTIVITY OF TANNINS AND THEIR EFFECTS IN RUMINANT AND MONOGASTRIC ANIMALS

Naturally occurring plant compounds including tannins, saponins and essential oils are extensively assessed as natural alternatives to in-feed antibiotics. Tannins are a group of polyphenolic compounds that are widely present in plants and possess various biological activities including antimicrobial, anti-parasitic, antiviral, antioxidant, anti-inflammatory, immunomodulation, etc. Tannins are widely distributed in plant kingdom, especially abundant in nutritionally important forages, shrubs, cereals and medicinal herbs. They are also found in many fruit species such as banana, blackberry, apple and grape as well as tea.

## Classification of Tannins

Tannins are primarily classified into three major groups: hydrolysable tannins (HT), condensed tannins (CT; or proanthocyanidins), and phlorotannins (PT) (Fig. 4.1A to C). The first two groups are found in terrestrial plants, while phlorotannins occur only in marine brown algae.

Hydrolysable tannins are susceptible to hydrolysis by acids, bases or esterases, thus can be easily degraded and absorbed in the digestive tract and may cause potential toxic effects in herbivores. Condensed tannins are oligomeric or polymeric flavonoids consisting of flavan-3-ol units that include catechin, epicatechin, gallocatechin and epigallocatechin. Only strong oxidative and acidic hydrolysis can depolymerise the condensed tannin structures that are also not susceptible to anaerobic enzyme degradation (McSweeney et al, 2001).

Condensed tannins are the most common type of tannin in forage legumes, trees and shrubs, while HT is often present in leaves of trees and browse shrubs in tropical areas. Generally, tannins are more abundant in vulnerable parts of the plants, e.g. new leaves and flowers. The PT are concentrated in the physodes located in the cytoplasm of cells within the outer cortical layers of the thalli.

## Biological Activity of Tannins

Tannins are plant secondary metabolites (PSM) that serve as a part of plant chemical

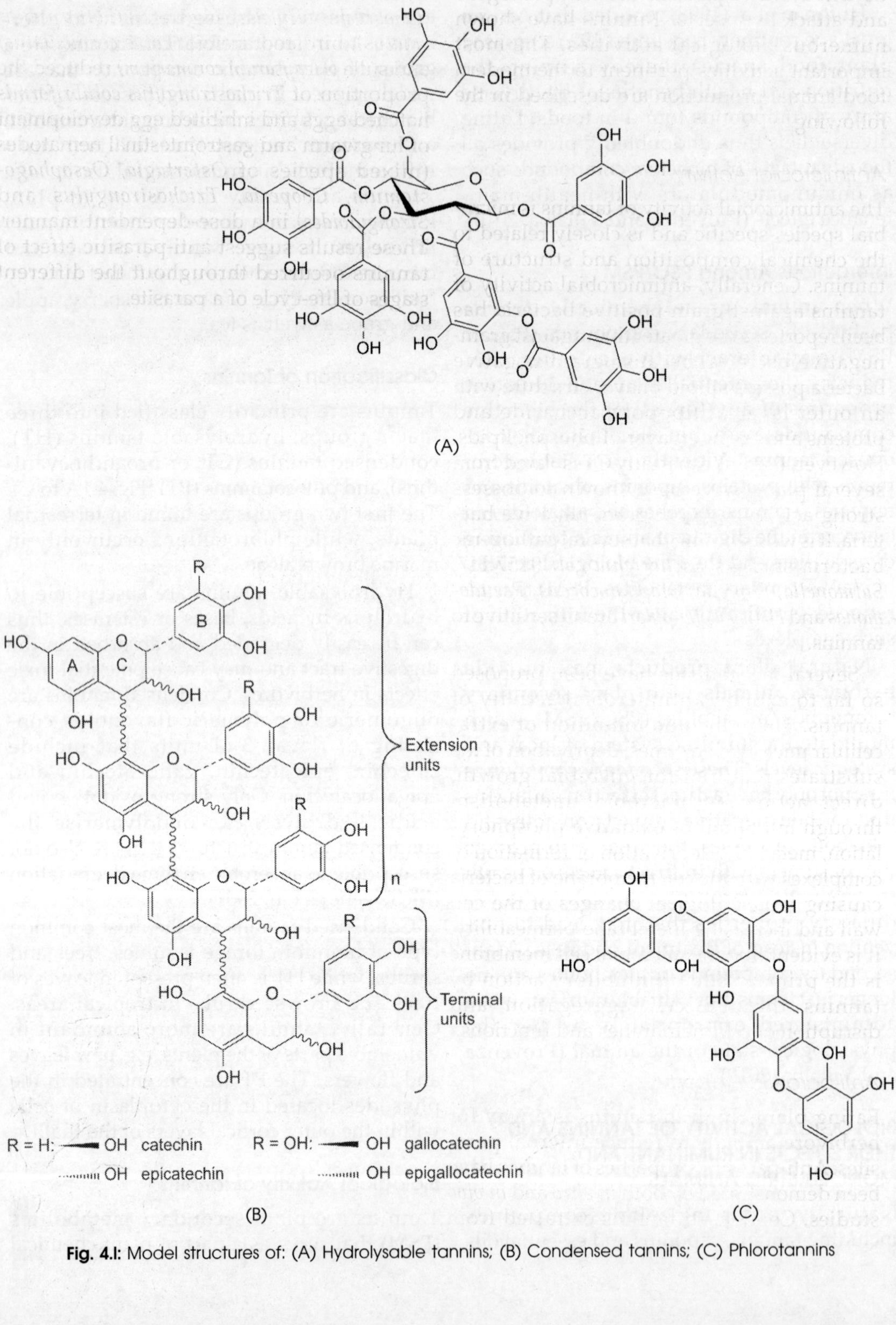
(A)
Extension units
n
Terminal units
R = H: OH catechin
OH epicatechin
R = OH: OH gallocatechin
OH epigallocatechin
(B)
(C)

**Fig. 4.I:** Model structures of: (A) Hydrolysable tannins; (B) Condensed tannins; (C) Phlorotannins

defence system against invasion by pathogens and attack by insects. Tannins have shown numerous biological activities. The most important activities pertinent to the modern food animal production are described in the following.

## Antimicrobial Activity

The antimicrobial activity of tannins is microbial species-specific and is closely related to the chemical composition and structure of tannins. Generally, antimicrobial activity of tannins against gram-positive bacteria has been reported to be greater than against gram-negative bacteria, because gram-negative bacteria possess a lipid bilayer structure with an outer layer of lipopolysaccharide and proteins and an inner layer of phospholipids. However, tannins especially CT isolated from several plants have been shown to possess strong activity against gram-negative bacteria. It is worth noting that several pathogenic bacteria such as *Escherichia coli* 0157:H7, *Salmonella, Shigella, Staphylococcus, Pseudomonas* and *Helicobacter pylori* are all sensitive to tannins.

Several mechanisms have been proposed so far to explain antimicrobial activity of tannins. These include inhibition of extracellular microbial enzymes, deprivation of the substrates required for microbial growth, direct action on microbial metabolism through inhibition of oxidative phosphorylation, metal ions deprivation or formation of complexes with the cell membrane of bacteria causing morphological changes of the cell wall and increasing membrane permeability. It is evident that the microbial cell membrane is the primary site of inhibitory action by tannins through cell aggregation and disruption of cell membranes and functions.

## Anti-parasitic Property

Eating plants high in tannins is a way for herbivore animals to reduce internal parasites. Anti-parasitic properties of tannins have been demonstrated by both *in vitro* and *in vivo* studies. Condensed tannins extracted from legume tanniferous forages such as sainfoin *(Onobrychis viciifolia)*, big trefoil *(Lotus pedunculatus)*, birdsfoot trefoil *(Lotus corniculatus)* and sulla *(Hedysarum coronarium)* reduced the proportion of *Trichostrongylus colubriformis* hatched eggs and inhibited egg development of lungworm and gastrointestinal nematodes (mixed species of *Ostertagia, Oesophagostomum, Cooperia, Trichostrongylus* and *Strongyloides*) in a dose-dependent manner. These results suggest anti-parasitic effect of tannins occurred throughout the different stages of life-cycle of a parasite.

## Antioxidant Property

Naturally occurring phenolic compounds have long been recognised as effective antioxidants (Rice-Evans et al, 1995, 1996). The antioxidant property of tannins has wide application in food industry and medical field to prevent oxidative stress related diseases such as cardiovascular disease, cancer or osteoporosis. It has been shown that CT and HT of relatively high molecular weight exhibited greater antioxidant activities than simple phenolics. The number of hydroxyl groups and the degree of polymerisation of tannins are considered to be correlated with their abilities to scavenge free radicals. Tannins with the most hydroxyl groups (see Fig. 4.1) are most easily oxidised and therefore possess greatest antioxidant activity. It has been demonstrated that effectiveness of tannins as natural antioxidants is due to their complex combinations of reducing and redox activities, which also contributes to their abilities to scavenge radicals.

Inclusion of forage containing CT improved the antioxidant status of both cattle and sheep by increasing serum antioxidant activity (Huang et al, 2015; Peng et al, 2016). Quebracho tannins in lamb diets improved the antioxidant status of muscle (Luciano et al, 2011), liver and plasma (Lopez-Andres et al, 2013) and enhanced meat colour stability by delaying myoglobin oxidation during refrigerated storage (Luciano et al, 2009).

Lopez-Andres et al (2013) found that quebracho tannins were not degraded or absorbed in the gastrointestinal tract, but increased the antioxidant capacity of liver and plasma in sheep. This demonstrated that CT may indirectly affect antioxidant status in animal tissues. The tannins-protein complexation has been shown to reduce but not eliminate the antioxidant activities of tannins (Arts et al, 2002). It has been speculated that dietary tannins may spare other nutritive antioxidants during digestive process or they may protect proteins, carbohydrates and lipids in the digestive tract from oxidative damage during digestion. However, the antioxidant mechanism of tannins in animal tissues is unknown. Hence, this is a fertile area of research, because **enhancing antioxidant status is suggested to be one of the most benefits of feeding tannins to animal well-being and performance** (Huang et al, 2015).

## Anti-inflammatory Property

Tannins possess varying anti-inflammatory activities (Park et al, 2014) that are positively associated with their antioxidant activities (Park et al, 2014). *In vitro* studies have showed that tannins from grape-seed lowered low-grade inflammatory disease such as obesity by modulating cytokine expression. Park et al (2014) demonstrated the anti-inflammatory activity of CT extracted from black raspberry seeds. Hydrolysable tannins from *Myricaria bracteata* showed a significant anti-inflammatory effect.

It is speculated that the mechanism of anti-inflammatory effects is related to the potent ability for scavenging free radicals rather than inhibitory effects of HT on nitric oxide and pro-inflammatory cytokines production.

Phlorotannins from *A. nodosum* and *Ecklonia cava* also exhibited potent anti-inflammatory effects based on their ability to inhibit cytokines release, nitric oxide and prostaglandin-$E_2$ production. The efficacy of the anti-inflammatory action of tannins in animal body needs to be evaluated further in *in vivo* model (Huang et al, 2015), since most of the studies are based on *in vitro* tests.

## Antivirus Property

Tannins have been shown to have significant activity against some virus, e.g. human immunodeficiency virus (HIV), bovine adeno-associated virus and noroviruses. Epigallocatechin from green-tea was reported to inhibit hepatitis C virus (HCV) entry. Hydrolysable tannins inhibited HCV entry and cell-to-cell transmission but did not interfere with intracellular HCV replication. Phlorotannins isolated from *E. cava* have been demonstrated to possess strong activity against influenza virus neuraminidase, porcine epidemic diarrhoea virus (PEDV) by inhibiting viral entry and/or viral replication.

All the aforesaid information demonstrated that tannins possess varying antivirus activities depending on chemical composition and structure. *In vivo* studies are needed to explore the potential of tannins as natural antivirus agents to be used in animal and poultry industries.

## Use of Tannins in Ruminants

Tannins especially condensed tannins are widely distributed in nutritionally important forages, trees, shrubs and legumes, which are commonly consumed by ruminants. In view of this, the effects of CT on ruminant nutrition, health and production have been extensively studied and reviewed (Mueller-Harvey, 2006; Waghorn, 2008; Patra and Saxena, 2011; Wang et al, 2015). Protein precipitation capacity, antimicrobial, antiparasitic and antioxidant activities are the most relevant properties of tannins to be considered for their use in ruminant animals.

**Important applications of tannin in ruminants:** Strong protein affinity is the well-recognised property of plant tannins that has successfully been applied to ruminant nutrition to (i) decrease protein degradation in the rumen. This improves protein utilisation and production efficiency. Tannin-containing forage in ruminant diets is incorporated to control, (ii) animal pasture bloat, (iii) intestinal parasite and (iv) pathogenic bacteria load.

Condensed tannins can have beneficial or detrimental effects on ruminants, depending on their amount consumed, their type and chemical structure as well as the composition of the rest of the diet, especially CP concentration of the diet (Mueller-Harvey, 2006). By summarising numerous researches, Waghorn (2008) has concluded that when forages are fed as a sole diet, the condensed tannins in *L. corniculatus* (about 30 g CT/kg DM) have been beneficial for ruminant production, but the CT in *sainfoin, Hedysarum coronarium* and *L. pedunculatus* (concentration generally greater than 50 g/kg DM) do not appear to benefit productivity other than mitigating the impact of parasites. The CT in browse from warm and hot climates are nearly always detrimental to ruminants in contrast to their counterparts from temperate climates, except for reducing internal parasite numbers (Waghorn, 2008).

Condensed tannins at low to medium concentrations benefit ruminant production efficiency because CT reduce protein degradation in the rumen and increase the amount of dietary protein reaching small intestine for absorption. At high concentration, however, CT would impede feed intake due to their astringent nature and reduce protein and other nutrients digestion by "over" protecting protein, decrease rumen microbial activity and inhibit endogenous digestive enzyme activities thereby negatively affect animal performance.

**Bloat:** The second application of tannins in ruminant production is to reduce frothy bloat. Bloat is a common digestive disorder in ruminants. The condition is characterised by an accumulation of gas in the rumen and reticulum that can impair both digestive and respiratory functions. The rapid lyses of plant cells and release of proteins from plant cells upon their entry into the rumen increase the viscosity of the rumen fluid. This is a major contributing factor to pasture bloat. Tannins by precipitating protein during chewing and rumination reduce protein solubility in the rumen thereby decrease bloat occurrence. Therefore, tannins-containing forage are regarded as "bloat free" and as little as 1.0 mg CT/g DM is needed to prevent pasture bloat. Incorporation of CT-containing forage such as *sainfoin* into alfalfa has been proved an effective method in controlling alfalfa pasture bloat.

**Control of digestive parasites:** The third application of tannins in ruminants especially in grazing ruminants is to control digestive parasites. Tannins in *sainfoin, sulla, L. pedunculatus, Sericea lespedeza, Acacia nilotica* and *chicory* had significant anthelmintic effects in digestive tract of sheep, goat and deer. External tannins such as that from mimosa (HT), chestnut (HT) and quebracho (CT) have been used to control various intestinal parasites in ruminant animals. It seems that dietary concentration below 20 g/kg DM of tannins is ineffective in controlling ruminant intestinal parasites.

**Control of pathogenic bacteria load:** It has been reported that sheep could detect the presence of internal parasites or associated symptoms and increase their preference for the tannin-rich feed (Lisonbee et al, 2009; Juhnke et al, 2012). These studies demonstrated that feeding plant tannins could be a practical method to effectively decrease the presence of *E. coli* 0157:H7 in ruminant digestive tract thereby **reduce the risk of carcass contamination** and, hence, **enhance the food safety.**

## Use of Tannins in Monogastric Animals

Tannins have traditionally been regarded as "anti-nutritional factor" for monogastric animals and poultry, with negative effects on feed intake, nutrient digestibility and production performance. However, recent research results changed this view positively. When applied in appropriate manner, low concentrations of several tannin sources improved intestinal microbial ecosystem, enhanced gut health status and thus increased productive performance in monogastric farm animals through their antimicrobial, antioxidant and anti-inflammatory activities. The mechanisms of growth promoting effects of tannins in monogastric animal are much less understood compared with those in ruminants.

The final impact of tannins on animal performance depends on the type of animals and their physiological status, composition of feed, type of tannins and their concentrations in the diets.

**Pigs seem to be relatively resistant to tannins in the diets:** They are able to consume relatively high quantities of tannin-rich feed-stuffs without presenting any toxic symptoms, when compared with other domestic animals. This is likely due to parotid gland hypertrophy and secretion in the saliva of proline-rich proteins that bind and neutralise the toxic effects of tannins (Cappai et al, 2010, 2014).

**Grape pomace feeding in poultry and swine:** Extracts of grape *(Vitis vinifera)* seed and grape pomace contain significant amount of polyphenolic compounds including CT. Grape pomace includes grape skins, pulp and contain significant amount of CT and other phenolic compounds. Grape pomace is the by-product of grape processing. Several studies evaluating the effects of grape pomace on swine and poultry performance indicated that addition of such tannin-rich product up to 10% of the diet had no effect on growth performance of broiler chicken, but **enhanced antioxidant status and increased intestinal populations of beneficial bacteria.** The grape pomace has also been found to improve antioxidant activity of pork and reduced the gastrointestinal absorption of mycotoxins in swine.

## PLANT POLYPHENOLS—THEIR POTENTIAL TO COMBAT OXIDATIVE STRESS AND INFLAMMATORY PROCESSES IN FARM ANIMALS

### Introduction

Plant polyphenols are part of the plant secondary metabolites (PSM). It has been well-established that polyphenols are able to act anti-inflammatory both *in vitro* and *in vivo* by inhibiting the activation of nuclear factor kappa B (NFκB) and to induce antioxidative and cytoprotective effects by inducing nuclear factor erythroid 2 related factor 2 (Nrf2) (Rahman et al, 2006). Among the polyphenols, resveretrol might be the most promising due to its well-established antioxidative and gene regulatory properties (Chuang and McIntosh, 2011).

These effects of plant polyphenols are well-established in humans and experimental animal models. However, in farm animals the effects of plant polyphenols with respect to their anti-inflammatory, antioxidative and cytoprotective effects have been less investigated. Gessner et al (2017) gave a comprehensive overview of polyphenols on their bioavailability, biotransformation, inflammation and oxidative stress in farm animals.

### Polyphenols and their Classification

Polyphenols are plant secondary metabolites (PSM) synthesised by plants to provide protection against invasive pathogens and to prevent damage to DNA and photosynthetic apparatus due to ultraviolet radiation. Phenolic compounds are characterised by having at least one aromatic ring with one or more OH groups attached. The polyphenols comprise more than 8000 different compounds with the phenol ring being the common structural feature. Polyphenols can be divided into the flavonoid-type and the non-flavonoid-type based on the number of phenol rings and the structural elements that bind these rings to one another.

### Flavonoid-type Polyphenols

The flavonoid-type polyphenols comprise the largest group of polyphenols with more than 4000 compounds identified and share as a common structure two benzene rings connected by three carbon atoms forming an oxygenated heterocycle. Based on the type of the heterocycle, the following flavonoid subclasses can be distinguished: flavonols, flavones, flavan-3-ols, flavanones, antho-cyanins and isoflavones.

Examples of frequently studied flavonoids are the flavonols (quercetin and myricetin), the flavones (orientin, vitexin and homo-orientin), the flavan-3-ols (catechin, epica-techin, epigallocatechin and their gallate esters), the flavanone (naringenin), the anthocyanin (cyaniding) and the isoflavones (genistein and daidzein). Isoflavones have an oestrogen-like structure and thus are able to bind to oestrogen receptors. Almost all dietary flavonoids exist in glycosidic form, mostly in O-glycosidic form, but C-glycosy-lated flavonoids, particularly flavones, are also abundant in plants. Flavonoids are widely found in fruits and vegetables.

## Nonflavonoid-type polyphenols

1. The nonflavonoid-type polyphenols are frequently present in cereals and can be subdivided into **cinnamic acids** (ferulic, caffeic, coumaric and sinapic acid) and the less abundant **hydroxyl benzoic acids** (gallic and vanillic acid). Typically, the cinnamic acids are bound to arabinoxylans of the plant cell wall, which impairs their bioavailability.
2. A second group of nonflavonoid-type polyphenols are the **lignans** (secoisolari-ciresinol, pinoresinol and syringaresinol) considered as phytoestrogens due to their oestrogen agonist and antagonist pro-perties.
3. The last group of nonflavonoid type poly-phenols is the **stilbenoids** (e.g. resveratrol). Resveratrol is the most famous compound due to its lifespan prolonging effects and it has two phenol rings connected by a two-carbon methylene bridge.

## Occurrence and Concentration of Polyphenols

The outer layers of plants contain higher polyphenol levels than the inner layers. Cell walls have insoluble polyphenolic com-pounds, whereas soluble ones are found in the cell vacuoles. Typical polyphenol-rich plant materials are fruits, vegetables, leaves, legume seeds and beans. Correspondingly, humans regularly consuming black and green tea, tropical fruits and berries, spinach, onion, soya beans, fruit juices and wine have a high intake of polyphenols. Due to economic considerations, relevant sources of poly-phenols for farm animals are agro-industrial byproducts from juice, wine and beer making, such as pomace, peels, seeds, stems and brewery waste and from processing of grains, seeds and nuts, such as hulls (e.g. soya bean, cottonseed, buckwheat, almond) and husks (e.g. paddy, grams).

It can be generally stated that the **concentration** of polyphenolic compounds in plant material **decreases with increasing storage time** because of the high susceptibility of polyphenols to oxidation. Accordingly, the concentrations and the type of polyphenols vary greatly in plants and the plant products (e.g. extracts) manufactured from.

## Bioavailability of Plant Polyphenols

Bioavailability of plant polyphenols is low. It is critically influenced by their chemical structure (e.g. glycosylation, esterification and polymerisation) and associations with other plant cell constituents (fibre, protein).

**Bioavailability of polyphenols in monogastric animals is only 5 to 10%:** The bioavailability of dietary compounds means the degree to which they become available in intact form to the target tissues following ingestion into the gastrointestinal tract. Faria et al (2014) estimated that less than 5–10% of plant polyphenols are absorbed in the small intestine:

1. This is due to the fact that polyphenols in plants exist as esters, glycosides or poly-mers and many polyphenols are associated with cell wall constituents (arabinoxylans), with proteins or with other organic compounds (organic acids) and lipids. The capacity for hydrolysis and liberation from the plant matrix is generally limited due to either lack of appropriate enzyme activity or the low microbial colonisation.

2. Polyphenolic compounds are recognised as xenobiotics by the body's biotransformation system. This is another reason for the low bioavailability of many polyphenols in target tissues following absorption.

As a result of low absorption, extensive biotransformation and excretion of metabolites, concentrations of polyphenols such as quercetin in plasma and tissues after supplementation remain relatively low. Even long-term supplementation of polyphenols does not lead to an accumulation in plasma or tissues.

## Biotransformation of Unabsorbed Polyphenols in the Colon

The unabsorbed polyphenols while passing through the colon get biotransformed by the gut microbiota to polyphenol metabolites. About 90 to 95% of ingested polyphenols are extensively biotransformed by classic detoxification pathways in enterocytes and liver to a large number of hydrophilic conjugated metabolites, which are excreted from the liver and enter the colon via the bile. These are biotransformed with the help of enzymatic activities of the colon microbiota to various polyphenol metabolites. For example, the conjugated polyphenol metabolites excreted via the bile are deconjugated by microbial glucuronidases and sulphatases into their aglycones, which can be further degraded by microbial enzymes leading to various metabolites (Fig. 4.2).

In the case of degradation of flavonols, flavones, flavanones and flavan- 3-ols, e.g. a large number of different metabolites, such as dihydroxyphenylacetic acids, phloretic acid, benzoic acid, phenyllactic acid and vanillic acid, are formed (Rechner et al, 2004).

The polyphenol metabolites in the colon can have three different fates
- One part is absorbed into the circulation after being conjugated once again in the enterocyte and the liver.

- Another part of polyphenol metabolites can serve as either growth-promoting substrates or antimicrobial substances for bacteria of the colon microbiota.
- The remaining part of non-absorbed and non-metabolised polyphenol metabolites is excreted via the faeces.

## Health Promoting Effects of Polyphenols

Polyphenol metabolites can modulate the composition of the colon microbiota in a desirable manner due to simultaneously promoting the growth of beneficial bacteria in a prebiotic-like manner, while inhibiting that of pathogenic bacteria (China et al, 2012). The resulting eubiotic microbiota contributes to gut health, intact gut barrier function and a properly working intestinal immune system. This modulation of the colon microbiota is considered a key mechanism for the overall health-promoting effects of polyphenols. This kind of two-way interaction between polyphenols and colon microbiota helps biotransformation of unabsorbed polyphenols that led to better healthcare. A schematic illustration of absorption and metabolism of plant polyphenols in farm animals is shown in Fig. 4.2.

## Bioavailability of Polyphenols in Ruminants

Limited studies performed on the bioavailability of polyphenols in ruminants indicated that at least a small part of polyphenols are absorbed from the diet in ruminants. Gohlke et al (2013) have shown that quercetin aglycon (upon intraduodenally administration in lactating dairy cows) is absorbed at a rate similar to that observed in pigs. In dairy cows, it has been shown that the administration of feedstuffs rich in isoflavones (genistein, daidzein) such as soya bean meal causes an increase in the concentrations of those isoflavones in blood and milk (Cools et al, 2014).

In sheep, it was observed that concentrations of different polyphenols, such as epicatechin, in plasma had increased following the administration of four different

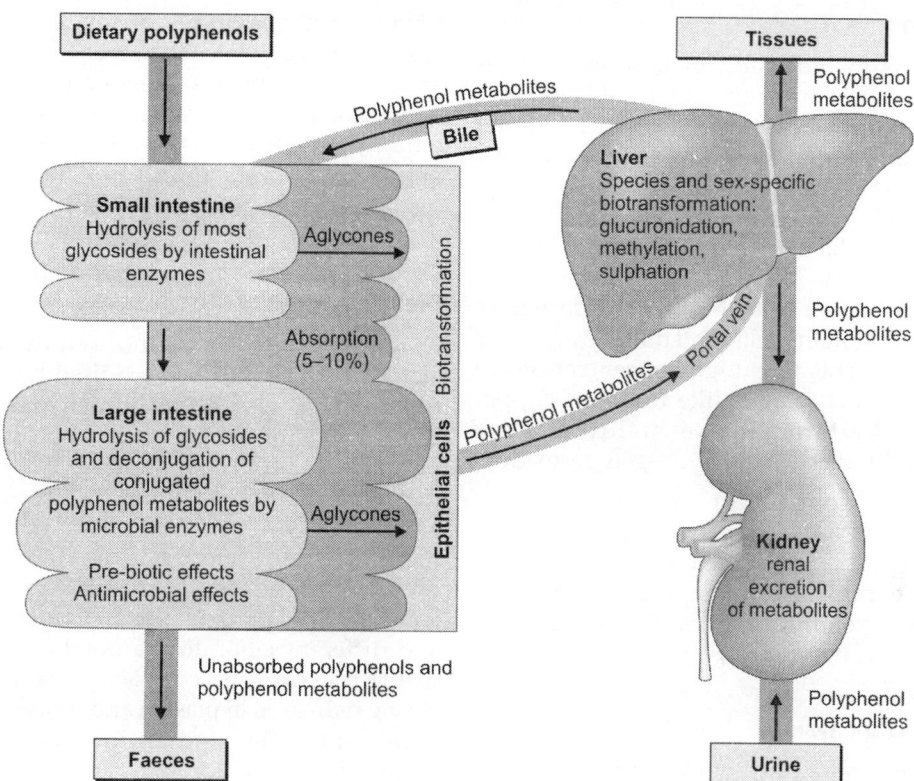

**Fig. 4.2:** Overview of absorption and metabolism of plant polyphenols in monogastric farm animals (*Source*: D.K.Gessner et al, 2017).

polyphenol-rich plant extracts (rosemary, grape, citrus, marigold) via a rumen cannula (Gladine et al, 2007). Those studies indicate that at least a part of the isoflavones present in the diet is protected against degradation in the rumen and is available in the small intestine, the site of absorption of polyphenols.

## Modulation of Rumen Microbiota Composition

With regard to the rumen bacterial community, it was reported that feeding a flavonoid-rich plant extract increases the numbers of lactate-consuming and propionate-producing bacteria (Balcells et al, 2012). Studies of De Nardi et al (2016) indicated that the composition of the microbiota in the rumen of ruminants is modulated by plant polyphenols. In ruminants, plant polyphenols are hydrolysed

and biotransformed by enzymatic activities of the rumen microbiota and the resulting aglycones and polyphenol metabolites are partially absorbed through the rumen epithelium. Non-absorbed polyphenols passing into the small intestine can be biotransformed like in monogastric animals.

## Oxidative Stress and Inflammation

Oxidative stress is due to the imbalance between the formation of oxidants and their detoxification by the antioxidant system. Oxidative stress is traditionally recognised as detrimental to the body because it can cause damage to the cell constituents including lipids, DNA, proteins and carbohydrates thus leading to tissue damage (Halliwell, 2007). Let us know about oxidants and antioxidant system briefly before going into details of oxidative stress.

## Oxidants

Oxidants include radicals and nonradicals and reactive oxygen species (ROS) and reactive nitrogen species (RNS). *See* **Chapter three for details.** The formation of oxidants can occur during normal metabolism (e.g. superoxide radicals are produced within the respiratory chain in the mitochondria), during inflammatory reactions (e.g. superoxide radicals are formed by NADPH oxidase from activated immune cells) and due to exogenous noxious agents (e.g. high concentrations of free transition metals like iron and copper induce the formation of highly reactive hydroxyl radicals from hydrogen peroxide).

Dietary sources for the generation of oxidants are undesirable substances in food such as pesticides, organic solvents or mycotoxins, because these compounds induce the hepatic xenobiotic system generating oxidants as byproducts.

## Antioxidant System

The antioxidant system is able to prevent oxidative stress through reducing the formation and/or scavenging of oxidants. Antioxidant system consists of three components:

i. Antioxidant enzymes, such as superoxide dismutase, glutathione peroxidase and catalase.

ii. low molecular mass antioxidants, such as tocopherols (vitamin E), ascorbic acid (vitamin C), carotenoids including β-carotene, uric acid, glutathione and polyphenols.

iii. Proteins that are able to sequestrate free transition metals. These proteins include storage and transport proteins for metal ions, such as ferritin, ceruloplasmin and metallothionein (Halliwell, 1996).

Amino acids and trace elements (copper, zinc, iron, selenium) are constituents of endogenous antioxidants (glutathione, superoxide dismutase, glutathione peroxidase and catalase) and different vitamins (thiamine, riboflavin, niacin, folic acid), which are involved as coenzymes in various antioxidant pathways. Hence an inadequate supply of these nutrients impairs the antioxidant defence system. This imbalance between oxidants and antioxidants cause oxidative stress (Evans and Halliwell, 2001).

## Oxidative Stress can be Induced by Dietary Factors

Oxidative stress can be induced by dietary factors, such as PUFA or oxidised fatty acids representing an oxidative burden to the body through the formation of lipid peroxidation products. In broilers, Eder et al (2005) found that feeding a diet containing 6% linseed oil as a source of PUFA in combination with a low dietary vitamin E supply (15 mg vitamin E/kg diet) strongly depletes vitamin E and increases lipid peroxidation in tissues. In pigs and different laboratory animals, feeding a diet rich in oxidised fatty acids also causes a strong reduction in plasma and tissue vitamin E concentrations and an increase in lipid peroxidation products in tissues.

## Oxidative Stress and Inflammation—Role of NFκB

Oxidative stress is directly linked with inflammation because oxidants are activators of nuclear factor kappaB (NFκB), the key or master or central regulator of inflammation. NFκB is a protein complex that is present in almost all animal cell types. It is bound to inhibitory proteins in the cytosol in the inactive state. Upon stimulation by oxidants and several other stimuli, such as cytokines, bacterial stimuli, viruses and ultraviolet radiation, the active NFκB is translocated into the nucleus and the transcription of a large set of genes involved in all aspects of inflammation (e.g. vasodilation, chemotaxis, cell adhesion, leucocyte extravasation, phagocytosis) are activated. The typical proteins encoded by NFκB target genes are pro-inflammatory cytokines, chemokines, inflammatory enzymes, adhesion molecules and various receptors (Barnes, 1997).

## Free Radical Diseases

Oxidants activate NFκB and NFκB-regulated proteins (cytokines and chemokines) stimulate the production of oxidants by activated neutrophils (respiratory burst) and in the mitochondria. Thus oxidative stress is promoted and a vicious cycle is triggered. If the vicious cycle cannot be broken due to sustained and overwhelming production of oxidants, the inflammatory process becomes chronic and the body's cells and tissues are damaged. This situation is the underlying cause of many free radical diseases (e.g. asthma, chronic obstructive pulmonary disease, inflammatory bowel disease (IBD), rheumatoid arthritis) in humans.

Such free radical diseases also occur in farm animals and examples are pneumonia, enteritis and sepsis in pigs, mastitis and pneumonia in ruminants and recurrent airway obstruction, exercise-induced pulmonary haemorrhage or joint disease in horses (Lykkesfeldt and Svendsen, 2007).

## Oxidants do have Health-promoting Effects in the Body

It has been recognised that low levels of oxidants have physiological functions for stress adaptation. This is explained by the role of many oxidants **as signalling molecules** of important intracellular pathways. For instance, several oxidants are activators of stress-sensitive transcription factors such as Nrf2. The nuclear factor erythroid 2 related factor 2 (Nrf2) is a relevant basic leucine zipper (bZIP) transcription factor that is essential in the regulation of cell cycle homeostasis, cytoprotection and innate immunity when cells are under stressful conditions. Upon activation of Nrf2, the expression of a great number of genes involved in cytoprotection is induced (Kim et al, 2010). These include antioxidant enzymes, several enzymes involved in the detoxification of xenobiotics and anti-inflammatory genes. Thus, physiological levels of oxidants are even useful for the adaptation of the body to cellular stress by way of improving defence and detoxification mechanisms.

## Mitochondrial Hormesis or Mitohormesis

It has been proved that moderate production of ROS in the mitochondria improves health and even extends the lifespan of different model organisms (*C elegans* and mice). This phenomenon has been named mitochondrial hormesis or abbreviated as mitohormesis (Yun and Finkel, 2014). See hormesis concept on page 148. It is known that physical exercise has health-promoting effects such as improvements of antioxidative defence and insulin sensitivity; during physical exercise substantial amounts of ROS are formed in skeletal muscle. Studies conducted by Ristow et al (2009) in humans demonstrate that supplementation with high doses of vitamins C and E prevents these health-promoting effects of physical exercise. This clearly indicates that ROS play an essential role for inducing health-promoting effects in the body.

The biological concept of mitohormesis also applies to farm animals as evidenced from a study with dairy cows showing that supplementation with vitamin E during the dry period increases clinical mastitis incidence postpartum through the induction of oxidative stress (Bouwstra et al, 2010a,b). This is likely due to resulting of suppression of the cows' own antioxidant and cytoprotective system. Thus, Gessner et al (2017) opined that the classic view of ROS as generally harmful products that destroy cellular structures is regarded as outdated, whereas **physiological ROS levels should be considered as protective by stimulating defence mechanisms that prevent cellular damage.**

## Effects of Polyphenols on Oxidative Stress and Inflammation in Studies with Farm Animals

**Oxidative stress activates NFκB:** Oxidative stress triggers pro-inflammatory pathways. Pro-inflammatory stimuli such as lipopolysaccharides (LPS), reactive oxygen species (ROS), viruses or cytokines activate the nuclear factor kappa B (NFκB). The activated NFκB translocates into the nucleus and initiates the transcription of a broad-spectrum of pro-inflammatory genes.

**Polyphenols suppress inflammatory processes:** A large number of studies with either cell cultures (e.g. intestinal cells, immune cells, endothelial and smooth muscle cells, adipocytes) or experimental animal models of inflammation (intestinal inflammation, systemic inflammation associated with obesity, metabolic syndrome and atherosclerosis) convincingly demonstrated that isolated polyphenolic compounds or polyphenol-rich plant extracts (e.g. green tea, hop, cocoa, grape) suppress experimentally induced inflammation processes (Romier et al, 2009). Effects of polyphenols against inflammation are mediated by complex cellular mechanisms, most of which are linked with an inhibition of NFκB (the master regulator of inflammation). Polyphenols are able to block the activation of NFκB by inhibiting phosphorylation and proteasomal degradation of IkB, an effect which is at least in part due to the antioxidant properties of polyphenols. Polyphenols are able to directly scavenge ROS.

**Polyphenols activate Nrf2:** Polyphenols induce the activation of Nrf2 that in turn leads to an activation of various antioxidant enzymes. Both, direct scavenging of ROS and activation of Nrf2 helps to prevent the development of oxidative stress. Moreover, polyphenols are able to activate transcription factors such as peroxisome proliferator-activated receptor γ (PPARγ), which is antagonising inflammation by blocking NFκB activation (Chuang and McIntosh, 2011).

### What is Hormesis Concept?

The activation of nuclear factor erythroid 2-related factor 2 (Nrf2) by polyphenols is one example of hormetic pathways, which are typically activated by polyphenols and many other phytochemicals. In the context of polyphenols, the hormesis concept states that

high doses of certain polyphenols are toxic, whereas subtoxic doses ingested by animals (by way of consuming plants) induce mild cellular stress responses, like activation of Nrf2, leading to the induction of so-called vitagenes, such as genes encoding antioxidant enzymes, biotransformation enzymes and heat-shock proteins, thereby preserving cellular homeostasis during stressful conditions and conferring resistance to a more severe stress (Calabrese et al, 2012).

Interestingly, the activation of the cytoprotective Nrf2 pathway in response to such unspecific stressors like ROS and reactive nitrogen species (RNS) stimulates autophagy. This 'self-digestion' pathway generates amino acids, fatty acids and nucleotides that can be recycled for protein synthesis and ATP generation during stressful conditions. Through this autophagic 'self-cleaning', the cell's ability to process damaged proteins, damaged mitochondria and to cope with the consequences of cellular stress is enhanced (Lee et al, 2012). As consequence of the activation of autophagy by hormetic phytochemicals, oxidative stress and inflammatory stress are reduced thus making autophagy an important biological process contributing to cellular and organismic health (Lee et al, 2012).

### Effects of Polyphenols on Oxidative Stress in Pigs

*Resveratrol*

Several studies have been conducted to know the effects of polyphenols on pathophysiological processes of various diseases in pigs as an animal model for humans. For example, it has been shown that resveratrol-rich grape extract lowers fat deposition, improves the lipid profile and glucose metabolism and prevents the development of atherosclerotic lesions in the aorta of pigs (Burgess et al, 2011). Other studies observed that resveratrol favourably influences risk factors for coronary heart disease and improves myocardial function in porcine models of metabolic syndrome and myocardial ischaemia

(Burgess et al, 2011). Resveratrol has well-established antioxidative and gene regulatory properties.

## Flavonol Quercetin

Supplementation of the flavonol quercetin (at a level of 10 mg/kg body weight/day) is able to increase plasma and liver concentrations of $\alpha$-tocopherol and reduce plasma lipid peroxidation products in growing pigs fed fish oil in combination with a low dietary vitamin E supply (7 mg/kg diet) (Luehring et al, 2011). These results indicate that quercetin exerts a tocopherol-sparing effect at a low vitamin E intake.

## Flavonol Ampelopsin

In pigs treated with subcutaneous LPS injection, supplementation of the diet with ampelopsin (dihydromyricetin), the most common flavonoid in dry tender stems and leaves (at a level of 400 mg/kg diet), ameliorated the antioxidative capacity in plasma and lowered the concentrations of malondialdehyde (MDA, marker of peroxidation) in the liver (Hou et al, 2014). This study suggests that the flavonoid ampelopsin improves the antioxidative status in pigs subjected to inflammation and oxidative stress.

## Isoflavones

In a study with gilts that were treated with zearalenone (a mycotoxin known to induce oxidative stress), supplementation of isoflavones lowered MDA concentration in plasma (Wang et al, 2012). This finding suggests that isoflavones are able to counteract oxidative stress induced by mycotoxin treatment.

The overall conclusion of these studies performed so far is that supplementation of polyphenols improves the antioxidative status and ameliorates oxidative stress in pigs subjected to prooxidative treatment. In pigs without prooxidative treatment (e.g. Gessner et al, 2013), polyphenols have either no or only marginal effects on the antioxidant status.

## Effects of polyphenols on gut health and inflammation in pigs

**Grape seed extracts:** Gessner et al (2013) reported that the diet containing grape seed and grape mart meal extract caused a downregulation of various pro-inflammatory genes in the duodenum of growing pigs. Supplementation of grape seed and grape mart meal extract also caused an increase in the villus height-to-crypt depth ratio, suggesting that plant polyphenols could influence intestinal microarchitecture in a beneficial manner.

**Plant extracts:** Studies of Fiesel et al (2014) with polyphenol-rich plant extracts (grape or hop) revealed that both the plant extracts were able to lower the expression of several pro-inflammatory genes in various parts of the intestine (duodenum, ileum, colon). These findings suggest that polyphenols exerted an antimicrobial effect on pathogenic bacteria in the intestine of pigs. In both of the aforementioned studies, feeding polyphenol-rich plant extracts caused an improvement of the gain-to-feed ratio in pigs, an effect which could be due to an inhibition of pro-inflammatory processes in the intestine or to antimicrobial effects.

**Flavanol-rich cocoa powder:** Jang et al (2016) also reported that feeding different doses of **cocoa powder** (2.5, 10 and 20 g) containing 51, 205 and 410 mg flavanols, respectively, to pigs for 4 weeks decreased gene expression of TNF-$\alpha$ and Toll-like receptors -2, -4 and -9 in the ileal Peyer's patches, mesenteric lymph nodes and the proximal colon. Since, the body weights of pigs were not influenced in the study of Jang et al (2016), this possibly indicates that the anti-inflammatory effects of the monomeric compounds (catechin and epicatechin) in cocoa powder dominated over the pro-inflammatory actions of procyanidins (D.K. Gessner et al, 2017).

Besides inhibiting pro-inflammatory gene expression in the intestine, this study revealed that feeding the cocoa powder increases the abundance of some beneficial bacterial strains, such as *Lactobacillus* and *Bifidobacterium* spp. in the proximal colon and faeces. These bacteria are known to inhibit the growth of pathogenic bacteria by the production of lactic acid through fermentation of sugars, reducing the intestinal pH and thus making the environment unfavourable for the growth of pathogens, competition for receptors on the intestinal epithelium and production of antimicrobial compounds.

**Cocoa husk meal:** The study conducted by Magistrelli et al (2016) found that feeding **cocoa husk meal** (a polyphenol-rich waste from agroindustry representing the integuments of the cocoa beans) at 75 g/kg diet to male pigs for 3 weeks increased faecal abundance of *Bacteroides—Prevotella* and *Faecalibacterium prausnitzii*. Both bacterial populations are considered beneficial for the intestine due to the production of large amounts of butyrate, which stimulates growth and differentiation of enterocytes and exerts anti-inflammatory effects.

## Polyphenols are Able to Suppress Inflammation and Enhance Gut Barrier Function

Published data suggest that polyphenols are able to suppress inflammation in the small intestine of pigs and enhance gut barrier function. Considering similar effects of polyphenol-enriched diets in laboratory animals (Larrosa et al, 2009), it can be postulated that polyphenol-rich diets in pigs exerts a prebiotic activity favouring the growth of beneficial bacteria, while inhibiting the growth of pathogenic bacteria (D.K. Gessner et al, 2017) and thus contributes to gut health.

It has been reported that the modulation of the colon microbiota by plant polyphenols correlated with reduced levels of systemic inflammatory markers, such as C-reactive protein (CRP) and decreased expression of inflammatory genes in tissues. With regard to the improvements of systemic antioxidative status and the reduction in ROS levels by polyphenol-rich diets observed in some studies with pigs, Gessner et al (2017)

postulate that these effects are due to the improvements of gut health and consequently less translocation of pro-inflammatory and prooxidative stimuli (into the circulation) rather than due to direct antioxidant effects of polyphenols because of their poor bioavailability.

**Plant polyphenols are helpful to attenuate both local and systemic inflammatory conditions:** Increasing evidence from studies with pigs, poultry and cattle indicates that plant polyphenols are helpful to attenuate both local and systemic inflammatory conditions, which are of particular relevance during the weaning phase in monogastric species and during the periparturient period in dairy cattle.

The main reason for improvements of animal's performance (increases in feed efficiency and milk yield) is due to attenuation of inflammation since the inflammatory condition reduces feed intake, increases energy requirement for the production of fever and induces several hormonal changes shifting the metabolism into a more catabolic state in farm animals.

Given the generally poor absorption of polyphenols from the intestine and the mutual interaction between polyphenols and gut microbiota (biotransformation of polyphenols to metabolites by the microbiota and modulation of the microbiota by polyphenols), it can be postulated (Gessner et al, 2017) that a key mechanism underlying the anti-inflammatory action of polyphenols is their contribution to a stable, intestinal microbiota and gut health, both of which are associated with enhanced gut barrier function and decreased translocation of bacterial components and prooxidative stimuli into the circulation (Mosele et al, 2015).

**Antioxidant effects of polyphenols is less due to their low rate of absorption:** It is well known that polyphenols have pronounced antioxidative properties *in vitro*, such as scavenging of ROS, chelating of metal ions and induction of antioxidant enzymes (Fraga, 2007). Nevertheless, supplementation of plant polyphenols has less effect on the antioxidant capacity, at least in healthy animals. The reason for this might be that, due to their low rate of absorption and their fast degradation in the body by the xenobiotic system, systemic concentrations of polyphenols are very low, when compared with other antioxidants in plasma such as ascorbic acid, tocopherols, albumin, uric acid and glutathione (Surai, 2014).

Direct antioxidant effects of polyphenols are expected to occur *in vivo* only in the gut, because of the markedly higher concentration of polyphenols in the intestinal lumen compared with systemic concentrations and the direct exposition of polyphenols to the intestinal epithelium following ingestion of polyphenol-rich diets.

Polyphenols cannot replace the unique antioxidant function of vitamin E, which due to its lipophilic structure is integrated in the biological membranes and there effectively neutralises fatty acid radicals and other ROS (Surai, 2014). Tocopherols are better bio-available antioxidants in the diet.

**Polyphenols have a different effect in unhealthy animals:** Unlike in healthy animals, improvements of systemic antioxidative status and the reduction in ROS levels by plant polyphenols were observed in some studies with challenged or stressed animals. These effects could be explained by the systemic anti-inflammatory action of polyphenols, which might be caused mainly by improvements of gut health and reduced translocation of pro-inflammatory and pro-oxidative stimuli into the circulation. More studies are necessary with farm animals to substantiate this hypothesis with experimental data (Gessner et al, 2017).

Polyphenols are secondary plant metabolites which have been shown to exert antioxidative and anti-inflammatory effects in cell culture, rodent and human studies. Based on the fact that conditions of oxidative stress and inflammation are highly relevant in farm animals, polyphenols are considered as promising feed additives in the nutrition of farm animals.

## RESVERATROL SUPPLEMENTATION MITIGATES THE TRANSPORT STRESS AND IMPROVES MEAT QUALITY

### Transport Stress Deteriorates Meat Quality

It is commonly reported that long duration transport, especially in summer, is detrimental to animal welfare and meat quality. Muscle lipid peroxidation and antioxidant enzyme [e.g. superoxide dismutase (SOD), catalase and glutathione peroxidase (GSH-Px)] defensive systems have significant effects on meat quality (Ma et al, 2010; Zhang et al, 2015b). Generally, decreasing lipid peroxidation and improving antioxidant status in muscle are beneficial to meat quality. However, long-term transport leads to free radical accumulation and decreased antioxidant enzyme activity. Hence, this transport stress accelerates muscle lipid peroxidation and cell membrane damage, which ultimately lead to meat quality deterioration of transported broilers (Kannan et al, 1997).

### Biomarkers of Transport Stress

Serum corticosterone concentration is a sensitive indicator that can be increased by many stress factors. Numerous previous studies showed that plasma corticosterone concentration in broilers was elevated by transport stress. Transport stress increases the activity of lactate dehydrogenase (LDH) enzyme in the muscle. Muscular energy metabolism and related enzymes affect many aspects of meat quality (Zhang et al, 2015b). Muscle LDH is one of the key enzymes in muscle for anaerobic glycolysis metabolism. It has been demonstrated that transport stress increased muscle glycogen anaerobic glycolysis, which leads to decreased muscle glycogen content and increased muscle lactate content and thus results in muscle pH reduction and further meat quality deterioration.

**Dietary supplementation of plant products is preferred:** Dietary supplementation with certain nutrients, e.g. creatine monohydrate, vitamin C, and chromium have been proven as effective ways to attenuate transport stress-impaired meat quality of broilers. With the advent on growth-promoting antibiotic ban and consumer preference towards natural plant products, numerous phytochemicals (e.g. isoflavones, carotenoids and polyphenols) are widely preferred in animal and poultry production to improve growth performance, product quality and immune function.

## Effect of Resveratrol on Transport Stress and Meat Quality

Resveratrol is a naturally occurring polyphenol compound found in various plants, including grape *(Polygonum cuspidatum)* and peanut. It has been well-investigated both at *in vitro* and *in vivo* level (Zhang et al, 2015b) for its biological activities, including antimicrobial, antioxidant, anti-inflammatory, energy metabolism and lipid metabolism regulating function. From the studies conducted to evaluate its functionality in poultry and pigs, resveratrol has been found as a safe and effective feed additive to improve pork quality (Zhang et al, 2015b) and quail egg quality (Sahin et al, 2010).

Published works of C. Zhang, L. Zhang and co-workers (2017) consistently indicated that the broilers in the transported group exhibited higher hormone concentration than those in the control group, indicating that the broilers in the transported group experienced more stress, which may induce various physiological and metabolic changes. C. Zhang et al, (2017) also found that a 3-hour transport decreased muscle glycogen content and increased muscle lactate content. Broilers transported with dietary resveratrol supplementation have a lower serum corticosterone concentration indicating that its dietary supplementation is helpful in weakening transport stress.

**Resveratrol can be used as an effective feed additive to improve meat quality:** The study of C. Zhang et al (2017) found that muscle SOD and GSH-Px activities were decreased by transport stress, along with increased malondialdehyde (MDA) content, which indicates a decreased body antioxidant capacity. Dietary resveratrol supplementation can beneficially increase antioxidant capacity (higher SOD and GSH-Px activities) and decrease lipid peroxidation [lower MDA content] in muscle of transported broilers and may partly explain why resveratrol can attenuate transport stress-impaired meat quality of broilers. Mechanisms of action may be partly attributed to the decreased muscle anaerobic glycolysis metabolism and the improved muscle antioxidant capacity induced by resveratrol.

# 5

# Immunomodulatory Nutrients to Support Gut Health

## GASTROINTESTINAL HEALTH AND FUNCTIONALITY

### Healthy Gut

A healthy gut is a proven solution for better health and feed efficiency. How to achieve a healthy gut? Nutritional approach for obtaining it is by reducing the antibiotic use in farm animals. It is reported that 60–80% of antibiotics are used for treating intestinal disorders. Hence reducing the antibiotic use can be achieved by aiming for a functional intestine that entails good integrity, immunity and stability.

### Definition of Gut Health

Effective functionality of the gastrointestinal tract (GIT) and its health are important factors in determining animal performance (growth, milk yield, meat and egg quality). Conway (1994) proposed three components of gut health namely the diet, the mucosa (GIT barrier) and the commensal flora (GIT microbiota). The mucosa is composed of the digestive epithelium with its specific structure, the gut-associated lymphoid tissue (GALT) and the mucous overlying the epithelium. The GALT, microbiota, mucous layer and host epithelium interact, forming a complex and dynamic equilibrium within the GIT that ensures efficient functioning of the digestive system. Therefore, Celi et al (2017)

propose the **definition of gut health** as "a steady state where the microbiome and the intestinal tract exist in symbiotic equilibrium and where the welfare and performance of the animal is not constrained by intestinal dysfunction". This definition combines the principal components of gut health, namely diet, effective structure and function of the GIT barrier and normal and stable microbiota, with effective digestion and absorption of feed and effective immune status.

### Functions of the GIT System

The functions of the GIT system are the digestion of feed and absorption of nutrients and maintenance of fluid and electrolyte balance and elimination of waste products. Further, it has also another important physiological role as a barrier against the entry of antigens and pathogens since, the GIT is the largest interface between the host and the environment. The GIT is considered to be the largest organ of the immune system as more than 70% of the cells of the immune system can call the GIT as their home (Vighi et al, 2008). Interestingly improved "gut health" usually results in improved digestion and absorption. Also, one needs to consider that intestinal inflammation (i.e. a proliferation in pathogens) negatively impacts gastrointestinal function, which is accompanied by reduced absorption of both macro and micronutrients. Malabsorption is most noticeable for micronutrients, especially iron and zinc (Davin et al, 2012, 2013), while amongst macronutrients, fat is the one that has impacted the most (Koutsos et al, 2003; Koutsos et al, 2006). Malabsorption can be ascribed to loss of integrity and function of the GIT barrier, to increase in passage rate of digesta along the GIT (hence reducing the time available for nutrients to be digested and absorbed) and finally to a direct response coordinated towards the pathogen by the immune system (Klasing, 2007).

## Diet and Gastrointestinal Functionality

As the ingested nutrients can play a significant role in the development and functionality of the GIT, diet composition (ingredients, nutrients and additives) can influence the development and function of the digestive system, including the immune system and the microbiota (Conway, 1994).

i.  Many dietary factors negatively impact the health of the GI tract in case of non-ruminant farm animals (Klasing, 1998). Such factors include certain types of dietary fibre (DF), trypsin inhibitor, phytate and lectins (antinutrients), undigested protein in the distal GI tract, mycotoxins, pathogenic and putrefactive microorganisms, diets with poor nutrient balance, temperature stresses and many others. These antinutrients and other factors potentially can compromise to various degrees the physiological, histological and consequently the functional integrity of the gut. However, some of the antinutritonal factors can be destroyed during feed processing and preparation, while the rest of factors can be controlled by feed enzymes and functional ingredients.

ii.  There are numerous functional ingredients (feed supplements, functional foods and nutraceuticals) that are known to enhance GIT development and could be strategically applied in starter diets for chicks and piglets to enhance digestive capacity and resilience to enteric pathogens (Kiarie, 2016) e.g. epidermal growth factors (EGF), yeast nucleotides and diet structure.

iii.  There are significant interactions between antioxidants, other dietary substrates and environmental conditions such as heat stress (Cottrell et al, 2015). Heat stress compromises the intestinal epithelial barrier integrity through mechanisms that may include oxidative stress. Higher dietary levels of selenium and vitamin E (greater than those usually recommended) reduced intestinal leakiness caused by heat stress. Indeed, supraphysiological levels of dietary antioxidants increased heat shock protein (HSP) gene expression (HSP70, HSP90) and decreased the expression of inflammatory genes NFκB and TNF-α (Chauhan et al, 2014b).

iv.  The diet can modulate immune function in the GIT by means of several distinct mechanisms. For example, it can influence the composition and the metabolic activity of the GIT microbiota (Yeoman et al, 2012; Yeoman and White, 2014). Dietary protein in particular seems to be an important nutritional factor for maintaining immune homeostasis in the GIT. Proteins and protein hydrolysates, originating from the digestion of various digestive enzymes, or from the processing of the GIT microbiota, are absorbed by the intestinal epithelial cells and can influence the GIT immune competence and immune homeostasis (van der Meer et al, 2016). Low crude protein-synthetic amino acids supplemented diets are better.

Moreover, the diet can modify the GIT microbiota composition and metabolism by modulating the production of antimicrobial peptides that can interfere with the growth and the adhesion of pathogens to the intestinal mucosa. The diet can also have a direct effect on the GIT epithelium by modulating cytokine production and regulating intestinal barrier function. Finally, the diet can have both local and systemic effect on the immune function by local activation of immune cells or by promoting the migration of immune cells in blood.

## Essential Characteristics of Gut-friendly Diets

The dietary nutrients, such as amino acids, amines, nucleotides and butyrate, can stimulate gut development (de Lange et al, 2010; Pluske, 2013; Onrust et al, 2015). Essential characteristics of gut-friendly diets include reduced levels of fermentable protein in the hindgut, minimal buffering capacity, negligible content of anti-nutritional factors (phytate, arabinoxylans, beta-glucans, lectins, protease inhibitors, saponins, tannins) and supply of beneficial compounds such as functional proteins and peptides (IgG, EGF, lactoferrin) and micronutrients such as vitamins and minerals (de Lange et al, 2010). If diet fails to provide adequate amounts of essential nutrients, a situation of immune-compromise may result.

## Dietary Fibre and Gastrointestinal Functionality

Dietary fibre (DF) includes cell walls, non-starch polysaccharides (NSP) and lignin. The main polysaccharides of NSP are cellulose, and a wide variety of noncellulosic polysac-charides, such as β-glucan, arabinoxylans, xylans, pectins. Other carbohydrates that have digestibility properties similar to NSP are non-digestible oligosaccharides and resistant starch. As a consequence of its resistance to endogenous enzymes digestion in the small intestine, DF is subjected to bacterial fermentation in the large intestine. Hence DF is well known for its prebiotic effect. In addition to the known effect on the GIT microbiota, DF can also interact with host mucosa at all sites of the GIT, modulating the immune function (Montagne et al, 2003).

After escaping the small intestine, both soluble and insoluble dietary fibres are fer-mented by the microflora in the large intes-tine. Stimulation of microbial fermentation is a desirable outcome as it is accompanied by an increase in short-chain fatty acids, which results in a decrease in intestinal pH. The stimulation of beneficial bacteria such as *Lactobacillus* (prebiotic effect) can sustain gastrointestinal health as the attachment of *Lactobacilli* to the GIT mucosa can protect animals from GIT infection (Jha and Berrocoso, 2015). However, these beneficial effects of fibre on gastrointestinal func-tionality can be easily offset by the fact that DF can decrease total tract digestibility as a result of increased bulk in the large intestine and in faeces (Freire et al, 2000). Therefore, it is important to establish the correct level of inclusion rate of dietary fibre in farm animal (monogastrics) diets.

## Diet form and Gastrointestinal Functionality

Diet form (e.g. structure: pellets vs crumbles vs mash) and particle size (coarse vs fine), type and size of the pellets and processing conditions (time and temperature during pelleting and hygiene) can influence GIT functionality (Celi et al, 2017).

In pigs, feed particle size and feed form not only influence the morphology of the gut mucosa but also the ability of pathogens like *Salmonella* to adhere to the ileal mucosa (Hedemann et al, 2005). When pigs are fed coarsely ground feeds the stomach acts as a barrier (Mikkelsen et al, 2004), which has been reflected in decreased prevalence of *Salmonella*. This effect could be ascribed to the lower pH in the stomach and small intestine content of pigs fed coarse mash diets. In contrast, finely grounded feeds can have a negative impact on pig's GIT health leading to higher incidence of stomach ulceration and other negative alterations of gastric mucosa (keratisation, erosions).

According to available data, optimal particle size of diets for pigs is in the range between 500 and 1600 μm, while particles smaller than 400 μm are considered as undesirable with high ulcerogenic capacity. It was shown that the most convenient grinding method is to combine roller mill and hammer mill. But nowadays pigs are mainly fed pelleted feed and pelleting causes strong additional grinding of feed particles and particle size distribution (PSD) get dramatically changed. Literature review (Vukmirovic et al, 2017) suggests modified extrusion process (i.e. processing using expander) followed by shaping element as an alternative for pelleting in order to obtain agglomerated pig feed with preserved PSD.

In poultry, reduction in particle size increases digestive efficiency in consequence of a greater interaction of the resulting larger surface of grains with the digestive enzymes in the GIT. There is evidence, however, that large particle size can promote GIT development and especially gizzard function (Choct, 2009). When the gizzard is well-developed an improvement in gut motility is also observed. Higher gut motility may reduce the risk of gut pathogens colonising the lower segments of the GIT (Bjerrum et al, 2005), thus reducing the risk of gut diseases including salmonellosis and coccidiosis (Engberg et al, 2004; Bjerrum et al, 2005).

*Feed Enzymes and Gastrointestinal Functionality*

Feed enzymes greatly improve the productive value of monogastric and ruminants' diets and improve the animal performance by hydrolysing feed substrates that are only partially or not broken down by the animal's endogenous enzymes. Feed enzyme supplementation is more useful in the case of young animals, since their GIT is relatively immature and unable to produce adequate amounts of endogenous enzymes. Exogenous enzymes increase nutrient availability by hydrolysing antinutrients resulting in overall improved energy utilisation. They can produce nutrient substrates for specific populations of bacteria through their action (Bedford and Cowieson, 2012).

Exogenous enzymes have been proposed as possible alternatives to antibiotic growth promoters (AGPs). Several possible mechanisms are suggested by which enzymes may contribute to the removal of AGPs and mitigate the risks associated with their use.

These mechanisms include shifting the site of digestion to anterior intestinal segments thereby 'starving' the microbiome of the posterior gut, producing fermentable oligosaccharides from previously largely inert fibrous material with a beneficial effect on intestinal pH and enterocyte proliferation and improved gut tensile strength and tight junction integrity. Thus, exogenous enzymes may improve the stability of the gut by reducing substrate for putrefactive organisms, increasing substrate for beneficial fermentative organisms and enhancing the ability of the intestine to defend itself against the pathogens.

Diet composition and formulation strategies will be pivotal for the development and maintenance of a functional and healthy gut, in addition to farm animal management and its genetics.

## GIT Microbiota and Gastrointestinal Functionality

The GIT microbiome is responsible for several functions including intestinal development and functionality (as evidenced by differences seen between gnotobiotic and conventional animals), nutrient digestion and absorption, mucous secretion, immune development and cytokine expression (Klasing, 2007).

### Job of Microbiota in the GIT

The intestinal microbiota contributes to the regulation of the host homeostasis by contributing to optimal digestion and absorption, regulation of energy metabolism, prevention of mucosal infections and modulation of the immune system (Willing and Van Kessel, 2010). It contributes to several physiological functions (Round and Mazmanian, 2009) such as protective functions (pathogen displacement, nutrient competition, receptor competition, production of antimicrobial factors), structural functions (GIT barrier fortifications, induction of IgA, apical tightening of tight junctions, immune system development) and metabolic functions (ferment non-digestible dietary residue and endogenous epithelial-derived mucous, synthesise vitamins, control intestinal epithelial cell differentiation and proliferation, ion absorption) (LeBlanc et al, 2013; Davila et al, 2013). Several of the metabolites produced by the microbiota also stimulate the neuroendocrine cells in the GIT and therefore, the microbiota plays an important role in the endocrine regulation of gastrointestinal functionality.

*Factors Influencing the GIT Microbiota Composition and Diversity*

Several factors such as changes in feeding practices, imbalanced diet (e.g. excess of protein in pigs, starch or fructose in ruminants), stress (e.g. thermal, weaning, transport, regrouping, overcrowding and poor management and hygiene conditions) can result in an impairment of the GIT microbiota. These factors, often negatively, impact the functionality of the host's local defence system. Therefore, a normal, stable and diverse GIT microbiota and an intact and effective GIT barrier are required to maintain optimal gastrointestinal functionality.

The microbiota composition and the metabolites produced by the bacteria are vital for the maintenance of optimal gut health. While high microbiota diversity has been linked to higher resilience in adult animals, low diversity has been associated with gut health problems (Yeoman and White, 2014). Lower microbiota diversity in young animals seems to be beneficial for developing towards an adult status over time (Yeoman and White, 2014). The absence of specific bacterial families can result in a decrease in metabolites, such as butyrate (Lee and Hase, 2014). Consequently, dietary manipulation of the GIT microbiota composition represents an attractive tool to prevent gut health issues and to promote animal performance.

*Tools to Characterisation of the GIT Microbiota*

While standard culture-based techniques may only be able to identify as little as 1% of the GIT microbiome, the development and availability of high-throughput techniques like 16S sequencing (phylogenetic composition), metagenomics (functional capability), metatranscriptomics (functional intent) and metabolomics (metabolic impact) are providing a more comprehensive and valuable information.

*Tritagonists in Animal Nutrition are Bacterial Strains used as Probiotics*

As a consequence of the plethora of uncharacterised microbial species in the GIT, it has been proposed that in order to broaden our understanding of intestinal ecology, a multi-species interaction approach should be adopted. Indeed, the term 'tritagonistics' has been proposed as a new term for uncharacterised microorganisms in environmental systems (Freimoser et al, 2016). Tritagonists can affect other microorganisms by means of direct physical interaction, exchange of signalling molecules, nutrient competition, metabolising of byproducts, environmental changes (e.g. pH) or modulation of host-immune responses. Well known relevant tritagonists in animal nutrition are bacterial strains used as probiotics whose mechanisms of action are yet to be fully characterised (Celi et al, 2017).

P. Celi and co-workers while reviewing the challenges and opportunities pertaining to GIT microbiota raised several questions on its impact on lifetime health and productivity. What is the role of the GIT microbiota in the relationships between animal nutrition (diet), physiology (digestion and absorption), health (immunology) and welfare (gut-brain axis)? It is imperative to address these questions by adopting a multidisciplinary system based approach as the answers might be able to provide some needed help in the development of alternatives to antibiotics as growth promotants.

## GIT barrier and Gastrointestinal Functionality

The GIT barrier separates the gut content from the host. A major challenge for the intestinal immune system is to balance the host response to pathogens and at the same time not respond to stimuli derived from commensal bacteria as well as food antigens.

The GIT barrier consists of an external or physical barrier and an inner or functional immunological barrier. The external barrier consists of the vascular endothelium, the epithelial cell lining and the mucous layer. The mucous layer is composed of a large variety of molecules, the major one being mucin synthesised by Goblet cells. The modulation of the protective role of the mucous is linked to mucin polymerisation and microbe trapping. The inner or functional immunological barrier consists of digestive secretions, immune molecules [dendritic cells, lymphocytes and macrophages constituting the gut associated lymphoid tissue (GALT)], cell products like cytokines, inflammatory mediators and antimicrobial peptides that are mainly produced by Paneth cells in the crypts of the small intestine (Bischoff et al, 2014) and trefoil factor family (TFF) proteins that have a protective effect on mucosal epithelium by actively triggering the repair process (Kim et al, 2009).

The function of the GALT is to respond to changes in environmental cues especially nutrition (Sanderson, 2007). Nutritional deficiencies such as lack of glycine in the diet, or intake of mycotoxin contaminated feed leads to changes in intestinal pro-inflammatory cytokines and alteration of the GIT barrier function in pigs (Lee et al, 2016). Early weaning stress results in disruption of the GIT barrier function and decreased mucosal innate immunity responses in piglets challenged with *E. coli*.

Trefoil factors family (TFF) proteins are protease-resistant and are able to maintain the epithelial continuity and therefore, play an important role in mucosal healing. Their synthesis can be activated by Toll-like receptors (TLR) in order to protect the mucosa from inflammation. In inflammatory diseases, a reduction in TFF can be observed leading to a decrease in mucous viscosity.

When an animal encounters pathogens the immune system is stimulated. The immune system responds by releasing pro-inflammatory cytokines.

At birth the newborn's **mucosal immune system** is relatively undeveloped. The neonatal pig is immunologically incompetent until about 4 weeks of age (Helm et al, 2007) and thus, the period from birth through weaning represents a critical time for pigs. During this early stage of their life, piglets are exposed to dietary and environmental antigens and their immune system needs to develop so that it cannot only tolerate these antigens but also can mount an adequate immune response, if needed.

Microbiota colonisation occurs in parallel with the development of the GIT. Nutrients intake and microbiota colonisation promotes GALT development resulting in a functional immune system. The GALT maintains GIT homeostasis by discerning non-pathogenic and pathogenic antigens and feed-borne threats to the host. This homeostatic orientation is continuously challenged by physiological events and accelerated productive performances, which can result in a dysregulation of the immune response in the GIT (Davis, 1998). The activity of the GALT and its requirements changes according to the physiological and health status of the animal.

When animals are challenged, it is critical to assure that nutrient supply is adequate not only to sustain animal productive performances but also to maximise GALT function and to maintain optimal animal welfare. There are several nutrient and feed additives that can play a key role in modulating the immune system. Innate immune responses can be modulated by feed additives. However, nutritional interventions alone cannot be the only solution to sustain gastrointestinal functionality. Nutritional interventions need to be integrated with husbandry and management practices, animal genetics (resilience to diseases), biosecurity practices and research in animal physiology, metabolism and immunology (Celi et al, 2017).

## Neuroendocrine and Motor Function of the Gut

The gut is also the frontline organ to gather environmental information in response to food intake and to communicate to several other organs including the brain. During the gastric and intestinal phase of digestion, the intraluminal content is sensed and, accordingly, neuroendocrine signals transmitted to match the digestive and absorptive capacity with the amount and composition of ingested food (Celi et al, 2017).

## The Gut-brain Axis

The GIT neuroendocrine function can be considered core communication mechanisms of the so-called 'gut-brain axis' that plays a critical role in animal welfare and performance. The recent recognition that the gut microbiota also influences neuroendocrine signalling pathways has led to the suggestion to extend the concept to the so-called **'microbiota-gut-brain axis'**(Cryan and Dinan, 2012).

## Gut Hormones

Besides neuroendocrine signalling, gastrointestinal peptide hormones are of particular importance. They are secreted in response to nutrient, neural or hormonal stimulation as well as by metabolic products of the gut microbiota from enteroendocrine cells that are widely distributed throughout the gut mucosa (Steinert et al, 2013). Gastrin, secretin and cholecystokinin (CCK) were the first gut hormones discovered more than 80 years ago. Now, there are more than 50 gut hormones and with a multitude of bioactive peptides identified, gut is the largest endocrine organ of the body (Rehfeld, 2012). Gut hormones are implicated in the digestive and absorptive function of the GIT, including the regulation of gastric acid and pancreatic secretion, release of bile from the gallbladder and gut motor activity. Gut hormones modulate GIT mucosal growth.

**Gut Hormones: (1) Cholecystokinin:** Cholecystokinin (CCK) released particularly in response to lipid and amino acid-rich food from enteroendocrine I cells in the mucosal lining of the duodenum and jejunum. It mediates digestion by inhibiting gastric emptying and decreasing gastric acid secretion. It further stimulates the release of pancreatic enzymes to catalyse the digestion of fat, protein and carbohydrates. It also increases the production of hepatic bile and stimulates contraction of the gallbladder resulting in the delivery of bile into the duodenal part of the small intestine to emulsify fats, aiding in their digestion and absorption. Finally, CCK controls small and large bowel motility and potentiates insulin secretion (Chao and Hellmich, 2012).

CCK is also the first hormone that has been implicated in the control of food intake. Its satiating effect has been studied in pigs extensively (Steinert et al, 2013), although there has been less work done in ruminants (Relling and Reynolds, 2007). In cattle, fasting reduces and nutrient repletion increases plasma CCK concentrations and, under some conditions, changes in plasma CCK concentrations have been associated with changes in food intake (Relling and Reynolds, 2007; Relling and Reynolds, 2008).

**Gut hormones: (2) Glucagon-like peptide-1 (GLP-1):** Glucagon-like peptide-1 is another gastrointestinal hormone that has been implicated in the control of food intake. In dairy cows, abomasal infusions of soya bean oil led to increased plasma GLP-1 concentrations and decreased dry matter intake (Relling and Reynolds, 2008). In contrast, **ghrelin** is an endogenous ligand for the growth hormone-secretagogue receptor and the only known or exigenic gastrointestinal peptide (Steinert et al, 2013). Plasma levels peak shortly before meals (i.e. ghrelin secretion is stimulated during fasting) and fall shortly after meals, which is consistent with an eating-stimulatory action. The effects of CCK, GLP-1 and ghrelin on eating in farm animals may be an appealing research target to optimise livestock growth and productivity (Celi et al, 2017).

**Gut hormones: (3) Glucagon-like peptide-2 (GLP-2):** Several gut hormones including gastrin, CCK, secretin, somatostatin, ghrelin, bombesin and GLP-2 also modulate GIT mucosal growth. GLP-2 is co-secreted with GLP-1 from entero-endocrine L cells mainly in the distal ileum and colon in response to nutritional and neural-endocrine stimulation as well as intestinal injury. Studies indicate that GLP-2 stimulates intestinal mucosal growth and cell proliferation, leading to an expansion of the GIT mucosal epithelium, to enhance gut barrier function, to stimulate intestinal nutrient transport, digestive enzyme activity and nutrient utilisation (Burrin et al, 2003; Connor et al, 2016).

Moran et al (2014) showed that stimulation of endogenous GLP-2 secretion (via sweet taste receptor activation by feeding artificial sweetener) increased digestive enzymes activity in ruminating calves and as a result tended to increase their feed conversion efficiency. Dietary monosodium glutamate supplementation in preterm pigs increased (dose-dependently) the plasma GLP-2 concentration (Bauchart-Thevret et al, 2013). Hence stimulation of endogenous GLP-2 (via activation of L cell taste receptors) may offer an attractive target to improve gut health and performance in animals.

Gastrointestinal hormones, therefore, contribute to the digestive and absorptive functions as well as gut barrier function. They are also involved in the control of mucosal health, the control of feed intake and other metabolic controls such as glucose homeostasis. However, majority of the data on gastrointestinal endocrine research comes from laboratory rodents and humans. Hence, further research is required in the animals.

## INTESTINAL BARRIER FUNCTION AND INTESTINAL PERMEABILITY

### Intestinal Health

Intestinal health is influenced by a complex set of variables involving the intestinal microbiota, mucosal immunity, digestion and absorption of nutrients, intestinal permeability (IP) and intestinal integrity. An increase in IP enhances bacterial or toxin translocation and this in turn activates the immune system and affects health. What causes this increase in intestinal permeability? The following description answers the question.

## Mucosal Barrier or Intestinal Barrier and its Functions

From the mouth to the anus, there is a mucosal barrier, which serves as the first line of defence against pathogens. The mucosal barrier also shows the body how to deal with food antigens, which may cause allergies and sensitivities. Mucosal barriers separate the external environment from the body's internal milieu. The intestinal mucosal barrier is also referred to as intestinal barrier. The term intestinal barrier refers to the ability of the intestinal epithelium to separate intraluminal substances from the rest of the animal body. The intestinal epithelium constitutes the largest and most important selective barrier against the external environment. That is why probably intestinal mucosal barrier is said to be the **body's second skin**. The gastric mucosal barrier is an example of superb natural engineering. It has to withstand a most hostile chemical environment of highly acidic and proteolytic gastric juice that rapidly kills the swallowed microorganisms and breaks down ingested feedstuffs.

The small intestine is the primary site for nutrient absorption and consists of a single layer of epithelial cells, interdispersed with goblet cells, stem cells and enteroendocrine cells. The epithelial layer, covering finger-like projections (villi), serves as a barrier between the harmful pathogens and sterile-blood circulation. Both small and large intestines are lined by a single layer of epithelial cells bound together by complex protein structures called tight junctions. The mucosal layer in the intestine prevents pathogenic adhesion. The intestinal epithelial cells are coated with a layer of viscous mucous to protect the epithelial cells against pathogens. The intestinal epithelial cells excrete, together with the underlying leukocytes, many defensive compounds into the mucosal layer, including mucins, defensins, antibodies and many more. However, once pathogenic bacteria are able to breakthrough the mucous layer, they are able to penetrate the tight junctions with, e.g. fimbria (enterotoxigenic *E. coli* [ETEC]), subsequently releasing toxins that trigger inflammation and post-weaning diarrhoea (PWD) in piglets (Pluske et al, 2002).

## Maintenance of Intestinal Barrier Function

The integrity of the intestinal barrier is controlled by different mechanisms such as intestinal permeability (IP) and the presence of commensal microbiota. The gut microbes (some pathogens) and their metabolites (e.g. lipopolysaccharide, peptidoglycan, other toxins) are known to affect the gut barrier permeability, induce inflammation in the gut and affect nutrient absorption and fluid retention (Petschow et al, 2014).

Maintenance of intestinal barrier function is dependent on the appropriate biological functioning of both the mucosal layer and the tight junctions.

The mucosal layer, which is the primary barrier between the internal environment and external environment, protects the epithelial layer against the microbes and antigens present in the intestinal lumen (Kim et al, 2012a). At the luminal surface of the epithelial layer, there is a mucous layer that consists of mucin glycoproteins. The mucous layer protects the epithelial layer. But the composition and functions of epithelial layer can be changed by environmental bacteria. Pathogens have to traverse the mucous layer before interacting and damaging the epithelial barrier (Naughton et al, 2014).

To maintain and regulate the integrity of the intestinal barrier, the epithelial cells are connected by tight junction (TJ) complexes consisting of TJ proteins. TJ proteins are integral transmembrane proteins that include occludin, claudins, junctional adhesion molecules and tricellulin. Intracellular proteins such as the zona occludens proteins (ZO-1, ZO-2 and ZO-3), cingulin and afadin are anchor proteins that connect transmembrane proteins to the actin cytoskeleton and maintain the TJ structure and function (Ivanov, 2013; Suzuki, 2013).

The structure of the intestinal epithelium maintains a selective barrier by forming interconnected protein networks between enterocytes. These protein networks (Fig. 5.1), known as desmosomes, adherens junctions,

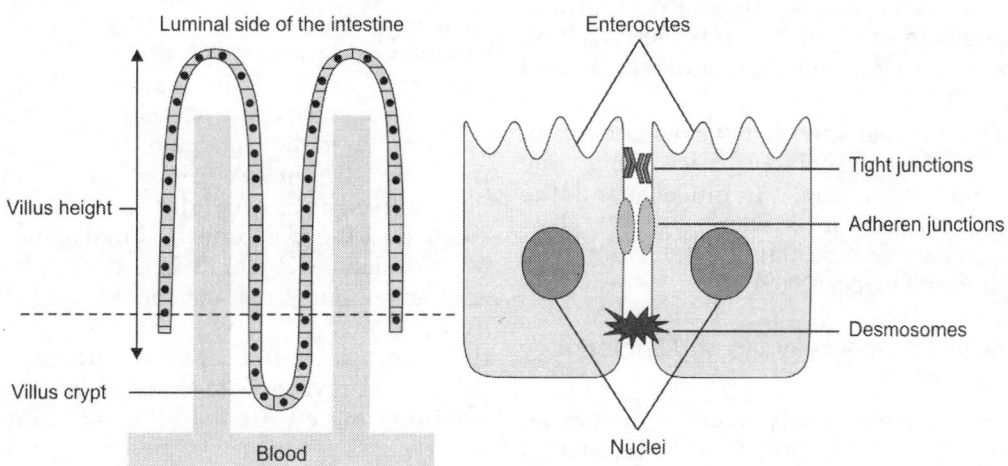

**Fig. 5.1:** Simplistic view of the intestinal villi and enterocytes with tight junctions, adherens junctions and desmosomes. (*Source:* Gilani et al, 2016)

and tight junctions, prevent the absorption of many potentially harmful substances (Andrade et al, 2015). **Absorption occurs by two pathways, transcellular and paracellular:** absorption of hydrophobic molecules mainly occurs by transcellular pathway, while passage via the paracellular route is regulated by tight junctions. Tight junction proteins form a physical barrier between two adjacent epithelial cells preventing paracellular absorption of undesired substances such as toxins or pathogens.

## Disturbances in the Intestinal Barrier

The mucosal or intestinal barrier can be disturbed by various factors like pathogens, pro-inflammatory agents, toxins, environmental and social stress factors. When the intestinal barrier integrity is disrupted, luminal substances (which are normally excluded by an intact barrier) can enter the body and cause an immune response such as inflammation or impaired health (Ivanov, 2013). **That means impaired intestinal barrier leads to increased intestinal permeability.** Such situation eventually lead to variation in feed intake and impaired functioning of the gut, which may lead to sudden changes in the microbial balance. A drastic change in microbial balance is often referred to as 'dysbiosis or dysbacteriosis'. Dysbiosis is characterised by abnormal changes in microbial counts, activity and changes in microbiota composition and diversity.

The mucosal/intestinal barrier consists of the mucosa-associated microbiota, the mucous layer, the gut mucosa and the embedded immune system (Fig. 5.2), all of which can be modulated by various feed additives (Hooper, 2009).

## Intestinal Permeability (IP) and Bacterial translocation

Intestinal permeability refers to the barrier properties of the intestinal mucosa that prevent harmful substances from penetrating the mucosa and entering the systemic circulation. Epithelial cells permit a small amount of luminal antigens, such as bacteria, to transcellularly cross the epithelium to extraintestinal sites (e.g. liver, spleen, kidney and bloodstream) via endocytosis, which is known as bacterial translocation (BT). Low levels of this bacterial translocation are normal and activate the host's immune system. However, when the intestinal barrier undergoes damage (due to heat stress or other stress conditions), it results in **increased intestinal permeability** (IP) and increased bacterial translocation (BT). This increased IP and BT can contribute to the release of systemic inflammatory mediators, induction of signalling transduction messengers and activation of immunological cells, leading to the development of inflammation and sepsis (Andrade et al, 2015).

## How Can Diseases or Other Stressful Conditions Damage Intestinal Barrier?

Now let us see how mycotoxins, e.g. impair intestinal barrier function. Mycotoxins pose a serious threat to animal production due to their negative impact on animal performance and health.

**Mycotoxins present in feed:** Once mycotoxins are taken up orally, the gastro-intestinal tract is the first target organ. Effects on epithelial cells include, among others, changed mucous production, altered cytokine production, decreased cell proliferation and compromised intestinal barrier function. After crossing the epithelial cells, mycotoxins are taken up in the blood and transported to the liver. In the liver, mycotoxins are metabolised into secondary metabolites. Aflatoxin B1, e.g. is converted into aflatoxin M1, zearalenone is mainly converted into α-zearalenone and β-zearalenone. Although the liver is known to detoxify toxic components, the liver does not always succeed in detoxifying mycotoxins. α–zearalenone, e.g. 100 times more toxic than the initial form. After passing the liver, mycotoxins are systemically distributed throughout the body impacting the immune system and all organs.

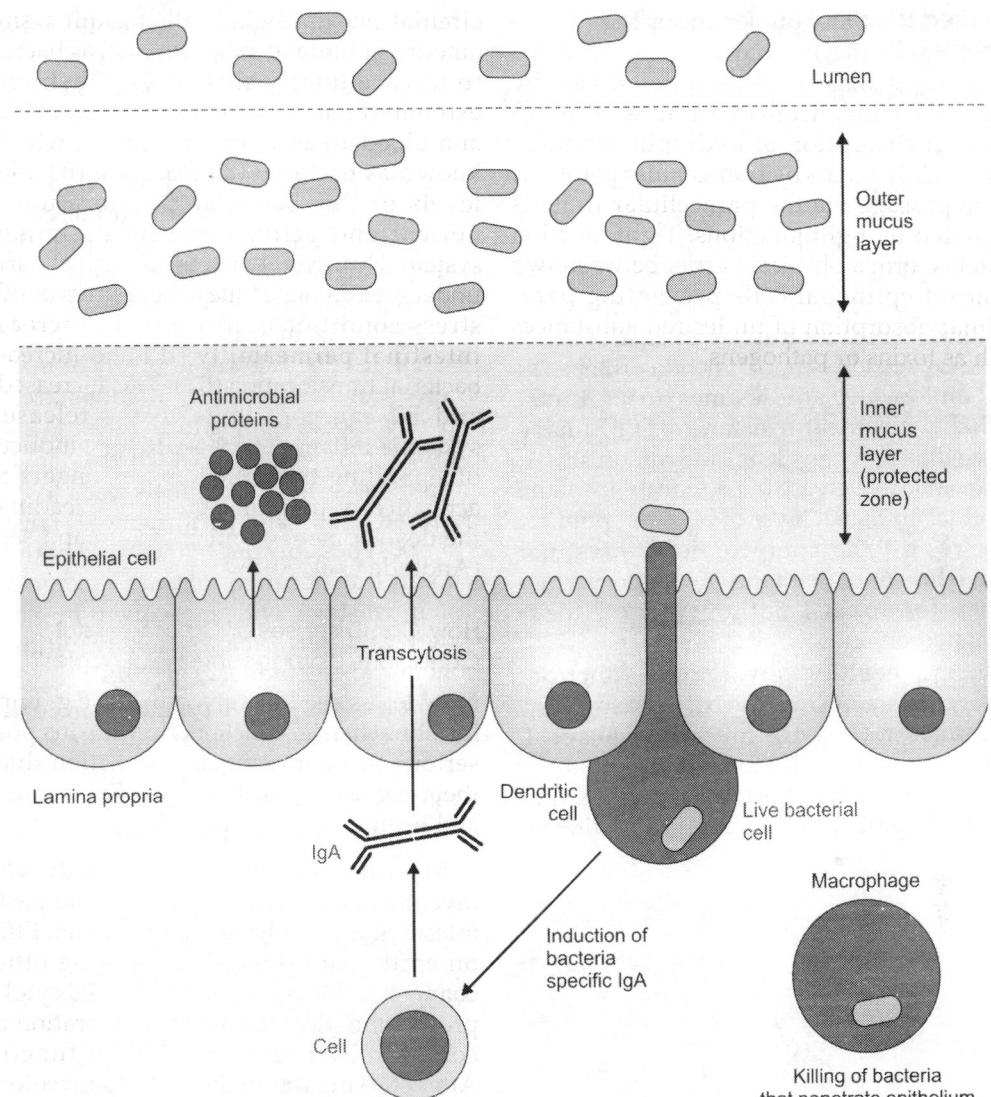

Lumen

Outer mucus layer

Inner mucus layer (protected zone)

Antimicrobial proteins

Epithelial cell

Transcytosis

Lamina propria

IgA

Dendritic cell

Live bacterial cell

Macrophage

Induction of bacteria specific IgA

Cell

Killing of bacteria that penetrate epithelium

**Fig. 5.2:** General components of Barrier function

**Induction of oxidative stress:** An important effect of mycotoxins is the induction of oxidative stress. Under normal conditions free radicals or 'reactive oxygen species' (ROS) are produced as part of standard metabolic processes. These highly unstable and chemically reactive molecules are rapidly eliminated by the natural antioxidant system in order to avoid potential damage. When exposed to mycotoxins, however, cellular ROS concentrations exceed the level of naturally occurring antioxidants resulting in oxidative stress. Excess ROS will induce a damaging chain reaction causing serious damage to nucleic acids, proteins and lipids. As these components are the basic molecules in all metabolic processes, higher oxidative stress levels result in lower feed intake and growth performance and have a negative effect on profitability.

## Impaired Intestinal Barrier Leads to Increased IP

After absorption or contact with epithelial cells, the gastrointestinal tract is highly impacted by the induction of oxidative stress by mycotoxins. Oxidative stress has a negative effect on the intestinal barrier function (Fig. 5.3) due to the modification of certain cellular proteins. This modification promotes production of pro-inflammatory cytokines, which in turn has a negative effect on the expression of tight junction proteins. *In vitro* and *ex vivo* studies measuring trans-epithelial electrical resistance (TEER) have shown that deoxynivalenol and fumonisin B1, e.g. are able to increase the permeability of the intestinal epithelial layer of pigs and poultry. As a result, the compromised intestinal barrier function results in increased permeability for toxins, pathogens and feed-associated antigens.

During healthy physiologic function, pathogens cannot cross the barrier. However, as a result of a disease or stress (Williams et al, 2013), intestinal barrier function is impaired, which can result in increased intestinal permeability (IP; Liu et al, 2010), initiating an immune response and, subsequently, inflammation. This inflammatory process and immune system activation consumes significant amounts of nutrients.

An increase in the production of pro-inflammatory cytokines such as TNF-α, IFN-γ and IL-6 is associated with an increase in intestinal permeability, while anti-inflammatory cytokines such as IL-10 are associated with a decrease in intestinal permeability (Hu et al, 2013). The increased cell turnover in the intestine results in lower numbers of mature enterocytes, where tight junctions are not fully developed, leading to an increase in the intestinal permeability (Wijtten et al, 2011).

An increase in IP in animals leads to compromised health and performance (Hanssen et al, 2004) possibly due to increased bacterial or toxin translocation, plasma leakage and protein wastage, with subsequent impaired growth and performance thus resulting in economic loss (Zuidhof et al, 2014).

Antibiotics as growth promoters have been used in chicken feed to ameliorate enteric inflammation. Their usage as growth promoters has been banned in the European Union since 2006. Other countries, such as

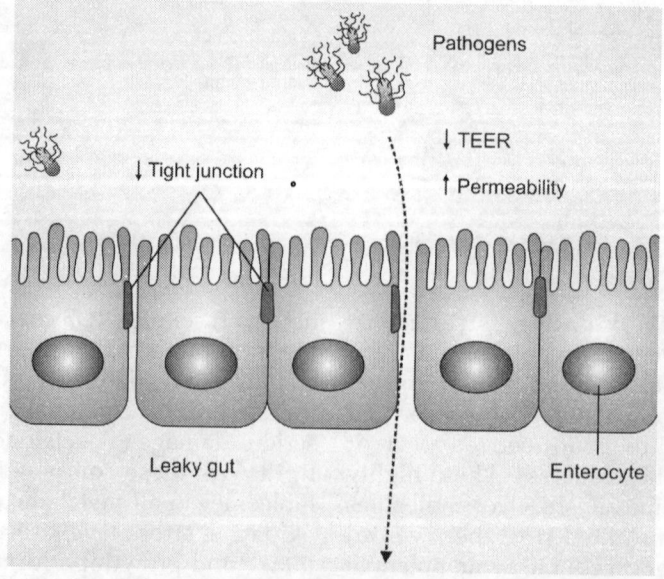

**Fig. 5.3:** Oxidative stress results in an impaired intestinal barrier function

Australia and the USA, are now also working to reduce the loads of these antibiotics in animal feed (Laxminarayan et al, 2015). This further highlights the importance of studying IP in chickens.

## Development of Potential Biomarkers to Measure Intestinal Permeability

Establishing a successful model of increased IP may help understand the mechanism of impaired intestinal barrier function and could lead to the development of reliable bio-markers of intestinal health. Gilani et al. (2016) reviewed to identify the knowledge gaps for increasing intestinal permeability as well as evaluating intestinal barrier function in chickens.

## Lipopolysaccharide is used to Increase Intestinal Permeability

Gram-negative bacteria have an outer layer made up of a lipid bilayer. The inner side of the lipid bilayer is composed of glycero-phospholipids and the outer layer is made up of lipopolysaccharide (known as endotoxin), which has also been used to induce systemic inflammation and to increase IP in rats, mice, pigs and chickens.

**Test to measure IP-lactulose, mannitol and L-rhamnose (LMR) sugar test:** Lactulose (L), L-rhamnose (R) and mannitol (M) are nondigestible and non-metabolisable carbo-hydrates (or sugars). These sugars have been used to assess increased IP in humans. Lactulose has a higher molecular weight (342 Dalton (D)) than L-rhamnose (164 D) and mannitol (182 D).

In healthy animals, lactulose passes through the stomach and small intestine undigested. If there is damage to the intestinal barrier, then it can pass through the tight junction (the paracellular pathway) in high quantity and enter the bloodstream, after which it is processed by the kidney and excreted from the body via urine (excreta in the case of chickens). Small molecular sugars (L-rhamnose and mannitol) are absorbed through the intestinal epithelium by simple diffusion, (the transcellular pathway). By measuring the ratios of these sugars through urine or blood, IP can be assessed.

A review by Jeurissen et al. (2002) suggested that using the LMR sugar method in chickens for measuring IP was impossible because this method was validated in urine samples only while chicken void excreta. A positive correlation was found between these sugars recovered in urine and blood samples in dogs (Sorensen et al, 1997), humans (Cox et al, 1999), rabbits and mice (Katouzian et al, 2005), suggesting that this technique could be used in serum or plasma as well as in urine. This further suggests that the LMR sugar test can be performed in chicken blood (plasma or serum). However, there has not been any published research on the recovery of these sugars in chicken blood and Gilani et al (2016) proposed that the sugar-recovery method may be optimal for application on chickens.

## INTESTINAL EPITHELIUM PROTECTS US AND PRESERVE OUR GI HEALTH

The gastrointestinal (GI) tract represents a unique challenge to the mammalian immune system. The intestinal epithelium is crucial for preserving gut homeostasis and acts both as a physical barrier and as a coordinating hub for immune defence and crosstalk between bacteria and immune cells. It protects the intestinal mucosa from harmful dietary antigens and invading pathogens.

Allaire et al (2018) reviewed the recent findings regarding communication between microbes and intestinal epithelial cells (IECs), as well as the immune mechanisms employed by distinct IEC subsets to promote homeo-stasis; they emphasised the central and active role that these cells play in host enteric defence. The recent discovery that each IEC type is actually comprised of multiple subsets highlights what we know is very little about these cells indicating that the functional integration the intestinal epithelium provides to protect us and preserve our GI health is much to be explored. Structure of intestinal epithelium, different functional subsets of IECs, their function and homeostasis, how they provide the first line of defence against pathogens are dealt in this chapter.

## The Structure of the Intestinal Epithelium

The intestinal epithelium is a single layer of cells that differs greatly in structure as well as cellular composition between the small intestine and colon. In the small intestine the epithelium extends over structures that protrude into the lumen, called villi, thereby increasing the mucosal surface area and nutrient absorption. Villi are absent from the colon, resulting in a relatively flat mucosal surface. The epithelium itself is not a straight layer of cells, but instead consists of invaginations termed 'crypts of Lieberkuhn'. Intestinal stem cells reside at the base of these crypts and give rise to transient proliferative cells that differentiate and mature as they travel up through the transition zone, with the intestinal epithelial cells (IECs) eventually shedding into the lumen at the apex of crypts (or villi in the small intestine). In this way intestinal crypts undergo constant cycles of IEC replenishment and renewal.

## Different Functional Subsets of IECs

Various differentiated cell types are found within the gut epithelium and each carries out unique and specialised functions. The distribution of these cell types is also different between the small intestine and colon. These cell types in small intestine include enterocytes, various secretory cells such as goblet cells, enteroendocrine cells and Paneth cells and M cells:

- Enterocytes are the most prominent cell type of the intestinal epithelium. These are responsible for nutrient and water absorption. Enterocytes are capable of secreting antimicrobial peptides (RegIIIg, β-defensins, cathelicidin).
- Goblet cells secrete mucins. Goblet cells also facilitate luminal antigen transfer to dendritic cells via goblet cell-associated antigen passages (GAPs).
- Enteroendocrine cells secrete hormones. Intestinal enteroendocrine cells comprise at least eight cellular subsets that are classified based on the hormones they produce. These include enterochromaffin cells (5-HT/serotonin), D cells (somatostatin) and G cells (gastrin).
- Paneth cells release antimicrobial factors (lysozyme, α-defensins) to protect nearby stem cells at the base of small intestinal crypts.
- There are tuft cells and M cells as well. The chemosensory tuft cells play a key role in defence against helminths.
- M cells are integral to the uptake and eventual presentation of luminal antigens to the immune system. M cells are located overlaying Peyer's patches.

In general, the majority of cell types located in the colon are also found in the small intestine; these include the enterocytes (also referred to as colonocytes in colon), enteroendocrine cells, goblet cells and tuft cells.

## Gut Microbes and Innate Signalling

Since, the first studies on germ-free mice it became clear that microbes play an important role in promoting normal intestinal structure and function. The intestinal mucosa of germ-free mice is very thin, displaying reduced IEC proliferation as well as impaired production of mucins and other IEC-derived mediators. This thinning of the protective mucin layer makes germ-free mice highly susceptible to the direct toxic effects of the colitogenic agent dextran sodium sulfate (DSS), reinforcing the importance of gut microbes in promoting intestinal tissue protection and repair. In 2004, groundbreaking studies showed that innate recognition of intestinal microbes protects the colon against DSS-induced injury by increasing IEC proliferation and repair (Rakoff-Nahoum, S. et al, 2004).

## Microbial Short-chain Fatty Acids are Responsible for IEC Homeostasis

Bacterial metabolites produced within the intestinal environment are important in maintaining normal IEC physiology in the small intestine and colon. There are approximately 100 trillion bacteria within the human gut, with the majority inhibiting the colon. Anaerobic bacteria, particularly those that can survive only in the absence of oxygen (i.e. obligate anaerobes), represent the majority of this microbial community. Together these commensal bacteria form a complex nutritional web that not only supports their own survival but also shapes the physiological environment and immune responses of the GI system. The intestinal microbiota generates a variety of compounds from ingested food products as a consequence of their metabolism and these metabolites have been shown to have direct effects on IECs.

**Butyrate-oxygen gradient along the crypt axis is life line for colonocytes:** Commensal microbes, such as *Clostridia* and *Bacteroides*, consume dietary fibre and are the major producers of the SCFA butyrate. Colonocytes at the apical tips of the crypts metabolise butyrate as their preferred energy source through β-oxidation that consumes local oxygen ($O_2$) delivered through underlying blood vessels. This establishes a butyrate-oxygen gradient along the crypt axis, reinforcing an anaerobic, butyrate-rich luminal environment at the apical tips, while the base of the crypt remains oxygen-rich, protecting stem cells from the inhibitory effects of butyrate on cellular proliferation.

**Colonisation resistance:** Colonic epithelial cells consume butyrate and oxygen through β-oxidation, creating a localised anaerobic microenvironment that favours the proliferation of butyrate-producers and this contributes to protection against pathogens via colonisation resistance, thus colon remains healthy.

**Dysbiosis due to disruption of the butyrate–oxygen gradient:** Disruption of the butyrate–oxygen gradient through antibiotic use or pathogen invasion produces a shift in intestinal epithelial cell (IEC) metabolism towards anaerobic glycolysis. This leads to an increase in luminal levels of nitrate and oxygen, which favours the proliferation of microaerophilic *Enterobacteriaceae* over anaerobic butyrate-producers, disrupting colonization resistance and culminating in 'dysbiosis'. Dysbiosis is an imbalance in the resident microbial population.

**Metabolic crosstalk between Paneth and stem cells:** In the small intestine lactate is vital for the maintenance of crypt stemness. Paneth cells produce lactate as an end-product of glycolysis, which can be converted by LGR5+ stem cells to pyruvate. This pyruvate fuels mitochondrial oxidative phosphorylation, leading to ROS signalling and activation of p38 that ultimately results in the regulation of stem cell self-renewal and differentiation.

**Lactate and acetate:** Other microbial metabolites that have been found to modulate IEC function are lactate and acetate. Microbe-derived lactate is a potent inducer of colonic hyperproliferation in mice. Lactate is an important energy source for small intestinal stem cells to sustain their proliferation and differentiation capacity. An important source of lactate may come from adjacent Paneth cells, which also produce vital signals for the maintenance of LGR5+ stem cells. Acetate, an SCFA produced by *Bifidobacterium*, has also been shown to influence goblet cell differentiation in a gnotobiotic rodent model. The presence of acetate-producing microbes as well as acetate itself increased goblet cell secretion of mucin and also promoted the terminal decoration of mucin glycans with sialic acid, whereas the presence of an acetate-consumer (*Fecalibacterium*) reduced these effects.

Germ-free mice, which lack these bacterial metabolites, displayed shorter Muc2 O-glycans and this correlated with a decrease in the expression of their respective glycosyl-transferase enzymes by IECs. These data support the concept that bacterial metabolites within the intestinal environment are important in maintaining normal IEC physiology in the small intestine as well as in the colon. Crosstalk between the microbiota and IECs has been developed as a means to prevent IEC dysfunction. Recent studies have shown that disruption of this crosstalk can also lead to aberrant changes in the resident microbial populations, termed 'dysbiosis'.

## IEC Function and 'Colonisation Resistance'

It has been known since the 1950s that the normal intestinal flora protects against incursion of foreign microorganisms. Since then considerable progress has been made towards understanding the basis behind this microbiota-mediated protection, also known as 'colonisation resistance' and the impact of specific microbial members on this key defence mechanism. The beginnings of colonisation resistance occur shortly after birth when microorganisms (a large number of which are facultative anaerobes) are transferred to the newborn from the mother and their surrounding environment. The makeup of the intestinal microbiota later shifts as the infant diet changes from maternal milk to a solid diet and over subsequent years it stabilises and becomes resistant to change within the individual. This resistance to change limits the ability of new microbes, including pathogens, to colonise the gut of the host. Thus, invading microbes must compete for limited space and nutrients against entrenched microbiota–host symbiotic relationships as well as resist against potent antimicrobial molecules produced by some resident gut microbes.

## IECs (M Cells and Goblet Cells) Provide the First line of Defence Against Noxious Luminal Stimuli Through a Variety of Innate Receptors

The intestinal epithelium is an integral component of innate immunity. It not only tolerates the presence of the luminal microbiota but also protects the intestinal mucosa from harmful dietary antigens and invading pathogens. The epithelium primes and signals professional immune cells to promote an effective inflammatory/immune response. IECs provide the first line of defence against noxious luminal stimuli and professional immune cells are only activated once these defences are overcome. Among the different IEC types, M cells and goblet cells play key roles in the establishment of intestinal tolerance and the induction of mucosal immune responses. They indiscriminately sample luminal contents and transcytose intact antigens to underlying dendritic cells for antigen processing and presentation.

**IECs express a variety of innate receptors** that detect microbes and endogenous danger signals, including the toll-like receptors (TLRs). Enterocytes are known to express TLR2, TLR3, TLR4, TLR5 and TLR9. Once activated at the basolateral membrane, TLR signalling initiates a signalling cascade cumulating in the nuclear translocation of NF$\kappa$B. This leads to the expression and secretion of various cytokines and chemokines, including TNF-$\alpha$, IL-6, IL-8, IL-18 and CCL20, which signal and prime underlying immune cells. Additional antimicrobial factors including $\beta$-defensins and iNOS are also induced following TLR activation.

While TLRs expressed by IECs play a key role in recognising nearby microbes and their products, the responses they elicit are primarily aimed at keeping microbes at a distance (mucin secretion and antimicrobial production) or recruiting immune cells (via chemokines) to the site of infection. Upon direct invasion of IECs by intracellular pathogens, a more vigorous means of host defence is triggered, by which enterocytes can physically expel themselves from the intestinal epithelial lining while still maintaining mucosal barrier function. They are excreted along with sloughed enterocytes.

This process prevents intracellular pathogens from breaching the epithelial barrier. This expulsion (of intracellular pathogen-invaded enterocyte) involves activation of the inflammatory caspases (e.g. caspase-1, -4, -8 and -11). The activation of the cell-specific 'inflammasome' may be due to various PAMP (pathogen-associated molecular pattern) and DAMP (damage-associated molecular pattern) cytoplasmic insults. Once the 'inflammasome' is activated, this triggers the processing and secretion of pro-inflammatory cytokine (PIC) IL-18 and the induction of inflammatory cell death (pyroptosis). This manifests in cell sloughing of IECs.

## ROLE OF IMMUNOMODULATORY NUTRIENTS IN SUPPORTING GUT BARRIER INTEGRITY AND FUNCTION

A substance that modulates the immune response is known as immunomodulator or immune modulator. It has been demonstrated that several immunomodulatory nutrients modulate host immune and inflammatory responses and restore the intestinal barrier after injury. Immunomodulatory nutrients include functional feed ingredients/nutrients that include organic acids, plant extracts, amino acids (glutamine, arginine, tryptophan and citrulline), fatty acids (short-chain fatty acids, omega-3 and conjugated linoleic acid) and probiotics.

### Functional Feed Ingredients that can be Applied to Modulate Intestinal Microbiota and Immunity

1. First and foremost is mild acidification (through organic acids) of water and/or feed to enhance the decrease in pH of the digesta in the stomach of pigs or the crop, proventriculus and gizzard of birds.
2. Second is strengthening the mucosal/ intestinal barrier function. Butyrate, but also specific plant extracts, may have pronounced protective effects on the mucosal/ intestinal barrier function by increasing mucous production, epithelial cell proliferation and modulation of the gut associated immune system.
3. A specific combination of organic acids, with butyrate, medium chain fatty acids (MCFA), probiotics, prebiotics, enzymes and a selected phenolic compound in both broiler chickens and piglets has worked well.

Plant-derived feed additives (PFAs) such as certain polyphenols have been documented to improve the intestine barrier function, e.g. via inhibition of the NFκB, modulation of protein kinase pathways (e.g., MAPK), regulation of the activity of key enzymes and reduction of reactive oxygen species, all resulting in beneficial effects on TJ integrity (Yang, et al, 2017). PFAs are applied as plant powders (often derived from culinary or medicinal herbs or spices) or as concentrated active ingredients (e.g. as essential oils, extracts or pure phytochemicals). PFAs are also referred to as "phytogenics" (Steiner and Syed, 2015).

Bachinger et al (2018) conducted *in vitro* tests to evaluate the influence of phytogenics on the barrier function recovery of intestinal porcine epithelial cells (IPEC-J2) after disruption, particularly on the abundance of tight junction proteins and found liquorice and angelica root extracts had potential beneficial effects. The increased transepithelial electrical resistance (TEER) caused by the liquorice root extract correlated with an increase in the abundance of the tight junction protein claudin 4.

### Amino Acids

Amino acids serve as important physiologic fuels for small intestinal mucosa apart from their essential monomeric role for synthesis of different nitrogenous compounds such as proteins. **Glutamine** is quantitatively the most important fuel for the intestinal tissue and immune cells. It is a key precursor for the intestinal synthesis of glutathione and is important for intestinal surface integrity. **Arginine** is required in higher quantity during metabolic stress, organ maturation and development. This amino acid is obtained from dietary proteins and can be metabolised in enterocytes. Nitric oxide (NO) and polyamines are metabolites of arginine. Nitric oxide is important for the maintenance of the intestinal barrier in different intestinal diseases. Polyamines (putrescine, spermidine and spermine) are important for the growth and repair of gastrointestinal mucosa. Arginine has been found to preserve intestinal barrier integrity in animals after intestinal obstruction. **Citrulline,** the precursor of arginine, also preserved gut barrier function and reduced bacterial translocation. Supplementation with **L-tryptophan** reduced intestinal permeability.

## Fatty Acids

**Short-chain fatty acids (SCFAs),** mainly acetate, propionate and butyrate are produced by bacterial fermentation in the large intestine and in the rumen in ruminants and in the large intestine in monogasrics. **SCFAs** are an important energy source for colonocytes. Butyrate is the preferred substrate for enterocytes. **SCFAs** are produced by bacteria through the fermentation of low-digestibility carbohydrates and proteins (Kong et al, 2014). *Bifidobacterium, Lactobacillus, Clostridium coccoides-Eubacteria rectal, Faecalibacterium prausnitzii* and *Prevotella* have been reported to produce SCFAs (Beards et al, 2010).

Enteral administration of **omega-3 fatty acids** reversed intestinal injury and stimulated intestinal recovery. This effect may be explained by increased cell proliferation and decreased cell death (Koppelmann et al, 2013).

**Conjugated linoleic acid** (CLA) is a mixture of positional and geometric isomers of linoleic acid. Beneficial effects of CLA supplementation have been observed in intestinal inflammation. Recent studies indicate that CLA exhibits anti-inflammatory activity by several pathways, including NFκB (an inflammatory transcription factor) and peroxisome proliferator-activated receptors (PPARs). Lipids bind and activate PPARs in the intestine and moderate anti-inflammatory effects by antagonising the actions of NFκB leading to the downregulation of pro-inflammatory cytokines and the upregulation of anti-inflammatory cytokines (Reynolds et al, 2008).

## Probiotics

The benefits conferred by the use of probiotics are diverse and include the activation of the immune system, enhanced mucosal/intestinal barrier function and prevention of infections. These systemic and local effects, especially in the intestinal mucosa, can provide benefits in the management of gastrointestinal diseases. Probiotic species commonly used commercially are *Bifidobacterium, Saccharomyces* and *Lactobacillus.*

Thus supplementation of immunomodulatory nutrients before and/or during intestinal injury has been shown to restore intestinal barrier homeostasis with respect to intestinal permeability and bacterial translocation and the balance of local and systemic immunological responses (Andrade et al, 2015). Further, the use of these agents in clinical practice could contribute to a reduction in hospital costs due to prolonged hospitalisation.

## CHITOSAN OLIGOSACCHARIDE AND INTESTINAL INFLAMMATION

### Immature Intestinal Barrier

The intestinal epithelium is continuously exposed to potentially harmful antigens, pathogens, toxins and air pollutants. Premature enterocytes are vulnerable to these exogenous and endogenous stimuli. An immature mucosal/intestinal barrier function and immune response are thought to make premature neonates particularly susceptible to intestinal inflammation, which can lead to mucosal damage and dysfunction such as necrotising enterocolitis.

### Chitin and its Derivatives

Certain nutrients such as glutamine, arginine, (n-3) polyunsaturated fatty acids and chitosan may play an active role in maintaining the barrier function of the intestine as well as in downregulating inflammation. There is substantial variation in the literature on the biological properties of chitosan and chitooligosaccharide (COS; Liu et al, 2006).

**Variance in MW of compounds:** This variation is most probably due to the widely different molecular weights (MW) of compounds used across studies. The supplementation of COS of molecular weight (MW) from 5–10 kDa upward range may act as effective substitute for in-feed antibiotics during the post-weaning period. The inclusion range of 10–50 kDa COS seems to be the optimum MW range to increase growth performance (Walsh et al, 2012) by enhancing small intestine structure, improving nutrient digestibility, modifying *E. coli* populations and reducing diarrhoea in pigs.

A possible reason for the higher-MW COS (5–10 kDa upward) exhibiting an antibacterial activity is that COS may interact with the membrane of the cell to alter cell permeability (Chung and Chen, 2008). The second mechanism is that COS penetrates the nuclei of the bacteria and interferes with RNA and protein synthesis (Liu et al, 2004).

## Chitosan Oligosaccharides

Chitosan oligosaccharides (COS) are hydrolysed products from chitosan with a mixture of oligomers of β-1,4-linked D-glucosamine residues. Due to their water solubility, biocompatibility, intestinal absorbability and bioactivity, COS have received considerable interest for potential application as a dietary supplement or nutraceutical. COS also may be a good source material for the development of a potent therapeutic agent against inflammatory responses that has been shown to have beneficial effects on inflammatory diseases in animal models and clinical trials.

## Mechanism of the Anti-inflammatory Effect of COS

Some studies have identified the direct target and molecular mechanism of the anti-inflammatory effect of COS. Nuclear transcription factor kappa B (NFκB) is one of the major signal transduction pathways that is activated in response to inflammation and regulates the expression of a variety of genes involved in the inflammatory response (Artis, D. 2008; Onizawa et al, 2009). It has been indicated that COS reduces inflammation through the suppression of NFκB activation in some cell and animal models (Qiao et al, 2010; Fang

et al, 2013; Fang et al, 2014). Study conducted by Muanprasat et al (2015) revealed that COS inhibited NFκB transcriptional activity (and the NFκB-mediated inflammatory response and barrier disruption) via adenosine monophosphate-activated protein kinase (AMPK)-independent mechanisms.

**Lipopolysaccharide (LPS) has been widely used to mimic features of inflammatory diseases:** LPS can interact with their respective receptors [toll-like receptor (TLR4), TNF receptors 1 and 2] and elicit the NFκB-mediated production of pro-inflammatory cytokines such as TNF-α, IL-1β, and IL-6 and induce extensive intestinal inflammation. In the present study (Huang et al, 2016), LPS induced higher serum concentrations of TNF-α, IL-1β, IL-6, and IL-8 and this was accompanied by significant growth impairment and intestinal histopathological injury. The LPS-induced production of these pro-inflammatory cytokines was suppressed by COS but was not observed in the normal piglets.

Studies of Yang et al, (2016) suggested that dietary supplementation with COS affects intestine and immune functions of weaned piglets.

## Chitosan Improves Intestinal Barrier Function

Intestinal barrier is mainly formed by a layer of epithelial cells covered with mucous. Tight junction proteins form a physical barrier between two adjacent epithelial cells to prevent paracellular absorption of pathogens or toxins. But the intestinal barrier gets damaged due to intestinal inflammation leading to an increase in intestinal permeability. Increased intestinal permeability has been shown to be closely associated with elevated pro-inflammatory cytokines in inflammatory bowel disease (IBD). Dietary supplementation of COS reduced the circulating pro-inflammatory cytokines. It also downregulated the expression of intestinal pro-inflammatory cytokines including TNF-α, IL-1α, IL-1β, IL-2, IL-8, IFN-γ and GM-CS in LPS-challenged piglets. This may reflect an improvement in intestinal barrier function and the prevention of subsequent infiltration of immune cells.

Huang et al (2016) have concluded that COS can act as an agonist of calcium-sensing receptor (CaSR) to exhibit intestinal anti-inflammatory effects. These findings indicate that COS may be able to reduce the intestinal inflammatory response, concomitant with the activation of CaSR and the inhibition of NFκB signalling pathways under an inflammatory stimulus. Further studies are needed to elucidate the mechanisms that regulate homeostasis and crosstalk between CaSR and the NFκB mediated inflammatory pathway in health and disease.

## HOW TO REDUCE WEANING-ASSOCIATED INTESTINAL DYSFUNCTION IN PIGLETS? ROLE OF MATERNAL NUTRITION TO STIMULATE GUT HEALTH

Gastrointestinal health is enormously important. Feed is not only supposed to help the animal to grow, but also to keep them healthy. Feed processing (grinding, rolling, pelleting) and form of feed (meal or pellet) have impacts on gut health. Particle size of feed influences stomach's health and function as well as animal welfare. The small intestine in pigs is about 22 meters long. This allows the animal to absorb nutrients. It is important that proteins are being digested in the small intestine. Details into these aspects give better understanding how nutrition strategies stimulate gut health and development. Before dwelling on these aspects, awareness on how maternal nutrition influences the immunity of piglets is imperative.

### Effect of Sow Nutrition on Composition of Colostrum

The colostrum and milk have the potential to deliver antimicrobial effects (Bauer et al, 2006a) and immune-enhancing properties to the piglet. Both colostrum and milk contain a lot of different antimicrobial substances such as glycoproteins, glycolipids, mucins and oligosaccharides (Bauer et al, 2006b). They also contain lactoferrin, which has bactericidal properties and prevents the induction of cytokines that can cause inflammation (Bauer et al, 2006b). Some of these components in milk can support the establishment of a beneficial commensal microbiota (Bauer et al, 2006a). The immunoglobulin IgA is an immunoglobulin in milk. It is important in the defence against intestinal pathogens and also serves an essential role in preventing bacterial translocation beyond the gastrointestinal tract (GIT). Higher levels of immunoglobulins in the colostrum and milk can improve the acquired passive immunity in newborn piglets. From studies that evaluated the effect of sow nutrition on colostrum and milk composition, it can be concluded that dietary manipulation affects the nutrient composition and immunoglobulin content of both colostrum and milk (Farmer and Quesnel, 2009).

### Development of GIT and Immune System

The development of both the GIT and the immune system of the pig are influenced by maternal factors throughout the gestation. The GIT develops early in embryonic life, during the process of gastrulation that occurs on about day 8 of gestation. The immune system has begun developing by day 16 of gestation, with the development of the lymphoid-cell population. The developing thymus and spleen are evident by day 22 of gestation. The first B cells can be detected in the liver at about day 30 of gestation, and surface IgM cells are found in the spleen at about day 50 (Sinkora and Butler, 2009).

The porcine foetus develops in the absence of maternal immunoglobulins, due to the specialised epitheliochorial placenta. Hence, B cells and the humoral component of the immune system are naive at birth, having developed without anti-idiotypic influences from the mother during foetal life. The number of circulating lymphocytes and their functional activity declines after birth and for a period of 14–21 days (Hammerberg et al, 1989). This period of decline in the circulating lymphocytes coincides with weaning and could potentially contribute to weaning dysregulation.

At birth, the GIT of pigs is sterile due to the sterile environment *in utero*. Immediately after birth, the GIT of the neonatal piglet is colonised by bacteria derived from the sow's vaginal tract and faeces and from other maternal and environmental sources. The process of microflora development can be influenced by diet, environmental factors and the genotype of the piglet itself. The establishment of the pig intestinal microbiota is a complex process, initially the intestine of the newborn is rapidly invaded by bacteria, followed by different successional steps where diverse groups become predominant. This process continues as the pig matures, the microbial patterns change in piglets within a few days, resulting in a characteristic and dynamic bacterial population for each individual. The microbiota establishment after birth plays an important role in the development of the neonatal intestinal and immune systems (Mukherjee and Hooper, 2015).

## Weaning age and Consequence of Weaning

It has been suggested to wean piglets at five to six weeks of age allowing the piglets to get used to dry (creep) feed more gradually. The younger the weaning occurs, the larger the risk for intestinal problems with piglets. But many farms in western countries wean their piglets somewhere between 22 and 26 days of age. This leads to post-weaning diarrhoea (PWD) caused by enterotoxigenic *E.coli* (ETEC). In India the weaning age, as per the ICAR, is eight weeks of age. But still diarrhoea remains a giant challenge.

Weaning is a major cause of stress to piglets due to multi-factorial stressors such as nutritional, environmental and physiological factors, resulting in an immediate drop in voluntary feed intake post-weaning (Lalles et al, 2007a). The decreased feed intake affects the intestinal health balance, inducing

undesired morphological, physiological and microbial changes in the GIT. Subsequently, these changes give pathogenic microbes an opportunity to colonise the intestinal tract and reduce the barrier function of the intestine (see page 164) and cause intestinal inflammation and PWD.

## Manipulation of Microflora in the intestinal Tract of Piglets

In their natural rearing, neonatal pigs are less exposed to potentially pathogenic bacteria and hence they have a lower chance of developing PWD (Bauer et al, 2006a, 2006b; Heim et al, 2014a). There are a few ways to manipulate the colonisation process in the newborn piglet's GIT.

Piglets are known to explore the farrowing crate and can ingest large quantities of faeces from the sow (Demeckova et al 2002). Hence, the maternal administration of probiotics containing beneficial bacteria can result in a higher colonisation of these bacteria in the piglet GIT, thereby reducing colonisation of pathogenic bacteria. Both Leonard et al (2012) and Heim et al (2014a) showed that supplementing pregnant-sow diets with seaweed extracts (SWE) containing laminarin and fucoidan during late gestation reduced the *Enterobacteriaceae* population in the sow's faeces, while also reducing colonic *Escherichia coli* numbers in the piglets at weaning. This indicates that manipulation of the microflora of the sow has the potential to reduce the abundance of pathogenic bacteria in the intestinal tract of her offspring.

## Maternal Supplementation of Yeast and Seaweed Extracts on GIT Health of Offspring

The use of feed additives such as short-chain fructo-oligosaccharides and β-glucans from different strains of yeast in sow diets result in improved immunoglobulin concentrations in colostrum. Heim et al (2014a) reported that seaweed extracts containing the bioactive compounds laminarin and fucoidan also increased immunoglobulin concentrations in colostrum and milk. Maternal seaweed extracts (SWE) supplementation increases piglet serum IgG concentration on day 14 of lactation (Leonard et al, 2012), while piglets suckling SWE-supplemented sows have improved leukocyte phagocytosis capacity (Leonard et al, 2010).

Maternal supplementation with SWE appears to have enhanced the immuno-globulin status of the piglets and the ability of the piglets to fight pathogenic bacterial challenges. Piglets suckling the sows supplemented with SWE containing laminarin and fucoidan have improved resistance to enterotoxigenic *E. coli* (ETEC) infections and reduced shedding of this pathogen post-weaning following an ETEC challenge (Heim et al, 2014a). More recently, it was shown that piglets suckling the sows supplemented with laminarin have improved resistance to an experimental *Salmonella* typhimurium challenge and reduced shedding of this pathogen post-weaning. The *IL-22* expression in the colon is reduced in pigs weaned from laminarin-supplemented sows. The presence of *S. typhimurium* is linked to the expression of *IL-22* in the intestinal tract, since IL-22 is involved in repair and protection of intestinal barrier surfaces, especially during microbial challenges. Indeed, IL-22 is thought to play a unique role in *S. typhimurium* infections.

Cytokines are produced in response to microbial threat and aid in the recruitment and activation of immune cells to protect the host. In response to epithelial damage or dysfunction, immune cells are activated to produce interleukin (IL)-22. Using comple-mentary *in vitro* and *in vivo* approaches, Ngo et al (2018) defined a critical IL-36/IL-23/IL-22 cytokine network that is instrumental for antimicrobial peptide (AMP) production and host defence. This cytokine network is activated in response to intestinal barrier damage and these are involved in providing critical host defence.

Pigs from laminarin- and fucoidan-supplemented sows [from day 87 of gestation and the offsprings were monitored until time of slaughter (~90 kg)] had greater nutrient digestibility and increased numbers of faecal

*Lactobacilli* spp., greater villous architecture at weaning and had higher daily gain than did control pigs of this long duration studies (Heim et al, 2015). These studies indicated that the ingredients used in the maternal diet can have a substantial influence on growth and gastrointestinal health of the offspring in postnatal life.

## Effect of Weaning on the Intestinal Health of the Piglet

The villi and crypts that line the epithelium of the small intestine are essential for the digestive and absorptive processes and their structure and function after weaning are affected by many factors (Pluske et al, 1997).

### Reduction in Nutrient Intake

Level of feed intake is the most important determinant of mucosal function and integrity. A continuous supply of nutrients is essential for maintenance of GIT integrity, as the absence of nutrients in the small-intestine lumen will have marked effects on the rate of cell differentiation and turnover (Pluske et al, 2003). Weaning is a critical period and is undertaken abruptly at an early age, normally 14–28 days after birth. Weaning induces transient and acute changes in the mor-phology and physiology of the GIT, which are most likely to be related to the post-weaning reduction in feed intake. Food deprivation in piglets leads to a lack of luminal stimulation and induces a reduction in villous height and an increase in crypt depth (Pluske et al, 1997). Villous height is minimised after 2–5 days post-weaning and is associated with cell loss and reduced absorption of nutrients. Inte-stinal villous height starts to recover in feed-deprived piglets at ~ 4 days after feeding is restarted, but can take more than 10 days to fully recover (Boudry et al, 2004).

### Change in Nutrient Source

Besides the intestinal morphology being affected by weaning, the activity of many enzymes of membranous phase of digestion is also reduced due to the reduced feed intake and reduced supply of nutrients. Part of this reduced supply can also be attributed to the change in nutrient source.

The sow milk is highly digestible, contains bioactive substances and the main energy sources are fat and lactose. The post-weaning feed is typically solid, has a much higher dry matter content, is less digestible and the main energy source is starch (Kim et al, 2012a). This reduced digestibility is partly due to the insufficient enzyme production in the piglet. The endogenous enzymes are adapted to the digestion of nutrients from sow milk. Therefore, sufficient amounts of lipase, amylase and other necessary enzymes needed to digest the post-weaning diet are not produced until ~3–4 weeks post-weaning.

The provision of creep feed supplemented with the necessary enzymes may be a useful tool to prepare piglets during weaning to the consumption of solid feed and to avoid the post-weaning anorexia.

*Impaired Intestinal Barrier Function and Increased Intestinal Permeability*

It has been reported that weaning stress results in an impaired intestinal barrier function and an increased intestinal permeability, as a result of a reduced energy uptake and increased inflammatory response in the GIT (Boudry et al, 2004; Wijtten et al, 2011). Therefore, it is very important to try and improve the small-intestinal morphology by improving feed intake in the immediate post-weaning period, so as to reduce the intestinal permeability and, thus, pathogenic susceptibility and intestinal inflammation. See page 160 for a detailed discussion on these topics, i.e. intestinal barrier function and intestinal permeability.

*Microbiological Changes in the GIT Post-weaning*

The balance between a healthy and unhealthy microflora can be easily changed towards a pathogenic profile immediately after weaning. The numbers of *Lactobacillus* spp. and other beneficial bacteria decrease in times of stress. This encourages the establishment of

pathogens. When lactic acid bacteria (harmless bacteria) are attached to the mucosal layer of the intestinal tract, they can prevent pathogens adhering to the enterocytes, thus preventing the multiplication of these pathogens and production of their toxins. This reduces the opportunities for pathogenic bacteria to increase their abundance and reduces the risk of the onset of PWD.

The gastric pH is an important first barrier against pathogens entering the intestine and influencing the intestinal microbiota. The conversion of lactose to lactic acid by microbes during the suckling period helps maintain this low gastric pH. However, the weaning-associated anorexia can result in an increased gastric pH and reduces the acidic protection against microbial pathogens. The introduction of a solid diet requires an increase in anaerobic bacteria in both number and diversity. Furthermore, reduced feed intake leads to rapid changes in the microbiota as substrates available for microbial fermentation are depleted.

Because of change of diet and lack of enough nutrients, the microbiota becomes unstable during the first week post-weaning, with a marked decrease in biodiversity, which will be restored after a reestablishment period of 2–3 weeks. Diarrhoea generally occurs in pigs 3–10 days post-weaning and is often associated with an over-population of ETEC bacteria carrying specific heat-labile and/or heat-stable enterotoxins (Lalles et al, 2007b).

## Impact of Nutrients on Gut Health and Development in Post-weaned Pigs

Extensive research studies have explored the impact of a wide range of feed ingredients and nutrients on various aspects of gut health and development in pigs during the post-weaning period (Lalles et al, 2007a). The value of selected nutrients and feed ingredients in stimulating gut health and development is discussed in the following.

### Amino Acids and Protein

In recent years, the recommended levels of amino acids have increased (NRC, 2012) in diets for weaned pigs, while the crude protein content is ~200–230 g/kg. This level of protein can be quite problematic to weaned pigs. Not all dietary protein is available for the newly weaned pig because the pig's ability to digest and absorb high protein diets is generally compromised post-weaning. This results in protein entering the large intestine to be fermented, which encourages the growth of N-utilising bacteria such as *E. coli*, producing potentially toxic substances such as ammonia, amines, indoles, phenols and branched-chain fatty acids; these are implicated in the pathogenesis of PWD (Pluske et al, 2002). The studies by several researchers proved that a reduced crude protein content reduces protein fermentation in the intestine but does not negatively affect growth performance.

## Lactose and other Fermentable Carbohydrates

The inclusion of dairy products and other highly digestible and palatable ingredients such as sugar, rolled oats, animal by-products and cooked rice is a common practice in piglet nutrition and this enhances feed intake in the immediate post-weaning period. Dairy products are known to have beneficial effects on feed intake, growth performance, feed efficiency and health in newly weaned piglets. This is due to the high palatability and digestibility of protein and energy in dairy products (Lalles et al, 2007a). Dietary inclusion of lactose results in rapid fermentation into lactic acid due to the presence of lactic acid bacteria. The subsequent lowering of the pH in the GIT may delay the multiplication of pathogenic bacteria thereby improves gastrointestinal health. The inclusion of other fermentable carbohydrates such as sugar-beet pulp, inulin and resistant wheat starch also promotes colonic microbial stability and diversity and stimulates gastrointestinal health (Lalles et al, 2007a). The inclusion of these fermentable carbohydrates results in an increased transient time of the digesta in the stomach and small intestine, giving the endogenous enzymes a better chance at hydrolysing the nutrients (Lalles

et al, 2007a). The inclusion of the right proportion of insoluble and soluble fibre reduces the abundance of *Enterobacteriaceae*.

## Leguminous Plant Proteins

Dietary components originating from leguminous plant proteins (e.g. soya bean meal and peas) are known to have negative effects on growth and health post-weaning due to antigenic effects associated with the feed. The inclusion of these legumes can result in a localised immune response, villous atrophy, crypt hyperplasia and decreased growth. However, high dietary concentrations of lactose allow for increased soya bean meal inclusion (>200 g/kg) in weaning pig diets, without affecting performance or health.

## Feed Additives in Post-weaning Diet

A diverse range of feed additives has been researched, so as to replace antimicrobial growth promotors (AGP; de Lange et al, 2010). Various (natural) materials have been investigated as efficient alternatives to AGPs, such as zinc oxide, copper sulphate, prebiotics such as galacto-oligosaccharides, yeast, β-glucans, mannanoligosaccharides, organic acids, probiotics, spray-dried plasma proteins, exogenous feed enzymes and essential oils. These feed additives can beneficially affect the microbiota composition and health and growth performance of pigs. However, only a limited number of feed additives are effective in stimulating gut development and health of pigs that are managed under wide-ranging conditions of housing, management, feeding and health status.

It is important to remember that these feed additives are now required on their own to improve digestive health in the absence of in-feed antibiotics. There is fundamental requirement to explore the underlying mechanisms of activity when evaluating the functional properties of feed ingredients and feed additives, so as to better understand under what conditions it is possible to achieve the optimal response to dietary interventions

(Pluske, 2013). Key aspects of gut functionality that should be considered to include are digestive capacity (activity of pancreatic and brush-border enzymes), absorptive capacity (villi architecture and nutrient-transporter expression), chemical and physical barriers, microbiota load and diversity and immune function (de Lange et al, 2010).

### Novel Bioactives in Post-weaning Diets

Terrestrial plants, marine macroalgae and marine organisms, including microorganisms, offers a valuable source of novel bioactives. Diverse organisms have evolved diverse chemical and molecular mechanisms for a variety of homeostatic activities, including cell-to-cell signalling, receptor sensitivity, inflammasome activity and gene activation (Sweeney and O'Doherty, 2016) and, hence, offer great potential as preventatives and prophylactics in mammals.

- Marine macroalgal extracts are showing a wide range of biological activities (i.e. antioxidant, anticancer, anticoagulant and anti-inflammatory activities, among others), with potential use in the food and nutraceutical markets. They are a rich source of structurally diverse bioactive compounds with valuable pharmaceutical and biomedical potential.

- Brown marine algae contain large amounts (~40% of the dry matter) of polysaccharides, particularly laminarin and fucoidan, which are resistant to hydrolysis by human endogenous enzymes and are, therefore, valuable dietary fibres for bacterial fermentation in the large intestine.

### Laminarin

Laminarin is a specific type of β-glucan extracted from seaweed species. In general, it has a low molecular weight of ~5 kDa and is soluble in water. It has been suggested that the immunoprotective effects are mediated through receptor-mediated interactions between β-glucans and epithelial microfold cells in the GIT.

The specialised microfold cells are primarily responsible for the transport of macromolecules within the Peyer's patches. The β-glucan is taken up by the Peyer's patches and is presented to underlying dendritic cells to influence cytokine production. Dietary supplementation of 50- day-old pigs with β-glucan from *Laminaria digitata*, *L. hyperborea* and *Saccharomyces cerevisiae* downregulated the expression of a panel of inflammatory cytokines in the colon and liver (Sweeney et al, 2012) and mucin gene expression in the ileum and colon. Similar observations were subsequently reported in the newly weaned piglet.

Beta-glucans can agglutinate certain bacterial species, inhibiting subsequent attachment and colonisation of epithelial mucosa' surfaces. β-glucan supplementation showed reductions in the faecal excretion of F4 *E. coli* and a reduced F4-specific serum antibody response, thus decreasing susceptibility to ETEC infection.

### Fucoidan

Fucoidan represents a class of fucose-enriched sulphated polysaccharides extracted from the extracellular matrix of brown algae. Research has indicated that fucoidan possesses antimicrobial, immunomodulatory, antioxidant and antiviral properties (Sweeney and O'Doherty, 2016). Fucoidan is thought to affect leukocyte recruitment following an infection and reduces tissue breakdown during inflammation. Fucoidan supplementation results in an increased *Lactobacillus* spp. abundance in colonic digesta in pigs (Sweeney and O'Doherty, 2016).

### LEAKY GUT—ITS CONTRIBUTION TO INEFFICIENT NUTRIENT UTILISATION IN KETOSIS AND HEAT STRESS

#### What is 'Leaky Gut'?

The intestinal barrier gets destroyed when intestine has inflammation. Intestinal permeability is increased. Intestinal luminal content is leaked inappropriately. This is referred to as 'leaky gut'. Leaky gut is a condition in which the small intestine lining becomes damaged, allowing molecules such as bacteria, pathogens (see page 164) and their toxins to pass in between epithelial cells, resulting in cell damage or inflammation of the intestine.

## How Leaky Gut Leads to Inflammation

Once the bacteria, pathogens or their toxins pass between cells, the immune system recognises them and triggers an immune response to destroy and remove the invaders. This inflammatory process and immune system activation consumes significant amounts of nutrients. The characteristics of leaky gut are shortened crypt depth, decreased villus height and decreased villus height to crypt depth ratio. This impedes nutrient utilisation.

Two well-known examples in an animal's life that markedly reduce production are heat stress and ketosis. In these situations nutrient utilisation is reprioritised. Decreased feed intake, experienced during both the diseases, is unable to fully explain the causes for decrease in the productivity. Additionally, both diseases are characterised by negative energy balance, body weight loss, inflammation and hepatic steatosis. The metabolism of ketosis and heat stress has been thoroughly studied for the last 40 years. Kvidera et al (2016) generated data implicating a metabolic disruptor, endotoxin, as the etiological culprit in each case.

## Reduction in Animal Performance: Heat Stress and Ketosis

### Heat stress

- Heat stress affects productivity indirectly by reducing feed intake. However, direct mechanisms also contribute as it is shown that reduced feed intake only explains approximately 35–50% of the decreased milk yield during heat stress (Rhoads et al, 2009; Wheelock et al, 2010; Baumgard et al, 2011).
- Direct mechanisms contributing to heat stress-milk yield losses involve an altered

endocrine profile, including reciprocal changes in circulating anabolic and catabolic hormones (Bernabucci et al, 2010; Baumgard and Rhoads, 2012).

Such changes are characterised by increased circulating insulin concentration, lack of adipose tissue lipid mobilisation and reduced adipocyte responsiveness to lipolytic stimuli. Hepatic and skeletal muscle cellular bioenergetics also exhibit clear differences in carbohydrate production and use, respectively, due to heat stress. Thus, the heat stress response markedly alters post-absorptive carbohydrate, lipid and protein metabolism through coordinated changes in fuel supply and utilisation across tissues in a manner distinct from commonly recognisable changes that occur in animals on a reduced plane of nutrition (Baumgard and Rhoads, 2013). Increase in plasma corticosterone concentration suppresses innate immune system of poultry, while decreased thyroid hormone triidothyronin affects lean tissue accretion and growth. The result of heat stress consequently is underachievement of an animal's full genetic potential.

**Ketosis:** The periparturient period is associated with substantial metabolic changes involving normal homeorhetic adaptations to support milk production. Ketosis is defined as an excess of circulating ketone bodies and is characterised by decreases in feed intake and milk production and increased risk of developing other transition period diseases. Traditionally, ketosis is thought to result from excessive adipose tissue mobilisation, which in turn contributes to fatty liver (hepatic steatosis) and excessive ketone body synthesis.

## Mechanisms Responsible for Altered Nutrient Partitioning During Heat Stress (HS)

The intestinal epithelial cells establish a barrier between luminal environments and the internal milieu and the tight junction proteins play key roles in forming the barrier by sealing the paracellular space (Turner, 2009). However, the intestinal barrier gets destroyed when the intestine has inflammation because the expression of tight junction proteins is inhibited by pro-inflammatory cytokines.

During heat stress, blood flow is diverted from the viscera to the periphery in an attempt to dissipate heat leading to intestinal hypoxia (Hall et al, 1999). Enterocytes are particularly sensitive to hypoxia and nutrient restriction (Rollwagen et al, 2006), resulting in ATP depletion and increased oxidative and nitrosative stress (Hall et al, 2001). This contributes to tight junction dysfunction and gross morphological changes that ultimately reduce intestinal barrier function. That means gut wall integrity is decreased and intestinal permeability (IP) is increased. As a result, luminal content is leaked into portal and systemic blood in heat stress situations (Hall et al, 2001; Pearce et al, 2013). Luminal content has abundant number of gram-negative bacteria. These bacteria have lipopolysaccharide (LPS; otherwise referred to as endotoxin) embedded in their outer membrane. LPS is a major inducer of inflammatory response. That is how LPS infiltration occurs during heat stress and thus systemic inflammation is initiated.

**Endotoxemia share metabolic similarities to heat stress:** It is remarkable how animals suffering from heat stroke or severe endotoxemia share many physiological and metabolic similarities to HS, such as an increase in circulating insulin (Lim et al, 2007). The possibility that LPS increases insulin secretion likely explains the hyperinsulinemia that has been repeatedly reported in a variety of heat-stressed models (Baumgard and Rhoads, 2013).

**Mechanisms responsible for altered nutrient partitioning during ketosis:** The inflammatory state following calving disrupts normal nutrient partitioning and is detrimental to productivity, and this assumption has been reinforced in recent times when TNF-α infusion decreased productivity. Additionally, in late lactation cows, injecting TNF-α increased (>100%) liver triacylglycerols

content without a change in circulating NEFA (Bradford et al, 2009). The data from Kvidera et al, (2016) demonstrated increased inflammatory markers in cows diagnosed with ketosis only and not other health disorders. In comparison with healthy controls, ketotic cows had increased circulating LPS prior to calving; postpartum acute phase proteins such as LPS-binding protein (LBS), serum amyloid A, and haptoglobin were also increased (Abuajamieh et al, 2015).

Endotoxin can originate from a variety of locations, the obvious sources in transition dairy cows include the uterus (metritis), mammary gland (mastitis) and the gastrointestinal tract (Mani et al, 2012). But intestinal permeability may be responsible for inflammation observed in the transition dairy cow (Kvidera et al, 2016). A transition dairy cow undergoes a postcalving diet shift from a mainly forage based one to a high concentrate based ration (see Chapter 11 for more details). This has the potential to induce rumen acidosis, which can compromise the gastrointestinal tract barrier (Khafi pour et al, 2009).

**Simulation studies to create 'leaky gut':** In order to further investigate the effects of intestinal permeability on production and inflammation, Kvidera et al (2016) intentionally induced intestinal permeability in mid-lactation dairy cows by using a gamma secretase inhibitor (GSI), a compound that specifically inhibits crypt stem cell differentiation into enterocytes via disrupting Notch signalling (van Es et al, 2005). Treatment with GSI decreased feed intake and altered jejunum morphology consistently with characteristics of leaky gut. Circulating insulin and LPS binding protein (LBP) were increased in GSI-treated cows relative to controls. In summary, inflammation is present during the transition period and likely contributes to changes in whole-animal energetics.

## Metabolism of Inflammation and Energetic Cost of Inflammation

*Pseudomonas aeruginosa, Klebsiella pneumoniae,* and *Escherichia coli* are three typical gram-negative LPS-containing pathogens. Lipo-polysaccharide is one of the main components of the external cell wall of gram-negative bacteria. LPS is a well-characterised potent immune stimulator in multiple species. Activation of the immune system occurs when LPS binding protein (LBP) initially binds LPS and together with CD14 and TLR4 delivers LPS for removal and detoxification, thus LBP is frequently used as a biomarker for LPS infiltration (Ceciliani et al, 2012).

LPS-induced inflammation has an energetic cost, which redirects nutrients away from anabolic process that support milk and muscle synthesis and thus compromises productivity and efficiency. Interestingly, immune cells become more insulin sensitive and consume copious amounts of glucose upon activation in order to support rapid proliferation and biosynthetic processes. In contrast, inflammation induces an insulin resistant state in skeletal muscle and adipose tissue. Recent data has also demonstrated a decrease in ketone oxidation during LPS infiltration (Suagee et al, 2011; Frisard et al, 2015), which may partly explain increased ketone body concentrations during the transition period.

### Warburg Effect

An activated immune system requires a large amount of energy and the literature suggests that glucose homeostasis is markedly disrupted (Leininger et al, 2000) during an endotoxin challenge. Upon immune system activation, immune cells switch their metabolism from oxidative phosphorylation to aerobic glycolysis, causing them to become obligate glucose utilisers in a phenomenon known as the Warburg Effect (Vander Hiden et al, 2009). This is explained in Chapter 2 page 42.

### Decreased Productivity

Kvidera et al, (2016) estimated approximately 1 kg of glucose is used by the immune system during a 12 hour period in lactating dairy cows. The amount of glucose utilised by LPS-activated immune system in lactating cows,

growing steers and growing pigs were 0.64, 1.0, and 1.1 g glucose/kg $BW^{0.75}$/h, respectively (Stoakes et al, 2015a, c, d). Increased immune system glucose utilisation occurs simultaneously with infection-induced decreased feed intake. This coupling of enhanced nutrient requirements with hypophagia obviously decreases the amount of nutrients available for the synthesis of valuable products (milk, meat, foetus, wool).

It has been demonstrated that both heat-stressed and ketotic animals have increased circulating markers of endotoxin and inflammation. The circulating LPS in both the maladies originate from the intestine and thus both likely have an activated immune system. This activated systemic immune response reprioritises the hierarchy of glucose utilisation and milk synthesis is consequently deemphasised (Kvidera et al, 2016).

Ketosis and heat stress are two of the most economically important pathologies which severely jeopardise the competitiveness of animal agriculture. LPS is the common culprit responsible for both the metabolic disorders and the literature suggests that LPS markedly alters nutrient partitioning and is a causative agent in metabolic disruption during heat stress and ketosis.

### How to Strengthen the Tight Junctions?

Livestock producers need to pay more attention to leaky gut, inflammation and the immune system. With more restrictions on the use of antibiotics, health conditions such as leaky gut and intestinal inflammation will likely become a more prominent production challenge within livestock and poultry operations.

- Follow best management practices that include reducing stock density in the sheds and implementing more detailed sanitation procedures.
- Feed a balanced ration.

Various research studies have shown that weakening of the tight junctions in the gastrointestinal tract becomes more serious when a zinc deficiency is present. Zinc is important for the formation of structural components of tissues, molecules and epithelial cells present in the intestine. It strengthens the bonds between the epithelial cells in the gastrointestinal tract, helping to maintain the tight junctions during a challenge and decreasing the occurrence of leaky gut and related intestinal inflammation. It enhances the leukocyte population in the animal. So when a challenge does occur, the immune system can respond in a more rapid and robust manner.

## MANIPULATION OF GUT MICROBIOME TO ENHANCE CHICKEN PRODUCTION

Aviculture is currently, the most efficient animal productive system. Broiler chickens convert feed into muscle mass efficiently. Its farming is an effective system for high-quality protein production. The gastrointestinal microbiota plays a crucial role in host immune system, its physiological development, health, nutrition and productivity. Hence manipulation of the microbial community plays a pivotal role to enhance chicken growth and control either human or animal pathogens.

## Microbiome

The microbiota is defined as the microbial community, including commensal, symbiotic and pathogenic microorganisms, which usually colonise an area of human and animal organisms and are around 2 times more plentiful than somatic and germinal cells of the host (Sender et al, 2016). The collective genome of these symbionts is known as the microbiome. The microbiome of the broiler chicken gastrointestinal tract (GIT) has been extensively studied (Wei et al, 2013). Clavijo and Florez (2018) reviewed the modulatory role that bacteriophages, probiotics, prebiotics and phytobiotics exert on the chicken GIT.

The microbiota is involved in reducing and preventing colonisation by enteric pathogens through the process of competitive exclusion and the production of bacteriostatic and bactericidal substances. The taxonomic composition of the microbiota is affected by different factors, such as the organ, the age of the animal, diet and the use of antimicrobials.

## Effect of Diet on Establishment of the Microbiota

Diet is the factor that has the major impact. Nutrients contained in the diet modulate the growth and establishment of the microbiota. The principal characteristics of feed that may affect the microbiota are (i) the form of cereal (whole or milled grains, or pellets), (ii) the kind of cereal, (iii) the quantity of water-soluble non-starch polysaccharides and (iv) the sources of fat, starch and proteins (Gabriel et al, 2006). It has been reported that chickens fed with diets containing soya oil have a lower abundance of *Clostridium perfringens* than birds fed with fats of animal origin (Luo et al, 2016).

## Composition of the Microbiota According to GIT Location

Each organ of the digestive system performs functions that are important to the digestive process and the absorption of nutrients. Microorganisms perform independent functions in each of the organs, and it has been suggested that there is a significant difference in the taxonomic composition of the different organs of the digestive tract. These are delineated briefly.

i. **Crop:** Different species of *Lactobacillus* predominate in the crop. These are believed to be responsible for the decomposition of starch and the fermentation of lactate. Organ crop also hosts several species of the *Clostridiaceae* family. The beak gathers feed, while the bifurcated tongue is used to drink and to moisten it. Crop is a temporary storage site of mucous-soaked feed, which undergoes pre-digestion by enzymes such as ptylin of the saliva. The food passes slowly to the proventriculus (glandular stomach), where feedstuffs are bathed in gastric juices, hydrochloric acid and digestive enzymes, beginning the process of nutrient breakdown and the construction of the food bolus. Bolus passes to the gizzard.

ii. **Gizzard:** Similar to crop, gizzard (masticatory organ) is dominated by the same two genera of bacteria. However, the principal difference between the crop and the gizzard is the presence of gastric juices, pepsin and hydrochloric acid in the gizzard, which acidifies the medium, resulting in lower bacterial and less fermentation activity.

iii. **Small intestine:** Small intestine has the highest concentration of bacterial cells, principally *Lactobacillus, Enterococcus* and various Clostridiaceae; *Lactobacillus* is the dominant genus accounting for almost 70% of the total (Han et al, 2016).

iv. **Caecum:** The caecum is made up of two loops, the caeca. It is described as the organ with greatest taxonomic diversity and abundance because food is retained here for the longest period (12 to 20 h). Other characteristics that make this organ an important niche for the microbiota are that it is the site of greatest water absorption, it is responsible for regulating urea and it carries out the fermentation of carbohydrates that are resistant to bacterial digestion in the small intestine. The microbiota of the caeca is associated with the digestion of feedstuffs rich in cellulose, starch and polysaccharides. This organ principally hosts *Firmicutes, Bacteroides, Proteobacteria* and *Clostridiaceae*. Oakley et al (2014b) reported that *Megamonas, Helicobacter* and *Campylobacter* are also abundant in the caeca.

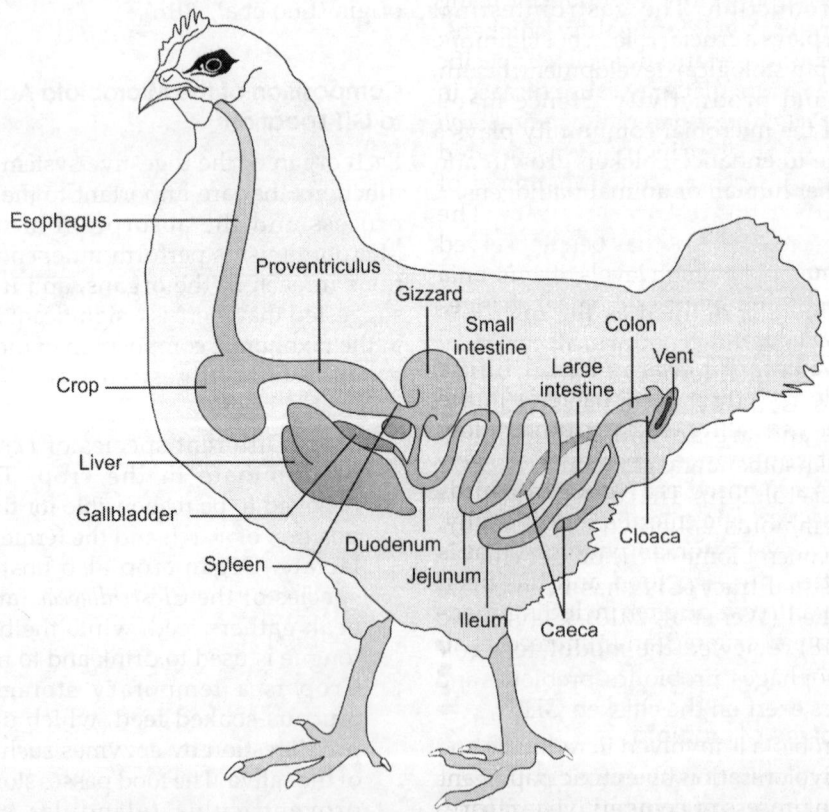

**Fig. 5.4:** Gastrointestinal tract in chickens and function. *Source:* Clavijo and Florez (2018)

## Presence of Pathogens in the Chicken Microbiota

The presence of pathogenic bacteria in the broiler chicken microbiota is important to animal and human health alike. Among the taxa that can cause illness in humans and that have been reported in the chicken microbiota are *Campylobacter* (principally *Campylobacter jejuni* and *Campylobacter coli*), *Salmonella enterica*, *Escherichia coli* and *Clostridium perfringens* (Oakley et al, 2014b). *Campylobacter* and *Salmonella* are principally responsible for gastrointestinal infections:

1. *Campylobacter* is generally accepted not to be pathogenic in birds, while.
2. *Salmonella enterica* can cause disease in chickens, depending on age, immune status and type of serovar.
3. On the other hand, *E. coli* is a gamma-proteobacterium present in the intestine, which is found in low abundance during the entire life cycle of healthy chickens. However, only certain strains have specific virulence factors that may cause disease in chickens; example avian pathogenic *E. coli* (APEC). APEC is principally associated with extra intestinal infections, most of which affect the respiratory tract. The pathogenicity of *E. coli* has been observed to be stimulated by high levels of ammonia in the sheds and by physiological changes in the host chicken.
4. *Clostridium perfringens* is found in the population of commensal bacteria in the intestines of healthy chickens at very low levels of abundance. However, *C. perfringens* is recognised as a pathogen in birds that causes necrotic enteritis. Additionally, *C. perfringens* is a human pathogen that is transmitted through food and has been traced to different origins, including foodstuffs of avian origin (Van Immerseel et al, 2004, 2009).

## Functions of the Microbiota

The digestive system is the most important reservoir of microorganisms. Therefore, various kinds of interaction have been found among broiler chickens and in their intestinal microbiota. Most important functions are four: these are 1. nutrient exchange, 2. modulation of the immune system, 3. the physiology of the digestive system and 4. the exclusion of pathogens.

### Nutrient Exchange

The commensal bacteria of the digestive system contribute nutrients that are both directly and indirectly important to the metabolism of chickens. These include short chain fatty acids (SCFAs), ammonium, amino acids and vitamins (Pan and Yu, 2014).

Most intestinal bacteria are capable of hydrolysing polysaccharides, oligosaccharides and disaccharides into primary sugars. Intestinal bacteria ferment these sugars and produce SCFAs such as acetate, propionate and butyrate. In the caeca, SCFAs are absorbed through the epithelium by passive diffusion.

Intestinal bacteria also contribute to the metabolism of nitrogen. For example, bacteria from the urogenital tract (these bacteria are capable of catabolising uric acid into ammonium) can travel from the cloaca to the caeca permitting the host to absorb ammonium. The absorbed ammonium is later used for synthesising amino acids.

The mucin produced by calceiform epithelial cells in the intestine is an important source of carbon, nitrogen and energy for commensal bacteria and pathogens alike (Tellez et al, 2006). The presence of mucin-degrading bacteria is associated with intestinal health, as they exert selection pressure on bacteria that cannot adhere to the mucosal surface (Pan and Yu, 2014).

### Immunological Modulation

The immunological system of chickens includes both the innate and the acquired immune response. The microbiota play an important role modulating the regulation and activation of both innate and acquired immune responses.

*Animal Nutrition and Immunity*

With reference to the innate immune response, the intestinal mucosa is considered the first line of defence against infection and a barrier that prevents commensal bacteria from penetrating the intestinal epithelium. This is achieved through glycoprotein mucin and antimicrobial peptides. The interior surface of the avian intestine is covered in a mucous layer made up of the glycoprotein mucin, secreted by calceiform epithelial cells (Brisbin et al, 2008). It has been found that mucins with sialic acid are more abundant in conventionally reared chickens when compared to mucins with sulphate, which are common in birds with low bacterial loads. These differences are observable from day 4 after birth and this suggests that the intestinal microbiota is involved in regulating the establishment of the mucous layer (Forder et al, 2007). The intestinal microbiota also regulates the production of antimicrobial peptides present on the surface of the intestinal epithelium, which are capable of rapidly killing or suppressing the activity of pathogens (Pan and Yu, 2014).

With reference to the acquired immune system, it would appear that the commensal bacteria provide protection to the mucosa membrane by modulating the immune response, by controlling the quantity of mediators secreted by the cells of the acquired immune system and stimulating the helper T cells (Oakley et al, 2014b). Using germ-free chickens, it was demonstrated that microbiota has a dramatic effect on the repertoire of intestinal T cells and their expression of cytokines (Oakley et al, 2014b).

*Physiology of the Digestive System*

The rapid development of the intestinal tract offers an ideal niche for colonisation by microorganisms and the microbiota also plays an important role in the development of the digestive tract (Uni et al, 1999). This process has been demonstrated in studies of germ-free chickens, which develop smaller intestines and caeca that weigh less and have thinner walls compared to conventionally reared

counterparts. It has been suggested that SCFAs increase the proliferation and growth of enterocytes, which would partially explain the difference (Mitsuhiro and Jun-ichi, 1994).

The activity of the digestive enzymes in chicken intestines may also be affected by the intestinal microbiota. When the activity of the alkaline phosphatase enzyme in germ-free chickens and conventionally reared chickens is compared, the latter display greater enzymatic activity. Diet can also stimulate the growth of certain bacteria such as *Bifidobacterium* and *Lactobacillus*, which help to increase the enzymatic activity of proteases, trypsin and lipases (Palmer and Rolls, 1983).

*Competitive Exclusion*

The ecological definition of competitive exclusion states that two species competing for the same resources cannot coexist stably. Therefore one of the competitors will always dominate the other, leading to an evolutionary modification, shift to another niche, or extinction. The intestinal microbiota compete with the colonising pathogenic bacteria and are able to reduce the adhesion and colonisation of pathogens in the intestine. This competitive exclusion process remains one of the most effective approaches to prevent intestinal colonisation by *Salmonella* in broiler chickens.

**Methods used to Modulate the Microbiota**

Different kinds of feed additives that regulate the microbial community include:

1. Probiotics (live microorganisms that when administered in adequate amounts confer a health benefit on the host).

2. Paraprobiotic or postbiotics (denote non-viable microbial cells, microbial fractions, or cell lysates. Postbiotics along with probiotics may improve the host health).

3. Prebiotics (ingredients that stimulate increased beneficial microbial activity in the digestive system in order to improve the health of the host).

4. Phytobiotics.

5. Phages may potentially provide an integrated solution to modulate the intestinal microbiome of chicken intestines; they reduce specific pathogenic microbial populations and permit the proliferation of beneficial microbiota. These are described in the following lines.

## Probiotics

The following benefits are expected from administering probiotics (Syngai et al, 2016): stimulation of the development of beneficial microbiota; reduction and prevention of colonisation by enteric pathogens; modulation of immunological activity; stimulation of epithelial health; increased digestive capacity and help in the maturation of intestinal tissue.

Probiotics can influence the immune system both directly and indirectly. Direct influence is exerted by different species of *Lactobacillus* that increase cytokine and antibody levels (Brisbin et al, 2011). Similarly, various studies have shown that chickens treated with probiotics produce a greater number of antibodies in response to a given antigen (Brisbin et al, 2010). Probiotics may also have indirect effects, promoting the growth of other bacteria. For example, *Lactobacillus agilis* and *Lactobacillus salivarus* have the ability to stimulate the butyrate-producing microbiota and to reestablish the balance of the microbiota.

Another benefit of probiotics is the reduction and prevention of colonisation by enteric pathogens, achieved through competitive exclusion mechanisms and the production of bacteriostatic and bactericidal substances (Pan and Yu, 2014). The inhibitory effects of probiotic bacteria on undesirable microorganisms might be the result of the production of different metabolites such as hydrogen peroxide ($H_2O_2$), diacetyl, bacteriocins and organic acids.

## Paraprobiotics or Postbiotics

The paraprobiotics or postbiotics have drawn attention because of their clear chemical structure, safety dose parameters, long shelf-life and the content of various signalling molecules, which may have anti-inflammatory, immunomodulatory, anti-proliferative and antioxidant activities. These properties suggest that postbiotics may contribute to the improvement of host health by improving specific physiological functions. Readers may refer 'Probiotics and Immunity' page 186 for more information.

## Prebiotics

The functions described for prebiotics are that they attach to pathogens, serve as substrates for fermentation, increase osmosis in the lumen of the intestine and may also indirectly stimulate the response of macrophages and the production of SCFAs and modulate the immune system (Patel and Goyal, 2012).

Two kinds of prebiotics have been described for aviculture. (i) Most of the currently used are non-digestible synthetic oligosaccharides that contain one or more molecules of a sugar, or a combination of simple sugars such as glucose, fructose, xylose, galactose and mannose. Mannose oligosaccharides found in the cell walls of yeasts have proved to be the most important as they contain compound proteins and glucan (Rehman et al, 2009). (ii) The other kind of prebiotic corresponds to lactose and lactose derivatives such as lactulose and lactosucrose (van Immerseel et al, 2002).

Several studies of prebiotics in chickens provide evidence of positive effects for oligosaccharides of mannose or fructose in the inhibition of the pathogens *Salmonella* and *E. coli*.

## Phytobiotics

Phytobiotics are primary or secondary components of plants that contain bioactive compounds, which exert a positive effect on the growth and health of animals. Primary components include the base nutrients, such as protein, fat and carbohydrates, while secondary compounds include essential and/

or volatile oils, bitterns, colorants and phenolic compounds (Grashorn, 2010). They may be classified into four groups:

i. Herbs (products from flowering, non-woody and non-persistent plants).

ii. Botanicals (whole plants or processed parts).

iii. Essential oils (hydro-distilled extracts of volatile plant compounds).

iv. Oleoresins (extracts based on non-aqueous solvents).

Properties such as the promotion of growth and health have been attributed to phytobiotics. These benefits are derived from improved intestinal health in the animal, including improved digestion, modification of digestive secretions and support to the histology of the intestine (Diaz-Sanchez et al, 2015).

The principal use of phytobiotics in aviculture has been the administration of essential oils as artificial flavours and preservatives in preparation of the feed. Most essential oils have been classified as generally recognised as safe (GRAS) by the US Food and Drug Administration (FDA). These oils are characterised as engaging in antimicrobial activities and having growth promoting properties. Several oils, including carvacrol and thymol obtained from oregano and eugenol from the clove plant, have been shown to inhibit a wide range of pathogenic bacteria (Dorman and Deans, 2000).

*Bacteriophages*

1. Virulent

2. Temperate

Bacteriophages (phages) are defined as specific intracellular parasites of bacteria that multiply using the metabolic machinery of their hosts. There are two large kinds of phages: virulent phages, with a lytic life cycle and temperate phages, with a lysogenic life cycle.

Phage therapy is defined as use of phages to treat bacterial infections and the term is restricted to the employment of virulent phages. Its application to humans was described almost as soon as these viruses were discovered in 1915. However, its use was displaced by the discovery of penicillin and continued only in some countries. Today, the problematic emergence of multidrug resistant bacteria has provided a new focus on bacteriophages as a natural, non-toxic alternative treatment of bacterial infections. Overall, bacteriophages represent a promising alternative for the control of *Salmonella* and *Campylobacter* in farms.

## PROBIOTICS AND IMMUNITY

### Antibiotic Growth Promoters in Animal Feeding

Antibiotics revolutionised the human medical world and are still often seen as the magic bullets to target pathogens without harming human body. Over the decades the use of antibiotics has been increasingly used in farm animals to treat diseases, to prevent diseases and to promote growth (by using at sub-therapeutic level). Sub-therapeutic antibiotics have been heavily used as antibiotic growth promoters (AGP) to overcome the stress of intensive animal production and to improve the performance in productivity.

This increased use of antibiotics in farm animals has been perceived to lead to 'antibiotic resistance' that hinders in treating the diseases. Hence, the European Union banned the antibiotics as growth promoters from the year 2006 and legislation against the use of antibiotics in livestock feed is now active in many countries across Europe, the USA (banned in early 2017) and the Asia Pacific. According to 2016 statistics from the OIE, 74% of the countries worldwide stopped using antibiotics as growth promoters and the remaining 24% of the countries still use antibiotics in farm animals. Impetus for alternative to AGP has come with increasing pressure from the consumers and regulatory agencies to reduce antibiotic use in commercial animal production because of increasing trouble due to antibiotic resistance.

## Antimicrobial Resistance (AMR)

Consider the three major sources of resistance: overuse of antibiotics by human beings, overuse in the veterinary sector and environmental antibiotic contamination due to pharmaceutical and hospital discharge. As far as veterinary use goes, India's 2017 National Action Plan on Antimicrobial Resistance did talk about restricting antibiotic use as growth promoters. India is yet to regulate antibiotic-use in livestock and poultry. Hence antibiotics are sold as growth promoters to poultry farmers (mostly antibiotics are used in poultry as growth promoters) in India legally. Similarly, there is no regulation of antibiotic levels in discharges from pharmaceutical firms. This has led to an explosion in resistance genes in the lakes, rivers and sewers.

Antimicrobial resistance is a present danger and future threat for human as well as animal health. The rapid development of AMR in human healthcare urges the need for effective strategies to reduce the antibiotic use in animal production. Wide application of selected feed additives and combinations thereof (e.g. short- and medium-chain fatty acids and other organic acids, prebiotic sugars and fibres, probiotics, botanicals with a wide range of plant extracts and microbial derived additives from yeasts and fungi) has been found successful for targeting intestinal microbiota and immunity. Probiotics are preferred being the natural residents of gastrointestinal tract.

## Probiotics Support three Core Benefits

The classical definition of probiotics indicates "they are live microorganisms which, when ingested in adequate amounts can provide health benefits to the host" (FAO/WHO, 2001). These benefits are provided due to interactions between the probiotics and the gastrointestinal microbiota and immunological system (Adams, 2010).

Probiotic cultures supplementation in poultry could encourage establishment of a protective barrier of bacteria in the digestive tract and prevent the colonisation of growth-depressing or pathogenic microorganisms (Grimes et al, 2008). Probiotics are believed to exert their effects through several ways that include production of antimicrobial substances, competition with pathogens for adhesion sites and nutrients, enhancement of mucosal barrier integrity and immune modulation. Thus probiotics can support three core benefits for the host: supporting a healthy gut microbiota, a healthy digestive tract and a healthy immune system.

In other words, the beneficial health effects provided by probiotics can be classified into three levels according to their site of action (Rijkers et al, 2010): (i) direct interaction with the intestinal microbiota or by enzyme activity within the GIT, (ii) direct interaction with the epithelium and the intestinal mucous layer, influencing the intestinal barrier function and the mucous immune system, (iii) action in the immune system and other organs such as the liver and brain.

## Benefits of Supplementation

The enhancement of growth performance and feed efficiency of probiotic-supplemented birds could be induced by the entire effects of probiotic action. Benefits of supplementation include the maintenance of beneficial microbial population, improving feed intake and digestion, altering gastrointestinal microflora, immune system modulation (Cox and Dalloul, 2015) and bacterial metabolism. Zhao et al (2017) evaluated the evidence from animal studies for the protective effects of probiotics administration on D-galactose-induced oxidative stress. Probiotics has significantly increased serum superoxide dismutase (SOD) and glutathione peroxidase (GSH-Px) activities and decreased malondialdehyde (MDA) and reduced oxidative stress in aged mice. This shows probiotics increased antioxidant enzymes and decreased lipid peroxidation.

## Paraprobiotics

Even though the classical definition of probiotics indicate that they should be alive in order to provide health benefits to the hosts, recent studies have proved that inactivated probiotic microorganisms can also provide such benefits. The non-viable probiotics have been known as "ghost probiotics", "postbiotics" and "inactivated probiotics", but recently the term "paraprobiotics" has been coined (de Almada et al, 2016). The term "postbiotics" has been proposed to define "non-viable bacterial products or metabolic by-products from probiotic microorganisms that have biologic activity in the host".

## Health Benefits Associated with Paraprobiotics

Paraprobiotics provide health benefits to the hosts through several pathways. For instance, paraprobiotics are known to modulate the immune system and to have increased adhesion to intestinal cells, which further result in inhibition of pathogens. Also, paraprobiotics can provide health benefits to hosts through secretion of metabolites by the dead cells.

Several reports can be found in the literature on the health benefits associated with the consumption of paraprobiotics. Paraprobiotics can be used for treatment of diarrheoa, colitis, liver diseases induced by alcohol, respiratory diseases, intestinal lesions, visceral pain, inflammation and to modulate the immune system, intestinal microbiota and bacterial translocation. Other effects include reduction of lactose intolerance, dental caries and ageing manifestations and cancer growth control.

## Route of Administration of Probiotics

An exclusive advantage of probiotics over other feed additives is their self-propagation ability in the digestive tract of the host. Although a rough phase feeding of probiotics to poultry is common practice recommended by many probiotics manufacturers, a full dose is given at the starter period and this decreases thereafter to a half dose (Habibi et al, 2013). The single-dose administration of probiotics is more effective in limiting feeding expenses, in contrast to the phase-feeding strategy provided a similar technical performance is maintained.

The most common route of administering probiotic preparations is in-feed supplementation. Production of the water dispersible probiotic products permits the probiotic administration in drinking water as a second popular method for probiotics usage (Karimi Torshizi et al, 2010).

Sheep red blood cells (SRBC; non-pathogenic antigen) are frequently used in experiments in order to evaluate the humoral immune response of birds. Probiotic administration in the hatchery slightly increased the anti-SRBC antibody titer. Similarly, continuous probiotic administration in feed only slightly improved antibody production against SRBC, while probiotic administration in drinking water improved cellular immune responses to phytohaemagglutinin-M and 1-chloro-2,4-dinitro-benzene (Karimi Torshizi et al, 2010).

## When to Administer Probiotics? Different Scenarios are Mentioned Here

1. Birds, whether free living or the farm-housed ones, are exposed to various environmental microorganisms immediately after hatching. In spite of traditional thinking that the intestinal tract of day-old chick is sterile, more recent studies using molecular techniques reveal the presence of complex community of bacteria in their intestinal tract originated from the prehatching phase, the environment at the hatchery, or in transport (Pedroso et al, 2005; Dibner et al, 2008). It is assumed that those microorganisms, which first established themselves in the host's gastrointestinal tract, would colonise and persist throughout the lifespan (Ducluzeau, 1993).

2. In commercial systems, chicks are hatched from fumigated eggs in hygienic hatcheries and grow in sanitised environments without any contact with established microbiota from adults. Under these circumstances, the establishment of microbial flora in the

chicks is delayed, which could result in the susceptibility of chicks to pathogens. The early administration of probiotics could fill the gap of delayed microflora establishment by introducing and establishing beneficial microbial flora in hatchlings. The concept of *in ovo* **administration** of probiotics extends this approach to pre-hatch embryonic life (Cox and Dalloul, 2015).

3. Commercial hatcheries are not sterile and microbial contamination of day-old chicks is possible during transportation from hatchery to farm. In addition, hatchlings' intestinal flora is not completely formed on the day of hatch. Therefore, early or **in-hatchery administration** of probiotics could be an appropriate way to accelerate establishment of flora and help protect against opportunistic and pathogenic bacteria. Seifi et al, (2017) suggested the spray method as a practical one applicable for mass probiotic administration over the Japanese quail birds at hatchery or when chicks arrive at the farm.

## Modulation of Immune System by Probiotics

Probiotics have an important role in the health of the host including modulation of the immune system. Through these probiotics, immune system of the gut protects the host from the different types of antigens (both dietary and microbial) that reach the lumen of the gastrointestinal tract (GIT). Both innate and adaptive immunity are affected by probiotics.

The adaptive immune response depends on the lymphocytes B and T, which are specific for particular antigens. The innate immune system, in turn, responds to structures known as pathogen-associated molecular patterns (PAMPs) present on the pathogens. The primary response of pathogens is unleashed by the pattern recognition receptors (PRRs) which will bind to the PAMPs. The toll-like receptors (TLRs) are the most studied PRRs. The PRRs are present in immune and epithelial cells (Bermudez-Brito et al, 2012).

Probiotics in general may modulate the intestinal microbiota composition and the immune system (Chaucheyras-Durand and Durand, 2010). Most commonly applied in pigs and poultry are *Bacillus* spp. based probiotics because of their heat stability of spores during pelleting. Another range of probiotics is based on live yeasts. These are mainly applied in dairy nutrition to improve rumen efficiency and prevention of rumen acidosis but also find their application in sow and piglet feed. In newly hatched or newborn animals, 'starter cultures', also other bacteria like specific *Lactobacilli* or *Enterococci* spp. are sometimes applied to steer the initial microbiota in a desired direction.

Specific sugars and fibre sources are able to modulate the intestinal microbiota and selectively stimulate specific groups of bacteria who are believed to be beneficial for animal health (Gaggia et al, 2010). Some sugars are able to block the binding of pathogens to the mucosa, e.g. mannose-based sugars can block the binding of some *Salmonella* spp. to the mucosa (Oyofo et al, 1988).

**Like probiotics, paraprobiotics also act on the immune system,** and there are various reports on their immunomodulation effects in the literature. Both probiotic and paraprobiotic *L. gasseri* TMC0356 show *in vitro* immunomodulation effects. Paraprobiotic *L. gasseri* TMC0356 induces a greater increase in the production of IL-12 in macrophages when compared to the probiotic, suggesting that the heat treatment may not negatively affect the ability of the strain to activate the production of IL-12 in macrophages (Miyazawa et al, 2011). Other examples are paraprobiotic *L. plantarum* L-137, paraprobiotic *L. casei* Zhang (LcZ), paraprobiotic *L. acidophilus* A2, *L. gasseri* A5 and *L. salivarius* A6; probiotic or paraprobiotic *L. rhamnosus* HN001; both probiotic and paraprobiotic *L. rhamnosus* HN001.

## Improvement in Innate Gut Immunity

Epithelial cells in the gastrointestinal mucosa create a selectively permeable barrier between the intestinal lumen (which contains harmful substances such as foreign antigens, microorganisms and toxic materials, as well as beneficial nutrients) and the internal environment of the body. This barrier is the first line of defence against the microbes in the GIT. It has a combined defence function, incorporating anatomical structures, immunological secretions consisting of mucous, immunoglobulins, e.g. IgA, antimicrobial peptides and the epithelial junction adhesion complex. Disease conditions that cause immunological disturbances disrupt this barrier (Turner, 2009), induce inflammation of the intestinal wall and intestinal disorders (Hooper et al, 2001; Sartor, 2006).

## Synbiotics

More recently, the concept of combining probiotics and prebiotics, i.e. synbiotics, for the beneficial effect on gut health of pigs has attracted major interest; benefits for pigs are pathogen inhibition and immunomodulation. Roselli et al (2017) reviewed the immunomodulatory effects of probiotics, either alone or in combination with prebiotics, based on *in vivo, in vitro* and *ex vivo* porcine experiments. A consistent number of studies showed the potential capacity in terms of immunomodulatory activities of these feed additives in pigs. But contrasting results were also noticed from the literature, which could be related to differences with respect to the probiotic strain used, experimental settings, diets, initial microbiota colonisation, administration route, time and frequency of administration of the probiotic strain and sampling for analysis.

Heshmati et al (2018) performed a systematic review and meta-analysis of the probiotics and synbiotics supplementation on biomarkers of oxidative stress. Oxidative stress parameters levels, including total antioxidant capacity (TAC), glutathione (GSH), superoxide dismutase (SOD) and nitric oxide (NO) were higher in probiotics (or synbiotics) group compared to controls, while malondialdehyde (MDA) level was lower than controls. This indicates that probiotic-synbiotic supplementation improve antioxidant resistance and increase the amount of antioxidant enzymes in the body.

## Probiotic Formulations Prevent Chronic Inflammation of the GIT

Probiotic formulations prevent chronic inflammation of the GIT through stimulation of innate immunity in the gastrointestinal epithelium (Galdeano and Perdigon, 2006; Pagnini et al, 2010). For example, a high dose $(50 \times 10^9$ cfu/day) of a probiotic formulation (VSL#3) containing four strains of lactobacilli *(L. casei, L. plantarum, L. acidophilus* and *L. delbrueckii* subspecies *bulgaricus);* three strains of bifidobacteria *(Bi. longum, Bi. breve* and *Bi. infantis)* and one strain of streptococcus *(S. salivarius* subspecies *thermophilus),* when fed to senescence-accelerated-prone mice for six weeks either completely prevented ileitis or significantly reduced the severity of inflammation (Pagnini et al, 2010). However, it was ineffective in treating the inflammation when administered to older mice that had already developed ileitis (Pagnini et al, 2010).

## Probiotics Improve Intestinal Barrier Function by Reducing the Permeability of the Intestinal Epithelium

Experiments in animal models have shown that improvement in intestinal barrier function by probiotics is due to a reduction in the permeability of the intestinal epithelium. Translocation of intestinal microbes out of intestinal sites and into sites such as the liver, spleen and mesenteric lymph nodes decreased in mice with induced colitis and pretreated with *Lactobacillus* probiotics (Mao et al, 1996; Pavan et al, 2003; Llopis et al, 2005). Translocation of enterotoxigenic *E. coli* (ETEC) to mesenteric lymph nodes was reduced in post-weaning piglets with dietary supplementation of probiotic *P. acidilactici* compared with the control group after ETEC challenge (Lessard et al, 2009).

Generally, timing of probiotic treatment is very important in maintaining intestinal barrier function. Administration of probiotics before the infectious or pathogenic agent is introduced experimentally, or before the pathogens enters the GIT and multiplies naturally, is the most effective time for probiotic introduction (Lodemann, 2010).

## Stimulation or Suppression of Immune Response by Probiotics

The immune response in the host should be sometimes stimulated (e.g. infection and immunodeficiencies) and sometimes suppressed (e.g. allergy and autoimmune diseases) based on the clinical condition (Borchers et al, 2009). Diets containing probiotics could modulate the host immune response. The responses are complicated as they vary with the probiotic strain or species, with the dose level and may differ in their effect pre- and post-weaning, and whether the antigen is a bacterium or a virus. The pattern of immune response-related blood plasma cells can vary between the ileum and jejunum lymph tissue. Probiotics can affect the expression of the anti-inflammatory cytokine or cell signalling proteins and may do so differentially depending on the cytokine.

**Immunostimulatory effects of probiotics:** Several studies have demonstrated the immunostimulatory effects of probiotics. Bai et al (2013) demonstrated that a probiotic containing *L. fermentum* and *S. cerevisiae* stimulated the intestinal T cell immune system as indicated by increased production of CD3+, CD4+ and CD8+ T-lymphocytes in the GIT of broiler chickens. Expression of CD3+, IL-2 and IFN-γ genes was significantly greater in the small intestine of neonatal chicks (day 3 and 7) fed with probiotics *L. jensenii* TL2937 and *L. gasseri* TL2919 than in the control without probiotics (Sato et al, 2009). Dalloul et al, (2003) found similar effects of probiotics on the intestinal immune system of broiler chickens. Probiotic supplementation increased population of intestinal intraepithelial lymphocytes (IEL) compared with control birds not given the probiotic. Similarly, administration of probiotic *E. faecium* to broiler chickens challenged with *E. coli* resulted in increased concentrations of

cytokines (IL-4 and TNF-α) and IgA in the small intestinal mucosa (Cao et al, 2013).

In the piglets, probiotic *L. fermentum* 15007 modulated immune function by enhancing T cell differentiation and upregulating ileum cytokine expression (Wang et al, 2009). Probiotic containing *P. acidilactici* and *S. cerevisiae* subspp. *boulardii* also increased T cells in ileum and IgA secretion in post-weaning piglets challenged with entero-toxigenic *E. coli* (Lessard et al, 2009).

**Probiotics also increase serum immunoglobulin levels:** A multi-strain probiotic containing *L. acidophilus*, *B. subtilis* and *C. butyricum* increased serum levels of IgA and IgM in chickens (Zhang and Kim, 2014). Likewise, addition of a commercial product (Gallipro) containing *B. subtilis* to broiler chicken diets increased the antibody response to sheep red blood cells (SRBC) administration (Afsharmanesh and Sadaghi, 2014). Antibody titre against the common poultry diseases newcastle disease, infectious bronchitis and infectious bursal disease was increased by the use of probiotic product Primalac (Landy and Kavyani, 2013).

## Immunosuppressive Action of Probiotics

*E. faecium* NCIMB 10415 had an immunosuppressive effect, delaying early immune response to antigens in post-weaning piglets (Siepert et al, 2014). Similarly, expression of intestinal immune-associated genes, especially during the post-weaning period, was reduced (Siepert et al, 2014). In the post-weaning period, expression of IL-8, IL-10 and CD86 (cluster of differentiation 86) genes in ileal Peyer's patches was significantly reduced in probiotic-treated piglets. In contrast, probiotic caused increased expression of IL-10 gene and CTLA4 (T cell inhibitory molecule) in Jejunal Peyer's patches in the post-weaning period. Blood serum inflammation-related cytokines IL-6 and IL-8 were not affected by the probiotic.

In an earlier study, supplementation of piglet diet with the same probiotic strain (*E. faecium* NCIMB 10415) had no effect on the lymphocyte populations in the jejunal Peyer's patches (Scharek et al, 2005). The serum level of immunoglobulin IgG was reduced in probiotic-treated piglets during the post-weaning period (28–56 days) but was not affected in the pre-weaning period (Scharek et al, 2005).

## Dose-dependent Responses

Oral administration of *L. brevis* ATCC 8287 at the high dose rate of $10^{10}$ cells per animal per day to weaned piglets reduced expression of IL-4, IL-6 and TGFβ1 genes in the ileum and increased expression of IL-4 and IL-6 genes in the jejunum, caecum and colon (Lahteinen et al, 2014). However, this change in cytokine gene expression in the intestine did not change the systemic humoral immune response. Levels of serum immunoglobulins IgA and IgG were the same in control and probiotic-treated piglets.

Drenching of *L. acidophilus* strain NCFM at low dose rates (up to $10^6$ cfu/dose × 5 doses) significantly increased the population of the antiviral interferon IFN-γ-producing T cells and reduced the regulatory T cells and production of TGFβ1 and IL-10 in intestinal lymphoid tissue of gnotobiotic piglets compared with untreated animals (Wen et al, 2012). In contrast, the same probiotic increased the regulatory T cells, when administered at a high dose rate (up to $10^9$ cfu/dose × 14 doses).

Such dose-dependent responses could be one of the reasons for variable results in different studies and with different probiotics. The gastrointestinal microbial profile of the host also could influence the immune response of the host against specific probiotic (Borchers et al, 2009).

## Impacts of Lactobacillus Isolates on immunological function

Studies of Zhang et al (2010) indicated that *Lactobacillus* isolates (LB1 and L3) can increase the intestinal immunological and defensive function of growing rabbits, especially in the caecum. Mast cells have long been recognised as the key cells in allergic reactions and they

are essential moderators to regulate T cells (Zhang et al, 2010). Many studies state that mast cells have important roles as the body's defence against bacterial and viral infections. This correlates with pathogen recognition mechanisms and inflammatory mediator release (Lu et al, 2006).

Some probiotics can produce elements with immune activities during the process of fermentation, for instance, peptidoglycan, lipopolysaccharide, etc. (Kandasamy et al, 2014). Both LB1 and L3 did not significantly affect the mast cells of jejunum and duodenum in 65-day rabbits, whereas the mast cells were remarkably increased in the caecum.

## A Systems-based Approach is Required to Address the Response to a Probiotic

Can probiotics "prime" the immune system in commercial operations to support response to animal and/or human bacterial and viral disease antigens and reduce their shedding in faeces (Yadav et al, 2016)? These are very complicated responses and the variation between probiotic strains means that there is no general "story" about the way probiotics might affect the immune system.

However, the significant outcome is that probiotic microbes can modulate the immune system and response to pathogen antigens; a systems-based approach is required to address the response to a probiotic in terms of host disease susceptibility, shedding of pathogens (both human and/or porcine), growth and feed use efficiency. Animal farmers may use this information as a guide while incorporating probiotics in the diets.

## PREBIOTICS PROMOTE GUT HEALTH

### Prebiotics

Prebiotics are defined as non-digestible carbohydrates (NDCs) including oligosaccharides, resistant starch (RS) and non-starch polysaccharides (NSPs) that are resistant to hydrolysis by digestive secretions. In species without forestomach, including humans and pigs, these NDCs resist digestion in the upper gastrointestinal tract (GIT) and reach the ileum and the colon where they usually undergo fermentation by resident microbes. Currently, prebiotics are more broadly defined as any type of food ingredient that has a favourable direct and/or indirect impact on the beneficial GIT microbiota and the intestinal homoeostasis (Hutkins et al, 2016) and consequently inhibit pathogenic infections.

## Categories of Prebiotics

The concept of prebiotics had its origin in monogastrics. Prebiotics were first identified and named by Marcel Roberfroid in 1995. The nature of prebiotic categorisation can be related to their source and function. Categories of prebiotics include fermentable/digestible and fermentation resistant.

### Fermentable/Digestible

Some examples are trans-galactooligosaccharide (GOS), inulin, fructooligosaccharide (FOS), lactulose. These groups of prebiotics include the following subcategories.

- Short-chain prebiotics, e.g. oligofructose, contain 2–8 links per saccharide molecule
- Longer-chain prebiotics, e.g. inulin contain 9–64 links per saccharide molecule
- Full-spectrum prebiotics provide the full range of molecular link-lengths from 2–64 links/molecule.

The length of molecule relates to the area of colonic fermentation: short chain prebiotics fermenting more rapidly in the right side of the colon, whereas the long chain one is being fermented more slowly, nourishing bacteria predominantly in the left-side colon or full-spectrum providing nourishment throughout the colon. This category of prebiotic is typically derived from plant sources. Their role in ruminant diets may be questionable since they could be digested in the rumen, and are more intended for monogastrics to modify lower gut populations of *Lactobacillus* and *Bifidobacterium*.

### Fermentation Resistant

This category of prebiotics support gut health in ruminants as well.

Some examples are mannan oligosaccharides (MOS) and beta glucans. These are immunosaccharides. These carbohydrate sources are typically not fermented in the rumen (deVaux et al, 2002) and play a role in modifying the balance of lower gut microbial populations and serve as immune-modulators at the intestinal mucosal level. This category of prebiotics is the focus of this chapter.

## General Aspects of Immune Function Modulation

There are two basic components of the mammalian immune system: innate and acquired (or adaptive). To understand how prebiotics function in mammalian systems, let us know some of the basics of the immune system. Readers are advised to see Chapter 2 for details of immune system.

**Leukocytes:** All white blood cells are known as leukocytes. Leukocytes are different from other cells of the body in that they are not tightly associated with a particular organ or tissue. Thus, they function similar to independent, single-cell organisms. Leukocytes are able to move freely and interact with and capture cellular debris, foreign particles, or invading microorganisms. Leukocytes cannot divide or reproduce on their own, but are the products of multipotent hematopoietic stem cells present in the bone marrow.

The innate leukocytes include natural killer cells, mast cells, eosinophils, basophils and the phagocytic cells including macrophages, neutrophils and dendritic cells. All these function within the immune system by identifying, presenting and eliminating pathogens that might cause infection.

Acquired immunity is triggered in vertebrates when a pathogen evades the innate immune system and (1) generates a threshold level of antigen and (2) "stranger" or "danger" signals activating dendritic cells.

**Dendritic cells (DC):** Dendritic cells are phagocytic cells present in tissues that are in contact with the external environment, mainly the skin and the inner mucosal lining of the nose, lungs, stomach and intestines (Janeway et al, 2005). They are named for their resemblance to neuronal dendrites, but dendritic cells are not connected to the nervous system. Dendritic cells are very important in the process of antigen presentation and serve as a link between the innate and acquired immune systems.

## Yeast Cell Wall Structure (MOS and Beta Glucan: Competitive Adhesion, Immune potential)

Yeast cell walls are a rich source of MOS and beta glucan, therefore it works as a prebiotic. In the yeast cell wall, mannan oligosaccharides (MOS) are complex molecules that are linked to protein moieties. The MOS component can be attached to the cell wall proteins as part of –O and –N glycosyl groups and also constitute elements of large $\alpha$-D-mannose polysaccharides ($\alpha$-D-Mannans); these are built of $\alpha$-(1,2)- and $\alpha$-(1,3)-D-mannose branches that are attached to long $\alpha$-(1,6)-D-mannose chains. Although mannose is present, it is not accessible because of physical/chemical orientation and association with other molecules.

### Mannan Oligosaccharides (MOS)

MOS is a high affinity ligand providing competitive binding site options for gram-negative bacteria, which possesses mannose-specific Type-1 fimbriae (Ofek et al, 1977). The immediate benefits are associated with pathogen removal from the digestive system without intestinal attachment and colonisation. This phenomenon elicits significant antigenic responses, thus enhancing humoral immunity against specific pathogens through presentation of the attenuated antigens to immune cells (Ferket, 2003; Spring et al, 2000).

In order for the pathogen to adhere to the mannose, the molecule must be physically exposed and accessible to the organism.

Therefore, processing to expose the mannose moieties is critical and supersedes quantity. The method of processing the cell wall could dictate the degree and consistency of exposure associated with the various moieties. Enzymatic processing of yeast cell wall at an optimal temperature, time and pH yields a more consistent exposure of binding sites than chemical or mechanical fractionation (Balasundaram and Harrison, 2006; Pitarch et al, 2008).

Although mannose is an important high affinity cell wall ligand, other cell wall carbohydrates exist (N-acetyl galactoseamine, d-galactoseamine, d-glucoseamine, d-glucose and d-galactose) and also possess other unique binding potential, i.e. N-acetyl galactoseamine with *Cryptosporidium parvum*.

### β-Glucans

* Beta glucans are known as "biological response modifiers" because of their ability to activate the immune system. Beta-glucan has been shown to exhibit immuno-modulatory effects when used as a supplement in aquatic, swine and poultry diets.
* The most active forms of β-glucans are those comprising D-glucose units with (1,3) links and with side-chains of D-glucose attached at the (1,6) position. These are referred to as β-1,3/1,6 glucans.
* Some researchers have suggested that it is the frequency, location and length of the side chains rather than the backbone of β-glucans that determine their immune system activity.
* Another variable is the fact that some of these compounds exist as single strand chains, while the backbones of other β-(1,3)-glucans exist as double or triple stranded helix chains.
* In some cases, proteins linked to the β-(1,3)-glucan backbone may also be involved in providing therapeutic activity.
* There are differing opinions on which molecular weight, shape, structure and source, β-(1,3)-glucans provide the greatest biological activity.

**Dectin-1:** Dectin-1 is an intestinal cell receptor that will bind with beta glucan. From that, it can stimulate inflammation to get the body start in fighting the infection. It also prepares macrophages from engulfing pathogens to destroy them. Lastly, beta glucan binding to Dectin-1 produces cytokines that help the T and B cells produce antibodies for more targeted defence of the infection, supporting the acquired immune system.

### Gut Health: Gut Microbiota, Gut Permeability and Mucosal Immunity form the Critical Trilogy

There is a complex and critical relationship among intestinal microbiota, gut permeability and mucosal immunity.

Intestinal epithelium plays a pivotal role to protect gut health. The intestinal epithelium is the most critical component of the innate immune system. Intestinal epithelium is the primary surface physical barrier separating highly immunogenic luminal agents (pathogens, toxins, antigens) from immune-reactive epithelial layer. Intestinal lining consists of intestinal epithelial cells with a primary function of intracellular nutritive absorption. However, transduction of inflammatory signals from luminal microbes by way of toll-like receptors is also critically important. The main controlling factor associated with inter (para) cellular transport is the bridging mechanism between cell bridges known as **tight junctions** (TJ) or **zona occludens** (Madara and Pappenheimer, 1987). The tight junction complex consists of transmembrane proteins with proteins from the **claudin** and **occludin** groups, which interact with the **actin** and **myosin** contractile elements to regulate paracellular transport. The control of these "gatekeepers" is critical to paracellular transport.

### Stress increases Intestinal Permeability leading to "leaky gut"

Psychological stress and corticotrophin-releasing hormone increase intestinal permeability in humans by a mast cell-dependent mechanism. It could be speculated that stress, therefore, be linked to increased paracellular intestinal permeability through a mast cell dependent release of zonulin. Zonulin is the only physiological modulator of intercellular tight junctions. Paracellular intestinal transport is a critical route of antigen, toxin and pathogen entry during stressful episodes.

### Critical Times of Maximum Susceptibility to Stress in Dairy Cattle

Critical times during the course of the cows' life are (1) neonatal calf: 1–35 days (2) transition cow 21 days before parturition to 35 days-in-milk [DIM] and (3) high producing cow, calving through 150 (DIM). Maximum susceptibility to stress is found during these three life stages that contribute to her susceptibility to compromised gut health and overall health.

Transition period is a good example to illustrate the potential for a compromised gut health scenario. Even in a well-managed programme, there is a dramatic change in the dietary regime from high roughage to high concentrate feed to meet the energy needs of milk production during this period. In addition, dry matter intake (DMI) naturally declines during the pre- and post-calving period. These episodes can result in a change of ruminal environment which will have an effect on the lower gut resulting in alterations of commensal microbiota. These changes subsequently invoke environments that promote pathogenic populations. The stress component will advance triggers (acetylcholine, mast cells, zonulin, etc.), which will alter intra- and para-cellular transport of bacteria and antigens leading to "leaky gut".

Both acute and chronic stress affects mucosal barrier dysfunction primarily through neuro-endochrinological factors. Impaired mucosal/intestinal barrier increases intestinal permeability. The consequence of this cascade of events can lead to clinical or subclinical toxicosis. However, mounting an immune response to stress or infection can be energetically expensive and prolongs negative energy balance at transition which further affects immunecompetence (Waldron et al, 2003; Goff, 2006) and predispose cows to infectious disease after calving.

## Prebiotics Play a Role in Supporting Gut Health in Cattle

Optimal management and stress reduction are critical factors in abating gut health problems. Yeast cell wall carbohydrates are prebiotic sources. Competitive agglutination assays, tissue adhesion determinations and clinical evaluations provide evidence that yeast cell wall carbohydrates play a role in supporting gut health naturally (Nocek, 2015):

Yeast cell wall carbohydrates (mannose, MOS, beta glucans) can play a role in reducing the implications of stressful situations and aid in improving gut health as mentioned below.

- Mannose: Used as a limited nutrient source for some commensal populations
- MOS: Competitive adhesion site for pathogens
- Beta glucans: Dectin-1 signalling of toll-like receptors and other signalling mechanisms of the innate immune system.

D. Baines and co-workers conducted series of experiments in dairy cattle and beef cattle to evaluate the ability of a prebiotic feed additive to modify the symptoms of jejuna haemorrhagic syndrome (JHS) and mycotoxicosis. Dairy cattle developed JHS after consuming feed containing several types of mycotoxigenic fungi. Shiga toxin producing *E. coli* (STEC) was colonised at the mucosa in the haemorrhaged tissues of the cattle and no other pathogens were identified. The inclusion of the prebiotic in the feed was associated with a decline in disease.

Calves consuming 1–3 ppb aflatoxin and 50–350 ppb fumonisin in calf feed ration promoted STEC associated haemorrhagic enteritis outbreaks (Baines et al, 2013). Application of a prebiotic and probiotic to the calves eliminated STEC shedding and the morbidity/ mortality losses.

## ROLE OF PREBIOTICS IN CONTROLLING INTESTINAL ENTEROPATHOGENS

### Enteric Bacterial Pathogens

Feed contamination is an important source for *Salmonella* infection in pig production. *Salmonella enterica* serotypes *(Salmonella spp.)* are the second cause of bacterial foodborne zoonoses in humans after campylobacteriosis. Pork is the third most important cause for outbreak-associated salmonellosis and colibacillosis is the most important disease in piglets and swine (Trans et al, 2016).

*Salmonella enterica* are hosted in the gut of most homoeothermic animals and include various serovars whose pathogenicity can differ widely. *Escherichia coli* is a common intestinal bacterium in humans and animals. Most *E. coli* strains are harmless commensals of the intestinal microbiome, but some serotypes are pathogenic, causing severe intestinal infections (Kalita et al, 2014). *E. coli* are ubiquitous commensals of the pig's gastrointestinal tract (GIT) with a prevalence of 100% (Rajkhowa and Sarma, 2014).

Among the taxa that can cause illness in humans and that have been reported in the chicken microbiota are *Campylobacter* (principally *Campylobacter jejuni* and *Campylobacter coli), Salmonella enterica, Escherichia coli* and *Clostridium perfringens* (Oakley et al, 2014b). *Campylobacter* and *Salmonella* are principally responsible for gastrointestinal infections. *Campylobacter* is generally accepted not to be pathogenic in birds, while *Salmonella enterica* can cause disease in chickens, depending on age, immune status and type of serovar.

Only certain strains of *E. coli* [example avian pathogenic *E. coli* (APEC)] have specific virulence factors that may cause disease in chickens. APEC is principally associated with extra intestinal infections, most of which affect the respiratory tract. Similarly, *Clostridium perfringens* is recognised as a pathogen in birds that causes necrotic enteritis. Additionally, *C. perfringens* is a human pathogen that is transmitted through food and has been traced to different origins, including foodstuffs of avian origin (van Immerseel et al, 2004, 2009).

## How the Pathogens Gain Entry and Establish in Animals?

Attachment to host cells, translocation of effector proteins into host cells, invasion and replication in tissues are the vital virulence steps of the pathogens that help them to thrive in the intestinal environment and invade tissues in the animals.

## Multiplication in the Host and Pathogenicity

To understand how to reduce the burden of the pathogens, let us know how they can invade the host successfully. Healthy and infected intestinal epithelium is depicted side by side for better clarity (Fig. 5.5). Several virulence factors are expressed that allow the pathogens to persist in the host and then cause disease through the attachment, translocation of effector proteins and replication and spread of the pathogenic bacteria into the host (Bhunia, 2008).

### Attachment to Host Cell Surface

Immediately following oral intake, bacteria that survive passage through the acidic stomach environment reach the small intestine in 2–3 hours in pigs (Nguyen et al, 2015). The pathogens must first get attached to the intestinal mucosa or intestinal epithelial cell surface to avoid washout by mucosal secretion and/or peristalsis (Kalita et al, 2014).

**Two mechanisms involve the adherence of these organisms to the intestinal mucosa and epithelium.**

1. Bacterial adhesins such as pili (*Salmonella* spp.), fimbriae or surface antigens (as per the *E.coli* pathotype) interact with their receptor on host cell. *Salmonella* spp. and *E. coli* use a syringe-like type-III secretion system (T3 SS, virulence central) to sense the presence of the host cell receptor (Fig. 5.5).

2. Pathogens translocate the bacterial adhesin and their receptor, e.g. intimin and intimin receptor via T3SS into host plasma membrane cells, which helps them in the

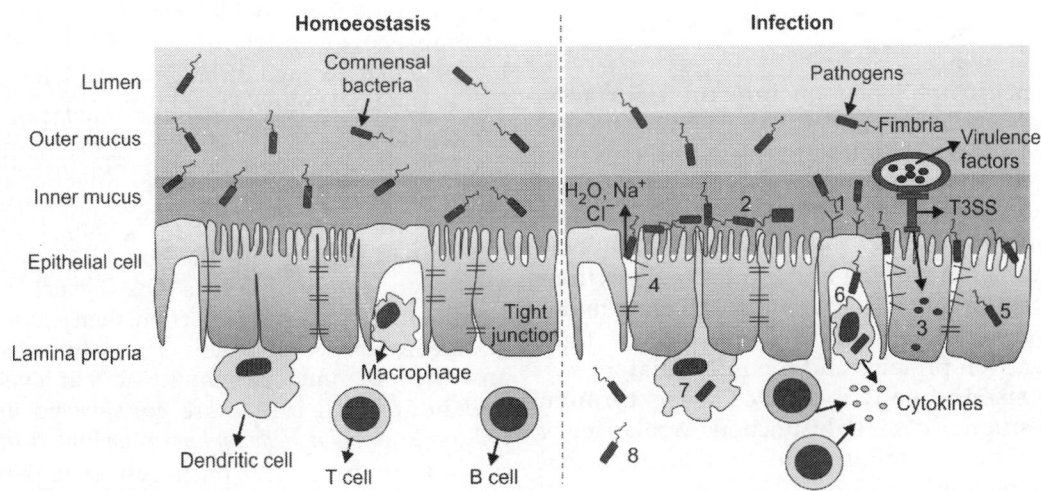

**Fig. 5.5:** Schematic representation of the colonisation ways and pathogenicity of *Salmonella enterica* and *Escherichia coli* into animal host (Sansonetti, 2004; Kalita et al, 2014 as presented by Trans et al, 2016): Bacterial adhesion on apical surface of epithelial cells thank to protein receptors (1); Biofilm formation (2); Via the type-III secretion system (T3SS), virulence factors of pathogens into the host cells (3); Then disruption of tight junctions between intestinal epithelial cells (4); Presentation of pathogens in intracellular cells (5); In macrophage (6); In dendritic cell (7); In lamina propria (8)

initial attachment. These virulence factors provoke an important mucosal inflammatory response that is associated with the secretion of inflammatory mediators such as interleukins (IL). Among those, the pro-inflammatory chemokine IL-8 is responsible for recruiting neutrophils to the epithelial mucosa without mucosal injury, and facilitates intestinal fluid secretion.

Moreover, biofilm formation (Fig. 5.5) on the surface of host's enterocytes is also another important adherence property of these pathogens. Pathogens may aggregate and recruit surrounding cells to form bacterial biofilms associated with the epithelium. These biofilms are multicellular structures held together by several factors such as fimbriae, pilus, curli, flagella and exopolysaccharide. Bacteria in biofilms adopt a starved state due to the undernutrition and waste accumulation. This change in physiological state increases their resistance to antimicrobial medication and host innate immune responses. In addition, pathogenic cells can detach from mature biofilms and spread to other organs.

*Translocation of Effector Proteins into Host Cells*

Once established on intestinal surfaces, *Salmonella* spp. and *E. coli* pathogens translocate bacterial effector proteins through T3SS (Fig. 5.5) to the extracellular space or the cytosol of target cells. These effectors will help them to fight back the immune response of the animal to survive in the intestinal environment or invade tissues by modulating multiple signalling pathways linked to the tight junction proteins and the inflammatory response to finally induce cell lysis through disruption of the tight junctions, weakening of the host response and loss of intestinal homeostasis.

**Disruption of intestinal epithelial tight junction:** Protein F secreted by *E. coli* pathotypes redistribute tight junction (TJ) proteins such as occludin and claudin from the villous membrane to the cytoplasm in colon epithelial cells. This disruption (Fig. 5.5) leads to a loss of transepithelial electrical resistance (Badia et al, 2013) and an increased **paracellular intestinal permeability** that cause local and systemic infections including haemorrhagic gastroenteritis, bacteremia, endovascular infections or cell inflammation. The consequence of disruption of this intestinal epithelial tight junction is weak host inflammatory response; that is the host innate immune responses and cellular processes (such as proliferation and differentiation) are negatively modulated.

Certain *E. coli* pathotypes release the host cell iron into the extracellular environment that can then be captured by the bacterium. An imbalance in intestinal homeostasis has been observed; intestinal intracellular osmotic pressure is increased resulting ultimately cell lysis. This local effect results in watery or bloody diarrhoea, especially in piglets.

*Pathogen Invasion and Replication in the Host*

*Salmonella* spp. predominantly colonise cell surfaces, mucous, basal membranes of intestinal mucosa. They cause a mucosal inflammation that provides a localised source of high-energy nutrients. The *Salmonella* bacteria use a range of chemical nutrients inside the host cell such as lipids, carbohydrates, amino acids, nucleosides and various pro-vitamins for their growth (Steeb et al, 2013). *Salmonella* can rapidly invade the lamina propria (enterocytes) (Fig. 5.5). They can spread throughout the body into gut-associated lymphoid tissues [GALT] such as tonsils quickly after oral infection, then jejunal and ileocaecal lymph nodes. They can cause an acute inflammatory stimulus so that fever and neutrophil influx are considered as hallmarks of *Salmonella typhimurium* infection.

Most of the *E. coli* pathotypes remain extracellular except one that can invade and proliferate within the host cells. The extracellular *E. coli* can replicate outside the cells, i.e. in the interstitial space, in the lumen of the respiratory tract and, obviously, in the intestinal tract from the mid jejunum to the ileum. They use the monosaccharides, mucosal glycoproteins and amino acids for their growth in the intestinal lumen. Thus attachment to host cells, translocation of effector proteins into host cells, invasion and replication in tissues are the vital virulence steps of these enteropathogens that help them to thrive in the intestinal environment and invade tissues.

**How to avoid the introduction of pathogens into the animals?**

1. **Feeding strategies—prebiotics are effective:** Many on-farm feeding strategies intervene to avoid the introduction of pathogens onto the farm by contaminated feeds or to reduce infection pressure when pathogens are present. Among the latter, prebiotics could be effective at protecting against these enteric bacterial pathogens. Prebiotics (e.g. non-digestible carbohydrates, NDC) can be effective by restoring or improving the resistance to colonisation, reinforcing the intestinal barrier function against invading pathogens (Bindles et al, 2015).

2. **Influence of feed characteristics on pathogen contamination:** The feed can potentially be an important vector to introduce pathogens, especially *Salmonella* onto the farm. Hence, strategies to reduce the load of pathogens on the farms can target this feed contamination. Further, the feed composition can also influence the in-host proliferation and transmission between pigs of *Salmonella* and pathogenic *E. coli* strains.

   i. **Physical properties and chemical composition of the feed** can influence the susceptibility of pigs to *Salmonella* and *E. coli* infection (Funk and Gebreyes, 2004). They influence not only the passage and absorption of nutrients in the GIT, but also the risk of colonisation and shedding in the pigs once infected (Berge and Wierup, 2012).

   ii. **Particle size:** Feeding a coarse meal to pigs results in lower growth performance and such feed protects animals against colonisation better than pelleted feed (Mikkelsen et al, 2004; Wilhelm et al, 2012). Coarsely ground feed mixture change the physico-chemical conditions in the stomach with higher concentration of organic acids and lower pH that promote the growth of anaerobic lactic acid bacteria and decrease the survival of *Salmonella* and *E. coli* during passage through the stomach (Mikkelsen et al, 2004). Moreover, larger feed particles are not digested as extensively as small feed particles. They enter the large intestine where they are fermented to produce short-chain fatty acids (SCFAs), which have beneficial effect on gut health leading to inhibition of pathogen infection (Wilhelm et al, 2012; Lebel et al, 2016).

   iii. **Level of fibre and protein:** The provision of high amounts of fibre and a low concentration of high-quality proteins in the diets may reduce the pathogen loads in the feed and the risk for intestinal disease in pigs. J.R. Pluske and coworkers published their research findings during 2008-2015 that indicated low protein diets can reduce the growth of one *E. coli* pathotype and the incidence of diarrhoea in piglets.

   iv. **Low digestible protein:** Pluske and coworkers also showed that diets made of poorly digestible proteins result in higher levels of undigested dietary proteins reaching the distal parts of the GIT. Undigested proteins are fermented into harmful metabolites (branched chain fatty acids [BCFAs], $NH_3$, etc.) by proteolytic bacteria. In turn, these putrefactive compounds can irritate the colonic epithelium, compromise the intestinal barrier function and the absorption capacity of electrolytes and fluids. Consequently, undigested proteins may selectively favour the growth of that *E. coli* pathotype leading to the incidence of post-weaning diarrhoea in piglets.

v. **Type of fibre:** The inclusion of some fibre such as cellulose, lignin, arabinoxylans or pectin into pig diets can increase mucous production and then increase the flow of undigested endogenous proteins to the large intestine (Jha and Berrocoso, 2016). Thus inclusion of some carbohydrate molecules can increase amount of proteins in the large intestine of pigs.

On the other hand, fermentable fibre can shift bacterial metabolism from proteins towards carbohydrates as the main energy source (SCFA) and then reduce harmful protein-derived metabolites from the protein feed. Indeed, proteolytic activity in the intestine decreases when the availability of indigestible carbohydrate sources increases (Pieper et al, 2012b). More interestingly, carbohydrates can also be involved in mechanism of the host's defence against pathogenic infections.

## Mechanisms of Action of Prebiotics on the Pathogen Infections in Pigs

Trans et al (2016) detailed the mechanisms on which prebiotics are likely to act in order to fulfil their protective action against these pathogens *(Salmonella* spp. and *Escherichia coli)* in pig production (Fig. 5.6). These mechanisms include an inhibition of adhesion sites, a modulation of the intestinal environment and a reinforcement of host immune system.

1. **Inhibition of pathogens adhesion sites:** Prebiotics can inhibit pathogen adhesion via several mechanisms. These are a coating of the host epithelial surface, promotion of beneficial bacteria and downregulation of adhesion in pathogens.

2. **Promoting beneficial bacteria:** Prebiotics such as lactulose regulate the intestinal microbiota by stimulating selectively the growth of a limited number of beneficial colonic bacteria, especially lactic acid bacteria. These beneficial bacteria can form biofilms (Fig. 5.6) attached to the intestinal epithelial cells locking out the adhesion of pathogens to the host's cells.

3. **Blocking the attachment of pathogens or coating the host epithelial surface:** Some prebiotics do not enrich beneficial bacteria as lactobacilli or enterococci, but they can act by blocking the attachment of pathogens and keeping them away from the gut

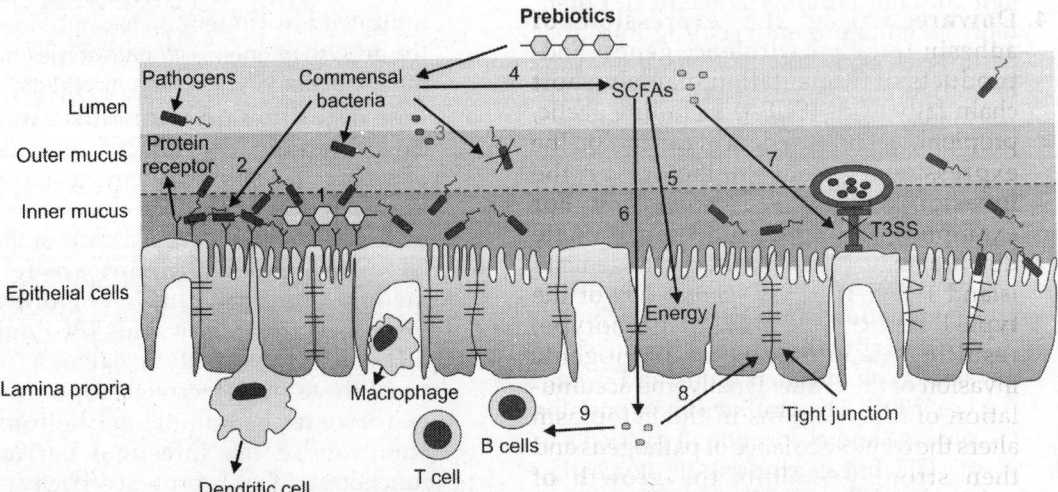

**Fig. 5.6:** Schematic representation of the mechanisms of prebiotics against pathogen infection: coating of the host surface receptors by adhesin analogs (1); By commensal bacterial biofilm formation (2); Bacteriocins (3); Short-chain fatty acids (SCFAs) (4); Produced by favourable bacteria; use of SCFAs as energy source for epithelial cells (5); Metabolic regulation (6); Inhibition of the type-III secretion system (T3SS) (7); Improvement of tight junction, mucin production (8); Immunomodulation (9); (Sansonetti, 2004; Kalita et al, 2014 as depicted by Trans et al, 2016)

wall due to similar structures to the glycosylated radical of the host's receptors. By the adsorption of prebiotics on the pathogen surface, they saturate the glycan-binding domains of pathogenic lectins and thus prevent binding to host glycoproteins, resulting in their excretion from the intestine (Molist et al, 2014). For example, casein glycomacropeptides, soluble extracts obtained from wheat *(Triticum aestivum)* bran, locust bean *(Ceratonia siliqua)*, locust bean gum and guar *(Cyamopsis tetragonoloba)* gum, chito-oligosaccharides or galacto-oligosaccharides (GOS) were used as antiadhesive candidates effective against the attachment of certain *E.coli* pathotypes to the surface of porcine ileal mucous.

**Studies of Roberts et al (2013) and Chen et al (2014) suggest that different cell types and pathogens respond differently to prebiotic exposure.** The prebiotics tested were soluble non-starch polysaccharide (NSP) from plantain bananas *(Musa paradisiaca)*, soya bean *(Glycine max)* hulls, sugar beet pulp *(Beta vulgaris)*, cranberry *(Vaccinium* spp.*)*, FOS, inulin, exo-polysaccharides (EPS), mannanoligosaccharides (MOS).

4. **Downregulating the expression of adhesin factors or virulence genes:** End-products of fermentation, namely short chain fatty acids (SCFA) including acetic, propionic and n-butyric acid can inhibit the expression of adhesin factors or the invasion genes of *S. Typhimurium*. For example, n-butyrate and propionate downregulate the *Salmonella* pathogenicity island 1 (SPI-1) of *S. Typhimurium* or the type-1 fimbriae of a *E. coli* pathotype, resulting in inhibition of pathogenic invasion of the tissue. Finally, the accumulation of SCFA anions in the cytoplasm alters the osmotic balance of pathogens and then strongly inhibits the growth of *Salmonella*.

5. **Modulation of ecology and physiology of the intestinal tract:** Prebiotics, as stated earlier, stimulate selectively the growth of beneficial intestinal bacteria and then regulate the intestinal microbiota. This microbial community affects host physiology and host health through the fermentation of indigestible carbohydrates to release the SCFA products. This SCFA production can lead to a decrease in pH, especially when lactate is produced because of the low pKa of this acid.

One cannot state that a low pH always correlates with the inhibition of pathogens (Fooks and Gibson, 2002). If the pH is below the optimal for the pathogen, it will inhibit its growth. Fooks and Gibson (2002) observed the inability of *E. coli* and *Salmonella enteritidis* to support an acidic pH ($\leq 5$) in bifidobacteria and lactobacilli cultures fermenting inulin, FOS, XOS, mixtures of inulin: FOS or FOS: XOS. This pH lowering effect of SCFA production contributes also to some extent to the protective effect of many lactic acid bacteria (Hopkins and Macfarlane, 2003). The effect of SCFAs on pathogen invasion depends also on the medium pH.

Despite the pH decrease, there was no reduction in pathogen growth, probably because pathogens can also compete with beneficial bacteria to use the NDCs (and produce SCFAs) and reduce the pH themselves (Fooks and Gibson, 2003; Patterson et al, 2009).

6. **Reinforcing the host immune system** Prebiotics have been shown to increase SCFA concentrations that can reinforce the host immune system. They increase the proliferation of epithelial cells and have stimulatory effects on both endocrine and exocrine pancreatic secretions in pigs. **Butyrate** acts as an energy source of colonocytes enhancing the barrier function of the colonic epithelial cells and helping in preventing the tissue breakdown and reducing oxidative DNA damage (Wang et al, 2012; Molist et al, 2014; Suryanarayana and Ramana, 2015).

**Prebiotics** that can change the physiology of epithelial cells have been associated with reductions in bacterial attachment without affecting the viability of pathogens. **Prebiotics**

may also enhance the cell-mediated immune response in early weaned piglets by modulating the production of antibodies. White et al (2002) described that the administration of mannanoligosaccharides (MOS) from the brewers dried yeast increased serum levels of immunoglobulin G (IgG) in piglets challenged with *E. coli* K88, associated with lower coliform counts.

## Conclusion

*Salmonella enterica* subspp. enterica and diarrhoeagenic *E. coli* strains are major intestinal pathogens in pigs causing foodborne infections in humans. Some potential prebiotics appear to be relevant to use in the feed for controlling these pathogens on the farms. These fermented carbohydrates can be included in diets of weaning piglets and fattening pigs at 0.2–1% for simple carbohydrate molecule (Andres-Barranco et al, 2015) or 14 –18% for fibre (Pieper et al, 2012a,b).

Several studies of prebiotics in chickens provide evidence of positive effects for oligosaccharides of mannose or fructose in the inhibition of the pathogens *Salmonella* spp. and *E. coli* (Rehman et al, 2009; van Immerseel et al, 2002).

Mechanisms by which these prebiotics might help chicken/pigs struggling against the pathogenic invasion are changes in intestinal ecology by SCFA production, inhibition of their adherence on gut epithelium and improvement of the host's immune system gene expression regulation by mainly *n*-butyrate.

# 6

# Amino Acids and Immunity

## AMINO ACIDS AND RELATED COMPOUNDS AND IMMUNITY

### Amino Acids play Important Roles in Immune Responses

Amino acids have been demonstrated to play important roles in immune responses by regulating (1) the activation of T lymphocytes, B lymphocytes, natural killer cells and macrophages, (2) cellular redox state, gene expression and lymphocyte proliferation, and (3) the production of antibodies, cytokines and other cytotoxic substances (Li et al, 2007; Kimet al, 2007). Functions of amino acids and their requirements in regulating the immune system are described here, since they provide great promise to improve health and to prevent infectious diseases in animals and humans (Tan et al, 2013).

The role of amino acids in regulating the immune function can be considered from two perspectives: (1) the enhancement of the immune response that protects individuals from infections and malignant neoplasms and (2)the reduction of over-responses such as inflammation and autoimmunity (Yoneda et al, 2009).

### Amino acids and enhancement of Immune response

The roles of glutamine, arginine, threonine, methionine, cysteine and tryptophan in enhancing the immune function in pigs have been well-established (Johnsona et al, 2006; Li et al, 2007b; Wang et al, 2006).

#### Arginine

Arginine synthesis occurs through a two tissue pathway. Dietary glutamine and glutamate can be used by enterocytes to generate citrulline. Arginine is synthesised from citrulline (Fig. 6.1), primarily in the kidney and is then released into the circulation to be taken up and used by other tissues. While arginine is also generated in large quantities by the liver, this arginine is recycled by the urea cycle within the hepatocyte, with little net production.

Arginine is a non-essential/a semi-essential amino acid in mammals and is involved in protein, urea and nucleotide synthesis and ATP generation. It is also the precursor of nitric oxide (NO), which is cytotoxic to tumour cells and to some microorganisms. Arginine is the precursor for synthesis of polyamines, which have a key role in DNA replication, regulation of the cell cycle and cell division. As a precursor for NO and polyamine synthesis, arginine profoundly influences immune function.

**Nitric oxide pathway of arginine metabolism:** Nitric oxide (NO) molecule has attracted more attention in 1990s than any other molecule. It is a potent immunoregulatory

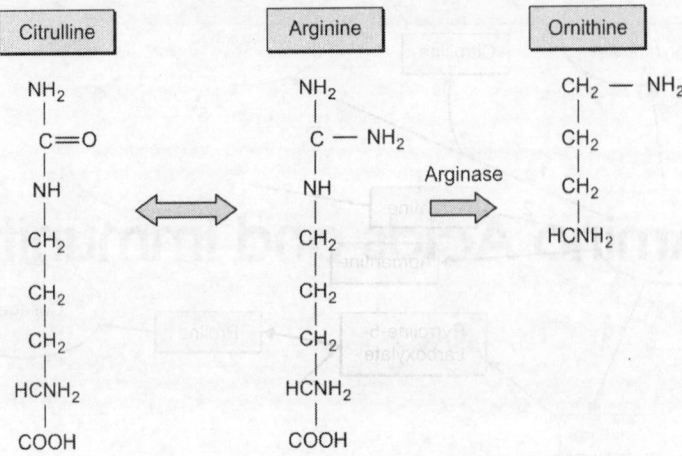

**Fig. 6.1:** The structures of citrulline, arginine and ornithine

mediator. This small molecule plays a pivotal role in a diverse range of functions, including vasodilatation, memory, peristalsis, penile erection, cytotoxicity and the control of various endocrine and exocrine secretions in the cardiovascular, reproductive, central nervous and immune systems (Nathan and Xie, 1994; MacMicking et al, 1997). NO is synthesised from arginine by nitric oxide synthase (NOS), with the formation of citrulline (Fig. 6.2).

**Nitric oxide synthase (NOS) is known to have three forms:** Neuronal, endothelial and inducible forms. Neuronal (nNOS) and endothelial cell (ecNOS) NO synthases are both constitutively expressed and calcium-activated. The inducible form (iNOS) is controlled at the transcriptional level and it is of most interest in the setting of the immune system. Therefore, this NO free radical is a key mediator of the immune system in animals.

The inducible form of NOS enzyme (iNOS) expression, and hence NO production, is induced in macrophages in response to a variety of stimuli, particularly the T-helper-1 cytokines [interferon (IFN)-γ and tumour necrosis factor (TNF)-α] and the gram-negative bacteria cell wall component [endotoxin or lipopolysaccharide (LPS)]. Inhibition of NO production increases the host susceptibility to viral, bacterial, fungal,

protozoal and helminthic infections. The mechanisms of NO cytotoxicity are complex, involving inhibition of DNA synthesis, mitochondrial inactivation, cell membrane lysis, cell cycle arrest, DNA strand break formation and induction of apoptosis (Burney et al, 1997).

NO can also react with superoxide to form peroxynitrite, a powerful oxidising agent capable of inducing cell injury and death (Samar et al, 1997). Apart from its cytotoxic effects, NO is involved in regulating the expression of major histocompatibility complex (MHC) II in antigen-presenting cells, in modulating T cell mitogenic responses and in the induction and suppression of many cytokines (Niedbala et al, 1999; Akaike and Maeda, 2000). However, the full extent of NO involvement in the functioning of the immune system has yet to be established (M.D. Duff and J.M. Daly, 2002).

**Arginine and immune function:** Arginine can become essential at times of growth and metabolic stress (trauma, sepsis or burn injuries). The most prominent effect of supplemental arginine is in abrogating (cancel or do away with) trauma-induced immuno-suppression. In the clinical setting, immunonutrition has been demonstrated to reduce infectious complications and length of hospital stay in critically ill patients.

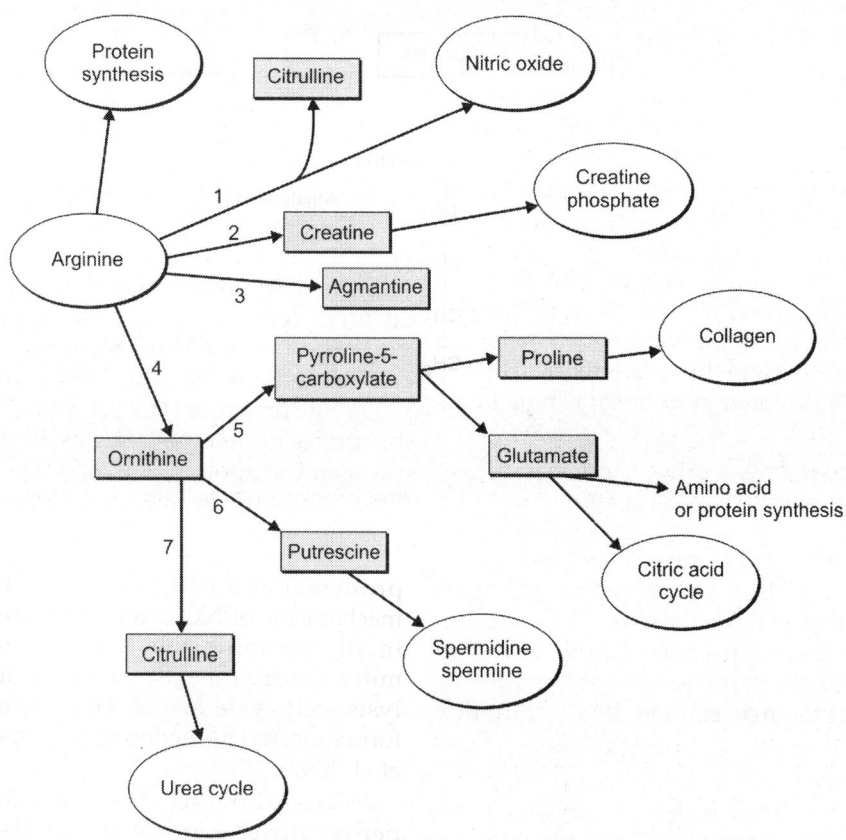

**Fig. 6.2:** An outline of arginine metabolism: 1. Nitric oxide synthase; 2. Arginine decarboxylase; 3. Argino-glycine amidinotransferase; 4. Arginase; 5. Ornithine aminotransferase; 6. Ornithine decarboxylase; 7. Ornithine transcarbamoylase

Immunonutrition comprises supplementation of arginine, nucleic acids and n-3 fatty acids.

In laboratory animals, arginine has been found to decrease the thymus involution associated with trauma, to promote thymus repopulation and cellularity, to increase lymphocyte proliferation, NK cell activity and macrophage cytotoxicity, to improve DTH, to increase resistance to bacterial infections and survival to sepsis and burns and to promote wound healing and the rejection of skin allografts (Evoy et al, 1998).

Arginine has been demonstrated to exert beneficial effects in pregnant sows and weaned pigs. This amino acid reduces morbidity and mortality in response to infectious pathogens. A large amount of NO synthesised from arginine by inducible NO synthase is cytotoxic to pathogenic microorganisms including virus. Dietary supplementation with the arginine enhances the immune status of milk-fed piglets (Kim et al, 2004) and pregnant sows (Kim et al, 2006). Administration of arginine increases thymus size. Arginine supplementation improves the development of digestive tract, prevents intestinal villous atrophy and decreases the expression of intestinal pro-inflammatory cytokines, thereby enhancing the mucosal immune status in early-weaned piglets and alleviating mucosal injury of lipopolysaccharide (LPS)-challenged pigs.

**Arginase/ornithine pathways of arginine metabolism:** *Arginase enzyme exists in two forms: Type I arginase or hepatic arginase and*

*arginase II*. While both forms catalyse the conversion of arginine to ornithine (Fig. 6.2), they are encoded by separate gene sequences. The two forms are located in different subcellular compartments and are expressed to varying degrees in separate tissues. Type I arginase or hepatic arginase is constitutively expressed in hepatocytes. It is a cytosolic enzyme and is a central component of the urea cycle. Its expression can be induced in macrophages by stimulation with T-helper-2 cytokines (especially by interleukins (IL)-4, -10 and -13) (Munder et al, 1999; Chang et al, 2000).

Arginase II, on the other hand, is localised to the mitochondria and is found in high concentrations in kidney, brain and small intestine. Arginase II can also be induced in macrophages but by different stimuli, namely, LPS and dexamethasone (Corraliza et al, 1995). The expression of both forms of arginase in macrophages is reduced by T-helper-1 cytokines, such as IFN-γ (Munder et al, 1999).

Following conversion to ornithine, a number of pathways may be followed for further metabolism. What directs a cell to choose one pathway over another is not yet understood (M.D. Duff and J.M. Daly, 2002). The reactions involved in the urea cycle occur primarily in the liver both in mitochondrion and cytosol. The function of the urea cycle is to clear nitrogenous waste, by converting ammonia to urea for excretion by the kidneys.

**Formation of proline and glutamate:** Ornithine aminotransferase catalyses the transfer of one amine residue to ornithine to form pyrroline-5-carboxylate, which can then either be reduced to proline or pass (via glutamate semialdehyde) to glutamate. Proline and its derivative hydroxyproline (formed *in situ* by the action of ascorbic acid) constitute 25% of the collagen molecule and therefore play a vital role in wound healing and tissue repair. Glutamate can be used by the cell for energy production through the citric acid cycle, or can be used for protein or amino acid synthesis.

*Glutamine*

The importance of glutamine to cell survival and proliferation *in vitro* was first reported by Ehrensvand et al (1949) but was more fully described by Eagle et al (1956). Glutamine is the most abundant amino acid (Fig. 6.3) in the blood and in the free amino acid pool in the body. It needed to be present at ten- to 100-fold in excess of any other amino acid in cell culture and could not be replaced by glutamate or glucose. Skeletal muscle is considered to be the most important glutamine producer (Fig. 6.4) in the body and it supplies glutamine to act as an interorgan nitrogen transporter (Fig. 6.5). The immune systen is considered to be an important user of glutamine.

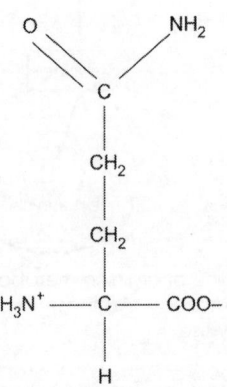

**Fig. 6.3:** The structure of glutamine

**Glutamine is a conditionally essential amino acid during stress:** Significant depletion of the skeletal muscle glutamine pool has been indicated as a characteristic of trauma. The lowered plasma glutamine concentrations that occur is most probably the result of demand for glutamine (by the liver, kidney, gut and immune system) exceeding the supply. It is proposed, therefore, that glutamine be considered a conditionally essential amino acid during stress. It has been suggested that the lowered plasma glutamine contributes to impaired immune function that accompanies such stress situations. Animal studies have reported that enrichment of diet with glutamine increases T-lymphocyte

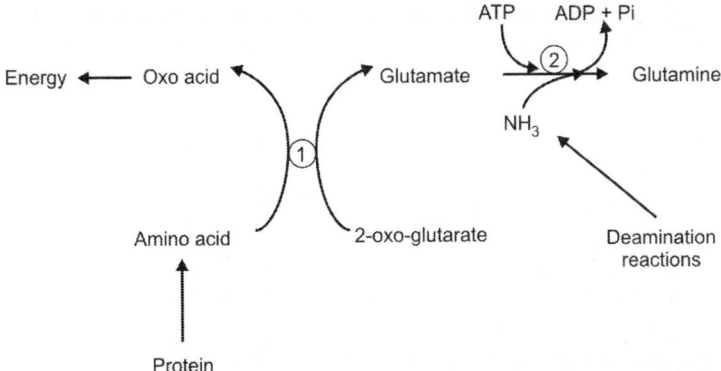

**Fig. 6.4:** The pathway of glutamine biosynthesis. Enzymes are indicated as: 1. Transaminase 2. Glutamine synthetase

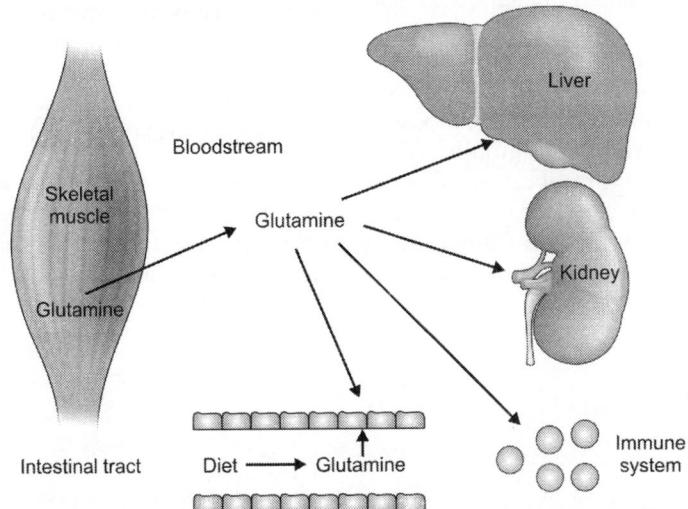

**Fig. 6.5:** Inter-organ transport of glutamine

proliferation and IL-2 production and increases the ability of rodents to survive infectious challenges (Wilmore and Shabert, 1998; Calder and Yaqoob, 1999).

Animal studies indicate that intramuscular and plasma glutamine concentrations are decreased in catabolic stress situations, e.g. sepsis and cancer cachexia and following burn injury and surgery.

**Glutamine depletion *in vivo* results in immunosuppression:** Evidence is now emerging that glutamine supplied orally or intravenously improves immune function *in vivo*, while additionally protecting against

infectious challenges. Thus, administration of glutamine or its precursors (N-acetylglutamine, 2-oxoglutarate, branched chain amino acids) should prove beneficial as a therapy for individuals, whose immune system is compromised by catabolic stress.

**Glutamine and the immune system:** Once released from skeletal muscle, glutamine acts as an interorgan nitrogen transporter (Fig. 6.5). Important users of glutamine include the kidney, liver, small intestine and cells of the immune system.

*Liver:* In the liver, the carbon skeleton of glutamine is an important precursor for glucose synthesis, glutamine itself can be used for the synthesis of other amino acids and proteins, while the excess nitrogen is disposed of via urea formation. Glutamine can also be used to synthesise glutathione.

*Kidney:* In the kidney, glutamine participates in acid–base balance, donating its amido and amino nitrogens to join with protons to form ammonium ions, which are excreted in the urine. The remaining carbon skeleton can be used to generate energy or as a precursor for glucose synthesis (gluconeogenesis).

*Small intestine:* Glutamine is the major energy source in the small intestine and is an important energy source for immune cells. Glutamine is a nitrogen donor for the synthesis of purines and pyrimidines (RNA, DNA). Since, these are the building blocks of RNA and DNA, this role of glutamine is likely to be a particularly important one in cells that have high rates of division and/or of protein secretion. These include cells of the immune system and cells of the small intestine, such as enterocytes.

**Glutamine metabolism by immune cells:** The high rate of glutamine utilisation by neutrophils, macrophages and lymphocytes and its increase when these cells are challenged suggests that supply of glutamine is required for the immune system to function optimally. See later the possible fates of glutamine carbon in Fig. 6.6.

Adding glutamine to the weaning diet of pigs has significantly modified the immune cells in the mesenteric lymph nodes (Johnsona et al, 2006). Glutamine is preferentially metabolised by the intestinal mucosa and by lymphocytes. As a precursor for glutathione (GSH), it helps in maintaining the antioxidant status of cells and improving the gut barrier function against bacterial infection. Hence glutamine supplementation is useful in reducing the weaning-related gastrointestinal infections (Ewaschuk et al, 2011).

**Pathway of glutamine utilisation:** One possible rate-determining step in the pathway of glutamine utilisation is that catalysed by the enzyme glutaminase (Fig. 6.6), which is found within mitochondria. The activity of

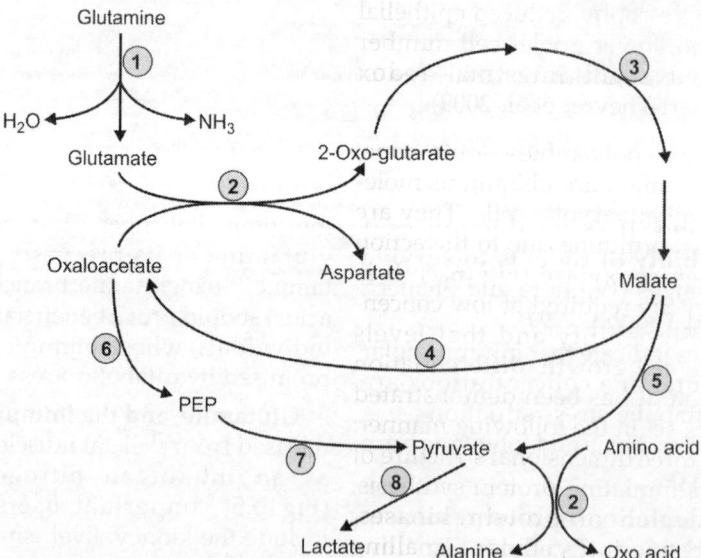

**Fig. 6.6.** The pathway of glutamine utilisation. Enzymes are indicated as: 1. Glutaminase; 2. Transaminase; 3. Enzymes of part of the citric acid cycle; 4. Malate dehydrogenase; 5. Malic enzyme; 6. Phosphoenolpyruvate carboxykinase; 7. Pyruvate kinase; 8. Lactate dehydrogenase PEP, phosphoenolpyruvate

glutaminase is high in all lymphoid organs examined, including lymph nodes, spleen, thymus, Peyer's patches and bone marrow, macrophages and in lymphocytes.

*Sulphur Amino Acids, Glutathione and Immune Function*

Sulphur amino acids, methionine and cysteine, have indeed been shown to be beneficial for the immune system, aside from their role in protein synthesis (Grimble, 2006). Additional dietary intake of methionine plus cysteine can reduce the adverse effects of immune system stimulation on whole body protein deposition in growing pigs. The availability of cysteine is a major factor that limits the synthesis of glutathione. Thus, dietary supplementation with N-acetylcysteine (a stable precursor of cysteine) is highly effective in enhancing immune functions under various disease states (Grimble, 2001).

Methionine and cysteine are precursors of important molecules and important for intestinal mucosal function. It has been demonstrated that a sulphur amino acid-free diet administered enterally to piglets for 7 days led to a reduced intestinal mucosal growth associated with villus atrophy, reduced epithelial cell proliferation, lower goblet cell number and diminished small intestinal redox capacity (Bauchart-Thevret et al, 2009).

**Polyamines:** The polyamines—putrescine, spermidine, spermine—are ubiquitous molecules found in all eukaryotic cells. They are synthesised from ornithine due to the action of ornithine decarboxylase (Fig. 6.2). It is known that they are required at low concentrations for cell viability and that levels increase during cell growth, differentiation and proliferation. It has been demonstrated that polyamines act in the following manner: (1) altering the three dimensional structure of tRNA thereby stimulating protein synthesis, (2) phosphorylation of protein kinases, thereby accelerating intracellular signalling pathways, (3) modulation of transcription and mRNA turnover and (4) DNA editing. Inhibition of polyamine synthesis, leads to a reduction in cell viability, cell-cycle arrest in S-phase and inhibition of cell differentiation.

Methionine is intimately involved in the synthesis of the **polyamines**: spermine and spermidine, in which the carbon chain of methionine is donated to a third polyamine, putrescine, which is derived from ornithine (Figs 6.2 and 6.7). The polyamines are present in high concentrations in rapidly dividing cells, such as those of an activated immune system. **Polyamines have been likened to 'molecular grease'**, in that they are permissive metabolites, ensuring the fidelity of DNA transcription and RNA translation (Grimble and Grimble, 1998). The first enzyme in the step from ornithine to putrescine (ornithine decarboxylase) is highly induced in rapidly dividing cells.

Methionine also acts as a methyl donor in the synthesis of creatine (Fig. 6.8), which is essential for muscle energy generation through its phosphorylation to creatine phosphate. Creatine phosphate can transfer its phosphate to ADP to restore cellular ATP supplies during periods of high metabolic activity.

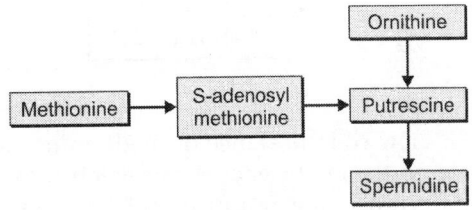

Fig. 6.7: Polyamine biosynthesis

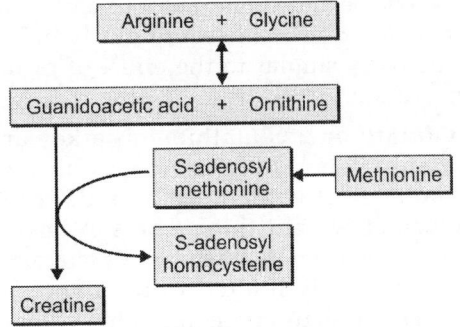

Fig. 6.8: Creatine biosynthesis

In addition to incorporation into proteins, cysteine can be incorporated into the key antioxidant glutathione (GSH), or converted to taurine and inorganic sulphate. The possession of an SH group by cysteine and GSH allows the formation of an S-S bridge between two molecules of cysteine or of GSH to form cystine and oxidised glutathione (GSSG), respectively. Taurine has many roles, including formation of the bile salt taurocholic acid and is a putative antioxidant and cell membrane stabiliser. Taurine is the predominant nitrogenous compound in immune cells.

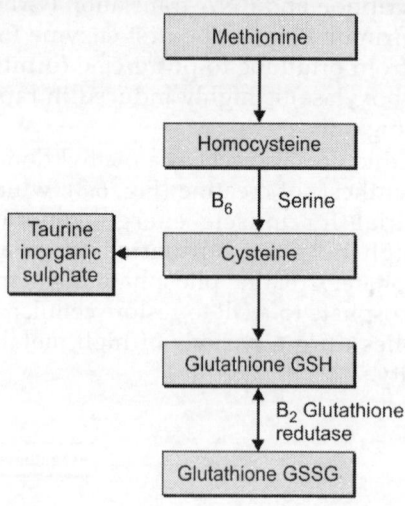

In view of importance of methionine and cysteine, their deficiency results in atrophy of the thymus, spleen and lymph nodes and prevents recovery from protein energy malnutrition. When combined with a deficiency of isoleucine and valine, sulphur amino acid deficiency results in severe gut lymphoid tissue, very similar to the effect of protein deprivation.

**Glutathione:** Glutathione is a key antioxidant tripeptide (glycine, cysteine and glutamate). It is the most abundant low-molecular weight thiol. The synthesis of glutathione from its three constituent amino acids is mainly limited to the liver. Two consecutive steps are required to synthesise glutathione, each step consuming one ATP

molecule (Fig. 6.9). The rate-limiting enzyme in the pathway is γ-glutamyl cysteine synthetase (step 1 of Fig. 6.9). That is, synthesis of glutathione is a 'demand-led' process, provided that cysteine is available. Thus, conversion of cysteine to GSH is strongly influenced by the rate of utilisation/transport of GSH within and between the cells of the body. Glutathione is transferred to the blood and transported around the body in both plasma and cells mainly in its reduced form (GSH).

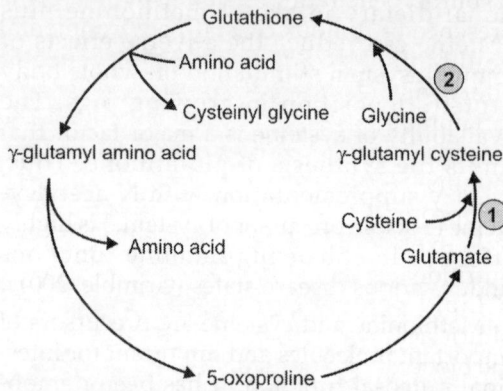

**Fig. 6.9:** Formation of glutathione and its role in the γ-glutamyl cycle; Enzymes: 1. γ-glutamyl cysteine synthase 2. Glutathione synthase

Glutathione concentrations in the liver, lung, small intestine and immune cells fall in response to inflammatory stimuli and this fall can be prevented in some organs by provision of cysteine in the diet. Glutathione itself can enhance the activity of human cytotoxic T lymphocytes and, hence, depletion of intracellular glutathione diminishes lymphocyte proliferation and the generation of cytotoxic T lymphocytes.

Apart from protein synthesis, sulphur amino acids are also involved as direct and indirect participants in pathways related to cell replication and stabilisation, antioxidant defence, assimilation of lipids and energy metabolism. Hence, the availability of sulphur amino acids has a major impact on immune function because the immune response involves major changes in cell replication, oxidant stress and lipid and energy metabolism.

**Response of the immune system to infection and injury:** Hostile environment is created to destroy the pathogens. Antioxidant defences are strengthened through immunonutrition.

The immune system has a great capacity for immobilising the invading pathogens by creating a hostile environment and brings about their destruction. The immune system can also become activated by a wide range of stimuli and conditions. These include: (1) burns, penetrating and blunt injury, (2) the presence of tumour cells, (3) environmental pollutants, (4) radiation, (5) exposure to allergens and (6) the presence of chronic inflammatory diseases. The strength of the response to this range of stimuli will vary. The immune response has a high metabolic cost; inappropriate prolongation of the response will exert a deleterious effect upon the nutritional status of the host.

Lipid peroxides and increased thiobarbituric acid reactive substances are present in the blood of patients with disorders/diseases such as diabetes mellitus and alcoholic liver disease. Peroxides also increase following cancer chemotherapy, bone marrow transplantation and haemodialysis. This enhances oxidant stress further and creates a pro-inflammatory effect.

**Many of the signs experienced after infection and injury are caused by PIC:** Pro-inflammatory cytokines (PIC) are essential for the normal operation of the immune system. They do play a major damaging role in many inflammatory diseases and in cancer. In conditions such as cerebral malaria, meningitis and sepsis, they are produced in excessive amounts and are important factors in increased mortality. Further, these inflammatory cytokines bring about a loss of lean tissue, which is associated with depleted tissue GSH (reduced glutathione) content and an increased output of nitrogenous and sulphur-containing excretion products in the urine.

The PICs interleukin (IL)-1, IL-6 and tumour necrosis factor (TNF)-$\alpha$ have widespread metabolic effects upon the body and stimulate the process of inflammation.

Many of the signs and symptoms experienced after infection and injury, such as fever, loss of appetite, weight loss, negative nitrogen, sulphur and mineral balance and lethargy are caused directly or indirectly by PIC. The indirect effects of cytokines are mediated by actions upon the adrenal glands and endocrine pancreas, resulting in increased secretion of the catabolic hormones: adrenalin, noradrenalin, glucocorticoids and glucagon.

The infected individual's immune system receives nutrients from within the body. Muscle protein is catabolised to provide amino acids for synthesising new cells, GSH and proteins for the immune response. Furthermore, amino acids are converted to glucose (a preferred fuel) and glutamine to meet the needs of immune system. Plasma concentrations of glycine, serine and taurine are greatly decreased following infection and injury because of production of substances rich in these amino acids such as GSH (which comprises glycine, glutamic acid and cysteine), metallothionein (the major zinc-transport protein with glycine, serine, cysteine and methionine) and a range of acute-phase proteins by the pro-inflammatory cytokines.

An increase in urinary nitrogen and sulphur excretion occurs as a result of this catabolic process. Cuthbertson as early as in 1931 reported that the urinary excretion of sulphur increases to a lesser extent than that of nitrogen, during the response to infection and injury, suggesting that sulphur amino acids are preferentially retained and so 'spared' from catabolism.

**Interaction between antioxidants is linked to maintain antioxidant defence:** Many of the components of antioxidant defence interact to maintain antioxidant status. Glutathione and the enzymes that maintain it in its reduced form (GSH) are central to effective antioxidant status. For example, when oxidants interact with cell membranes, the oxidised form of vitamin E that results is restored to its reduced form by ascorbic acid. The dehydroascorbic acid formed in this process is reconverted to ascorbic acid by interaction with the reduced form of glutathione. Subsequently, oxidised glutathione (GSSG) formed in the reaction is reconverted to the reduced form of glutathione by glutathione reductase (Fig. 6.10). Vitamins E and C and glutathione are thus intimately linked in antioxidant defence.

**Vitamin B$_6$:** Vitamin B$_6$ and riboflavin (which have no antioxidant properties *per se*), also contribute to antioxidant defences indirectly. Vitamin B$_6$ is the cofactor in the metabolic pathway for the biosynthesis of cysteine (Fig. 6.10). Cellular cysteine concentration is rate-limiting precursor in glutathione synthesis (Figs 6.10 and 6.11). Riboflavin is a cofactor for glutathione reductase, which maintains the major part of cellular glutathione in the reduced form (Fig. 6.10). Vitamin B$_6$ deficiency causes thymic atrophy and lymphocyte depletion in lymph nodes and spleen. Various aspects of cell-mediated immunity are also influenced by vitamin B$_6$ deficiency.

**Ascorbic acid:** High concentrations of vitamin C are found in phagocytic cells. The role of vitamin C as a key component of antioxidant defence is well-established (Fig. 6.10). It is important in GSH metabolism, though it has only minor effects upon a range of immune functions. Unlike deficiencies in vitamins B$_6$, E and riboflavin, deficiency of vitamin C does not cause atrophy of lymphoid tissue. The interrelationship between gluta-

thione and ascorbic acid may, therefore, play a role in the effect of exercise on immune function.

**Antioxidant defences get depleted following infection and injury:** Observations in experimental animals and human patients indicate that antioxidant defences such as vitamins C and E and glutathione become depleted during infection and after injury, though the body strives to maintain them.

**Effect of antioxidants on inflammation and immune function:** There is a growing body of evidence that antioxidants suppress inflammatory components of the response to infection and trauma, while enhancing components related to cell-mediated immunity.

**Oxidant stress activates NFκB and API:** The oxidant molecules produced by the immune system (to combat infection/injury) to kill invading organisms may activate at least two important families of proteins that are sensitive to changes in cellular redox state. The families are nuclear transcription factor kappa B (NFκB) and activator protein 1 (AP1). These transcription factors act as 'control switches' for biological processes. NFκB is present in the cytosol in an inactive form. Activation of it can be brought about by a wide range of stimuli, including PIC, hydrogen peroxide, mitogens, bacteria and viruses and their related products, UV and ionising radiations. The active NFκB is translocated to the nucleus, where it binds to response elements in the

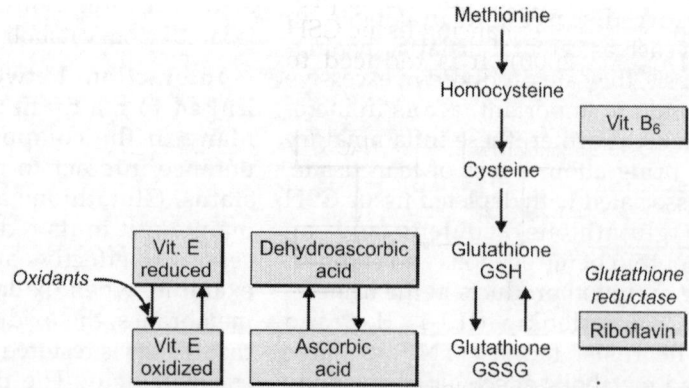

**Fig. 6.10:** The interaction between antioxidants in maintaining antioxidant defence

promoter regions of genes. A similar translocation of AP1 from cytosol to nucleus also occurs in the presence of oxidant stress. Binding of the transcription factors is implicated in the activation of a wide range of genes associated with inflammation and the immune response (Schreck et al, 1991).

Oxidant damage to cells will indirectly create a pro-inflammatory effect by the production of lipid peroxides. This situation may lead to upregulation of NFκB activity, since the transcription factor has been shown to be activated in endothelial cells cultured with linoleic acid (n-6 fatty acid), an effect inhibited by vitamin E and N acetyl cysteine (NAC) (Hennig et al, 1996). The interaction between oxidant stress and an impaired ability to synthesise glutathione results in enhanced inflammation. **Addition of anti-oxidants might act to prevent NFκB activation** by quenching oxidants.

**Strategies for modulating tissue GSH content and improving immune function:** A number of strategies are evolved to raise levels of glutathione in depleted individuals (Fig. 6.11). There are three potential ways of enhancing cellular GSH content: (1) administration of the three amino acids (cysteine, glutamic and glycine) that comprise the tripeptide, (2) administration of cofactors (vitamin B$_6$, riboflavin and folic acid) for the metabolic pathways leading to GSH production and (3) administration of synthetic compounds that become converted to precursors of GSH. Alpha-lipoic acid provides a good means of enhancing tissue GSH content (Deneke, 2000). It is reduced to

dihydrolipoic acid that converts cystine to cysteine. N acetyl cysteine (NAC) and L-2-oxothiazolidine-4-carboxylate (OTZ) deliver cysteine directly to cells.

*Taurine and Immune Function*

Taurine possess antioxidant properties and plays a role in immune function. Taurine is the end-product of cysteine metabolism. It is the most abundant free nitrogenous compound in cells. It is a membrane stabiliser and regulates calcium flux, thereby control cell stability. Studies in laboratory animals and humans showed that it regulates the release of pro-inflammatory cytokines (Grimble, 1994; Kontny et al, 2000). Taurine is an essential nutrient in cats (obligate carnivore). Substantial impairment of immune function occurs in cats that are deprived of taurine (Grinible, 1994).

**Taurine chloramine and taurolidine:** Taurine interacts with hypochlorous acid (produced during the 'oxidant burst' of stimulated macrophages) to produce taurine chloramine. This compound may have important immunomodulatory properties. Taurine chloramine has been shown to inhibit nitric oxide, PGE$_2$, TNF-α and IL-6 production from stimulated macrophages. Taurolidine (a derivative of taurine) has been used as a bactericidal and anti-lipopolysaccharide agent. Taurolidine may also have an immuno-modulatary influence.

*Tryptophan and Immune Function*

In addition to its indispensable role in protein synthesis, the essential amino acid

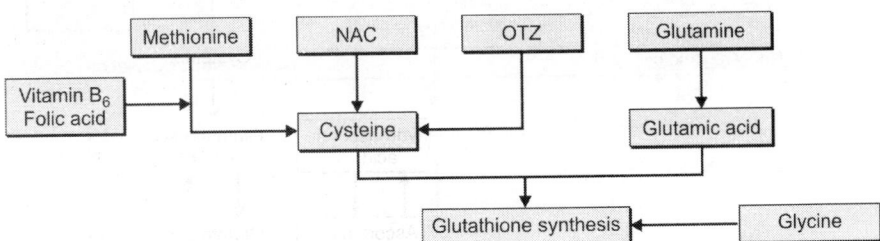

**Fig. 6.11:** 'Strategies to enhance glutathione synthesis: Role of nutrients and drugs'; NAC, N acetyl cysteine; OTZ, L-2-oxothiazolidine-4-carboxylate

l-tryptophan is the precursor of many physiologically important metabolites produced during the course of its degradation along four pathways. Three pathways are of quantitatively minor significance and the fourth one the kynurenine pathway (KP) accounts for ~95% of overall tryptophan degradation. The 3 minor pathways (and their important products) are (1) hydroxylation (serotonin, 5-hydroxytryptamine or 5-HT in brain and melatonin in the pineal), (2) decarboxylation (tryptamine) and (3) transamination (indolepyruvic acid).

**Kynurenine pathway (KP):** Tryptophan plays an important role in the defence of the body and immune response modulation (Le Floc'h and Seve, 2007), in relation with the kynurenine pathway (KP). In pigs this metabolic pathway is involved in tryptophan metabolism disturbances associated with an inflammatory response. There is a progressive decline in plasma levels of tryptophan in pigs suffering from chronic lung inflammation with higher indoleamine 2,3-dioxygenase (IDO) activity in lungs and associated lymph nodes. Here an understanding of kynurenine pathway (KP) of tryptophan degradation is helpful (Fig. 6.12).

**Kinurenic acid has anti-inflammatory properties:** The KP produces many biologically active metabolites that play important roles in health and disease and, in particular, conditions associated with immune dysfunction and central nervous system

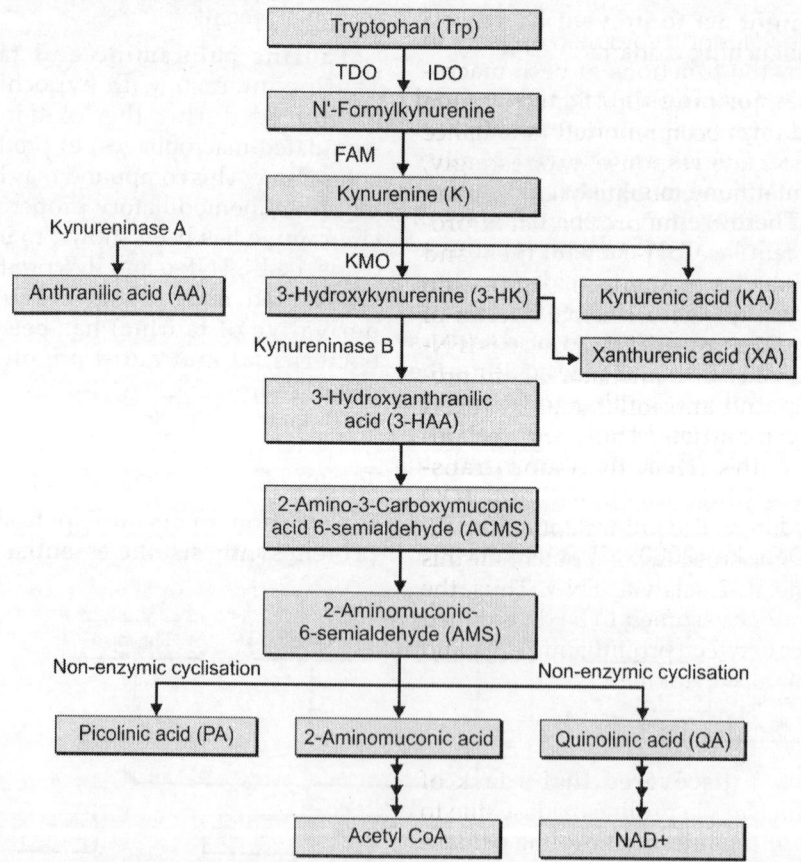

**Fig. 6.12:** The kynurenine pathway of tryptophan degradation; TDO, Trp 2,3-dioxygenase; IDO, Indoleamine 2,3-dioxygenase; FAM, N'-Formylkynurenine formamidase; KMO, Kynurenine hydroxylase (monooxygenase)

disorders. Tryptophan (Trp) is converted to N2-formylkynurenine by the action of either Trp 2,3-dioxygenase (TDO) mainly in liver or indoleamine 2,3-dioxygenase (IDO) extrahepatically. N2- formylkynurenine is then hydrolysed to kynurenine (K) and it is metabolised mainly by hydroxylation to 3-hydroxykynurenine (3-HK). This is hydrolysed to 3-hydroxyanthranilic acid (3-HAA) by kynureninase. This latter enzyme can also hydrolyse kynurenine to anthranilic acid (AA). These metabolites [(3-HK, 3-HAA, quinolinic acid (QA) and picolinic acid (PA)] are immunosuppressive kinurenine metabolites (Fig. 6.12). Modulation of immune function has been established for these metabolites. Kinurenic acid (KA) modulates immune function. It has anti-inflammatory properties. This is likely to influence IDO activity.

Thus catabolism of tryptophan appears to be critical for the functions of both macrophages and lymphocytes. Oral administration of tryptophan has been reported to enhance the innate immune response. Interestingly, anthranilic acid (a metabolite of tryptophan via the IDO) inhibits the production of pro-inflammatory T-helper-1 cytokines and prevents autoimmune neuroinflammation (Platten et al, 2005). The principal effector of IDO is IFN-γ and a less efficient inducer is IFN-α. Other cytokines and mediators (both pro-inflammatory and anti-inflammatory) exert various effects on IDO. Thus, anti-inflammatory cytokines (IL-4, IL-10 and transforming growth factor β) inhibit IDO induction by IFN-γ. The pro-inflammatory IL-1β and tumour necrosis factor α potentiate this induction and IL-2 acts via IFN-γ. Thus, the IDO status can be assumed to be determined by the balance between pro-inflammatory and anti-inflammatory cytokines.

## Proline and Immune Function

Ha et al (2005) discovered that a lack of proline catabolism via proline oxidase due to a deficiency of the intestinal proline oxidase impairs gut immunity. The major mediator derived from proline oxidation is $H_2O_2$, which is cytotoxic to pathogenic bacteria and is also a signalling molecule. It can be conjectured that a high activity of proline oxidase in the porcine placenta (Wu et al, 2005) and the piglet small-intestine (Wu, 1997) may play a crucial role in protecting these organs from infections during the critical periods of foetal and neonatal development.

## Threonine and Immune Function

Besides protein synthesis, the major functions of threonine include maintenance of gut integrity and immunity (Ruth and Field, 2013). A significant part of the threonine intake is utilised by the gut itself and is used for the synthesis of endogenous secretions, particularly mucous, which is important to maintain the gut barrier. Considering the importance of digestive secretions for gut health and for the digestive process, an adequate dietary threonine level is the key to allow proper gut function.

Threonine plays an important role in the production of antibodies and in providing overall immune system support. Because of the high threonine content of immunoglobulins, dietary threonine deficiency may affect immunoglobulins. Dietary supplementation with threonine also has been demonstrated to promote serum levels of IgG in sows and increase antibody production, serum IgG levels and jejunal mucosal concentrations of IgG and IgA, while decreasing jejunal mucosal concentrations of IL-6 in young pigs challenged with E. coli (Wang et al, 2006).

## IMMUNE SYSTEM NEEDS FOR AMINO ACIDS

### Porcine Immune System

The primary immune responses to microorganisms and their antigens are generated by the (1) innate and (2) acquired or adaptive immune systems. The two immune systems interact intimately and fulfil the different needs of the host to control microorganisms. The reader may refer Chapter 2 for the details of these immune systems.

The porcine immune system differs in many aspects from that of humans and mice, including morphological differences in the lymphatic system and phenotypic differences in immune cells as well as functional differences in immune cell populations (Rothkotter et al, 2002). Unlike other most species, the lymphocytes enter into the lymphoid organs through the lymphatic vessels and exit directly into the blood in the pig. These differences might contribute to the predisposition to and outcomes of bacterial infections such as *Salmonella serovars* (Scharek and Tedin, 2007).

In modern, high-density production systems, swine (and other animals) are challenged by pathogenic microorganisms-bacteria, viruses and parasites that can cause infectious disease or pathology, especially for neonatal and weaned piglets (Zhang et al, 2012). Immune system is not well-developed in the first four weeks of life in weaned piglets.

The gastrointestinal tract (GIT) is one of the largest immunological organs of the body. It contains greater than $10^{12}$ lymphocytes and has a greater concentration of antibodies than any other site in the body (Mayer, 2000). With respect to immune function within the GIT, it may be equally important to achieve a homeostatic balance between immune tolerance and immune responsiveness (Artis, 2008). Both birth and weaning are associated with major changes in the development and metabolism of GIT and the gut-associated lymphoid tissue (GALT). Prenatally, the GALT is immature but after birth the GALT begins to develop rapidly, although some processes may take up to 6 weeks to mature.

## Mucosal Immune System Development in Piglets

The mucosal immune system is adequately equipped to generate a protective immune response directed at harmful pathogens. It also has the capability to be tolerant of the ubiquitous dietary antigens and normal microbial flora, while maintaining the ability to permit the absorption of nutrients. There-fore, the development of the gastrointestinal immune system is important for establishing an effective immunological response to a diverse milieu of dietary and microbial antigenic components (Burkey et al, 2009).

## The Processes of the Immune Response in Piglets

The immune protection for piglets comes primarily from (1) passive immunity through colostrum and (2) active immunity from auto-development of immune system of the piglets. Due to incomplete development of the immune system of the newborn piglets, the immune protection is mainly from the antibodies transferred through maternal colostrum (passive immunity), rather than the cell-mediated immune response, until about 4 weeks of age.

It is now well-accepted that the animal's immunological reaction to immune stimulants is the cause of decreased growth and rate of development (Klasing, 1988; Roubenoff, 1997). It is challenging to nutritionists to seek nutritional means of improving the immune system.

Birth (natural farrowing) and suckling are associated with the initial introduction of microbes into the sterile GIT of the newborn. Since, the pig placenta does not transfer immunoglobulins, the consumption of colostrum represents the initial transfer of immunity to the neonate during the first two days before the 'intestinal closure' occurs. Thus piglets receive the passive immunity via colostral immunoglobulins intake. As time progresses up to weaning, the active mucosal system gradually gathers the ability to generate its own antibody molecules in the gut wall. In the first 2 weeks of life, the intestine rapidly becomes colonised with lymphoid cells. Between 14 and 28 days of age the intestinal mucosa becomes colonised with CD4+ cells, while CD8+ cells begin to appear at 35 days age. The immunological architecture of piglet cannot be considered fully mature until 7 weeks of age (Sinkora and Butler, 2009).

## Early Weaning of Piglets—GALT Development

In commercial practice, piglets are weaned at 3–4 weeks of age. This early weaning of piglets inflicts considerable stress on the entire gastrointestinal tract and this result in an increased susceptibility to bacterial infection leading to acute diarrhoea and high mortality rates. Major causes for this are change in feed and its after effects.

During suckling the piglet is consuming a highly palatable, high fat milk diet that is relatively easy to digest. However, weaning diet is relatively high in carbohydrate and more complex, which is not only more difficult to digest but it is also associated with a dramatic change both in the number and variety of ingested microbes.

Such early weaning is associated with low feed intake. There is a loss of body weight, excessive diarrhoea and lower feed efficiency. These problems are associated with major morphological changes in the structure of the small intestine such as decreased villus height and overall loss of function. It is critical to develop the GALT to avoid undue systemic infections and to limit the incidence of diarrhoea. Ultimately, the GALT becomes the largest immune organ in the body and it is well established that protein deficiency is associated with immune deficiency and specific amino acids have major effects on both gut integrity and GALT function (Ruth and Field, 2013).

## Amino Acids Needs of Immune Cells

Amino acids do affect immune system function usually through actions at several levels in the gastrointestinal tract, thymus, spleen, regional lymph nodes and immune cells of the circulating blood (Cunningham-Rundles, 2002). The utilisation of amino acids by immune cells plays an important role in the function of the immune system.

**Glutamine:** Glutamine is required to support optimal lymphocyte proliferation and production of cytokines by lymphocytes and macrophages (Calder and Yaqoob, 1999).

This amino acid also enhances the phagocytic activity of macrophages, cytokine production by T lymphocytes and antibody generation by B lymphocytes (Field et al, 2002). Glutamine utilisation has been linked to functional activities of immune cells such as cytokine production, nitric oxide production, super-oxide production and phagocytosis. Many cells of the immune system including lymphocytes, macrophages and neutrophils utilise glutamine at high rates, which is related to the specific function of these cells in the inflammatory response.

**Branched chain amino acids:** A branched-chain amino acid (BCAA) is an amino acid having an aliphatic side-chain with a branch. For example, leucine, isoleucine and valine. Cell culture studies have showed that branched chain amino acids (BCAA) are absolutely essential for lymphocytes to synthesise protein, RNA and DNA and to divide in response to stimulation (Calder, 2006). Immune cells are able to incorporate BCAA into proteins and are able to oxidise them.

**Arginine:** Arginine is another important immuno-enhancing amino acid. As a precursor for nitric oxide (NO) and polyamine synthesis, arginine profoundly influences immune function. It is metabolised either by inducible nitric oxide synthase (iNOS) or by arginase 1 in immune cells. These enzymes are stimulated by T helper 1 or 2 cytokines, respectively. In the absence of immune stimulation, little arginine is used by immune cells due to a lack of expression of major arginine metabolising enzymes, iNOS and arginase 1 (Bernard et al, 2001).

**Deficiency of dietary protein:** A deficiency of dietary protein or amino acids has long been demonstrated to impair immune function and increase the sensitivity/susceptibility of animals to infectious challenges or stressful conditions. (i) For example, deficiency of branched chain amino acids and of arginine + lysine increased splenocyte proliferation, but sulphur amino acid deficiency decreased splenocyte and lymphocyte proliferation (Konashi et al, 2000). (ii) The study with piglets has shown that threonine deficiency caused higher nitrogen excretion, blood urea and lower number of acidic mucin-producing goblet cells in the small intestine.

**Dietary supplementation:** Dietary supplementation with amino acids beyond their requirements for growth deposition is useful depending on environmental conditions particularly during periods of stress and when the immune system is challenged.

## Immune System Stimulation Require Higher Quantity of Amino Acids

It is now clear that immune system stimulation (ISS) can cause morphological and physiological changes in the gastrointestinal tract and impact nutrient utilisation in pigs (Mani et al, 2012). During immunological stress, amino acids are redistributed away from protein production towards tissues involved in inflammation and immune response. They are used for the synthesis of inflammatory and immune proteins, to support immune cell proliferation and for the synthesis of other compounds important for body defence functions (Webster et al, 2002).

a. Immune activation appears to alter glutamine and arginine metabolism. During the peak of an immune response, the requirement for these nonessential amino acids (glutamine, arginine, cysteine, and so on) increases 2- to 3-fold and may become potentially limiting.

b. ISS does not change the apparent ileal digestibility (AID) of amino acids but alters the partitioning of sulphur amino acids in favour of nonprotein body stores in growing pigs. These findings reflect an increased need for dietary sulphur amino acids to support the immune response during immune system stimulation in growing pigs (Rakhshandeh et al, 2010).

c. Pigs injected with turpentine increase plasma fibrinogen concentrations by 30% and fibrinogen synthesis by 140%. Pigs

with a lung inflammation (induced by intravenous injection of complete Freund's adjuvant) show declined plasma tryptophan concentrations for 10 days (see page 214). Therefore, the increase in protein synthesis may require a higher quantity of tyrosine, phenylalanine and tryptophan.

d. Li et al (1999) reported that although maximum growth rate of 17–31 kg pigs occurred at a dietary threonine level of 6.8 g/kg, **higher threonine** levels were needed to maximise humoral antibody production and IgG levels. To optimise immunity of 10–25 kg pigs, 6.6 g per day of true ileal digestible (TID) threonine should be fed (Wang et al, 2006). Li et al (2007) showed that the ideal amino acid pattern of lysine/methionine/threonine/tryptophan on the digestible basis was 100:27:29:59 for 10 kg pigs under immune stress and 100:30:21:61 for piglets under normal conditions.

## FUNCTIONAL ROLES OF GLUTAMINE AND ARGININE IN THE DEVELOPMENT AND MAINTENANCE OF INTESTINAL IMMUNE FUNCTION IN THE NEONATAL PIG

### Functional Amino Acids

Traditionally dietary amino acids have been described as essential (non-dispensable) or non-essential (dispensable) on the basis of synthesis in sufficient amounts to support maximal growth or maintain nitrogen balance. But now dietary amino acid requirements are increasingly being assessed in terms of their non-protein roles. Some non-essential amino acids are being reclassified as functional amino acids (Wu, 2010 and 2013).

The important non-protein roles of such functional amino acids are (1) to maintain intestinal integrity (barrier function) and (2) to support the immune system. These functions are linked in that the epithelial cells of the gut are considered to be part of the innate immune system and thus comprise part of the gut-associated lymphoid tissue (GALT) (Ruth and Field, 2013). Here the functional roles of glutamine and arginine in the development and maintenance of GALT in the neonatal pig from birth through weaning are discussed.

## Functional roles of Glutamine

**Glutamine—Glutamate:** Glutamine and glutamate represent the most abundant amino acids in milk and most commercial feedstuffs. Often these two amino acids are expressed simply as "glutamate" since acid hydrolysis of proteins effectively hydrolyses all glutamine to glutamate and thus, the final estimate of "glutamate" in feedstuffs usually refers to the sum of glutamate plus glutamine.

*Metabolic Role*

Within the body, glutamine is the most abundant free alpha amino acid. It is also the most abundant alpha amino acid in blood plasma of most mammals studied to date (Watford, 2014). In contrast, intracellular glutamate concentrations are relatively high in most cells, while its concentration in plasma is much lower. Thus glutamine serves as a major transport form of nitrogen, carbon and energy between tissues, while glutamate plays a more direct role in intracellular intermediary metabolism.

Glutamine is required for the synthesis of NAD, NADP, purines, pyrimidines and glucosamine, all substances required by differentiating and growing cells. Glutamine is the major respiratory fuel for immune cells (macrophages, B and T lymphocytes, neutrophils, granulocytes); anything that stimulates these immune cells to proliferate, mature and produce cytokines or undergoes phagocytosis (macrophages) enhances the utilisation of glutamine (Colder and Yaqoob, 1999; Li et al, 2007).

In addition, after food consumption, enterocytes use both glutamine and glutamate derived from the diet as their major fuels and effectively these two amino acids do not enter the circulation (Wetford and Reeds, 2003). Enterocyte glutamine and glutamate metabolism also give rises to citrulline, alanine, proline, lactate, glutathione and ammonia. The major site of glutamine

utilisation of circulating glutamine is the small intestine, where glutamine serves as the major respiratory substrate for the epithelial cells (enterocytes). Because of these functions probably, glutamate cannot completely replace the use of glutamine by enterocytes and other cells.

*Glutamine Exhibits Specific Signalling Properties*

In addition to its metabolic roles, glutamine has been shown to exhibit specific signalling properties including changes in expression of key genes encoding metabolic and cryoprotective processes (e.g. heat shock proteins) and acting overall in an anabolic sense in most cells, that is increased proliferation and differentiation, increased protein synthesis, decreased proteolysis, decreased apoptosis (Rhoads and Wu, 2009). Thus glutamine and glutamate play essential and quantitatively important roles in the metabolism and function of both the epithelial barrier of the GIT and of the GALT in general.

In catabolic states (burn, infections, etc.), there is a release of glutamine from the skeletal muscle and a decrease in the free glutamine pool within that tissue. Concomitantly, there is an increase in muscle net proteolysis that provides the substrate for continued synthesis and release of glutamine to fuel immune cells, aid in wound repair, correct metabolic acidosis and provide the carbon substrate for both hepatic and renal gluconeogenesis (Colder and Yaqoob, 1999).

## Effects of Glutamine Supplementation

The benefits of enteral glutamine have mainly been the preservation of intestinal function in severely ill patients particularly in those receiving total parenteral nutrition. Supplementary effect of glutamine in suckling piglets and sow are furnished hereunder.

*Suckling Piglets*

Although glutamine/glutamate concentrations are high in milk, it appears that these may be insufficient for maximal growth of the piglets. Haynes and colleagues (2009) fed glutamine or alanyl-glutamine by gavage two times a day for 7 days (from 7th day of age) to piglets that were still nursing on the sow. The piglets then received injections of *E. coli* endotoxin and were sampled 24 and 48 h later. They found that extra glutamine decreased the expression of Toll like receptor 4 (TLR4), active caspase 3 and NFκB (all increased in response to endotoxin), with an overall amelioration of intestinal injury, a decrease in rectal temperature and enhanced piglet growth performance. However, treating individual piglets by twice daily gavage is not practical in a commercial pig rearing facility.

An alternative approach is to use creep feeders (Cabrera and co-workers, 2013). Supplementation of glutamine (1%) or a mixture of glutamine plus glutamate (0.88% Aminogut) in creep feed from days 14 to 21 resulted in improved intestinal villus height and feed conversion through six weeks of age.

Studies from C.J. Field and colleagues (1997 and 2006) also showed that (1) glutamine (4.4%) could prevent the drop in skeletal muscle glutamine content in recently weaned piglets, (2) had beneficial effects on immune cells in mesenteric lymph nodes and (3) could normalise lymphocyte function in *E. coli*-infected piglets.

More recently field and coworkers reported the effect of glutamine (4.4%) on intestinal barrier function in *E. coli* infected piglets and found that glutamine attenuated catabolism, suppressed inflammation and cytokine release and maintained tight junction protein expression and epithelial barrier function (Ewaschuk et al, 2011).

C. Domeneghini and colleagues found a positive effect on the barrier function, an increase in epithelial cell number and an increase in mitotic cells in epithelium.

### Lactating Sow

Providing glutamine supplement to the lactating sow with the aim of increasing milk glutamine content is an alternative to individually feeding the suckling piglets. It is shown that lactation in pigs and other species, is accompanied by a mild catabolic state as indicated by a loss of lean body mass and a decrease in intramuscular glutamine content (Manso et al, 2012) and thus supplemental glutamine to the sow may alleviate such losses. Kitt et al (2004) found that feeding 2.5% glutamine to sows increased glutamine content of milk.

Thus glutamine and/or glutamate supplementation to early weaned, suckling (creep feeders), or the lactating sow, may improve intestinal health and immune function and so alleviate some of the stress of abrupt early weaning.

**Molecular mechanisms responsible for the protective effects of glutamine in early weaning:** Wang et al (2008) used microarray analysis of gene expression in small intestine to investigate the molecular mechanisms responsible for the protective effects of glutamine in early weaning. They compared weaning at day 21 to a commercial diet with or without glutamine, with sampling at day 28, with piglets that had been allowed to nurse through day 28. Early weaning (without glutamine) resulted in a marked decrease in body weight gain, small intestinal weight, length and villus height, together with less glutathione and a more oxidised glutathione ratio. This was accompanied by increased expression of genes involved in oxidative stress and immune activation but decreased expression of genes related to macronutrient metabolism and cell proliferation in the small intestine.

When the piglets were weaned to a diet supplemented with 1% glutamine, there was some alleviation of the effects on body weight gain and intestinal weight, villus height, glutathione levels and an overall enhancement of oxidative-defence capacity. Furthermore, glutamine supplemented-piglets showed increased intestinal expression of genes involved in cell growth and removal of oxidants and decreased expression of genes coding for factors that promote oxidative stress and immune activation.

## Functional roles of arginine

i. Arginine is a basic amino acid that is recognised as being essential in the neonate for most mammalian species. In most adult mammals, arginine is considered a dietary non-essential amino acid as it can be synthesised from glutamine, glutamate and proline, but becomes conditionally essential during periods of stress (Li et al, 2007). Exceptions are carnivores such as cats and ferrets that are unable to synthesise arginine, apart from that used in the hepatic urea cycle. Hence cats and ferrets have an absolute requirement for dietary arginine throughout life.

ii. There is, however, evidence that dietary arginine deficiency impairs fertility in both humans and boars.

iii. Arginine metabolism in the liver is limited for urea synthesis only and can be ignored with regards to extra-hepatic arginine metabolism. Arginine synthesis occurs through a two tissue pathway whereby in the intestine glutamate, glutamine or proline are used to synthesise citrulline. This citrulline is taken up by the kidney, where it is converted to arginine. Arginine (and citrulline), from the diet and that synthesised in the intestine and kidney, are not taken up by the liver (and thus not used for urea synthesis) and are available for extrahepatic functions.

iv. Arginine is the only precursor of nitric oxide (through the action of nitric oxide synthase), which has important roles in both vasodilation and immune cell killing of pathogenic microbes. Thus, it is not surprising that arginine is essential for the function of the GALT.

v. Arginine is a precursor for the synthesis of creatine, proline, glutamate and agmatine.

vi. Arginine stimulates expression of heat shock protein (HSP) 70 for cytoprotective roles in times of stress (Wu et al, 2013). It has been demonstrated that HSP70 expression get increased (in the liver) by feeding 6g arginine/kg feed thrice a day to early weaned pigs and this is accompanied by decreased expression of inflammatory cytokines.

vii. Arginine is also a powerful stimulator of both insulin and growth hormone secretion and positively regulates expression of genes related to growth and mitochondrial proliferation (G.Wu and coworkers, 2009). Similar to glutamine, arginine acts in an overall anabolic nature with respect to the GIT and GALT.

**Arginine is limiting in suckling piglets:** J. Leibholz (1982) has reported that only 55% of arginine could be synthesised endogenously; hence arginine is essential in young piglets. Although arginine is relatively high in most of the proteins found in feedstuffs (usually 3–5% of the amino acids), it is low in 'low protein-foods' such as grains. Surprisingly the arginine content in porcine milk is low and actually decreases as lactation progresses. Equally surprising is the fact that, the endogenous pathway of arginine synthesis is poorly developed in neonatal piglets.

Kim and Wu have reported that arginine deficiency resulted in growth retardation, intestinal, reproductive and immune dysfunction, impaired neurological development, impaired wound healing and higher circulating ammonia concentrations. In 2004 they reported that 0.2 to 0.4% arginine supplementation to very early (day 7) weaned piglets lowered plasma ammonia and enhanced body weight gain, unequivocally showing that arginine is limiting in suckling piglets.

There are also indications that arginine supplementation, possibly through nitric oxide formation and improved vascularisation, improves reproductive performance with more piglets born alive, heavier litter weights, etc. (G.Wu et al, 2009). The optimal amount of arginine supplementation for pigs seems to be between 0.5 and 1.0% of the diet. Some studies have reported adverse effects at higher concentrations, which may be related to inappropriate arginine: lysine ratios resulting in amino acid imbalance and/or antagonism in absorption from the gut (Ball et al, 2007).

## Conclusion

The gastrointestinal tract and the gut associated lymphoid system are critical to maintain both adequate nutrient absorption and defence against pathogenic microbes. Glutamine (and glutamate) and arginine are required by both intestinal and immune cells for many vital functions. With regard to the maintenance of GIT and GALT function, glutamine (glutamate) and arginine have been proven to be beneficial. They are required in the diet in sufficient amounts to achieve optimal performance in both early weaned piglets and possibly for the sow to maintain lean body mass during lactation. Thus at least, glutamine and arginine should be reclassified a functional amino acids.

## IMMUNE MODIFYING EFFECTS OF AMINO ACIDS ON GUT-ASSOCIATED LYMPHOID TISSUE (GALT)

It is well-established that protein deficiency suppresses the immune response and increases susceptibility to infection. In fact, protein energy malnutrition (PEM) is hypothesised to be the leading contributor to immune deficiency globally.

## Dietary NEAAs Could Become Essential During Critical States of Health or Life Stages

Research trials conducted by C.J. Field, G. Wu and coworkers since 1990s revealed that amino acids are important energy substrates for immune cells, critical in health states of burns, trauma and perenteral feeding or periods of development such as weaning, pregnancy. Now, it is accepted that some dietary non-essential amino acids (NEAA) could become conditionally essential during these situations. These include arginine, glutamine, glutamate, glycine, proline, taurine and cysteine. This change in need for these amino acids in the diet may be due in part because of their effects on immune function. Each of these amino acids have unique properties that include, maintaining the integrity, growth and function of the intestine, as well as normalising inflammatory cytokine secretion and improving T lymphocyte numbers, specific T cell functions and the secretion of IgA by lamina propria cells.

## Amino Acids and Functions of Intestinal Epithelium

The intestinal epithelium facilitates nutrient absorption. It also has a major role in protecting the host from oral pathogens, inducing oral tolerance and maintaining a healthy interaction with commensal bacteria. It is known that both protein and single amino acid deficiencies impair the physical integrity and growth of the intestinal epithelium, as well as alter the immune response (Ziegler et al, 2003). Ruth and Field (2013) reviewed the current understanding of gut-associated lymphoid tissue (GALT) and the immuno-modulatory effects of specific amino acids on immunity that occurs or originates in the intestine.

### Gut-associated Lymphoid Tissue

GALT contains a variety of immune cell types from the innate and acquired immune systems. Because of the proximity to the microbiome and the immediate contact with food, it is continually exposed to both 'normal' and potentially dangerous antigens. Accordingly, GALT develops in a manner that allows non-pathogenic commensal bacteria to survive and enables tolerance to food antigens, while protecting the host from pathogenic organisms and other potentially toxic substances.

GALT is considered a component of the mucosal immune system. It consists of aggregated tissue including Peyer's patches (PPs) and solitary lymphoid follicles and nonaggregated cells in the lamina propria, intestinal epithelial cells (IECs), intraepithelial lymphocytes (IELs), as well as mesenteric lymph nodes (MLNs). Collectively, GALT plays a critical role in the development of the systemic immune response. As a primary site of antigen exposure, it primes naive T and B lymphocytes that develop into effector cells. They migrate from the intestine to other sites of the body to protect against immune challenges, such as invading pathogens (Fig. 6.13).

GALT has an important role in first line mucosal defences. The epithelium is protected from large pathogens or particles by a layer of mucin, a glycoprotein secreted from the specialised goblet cell within the endothelium (Turner, 2009). The intraepithelial lymphocytes (IEL) are dispersed among the intestinal epithelial cells (IEC) that line intestinal villi and both cell types play a role in gut immune function (Fig. 6.13). Tight junction proteins, such as claudin, occludin and ZO-1, determine the mucosal permeability and regulate the flow of solutes between the intestinal epithelial cells (Turner, 2009).

The Intraepithelial lymphocytes (IEL) are **primarily T cells** but have functions distinct from **peripheral T cells**. The Peyer's patches are lymphoid aggregates that line the small intestine and colon and are the primary inductive sites of the mucosal humoral immune response. The epithelium layer of the Peyer's patches contains highly specialised cells called **microfold or M cells** that continually sample the intestinal contents bringing them in contact with the **resident immune cells** (primarily B cells and small numbers of macrophages, dendritic cells and T cells). Dendritic cells can also extend through the intestinal epithelial cells to directly sample antigen. Antigen presenting cells (APC), particularly dendritic cells, migrate from the Peyer's patches or epithelium to the mesenteric lymph nodes where they educate naive T cells.

The mesenteric lymph nodes act as the interphase between the peripheral immune system and the gut and it is believed that they are the primary sites of oral tolerance induction. In rats, mesenteric lymph nodes are composed primarily of T-helper cells (55%),

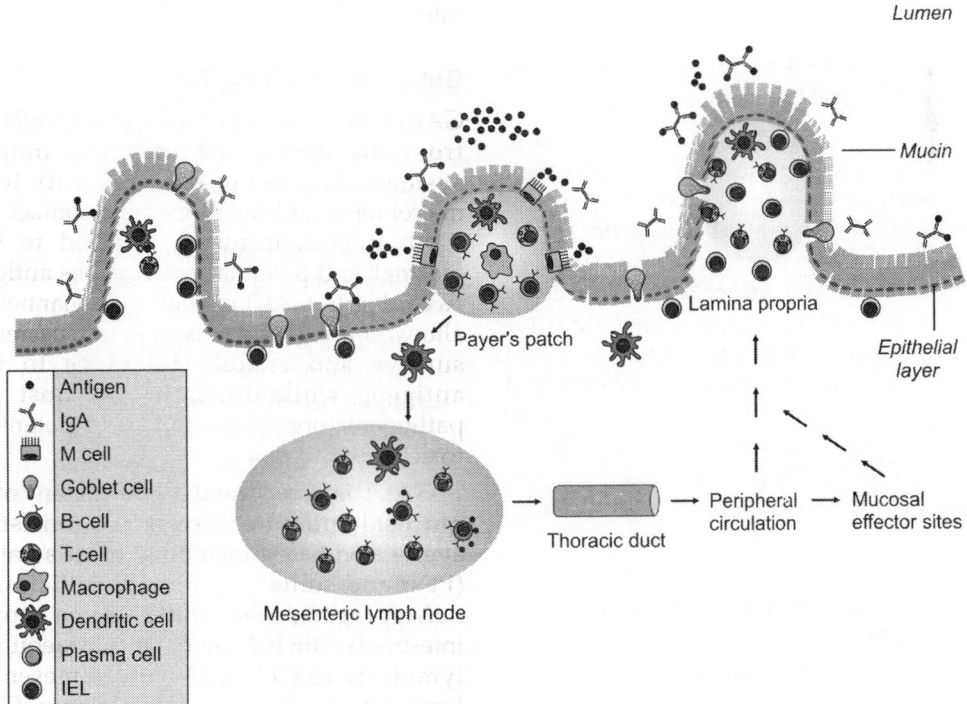

**Fig. 6.13:** Diagram of the gut-associated lymphoid tissue. *Source*: Ruth and Field, 2013

but also contain cytotoxic T lymphocytes (15%), B cells (25%) and dendritic cells (5%) (Ruth et al, 2009). Pigs have slightly different phenotypes, with approximately 12% CD4+ CD8+, 25–28% CD4+ (single positive), 27-32% CD8+ (single positive) and the rest composed of B cells and other antigen presenting cells.

After exposure to antigen in the Peyer' patches and mesenteric lymph nodes, immune cells circulate in the periphery and migrate to other mucosal effector sites and home back to the lamina propria (Fig. 6.13; Brandzaeg, P, 2009). This is the major effector component of GALT as these cells are antigen mature and primed to respond to foreign antigens. The lamina propria is comprised primarily of IgA secreting plasma cells and effector T cells (50% T-helper and 30% cytotoxic T lymphocytes). Secretory IgA (sIgA) is the most abundant immunoglobulin in the mammalian intestine and acts by binding pathogens and facilitating the entrapment in mucous and removal from the intestinal track. Indeed a deficiency or inability to produce IgA results in frequent intestinal infections.

## Supplementary Feeding of Amino Acids on Gut Function and the Immune System

The importance of individual amino acids to gut function and immunity is based on their supplementary feeding to animals: (1) intravenous (total parenteral nutrition, TPN) feeding demonstrates the importance of GALT and immune functions beyond the intestine (2) supplementary feeding after weaning demonstrates the importance of these amino acids to the normal growth and development of the intestine and GALT of weaned animals and (3) feeding the suffering animals during infection or chronic inflammation for their role in regulating inflammation and infectious challenges.

## Glutamine is a Lifeline for Immune Cells and Enterocytes

Glutamine is a lifeline for immune cells and enterocytes. It has been the most extensively studied amino acid with regards to its effects on GALT and the intestine. Glutamine is categorised as a non-essential amino acid in healthy animals and represents the amino acid in highest proportions in the body. However, during periods of stress and during critical stages, it supports growth and health in young animals.

Glutamine is an important energy substrate and precursor for other amino acids and derivatives in immune cells and enterocytes. In fact, both the cell types cannot function without at least some exogenous glutamine. In immune cells, particularly lymphocytes, neutrophils and macrophages, glutamine is used rapidly and metabolised to glutamate, aspartate, lactate and $CO_2$. Wu et al (1995) demonstrated the main metabolic fates of glutamine in enterocytes from weaning piglets are ammonia, glutamate, alanine, aspartate and $CO_2$. As a precursor for glutamate, glutamine facilitates the production of glutathione (GSH). It also provides nitrogen for the synthesis of nucleic acids and proteins that are needed for lymphocytes to proliferate and produce signals such as cytokines (Calder and Yaqoob, 1999).

In addition to its role as an energy substrate, glutamine is important for intestinal development and function, including maintaining the integrity of the gut barrier, the structure of the intestinal mucosa and redox homeostasis.

**Glutamate:** Glutamate is one of the most abundant dietary amino acids, but is found in very low concentrations in plasma (Blachier, F. et al, 2009). This is likely the result of glutamate being a major energy substrate for intestinal epithelial cells. It also serves as a precursor for other amino acids (L-alanine, L-aspartate, L-ornithine and L-proline) and for GSH in the intestine. GSH is essential to maintaining the thiol redox state, which is vital to adequate functioning of enterocytes and immune cells.

**Arginine:** Arginine is the most plentiful nitrogen carrier in animals. It is essential for the function of the GALT.

**Threonine:** Threonine is a dietary essential amino acid that has been shown to have a particularly high retention rate in the intestine, which suggests its role in maintaining GIT and GALT function. Threonine has a major role in mucin synthesis, a glycoprotein that is required to protect the intestinal epithelium (G.K. Law et al, 2007).

**Other amino acids:** Similarly, methionine (and cysteine) through their roles in taurine and glutathionine production may also be beneficial to the GALT. Other amino acids such as glycine and proline have been hypothesised to be beneficial to the GALT.

## Conclusion

The intestine and the GALT are essential components of immune defence, protecting the animal from foreign antigens and pathogens, while allowing the absorption and tolerance of dietary nutrients. With regard to the maintenance of GIT and GALT function, glutamine (glutamate), arginine, threonine, methionine and cysteine, glycine and proline have been proven to be beneficial. The studies conducted using the feeding regimens such as total parenteral nutrition (TPN) (that bypass the oral route) suggest that amino acids delivered in the blood from other parts of the body are important for maintaining GALT.

## AMINO ACIDS AND INTESTINAL HEALTH IN POULTRY AND PIGS

### Healthy Intestine

A healthy intestine has a well-coordinated immune system that must accommodate commensal microbiota, while inhibiting the colonisation and proliferation of harmful pathogens.

### Nutrient Requirements of Intestinal Tissue

Intestine represents a small proportion (about 5%) of body weight. But its requirement for nutrients is high. It consumes 15 to 30% of the $O_2$ and proteins in a live organism (Gaskins, 2001) and 20% of the energy (McBride and Kelly, 1990) due to its rapid turnover rate and intense cellular metabolic activity. Animals or birds raised under different sanitary conditions have varied microbial (pathogenic) load and consequently, to that extent, cascade of events rolled out such as activation of immune system, increased metabolic activity, so on. The activation of the immune system with moderate levels of inflammation is essential for survival following an infection.

For example, pigs with enhanced microbial load are continuously being challenged by their immediate environment, which can cause an immune response to be mounted. Such a process results in enhanced rate of protein turnover associated with the production of immune cells, antibodies and acute-phase proteins (APP) increasing energy expenditure by 10–15% of maintenance needs and protein requirements by 7–10%. The requirements for lysine, tryptophan, sulphur-containing amino acids and threonine can be increased by a further 10% (Pluske et al, 2018).

Hence, the intestinal tissue may have increased nutritional requirements during an intestinal challenge to maintain its cellular proliferation. These additional needs are to be supplied to the animals or birds to obtain optimum performance from the feed. However, in practice, nutrient profiles used in feed formulations for animals or birds are typically based on economically important production parameters such as weight gain, feed intake, feed conversion ratio and carcass yield (Kidd, 2004).

### Intact Intestinal Mucosa Protects the Animal from Invasion by Pathogenic Microbes

An intact intestinal mucosa protects the animal against the uptake of toxic substances present in the feed, as well as from invasion by pathogenic microorganisms and the antigens they secrete. Accordingly, the mucosa must accommodate a variety of immune cell types, including macrophages, polymorphonuclear cells, dendritic cells and T and B lymphocytes to protect the intestinal barrier. When the immune system is activated, the organism prioritises proliferation of defence cells, expression of receptors to recognise non-self antigens, and production of cytokines and antibodies. This increased metabolic activity, due to the activation of the immune system, may be responsible for the impaired growth and productive performance that is often observed during periods of intestinal challenge.

## Importance of Intestinal Microbiota

In coordination with the intestinal mucosa, the intestinal microbiota are responsible for the first line of defence in an animal and work by regulating cellular permeability, altering the expression of genes in goblet cells for increased mucous production and stimulating secretion of antimicrobial peptides (Laparra and Sanz, 2010). Hence, a well-established intestinal microbiota brings benefits to the host due to production of vitamins, immune modulation and inhibition of pathogens.

## Maintenance of the Intestinal Mucosa Integrity

Microbial imbalance may contribute to the development of metabolic and immunologic diseases (Jeurissen et al, 2002), increase competition for nutrients with the host and cause morphological damage. Further, diseases such as coccidiosis and necrotic enteritis (NE) can decrease the abundance of desirable groups of bacteria, particularly segmented filamentous bacteria that play a role in the modulation of the host immune system. Microbial imbalance in the GIT increase competition for nutrients with the host resulting in impaired productive performance that is often observed during the periods of intestinal challenge. Hence maintenance of intestinal mucosal integrity is essential.

**Two main components are responsible for maintaining the intestinal mucosa integrity. Mucosal layer:** The first is the mucosal layer, which serves as a barrier between luminal contents and enterocytes lining the intestine. Mucin-type glycoproteins that make up the mucosal layer can aggregate different bacterial species and in some cases, prevent the attachment of pathogens to the intestinal epithelium. The intestinal mucosal layer is a key component of the innate immune response; the development of the immune system of the animal or bird varies according to age and section of intestine, which appears to be faster in proximal than in distal intestinal segments (Zhang et al, 2015).

**Enterocyte layer:** The second barrier component of the intestine is the enterocyte layer. The intestinal epithelium of the animal or bird is constantly renewed as proliferating cells in the mucosal crypts differentiate, predominantly to enterocytes and migrate to the upper part of the villus, where they are eventually lost through desquamation. This turnover rate increases considerably during an intestinal challenge, but the magnitude and duration of this response varies among intestinal regions and intensity of the challenge.

## Amino Acids may Become Limiting Factors for Appropriate Immune Function

Enteric challenges such as coccidiosis or necrotic enteritis (NE) may alter the development of the immune response and certain nutrients such as amino acids may become limiting factors to produce key proteins required for appropriate immune function. Increasing the dietary levels of highly digestible protein sources or amino acids may help compensate for malabsorption during the periods of intestinal challenge. For example, coccidiosis has been shown to be detrimental to amino acid digestibility; decreased ileal digestibility is observed; absorptive capacity of intestine is impaired. Improved feed efficiency in broiler chickens (normal and disease-challenged) fed on higher concentrations of amino acids may reflect better development of intestinal mucosa.

## Dietary Supplementation Improve Intestinal Recovery Following an Infection or Injury

Trophic amino acids, such as threonine, arginine and glutamine, play a very important role on the intestinal mucosa and may support increased epithelial turnover rates to improve intestinal recovery following an infection or injury. Furthermore, these amino acids may help to minimise over-activation of the innate immune system, which is the most expensive in terms of nutrients and energy, as well as modulate the intestinal microbiota.

For instance, studies in mammals have shown that dietary supplementation of arginine and glutamine increased the expression of antioxidant genes and reduced mRNA of pro-inflammatory genes in the small intestine and adipose tissue (Wang et al, 2008). Supplementation of amino acids also promote intestinal repair through induction of enzymes needed for the mitotic process, such as ornithine-decarboxylase required for the synthesis of polyamines. Accordingly, amino acid manipulation of diets appears to be an important nutritional strategy to enhance the capacity and responsiveness of the GIT to cope with a pathogen.

## Amino Acid Manipulation of Diets

Amino acids regulate expression of genes and the production of molecules, including poly-amines and nitric oxide (Fernandes and Murakami, 2010). Indeed amino acids are needed for a well-functioning gastrointestinal tract (GIT; Li et al, 2007). In particular, threonine, arginine and glutamine have been studied for their roles in mucin production (Fernandez et al, 1994), immune function (Tan et al, 2014a,b; Chen et al, 2016) and epithelial proliferation (Scheppach et al, 1996), respectively.

## Role of Threonine on the Development and Immunity of GIT of the Host under Both Normal and Disease-challenged Scenarios

Threonine is a major component of intestinal mucin and immunoglobulins (IgA). Threonine participates in the synthesis of proteins. Its catabolism generates glycine, acetyl CoA and pyruvate that are important for metabolism. Compared with other amino acids, broiler chickens have a high threonine requirement for maintenance due to its rapid

turnover rate and high abundance in intestinal secretions. As the major component of intestinal mucin in animals, threonine represents approximately 30% of its total amino acid content. Due to its importance in maintaining barrier function, mucin is not digested by the normal mechanisms within the GIT and is eventually lost in the excreta or fermented by caecal microorganisms.

Mucin-type glycoproteins prevent the attachment of pathogens to the intestinal epithelium. Hence during disease-challenged scenarios (infections) mucin secretion is increased. Faure et al (2007) reported increased utilisation of threonine for protein synthesis in the small intestinal wall, mucosa and mucin in infected rats. Therefore, factors that induce mucin secretion may increase dietary threonine requirement. These include bacterial load, due to intestinal as well as systemic infections, which can influence endogenous amino acid flow through mucin production (Adedokun et al, 2012).

Studies have indicated that the components of the immune system are responsive to manipulations in dietary threonine (Wang et al, 2006; Chen et al, 2016). As a major component of immunoglobulins (Ig), particularly IgA, threonine is secreted by the intestinal mucosa and accounts for more than 2/3 of all immunoglobulins in the body. IgA is essential for maintaining intestinal homeostasis by preventing the attachment and entry of bacteria in intraepithelial cells (IEC), or eliminating bacteria from the basolateral space to the lumen (Brisbin et al, 2008). Threonine is essential for the well-functioning of the local immune system.

Threonine supplementation changes the microbial balance in the intestine and modulates the immune system by increasing IgA secretion and downregulating the expression of the inflammatory genes INF-y and IL-1β (Chen el al, 2016). Decreased expression of IL-1β has been observed in coccidiosis-infected broilers upon feeding higher dietary threonine. In pathological situations, the defence and repair will increase the demand for amino acids, especially threonine (Faure et al, 2007).

Chen et al (2016) reported that feeding higher dietary threonine (26% higher than the recommended by NRC, 1994) decreased *Salmonella* and *Escherichia coli* colonies and increased *Lactobacillus* in broiler chickens. The reduction of *Salmonella* and *E. coli* observed with this higher threonine concentration may be due to its indirect effect on the host, as observed by higher mRNA expression of MUC2, lower expression of the pro-inflammatory cytokine IL-1β and reduced inflammation (Chen et al, 2016). This implies that threonine has immunomodulatory effects on the host and either directly or indirectly influences beneficial microbiota, rather than altering nutrient supply in the lumen.

### Role of Arginine on the Development and Immunity of GIT of the Host Under Both Normal and Disease-challenged Scenarios

Poultry lack key enzymes involved in *de novo* arginine synthesis thereby they have a unique and essential dietary requirement for arginine.

The genetic material of birds does not encode for the enzyme carbamoyl phosphate synthetase, which catalyses the first step of ammonia detoxification involved in the production of citrulline from ornithine. Citrulline can ultimately be converted to arginine through urea cycle (Fig. 6.14) enzymes and as such, citrulline can spare dietary arginine in chickens.

Additionally, chickens lack the enzymes necessary for citrulline production in the small intestine, precluding the supply of intestinal citrulline for arginine production in the liver or kidney as occurs in mammals. Furthermore, chickens have a very high activity of kidney arginase compared with mammals, so dietary supply must account for this degradation as well.

Arginine is a precursor for the synthesis of creatine, polyamines (see page 209) and nitric oxide (NO) and stimulates secretion of insulin-like growth factors (IGF; Fernandes and Murakami, 2010). Arginine is converted into citrulline and NO by the action of a group of enzymes called NO synthetases, which is the only path for production of NO

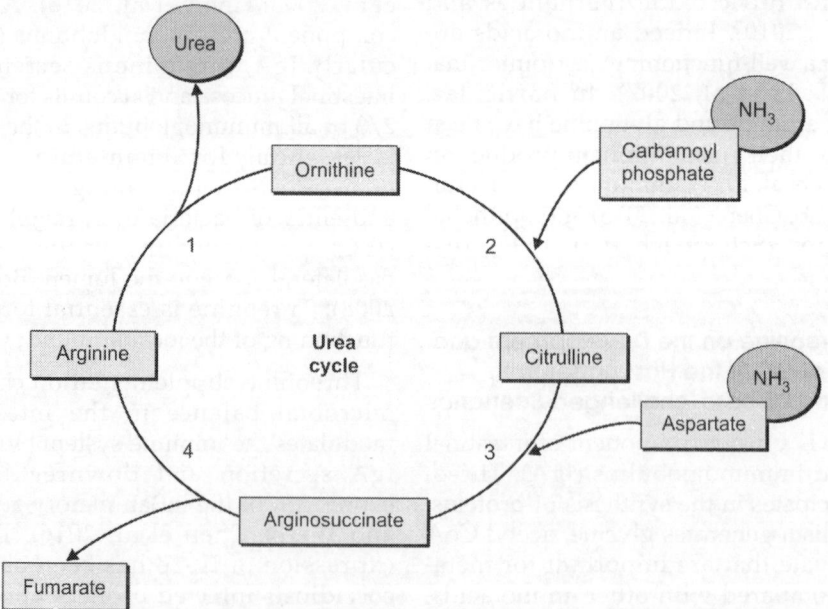

**Fig. 6.14:** The urea cycle:1. Arginase (cytosol); 2. Ornithine transcarbamoylase (mitochondrion); 3. Arginosuccinate synthase (cytosol); 4. Arginosuccinate lyase (cytosol)

(Fernandes and Murakami, 2010). Nitric oxide has several biological functions, but it primarily acts as a cytotoxic mediator of immune-activated cells and regulator of the immune system (Hibbs et al, 1988).

Polyamines are important for the development of the intestine in newborns, which may explain the positive effects of arginine supplementation on performance and small intestine morphology of one-week-old broiler chickens (Murakami et al, 2012). Polyamines can stimulate proliferation, migration and apoptosis of intestinal cells. Therefore, arginine may be considered as a trophic substance by supporting the mitotic process in the crypt-villus region to increase the number of cells and the size of the villus.

The effects of dietary L-arginine on the immune system of broiler chickens also have been investigated during periods of inactive (Murakami et al, 2012) and active immune stimulation (Tan et al, 2014a,b). Tan et al (2014a) showed that coccidiosis-induced jejunal inflammation is characterised by villus damage, crypt dilation and goblet cell depletion. Further, coccidiosis downregulated the expression of MUC-2 and IgA, while upregulating β-Defensin-8 and inflammatory genes (iNOS, IL-1β, IL-8, TLR4) mRNA expression. Dietary L-arginine linearly diminished the expression of TLR4, suggesting that the anti-inflammatory effect of arginine is via suppression of the TLR4 pathway (Tan et al, 2014b).

Xu et al (2018) reported that dietary arginine supplementation in excess of the 1994 NRC requirement enhanced the growth performance and immune status of broiler chickens. Extra arginine supplementation can promote secretion of growth hormone (GH) and insulin-like growth factors-1 (IGF-1) in broiler chickens and regulate immune response. Thus, it can be used as a potential growth promoter and immunomodulating agent in broiler chickens.

## Role of Glutamine on the Development and Immunity of GIT of the Host Under Both Normal and Disease-challenged Scenarios

Glutamine is supplemented because of its effects on both intestinal structure and function (Wang et al, 2008; Soares et al, 2014). Glutamine serves as an important source of energy for enterocytes, particularly during periods of increased proliferation. As such, glutamine may reduce the intestinal atrophy and support mucosal repair following an injury. That is why probably, the intestinal mucosa has a high capacity to remove glutamine from both arterial blood and dietary supply; the intestine competes with other organs for glutamine. Glutamine is also a component of glutathione, a key molecule in the defence against free radicals (Kidd, 2004).

Glutamine may be considered an essential amino acid under inflammatory conditions, disease challenge, or surgery (Newsholme, 2001) and dietary supplementation at 1% has beneficial effects on small intestinal morphology at 3 and 14 days of age in broiler chickens. The higher villus height reflected in enhanced growth performance.

Using mice under heat stress conditions, Soares et al (2014) showed that the supplementation with dietary glutamine improved intestinal barrier function, thereby preventing the increase in the intestinal permeability and limiting the bacterial translocation induced by the heat stress. Other studies confirmed that glutamine reduced intestinal permeability and bacterial translocation to physiological levels and preserved mucosal integrity.

Early weaned piglets had higher expression of genes that promote oxidative stress and immune activation. However, 1% dietary glutamine supplementation restored the function of the small intestine by increasing the expression of genes that prevent oxidative activity and stimulation of cell growth (Wang et al, 2008).

# Fatty Acids and Immunity

## DIETARY FAT AND IMMUNITY

Fats are greasy in texture and taste and not miscible with water. Fats are an important source of energy in the diet. Chemically, they are composed of esters of glycerol with fatty acids.

## Types of Fatty Acids in the Diet

Dietary fat, depending on the source, contributes varying amounts of fatty acids. Vegetable oils (sunflower, safflower) are rich in n-6 polyunsaturated fatty acids (PUFAs), while marine or sea foods are rich in n-3 PUFAs. Olive oil and butter are rich in monounsaturated fatty acids (MUFAs), while fats from animal sources have high concentrations of saturated fatty acids (SFAs) and low levels of PUFAs. There is now convincing evidence that the type of fat in the diet has a major impact on inflammation and other aspects of immune function, and this has formed the basis for interventions with fish oil (rich in omega-3 fatty acids) in diseases characterised by immune dysfunction.

Mammalian cells are able to synthesise (from non-fat precursors) saturated fatty acids and unsaturated fatty acids of the n-9 and n-7 series but lack the delta-12 and delta-15 desaturase enzymes (found in most plants; Fig. 7. 2) for insertion of a double bond at the n-6 or n-3 position (Fig. 7.1). Thus, mammalian cells cannot synthesise n-6 or n-3 PUFAs *de novo*.

The n-6 and n-3 fatty acids are essential (as they cannot be synthesised in the body) substrates for many of the major regulatory lipids in the body and, the body must obtain them from the diet. The commonly consumed PUFAs are linoleic acid (18:2n-6) and α-linolenic acid (18:3n-3). Once consumed, these fatty acids can be converted to the longer-chain, more unsaturated derivatives. Thus linoleic acid is converted via γ-linolenic (18:3n-6) and dihomo-γ-linolenic (20:3n-6) acids (DGLA) to arachidonic acid (20:4n-6) (Fig. 7.2). Likewise, α-linolenic acid is converted to eicosapentaenoic acid (EPA) (20:5n-3) and docosahexaenoic acid (DHA) (22:6n-3).

EPA and DHA are found in high quantities in many marine (e.g. herring, mackerel, fresh tuna, sardines) oils and in the oils extracted from the livers of fish that live in warmer waters (e.g. cod). EPA and DHA comprise 20–30% of the fatty acids in a typical preparation of fish oil. In the absence of oily fish or fish oil consumption, α-linolenic acid is the main dietary n-3 PUFA.

**Amount of dietary fat and cell-mediated immune function:** Animal studies indicate that high-fat diets diminish lymphocyte proliferation and natural killer (NK) cell activity compared with low-fat diets. A

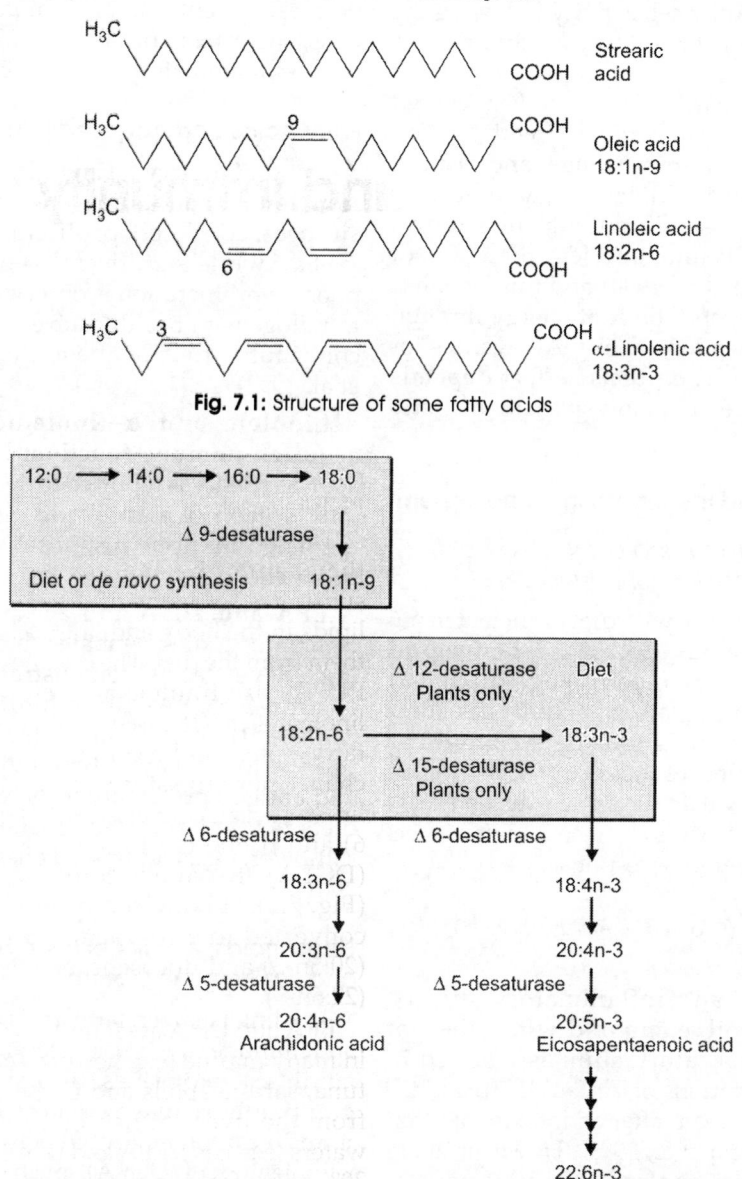

**Fig. 7.1:** Structure of some fatty acids

**Fig. 7.2:** Biosynthesis of polyunsaturated fatty acids

reduction in total dietary fat intake (from 40 to 25% of total energy) resulted in greatly enhanced human blood lymphocyte proliferation in response to mitogens. These data suggest that a high-fat diet suppresses the activity of cellular components of both natural and cell-mediated immunity in humans.

**Amount of dietary fat and innate immune function:** Most studies have found that high-fat diets result in diminished innate immune responses. Animal studies have reported lower natural killer cell activity following the feeding of high fat including oils rich in linoleic acid (maize, sunflower or safflower oil) or oils rich in α-linolenic acid (e.g. linseed (flaxseed) oil), when compared with feeding high saturated-fat diets (Kelley and Daudu, 1993; Calder, 1998a, b). Human natural killer cell activity was significantly increased by a reduction in fat intake to less than 30% of energy (Hebert et al, 1990) and this level has been taken as upper limit of energy through fat in Recommended Dietary Allowances for human beings. The precise effect depends upon the source of fat and specially the fatty acids present in it.

## Fatty Acids and the Innate Immune System

### Linoleic Acid (n-6) and a-linolenic Acid (n-3) and innate immune function

Feeding rats or mice with diets deficient in n-6 or n-3 fatty acids decreased neutrophil chemotaxis and macrophage-mediated phagocytic and cytotoxic activity, as compared with animals fed diets containing adequate amounts of these fatty acids (Kelley and Daudu, 1993). In the same way, an excess of essential fatty acids can also impair aspects of the innate immune response.

### EPA and DHA (n-3 Fatty Acids) and Innate Immune System

Fish oil has anti-inflammatory effects. Feeding fish oil, compared with other fat sources, to laboratory animals resulted in lower concentrations of TNF-α, IL-1β and IL-6 in the bloodstream after endotoxin injection or burns (Sadghi et al, 1999). However, there are reports that contradict these findings, which only indicate the effect is fatty acid-specific. Parenteral nutrition supplemented with fish oil decreased serum TNF-α and IL-6 concentrations in patients following major abdominal surgery, compared with n-6 fatty acid-rich parenteral nutrition (Wachtler et al, 1997). Thus studies in animals and humans have demonstrated that high levels of fish oil or its component n-3 PUFAs in the diet exert potent anti-inflammatory effects, particularly decreasing neutrophil and monocyte chemotaxis, superoxide production and production of pro-inflammatory cytokines.

## Fatty Acids and Acquired Immune System

**Amount of dietary fat and acquired immune function:** High fat-diets are associated with suppressed T cell proliferation (Calder, 1998a), while significantly enhanced lymphocyte proliferation is observed in response to mitogens in healthy subjects when the fat contributed to 25% of energy intake (Kelly et al, 1992).

**Linoleic and α–linolenic acids and acquired immune function:** Essential fatty acid deficiency is reported to decrease thymus and spleen weights and suppress cell mediated immune responses and antibody production.

**EPA and DHA and acquired immune function:** Studies in rabbits, chickens, rats and mice have clearly demonstrated that long-chain n-3 PUFAs can inhibit lymphocyte proliferation, IL-2 and interferon (IFN)-γ production, delayed-type hypersensitivity and antigen presentation, as compared with diets rich in lard, or hydrogenated coconut, safflower, maize or linseed oils (Wallace et al, 2001).

## Eicosanoids: A Link Between Fatty Acids and the Immune System

A key link between fatty acids, inflammation and immune function is eicosanoids (prostaglandins, leukotrienes, thromboxanes). This group of bioactive mediators is synthesised from 20-carbon PUFAs, in particular dihomo-γ-linolenic acid (DGLA), arachidonic acid and eicosapentaenoic acid (EPA) (Figs 7.2 and 7.3). Since membranes of most cells contain large amount of arachidonic acid compared to DGLA and EPA, arachidonic acid is usually the principal precursor for eicosanoid synthesis.

Arachidonic acid (n-6 fatty acid) in cell membranes can be released by various phospholipase enzymes, most notably

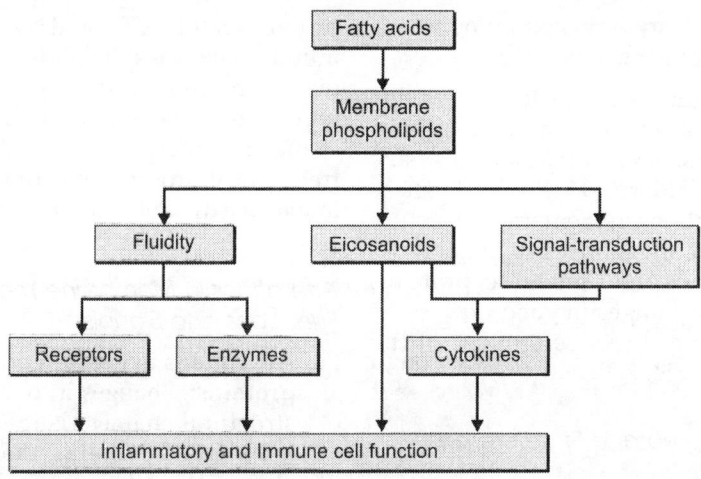

**Fig. 7.3:** Mechanisms whereby fatty acids might exert effects on immune cell function. *Source*: CABI (2002)

phospholipase $A_2$. The free arachidonic acid can subsequently act as a substrate for cyclooxygenase (COX), forming prostaglandins and related compounds or it can be a substrate for one of the three lypoxygenase (LOX) enzymes, forming leukotrienes and related compounds (Fig.7. 4). These compounds are involved in regulating inflammation and the functions of neutrophils, monocytes/macrophages, T cells and B cells. The capacity of inflammatory cells to produce arachidonic acid-derived eicosanoids can be decreased by the increased availability of n-3 fatty acids, especially EPA from fish oil. The reduction in generation of arachidonic acid-derived mediators that accompanies fish oil consumption has led to the idea that fish oil is anti-inflammatory. It is clear that fish oil protects against the deleterious effects of endotoxin and is a useful adjunct to existing therapies for inflammatory diseases, such as rheumatoid arthritis (Calder, 2001).

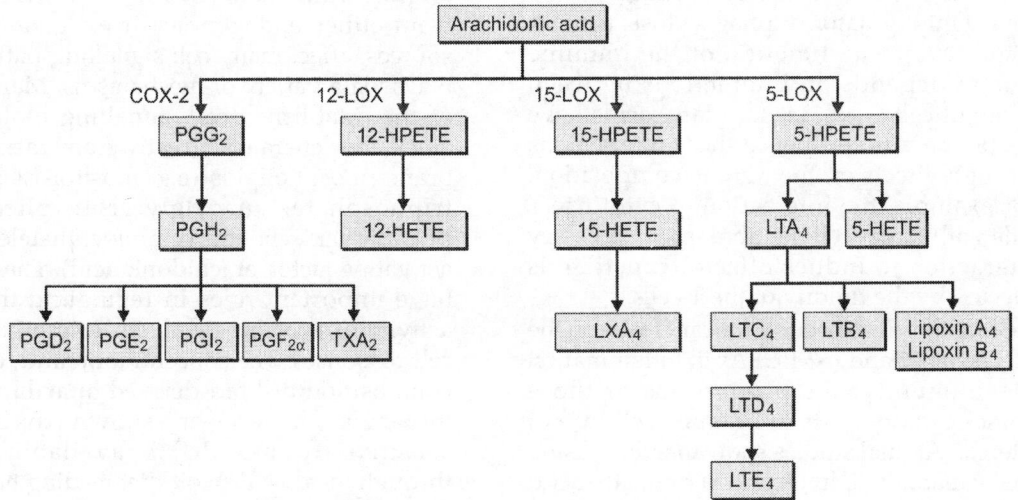

**Fig. 7.4:** Synthesis of eicosanoids from arachidonic acid. COX, cyclooxygenase; LOX, lipoxygenase; LT, leukotriene; PG, prostaglandin; TX, thromboxane; HETE, hydroxyl-eicosatetraenoic acid; HPETE, hydroperoxy-eicosatetraenoic acid

## Effect of Dietary Fatty Acids on Immune Function: Mechanisms

It is widely recognised that dietary fatty acids can potentially alter immune and inflammatory responses. Several mechanisms have been proposed (Calder and Field, 2002). These include (a) alterations in membrane structure and composition, (b) changes in membrane-mediated functions and signals (i.e. proteins, eicosanoids), (c) changes in gene expression and (d) effects on the development of the immune system (Fig. 7.3).

### Alterations in Membrane Structure and Composition

Immune cell activation results in both *de novo* synthesis and an increased turnover of membrane phospholipids. Therefore, essential fatty acids would be required for the synthesis of new membranes during immune cell responses, especially those involving increased membrane synthesis and turnover (e.g. cell proliferation, phagocytosis).

The fluidity of the plasma membrane or of regions of the plasma membrane is important in the functioning of cells (Stubbs and Smith, 1984). The fluidity of a membrane is determined by its lipid components and their fatty acid composition. Membrane fluidity is an important regulator of phagocytosis (Calder et al, 1990). The function of the immune system depends on interactions between different cell types. Dietary fatty acids have the potential to influence these interactions through effects on membrane composition. For example, the interaction of cytotoxic T cells with target cell membranes, a necessary interaction to induce effector function, is affected by the fluidity of the T cells.

Since there has been significant focus on the effects of n-6 and n-3 PUFAs in inflammation and immunity, the proportions of those classes of fatty acids in immune cells are of interest. Animal studies show that decreasing the availability of linoleic acid (n-6 fatty acid) in the diet, especially by replacing it with n-3 fatty acids (either alpha-linolenic acid or long-chain n-3 fatty acids) results in decreased proportions of DGLA and arachidonic acid, in immune cell-phospholipids. Since n-3 PUFAs oxidise more readily than n-6 PUFAs, they may increase susceptibility of cellular membranes to lipid peroxidation. The increased free radical production can be minimised by intake of extra antioxidants such as vitamin E.

### Alterations in Membrane-mediated Functions and Signals

i. **Alterations in the function of membrane proteins:** Changes in plasma membrane structural characteristics can change the activity of proteins that serve as ion channels, adhesion molecules, transporters, receptors, signal transducers or enzymes (Stubbs and Smith, 1984; Clandinin et al, 1991). Many membrane-associated proteins in immune cells have been shown to be modulated by membrane lipid changes. For example, feeding 5% w/w long-chain n-3 PUFAs to rats resulted in a higher proportion of T and B cells and macrophages expressing the transferring receptor (CD71) after stimulation with mitogen (Robinson and Field, 1998).

ii. **Changes in membrane-mediated signals (signal transduction):** Lipids, derived from either endogenous or exogenous sources, affect many cell signalling pathways via a variety of mechanisms. Many of the established cell signalling molecules are generated directly from membrane phospholipids (e.g. inositol-1,4,5-triphosphate, diacylglycerol, phosphatidic acid, choline, ceramide, platelet-activating factor, arachidonic acid). These have important roles in regulating the activity of proteins involved in immune cell responses. The concentration and/or composition of lipid-derived signalling molecules have been shown to be sensitive to n-3 PUFA availability through the diet. Fish oil-diet feeding has led to the decreased generation of signalling molecules (Sanderson and Calder, 1988b).

There is evidence that arachidonic acid released from the plasma membrane has a direct role in regulating some immune cell functions, such as natural killer cell granule release and cell-mediated toxicity. Further, arachidonic acid is an intracellular activator of the nicotinamide adenine dinucleotide phosphate (NADPH) oxidase enzyme in neutrophils (Sakata et al, 1987) and enrichment of arachidonic acid in neutrophil membranes is reported to increase the oxidative burst of neutrophils (Badwey et al, 1981, 1984; Hardy et al, 1991). Dietary lipids have been demonstrated to influence the pattern of fatty acids released from lymphocytes (Sanderson et al, 2000).

iii. **Changes in eicosanoid synthesis:** Prostaglandins (PG), leukotriene (LT) and thromboxane (TX) are a group of bioactive mediators termed eicosanoids. These are synthesised from 20-carbon PUFAs particularly DGLA, arachidonic acid and EPA. Eicosanoids provide a key link between fatty acids, inflammation and immune function. The two major pathways for eicosanoid synthesis are via the enzymes cyclooxygenase (COX) and lipoxygenase (LOX). Enzyme COX initiates pathway that result in the production of prostaglandins/thromboxanes, while enzyme LOX produce leukotrienes/hydroxyeicosatrienoic acids/lipoxins. See page 251 for the cardioprotective effects of n-3 fatty acids.

Arachidonic acid present in the cell membranes is the main precursor of these mediators, giving rise to dienoic prostaglandins (e.g. $PGE_2$) and thromboxanes ($TXA_2$) and tetraenoic leukotrienes (e.g. $LTB_4$) through cyclooxygenase enzyme and one of the three lypoxygenase enzymes (Fig. 7.4).

There are at least 16 different 2-series PG and these are formed in a cell-specific manner. For example, monocytes and macrophages produce large amounts of $PGE_2$ and $PGF_2$, neutrophils produce moderate amounts of $PGE_2$ and mast cells produce $PGD_2$. The LOX enzymes have different tissue distributions, with 5-LOX being found mainly in mast cells, monocytes, macrophages and granulocytes and 12- and 15-LOX being found primarily in epithelial cells. Metabolism of arachidonic acid by the 5-LOX pathway gives rise to hydroxyl and hydroperoxy derivatives (5-hydroxyeicosatetraenoic acid, 5-HETE; 5-hydroperoxy-eicosatetraenoic acid, 5-HPETE) and the 4-series LT (Fig. 7.4).

## Immunoregulatory Roles of $PGE_2$

Eicosanoids (particularly $PGE_2$ and 4-series LT) are involved in modulating the intensity and duration of inflammatory and immune responses (Tilley et al, 2001). The pro-inflammatory effects of $PGE_2$, include inducing fever, increasing vascular permeability and vasodilatation and enhancing pain and oedema caused by other agents, such as histamine.

Additionally, $PGE_2$ suppresses lymphocyte proliferation and natural killer cell activity and inhibits production of TNF-$\alpha$, IL-1, IL-6, IL-2 and IFN-$\gamma$. Thus, in these respects, $PGE_2$ is immunosuppressive and anti-inflammatory. $PGE_2$ does not affect the production of T-helper 2 (Th2)-type cytokines IL-4 and IL-10, but promotes immunoglobulin E (IgE) production by B lymphocytes.

## Immunoregulatory Roles of $LTB_4$

$LTB_4$ is a potent chemotactic agent for leukocytes. $LTB_4$ increases vascular permeability, enhances local blood flow, induces release of lysosomal enzymes, enhances generation of reactive oxygen species, inhibits lymphocyte proliferation and promotes natural killer cell activity. In addition, 4-series LT regulate the production of pro-inflammatory cytokines, e.g. $LTB_4$ enhances production of TNF-$\alpha$, IL-1, IL-6, IL-2 and IFN-$\gamma$. 15-HETE inhibits lymphocyte proliferation, while 5-HETE enhances it. Thus, arachidonic acid gives rise to a range of mediators that have opposing effects to one another, so the overall physiological effect will be the result of the balance of these mediators, the timing of their production and the sensitivities of target cells to their effects.

## Shifting Towards n-3 Fatty Acids

Dietary fatty acids can influence eicosanoid synthesis by affecting the supply of substrates. Feeding animals on increased amounts of fish oil results in a decrease in the amount of arachidonic acid in the membranes of most cells in the body, including those involved in inflammation and immunity, such as monocytes, macrophages, neutrophils and lymphocytes. This means that there is less arachidonic acid available for the synthesis of eicosanoids. There is a shift in fatty acid synthesis on fish oil supplementation. Dietary fish oil decreases the production of arachidonic acid-derived eicosanoids from animal immune cells (Calder and Field, 2002).

EPA (n-3 fatty acid) is also a substrate for the COX and LOX enzymes, resulting in the synthesis of the trienoic prostanoids (e.g. $PGE_3$) and pentaenoic leukotrienes (e.g. $LTB_5$; Fig. 7.2). The eicosanoids produced from EPA are often less biologically potent than the analogues synthesised from arachidonic acid. For example, $LTB_5$ is only about 10% as potent as $LTB_4$ as a chemotactic agent and in promoting lysosomal enzyme release (Kinsella et al, 1990). Since dietary fish oil leads to decreased $PGE_2$ production, it is often stated that feeding n-3 lipids should result in a reversal of the effects of $PGE_2$. Thus, fish oil is expected to result in less inflammation, enhanced cytokine production by monocytes/macrophages and Th1 lymphocytes and enhanced lymphocyte proliferation.

The reduction in the generation of arachidonic acid-derived mediators that accompanies fish oil consumption has led to the idea that fish oil is anti-inflammatory and might enhance immune function (Fig. 7.5). However, the *in vivo* situation is likely to be more complex than this. EPA will give rise to mediators with varying actions (Fig. 7.2), some of which may actually be the same as those of the analogues produced from arachidonic acid. Thus, the overall effect of fish oil feeding cannot be predicted solely on the basis of revocation of $PGE_2$-mediated effects. Furthermore, a number of the effects of n-3 PUFA have been shown to occur inde-

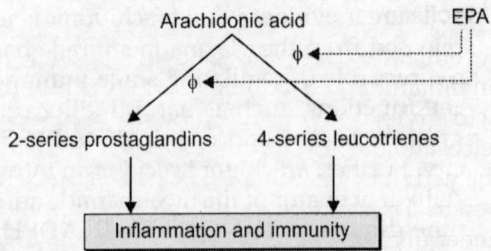

**Fig. 7.5:** Theoretical basis for the immunoregulatory effects of eicosapentaenoic acid (EPA).∅-inhibits

pendent of changes in eicosanoid production (Calder et al, 1992).

### Changes in Gene Expression

Fatty acids, especially PUFAs, are known to modulate the expression of a variety of genes coding for key regulatory proteins in numerous metabolic pathways in hepatocytes and adipocytes (Clarke and Jump, 1994). These effects are mediated by both indirect mechanism (e.g. by eicosanoids, hormones) and direct effects on gene expression. There is now emerging evidence that PUFAs regulate the expression of genes for cytokines, adhesion molecules, cyclooxygenase, inducible nitric oxide synthase and other inflammatory proteins (Wallace et al, 2001). PUFAs also have the ability to regulate the expression of genes involved in inflammation through transcription factors (1) nuclear factor kappa B (NFκB) (2) peroxisome proliferator-activated receptors (PPARs).

### Effects on the Development of the Immune System

Little work has been done on the effects of dietary PUFAs on T cell development in the infant or young animal (Calder and Field, 2002). Field et al (2000) examined the effect of altered long-chain PUFA availability on the functional indices of immune development during the first 42 days of human life. The data suggest that adding DHA and arachidonic acid to preterm formula may have assisted in the maturation of peripheral CD4+ cells. This work supports an effect of dietary lipids, particularly long-chain PUFAs on immune development.

## Conclusions

Several fatty acids can potentially exert effects on inflammation and immunity. Arachidonic acid gives rise to inflammatory mediators (eicosanoids) and through these, it regulates the activities of inflammatory cells, the Th1 versus Th2 balance and B cell function. It is generally considered that n-3 PUFAs act as arachidonic acid antagonists. As such, among the fatty acids, it is the n-3 PUFAs that are believed to possess the most potent immuno-modulatory activities and, among the n-3 fatty acids, those from fish oil (EPA and DHA) are more biologically potent than $\alpha$-linolenic acid. Components of both natural and acquired immunity, including the production of key inflammatory mediators, can be affected by n-3 PUFAs.

## IMMUNOMETABOLISM – ROLE OF FREE FATTY ACID RECEPTORS AS A MEANS TO SENSE NUTRIENT AVAILABILITY

### Association of Low Grade Chronic Inflammation with Obesity

The diet of a high-income group population is based substantially on high fat- and high sugar-content. This dietary regimen undoubtedly triggered what is now considered an epidemic of obesity that has consequently resulted in an increase in serious, chronic conditions associated with dysfunctions of energy balance, including type 2 diabetes and cardiovascular diseases (Thorbum et al, 2014). Furthermore, it is now widely accepted that low grade chronic inflammation associated with obesity may be directly connected to other inflammatory related pathologies such as asthma, colitis and, potentially, some forms of cancer, including colon cancer (Lackey and Olefsky, 2016; Murray et al, 2015).

### Immunometabolism

These effects have triggered a major increase in interest with regard to the role of metabolite sensing and how this may affect physiology in health and disease, with concepts including the interface between the metabolic and immune systems, i.e. immuno metabolism, coming to the front of scientific discussions (Lackey and Olefsky, 2016). There has been particular interest in free fatty acid (FFA) sensing and its association with the mode of signalling of a number of recently de-orphanised G protein-coupled receptors (GPCRs) (Rasoamanana et al, 2012). This is a fast moving and exciting area of research focusing the interest of pharmacologists, chemists, immunologists and physiologists in an interdisciplinary manner (Alvarez-Curto and Milligan, 2016).

### Free Fatty Acids (FFAs) are Critical Signalling Molecules

Free fatty acids, including health boosting omega-3 fatty acid containing oils, are no longer considered only as metabolic intermediaries but also as critical signalling molecules due to their role as agonists for different members of the family of free fatty acid receptors (FFARs) (Hara et al, 2013, 2014). Their presence on key cell types regulating both metabolic and immune health acts to link the regulation of energy homeostasis with the control of inflammatory responses. Therefore, FFARs are considered very attractive targets for the development of novel medicines/strategies to treat both metabolic and inflammatory pathologies. Alvarez-Curto and Milligan (2016) details the key players and connections between FFAs that are obtained through the diet or as a result of the actions of the gut commensal microbiota and the immune system. They propose how further understanding of these systems might be used to limit or treat disease.

Free fatty acid is a carboxylic acid linked to an aliphatic chain of variable length that may be saturated or unsaturated. It is non-esterified within larger species such as triglycerides or phospholipids. Fatty acids are widely classified based on the length of their carbon chains and grouped into short chain fatty acids (SCFAs, C2–C6), medium chain fatty acids (MCFAs, C7–C12) and long chain fatty acids (LCFAs, >C12).

These may have a number of different origins. Most of the 'essential' fatty acids such as linoleic acid (18:2, n-6) or alpha-linolenic acid (18:3, n-3) and other LCFAs and MCFAs, are generally obtained through the diet. Some other FFAs are obtained through the breakdown of fats (triglycerides) in adipose tissue and the liver. By contrast, the vast majority of SCFAs including acetate (C2) and propionate (C3) are derived from the fermentation of fibres and breakdown of dietary carbohydrates by the bacteria present in the gut. There is mounting evidence to support a central role for the gut microbiota in the regulation of energy homeostasis and its impact in inflammatory processes (Maslowski and Mackay, 2011).

## Free Fatty Acid Receptors

Free fatty acid receptors (FFARs) are members of the 'rhodopsin-like' GPCR family and currently four receptors (FFAR1-4) are so classified. FFAR 1, 2 and 3 are closely related in terms of sequence. The FFAR1, 2 and 3 (formerly GPR40, GPR43 and GPR41, respectively) are co-located on chromosome 19 (19q13.12) in humans, while the FFAR4 (formerly GPR120) located on chromosome 10 (10q23.33) in humans. There are significant numbers of nutrient sensing G protein-coupled receptors (GPCRs) that can be found in cells of the immune system and in tissues that are involved in metabolic function, such as the pancreas or the intestinal epithelium. For this reason, the family of free fatty acid receptors (FFAR1-4, GPR84), plus a few other metabolite sensing receptors (GPR109A, GPR91, GPR35) have been the focus of studies linking the effects of nutrients with immunological responses.

## Signal Transduction and Expression of FFARs

The most common feature of GPCRs is their ability to signal through the activation of heterotrimeric G proteins. The four FFARs are no exception and show diverse coupling preferences to G proteins as well as also promoting a variety of G protein-independent pathways. **FFAR2** is heavily expressed in two key populations of immune cells: neutrophils and mesenteric and small intestine dendritic cells (DC). **FFAR1** is found in pancreatic islets, with particularly enriched expression in the β cells that produce and release insulin and, therefore, its function has been linked to the modulation of glucose-stimulated insulin release. This receptor is expressed together with FFAR4 in enteroendocrine cells of the gastrointestinal tract where it mediates FFA-stimulated incretin secretion. FFAR4 is also found in the pancreas (δ cells), in adipocytes, lung, and in (selective) immune cells. Expression of **FFAR4** in different types of macrophages (monocytes, Kupffer cells in the liver, osteoclasts in the bone, resident macrophages in the lung) and its potential to regulate inflammation make this receptor a very exciting target for the development of novel compounds to treat metabolic syndrome and its many ramifications.

## The Role of Free Fatty Acid Receptors in Metabolism and Immune Responses

### Short-chain Free Fatty Acid Receptors in Immune Cell Signalling and Regulation

Short-chain free fatty acid (SCFA) receptors, FFAR2 and FFAR3, are co-expressed in certain cells and tissues, such as pancreatic α and β cells and some enteroendocrine cells such as K cells (gastric inhibitory polypeptide (GIP) release), I cells (cholecystokinin (CCK) release) and L cells (glucagon-like peptide-1 and peptide YY (GLP-1 and PYY) release). FFAR2 is more pleitropic than FFAR3. FFAR2 in particular is also highly expressed by a number of white cell types, including neutrophils, eosinophils, monocytes and, quite importantly, epithelial colonic cells, where it may play a role in maintaining epithelial integrity and in intestinal Treg cells.

### Roles of FFAR2 Receptor in Inflammatory Processes Related to the Gut and Other Tissues

A growing number of studies are linking general well-being and healthy gut function because of highly diverse intestinal microbiota and intake of fibre in the diet (Le Chatelier et al, 2013). With this there is a growing belief that a healthy gut microfloral population can positively influence immune responses such that the individual might be protected from the development of inflammatory pathologies such as ulcerative colitis, arthritis or even asthma. Bacteria belonging to the *Bacteroidetes* and *Firmicutes* phyla have been found to produce high levels of the SCFAs C2—C4, which are the main agonists for FFAR2. Levels of these SCFAs in the intestinal tract can vary depending on the bacterial composition within individuals and dietary habits but they reach the systemic blood circulation in sufficiently high levels to activate these receptors. However, the molecular link between microbiota SCFA production, FFAR2 function and immune regulation had not been clear until recently. In the studies carried out using FFAR2 knockout and germ-free mice, Maslowski and colleagues (2009) showed that FFAR2 was necessary for the resolution of a number of inflammatory responses in models of colitis, asthma and arthritis.

### FFAR3 is a Key Player in Airway Inflammation

FFAR3 may be a key player in inflammatory processes. In airway inflammation the intestinal microbiota composition, fibre content of the diet and subsequent SCFA production can have a profound impact on the immunological makeup of the lungs and has been suggested to regulate inflammation during induced allergic asthma by the administration of house dust mite (Trompette et al, 2014). The animals maintained on low-fibre diets displayed an increase in white cell infiltration in the lungs as well as the production of a variety of cytokines (IL-4, IL-13, IL-5, IL-17A) following the airway inflammation. These effects were reversed by changing to high-fibre diet with highly fermentable fibre pectin.

It is already clear that FFAR2 and FFAR3 provide the molecular targets within an emerging **gut-lung axis** that regulates the balance between pro- and anti-inflammatory

processes between the two mucosal tissues and this may be influenced greatly by the diet and composition of the intestinal microflora (Alvarez-Curto and Milligan, 2016).

### Medium and Long-chain Free Fatty Acid Receptors in Immune Cell Signalling and Regulation

The MCFA receptor GPR84 is found mostly on cells of the immune system such as neutrophils, T cells, macrophages, including glial cells. GPR84 expression is also found in adipocytes, in the spinal cord and sciatic nerve of mice. GPR84 is the least studied of the FFA-regulated GPCRs. Although still poorly defined, its function has been linked to pro-inflammatory phenotypes; some report that the role of GPR84 is directly connected to immune function and metabolic dysregulation. GPR84 expression is upregulated in macrophages by the presence of lipopolysaccharide (LPS), where it also seems to mediate the release of the pro-inflammatory cytokine IL-12.

FFAR1 and FFAR4 can be activated by a broad range of both saturated and unsaturated LCFAs but there has been a special focus on FFAR4 and the actions that both omega-3 and omega-6 PUFAs may exert via this receptor. Omega-3 fatty acids, such as docosahexaenoic acid (DHA) present in high levels in fish oils and α-linolenic acid present in some vegetable and nut oils, have increasingly been promoted as healthy supplements. This has been supported by a number of studies that suggest a link between inflammation and saturated fats, as these promote inflammation via Toll-like receptors, and the protective, anti-inflammatory effects of omega-3 fatty acids such as DHA on adipocytes and macrophages.

### FFAR4 Receptor: The Paradigm of an Anti-inflammatory Mediator with Important Metabolic Consequences

The role of FFAR4 in metabolic function has been analysed in detail using FFAR4 deficient mouse models (Suckow et al, 2014; Ichimura et al, 2012). When FFAR4 knock-out mice were subjected to a high fat-diet, they developed obesity, glucose intolerance and fatty liver to a higher degree than wild type animals. These mice displayed exacerbated insulin resistance and, furthermore, they had a higher proportion of pro-inflammatory infiltrated macrophages in the adipose tissue. These findings suggest a potentially causative link between obesity, the development of insulin resistance and a fundamental role for the nutrient-sensing FFAR4 as a protective element (Ichimura et al, 2012).

Relatively recent studies of Oh et al (2010) and Oh da et al (2014) show that inflammatory processes in macrophages are regulated via the activation of FFAR4 with the help of omega-3 fatty acids.

Further supporting a central role of FFAR4, and of FFAR1, in anti-inflammatory processes there have been many studies that describe the mechanisms by which omega-3 fatty acids suppress inflammation by inhibiting the activation of the NLRP3 inflammasome acting predominantly via 'an arrestin-FFAR4 dependent pathway' (Yan et al, 2013). A number of the beneficial anti-inflammatory effects credited to dietary fats such as omega-3 fatty acids are attributed to their actions on FFAR4. This might play an important protective role in the development of obesity, insulin resistance or asthma (Alvarez-Curto and Milligan, 2016).

Now, it is clear from studies on the expression profiles in various immune cell populations of each of the SCFA receptor FFAR2, the MCFA receptor GPR84 and the LCFA receptor FFAR4, that these receptors would likely play important roles in immune cell function. In concert with improved understanding of the roles that these and the other FFARs, play in other cell types and tissues in providing a means to sense metabolite availability then an emerging view is that they act to regulate the metabolic-inflammatory axis.

Given that aspects of inflammation underlie many chronic and comorbid diseases, including type II diabetes and obesity, there is considerable anticipation that agonist and/or antagonists of these receptors may play important roles in further understanding this interface and potential in the therapeutic treatment of such diseases (Alvarez-Curto and Milligan, 2016).

## IMMUNOMODULATORY EFFECTS OF CONJUGATED LINOLEIC ACID

Before dwelling on immunomodulatory effects of it, let us know about conjugated linoleic acid.

### Conjugated Linoleic Acid: Definition and Occurrence

Conjugated linoleic acid (CLA) refers to a group of positional and geometric conjugated dienoic isomers of linoleic acid, of which cis-9, trans-11 (c9, t11) and trans-10, cis-12 (t10, c12) CLA predominate. The predominant geometric isomer in foods is the c9, t11 that amounts to as much as 90% of the total CLA content, while the other 10% isomers are t7, c9-; c11, t13-; c8, t10 and the t10, c12-CLA isomer. CLA is naturally present in the milk and meat of ruminants and can be produced industrially by partial hydrogenation of linoleic acid.

### Physiological effect of CLA

Most of the physiological effects of CLA are observed when feeding animals with mixtures of CLA isomers that contain mostly c9, t11-CLA and t10, c12-CLA in roughly equal amounts. The physiological effects of CLA include anticarcinogenic, antiatherosclerotic, antidiabetogenic and to be able to change the body composition. CLA also altered the concentration of insulin-like growth factor in bone tissues to increase bone formation and muscle mass but decrease subcutaneous fat tissue. Furthermore, the results of studies that used animal models indicate that CLA enhances immune function, while ameliorating immune-mediated catabolism. In feeding industries, the study of CLA is important being as additive to animal diets to enhance immune function and relieve stress. Lai et al (2006) reviewed the immunomodulatory effect of CLA and possible mechanisms of action in piglets (C.H. Lai et al, 2006).

## Immune Cytokines—Need for Nutritional Means of Improving Nonlymphoidal Tissue Resistance

It is now well-accepted that the animal's immunological reaction to immune stimulants is the cause of decreased growth and rate of development (Klasing, 1988; Klasing and Johnstone, 1991).

Immune cells of the monocyte/macrophage lineage (encountering non-self-immune stimulants) release cytokines, which communicate with other cells in the immune system and the host. Interleukin (IL)-1, IL-6 and tumour necrosis factor (TNF)-$\alpha$ are among the most important cytokines produced by monocytes and macrophages and induce a number of effects in immune cells including the inflammatory response (Lewis, 1983). These cytokines are not only essential in upregulating the immune system, but also have pronounced effects on other nonlymphoidal target tissues and induce a host of metabolic changes (Klasing, 1988). Therefore, it would be beneficial for animal nutritionists to seek nutritional means of improving nonlymphoidal tissue resistance to immune cytokines (Lai et al, 2006).

## Immunomodulatory Properties of CLA

*Numerous Studies Indicate that CLA Enhances the Non-specific Immune Response*

1. Serum immunoglobulin (Ig) G concentration in piglets was increased when fed with 0.5% or 1.0% CLA in dietary supplement (Corino et al, 2002). Sugano et al (1998) observed that CLA increased serum IgA, IgM and IgG, but decreased IgE in rats. Lipopolysaccharide stimulation of mesenteric lymphoid lymphocytes showed that dietary CLA also reduced IgE concentration in rats. The type switch of the immunoglobulins from IgM to IgG and IgE requires IL-4, a potent Th2 cytokine, which suggests that CLA may downregulate the Th2 immune response and/or upregulate Th1 activities.

2. The studies on nutrition and immunity have found that dietary CLA improves lymphocyte proliferation. In piglets, lymphocyte proliferation induced by conconavalin A (endotoxin) increased quadratically as dietary CLA concentration increased from 0 to 3%.

3. The amount and function of CD4 and CD8 are also regulated by dietary CLA. With an *in vivo* vaccination and challenge to the porcine peripheral lymphocytes, dietary CLA enhanced the cytotoxic T lymphocytes function and stimulated T cell receptor lymphocytes and natural killer cell subset proliferation. Lai et al (2006) speculated that dietary CLA could enhance cellular immunity by modulating phenotype and effector functions of CD8$^+$ cells involved in both adaptive and innate immunity.

4. **CLA can improve immune function and suppress the inflammatory response:** The modulatory effect of CLA on cytokine production is different. Cytokines are hormone-like mediators of immunity and inflammation that are produced by macrophages and other immune cells under the stimulation. Dietary CLA has inhibited the production of TNF-$\alpha$ by pig peripheral blood mononuclear cells (PBMC) both at the mRNA expression and protein levels (Zhao et al, 2005). These results suggest that CLA can improve immune function and suppress the inflammatory response.

5. **CLA modulates the immune system and prevents immune-induced wasting** (Miller et al, 1994). Chicks fed CLA gained weight after endotoxin injection, whereas those fed the control diet either lost weight or failed to grow. Additional experiments were conducted in rats (Cook et al, 1993) and

mice (Miller et al, 1994) to determine whether the protection against immune-induced wasting was conserved across several animal species. Both rats and mice were responsive to the protective effects of CLA against immune stress. Mice fed CLA also showed significantly less immune-related anorexia (Miller et al, 1994). When male broiler chickens were fed control or CLA-supplemented diets, the CLA diet partially prevented reductions in body weight gain and the weight gain to feed intake ratio caused by repeated injections of LPS and Sephadex (Takahashi et al, 2002). A study on weaned piglets has also shown that growth depression due to LPS injection is alleviated by supplementation of 2% CLA.

6. **CLA individual isomers, c9, t11-CLA and t10, c12-CLA, have also been found to have immunomodulatory properties.** DeVoney et al (1999) provided evidence indicating that the t10, c12-CLA isomer alters lymphocyte blastogenesis. In this regard mixtures of CLA isomers (mostly c9, t11-CLA and t10, c12-CLA) have been shown to enhance the immune system, reduce the catabolic effects of immune stimulation and reduce the release of prostaglandin $E_2$ ($PGE_2$) and leukotriene $B_4$ ($LTB_4$) from antigen-challenged lung, trachea and bladder in the guinea pig.

In mice, c9, t11-CLA regulates CD8+T cells numbers, while t10, c12-CLA modulates B cells function to some extent. The t10, C12-CLA has increased splenic lymphocyte IgA content in mice, while C9, t11-CLA did not affect any Ig subtype but stimulated TNF-$\alpha$ production in lymphocytes. In *in vitro* studies, both c9, t11-CLA and t10, c12-CLA decreased the production of IL-1$\beta$, IL-6 and TNF-$\alpha$ in porcine peripheral lymphocyte. Moreover, the inhibitory effects of t10, c12-CLA on these cytokines was greater than those of c9, t11-CLA. However, c9, t11-CLA reportedly inhibited TNF-$\alpha$ production in rat macrophages. These results indicate that both CLA isomers have immunomodulatory properties,

but some of the effects of CLA on the immune system appear to be due to t10, c12-CLA.

**Possible Action Mechanisms of CLA**

Several mechanisms are proposed as underlying the modulating effects of CLA on the immune system. Lai et al (2006) proposed two mechanisms though there is no definitve molecular evidence.

1. An earlier hypothesis was that **CLA could modulate the immune response by altering eicosanoid signalling** (Pariza et al, 2000). Considering the structural similarities between the CLA isomers and linoleic acid, it is speculated that some of the effects of CLA may be mediated by modification of intracellular signalling by eicosanoids and other lipid mediators. Moreover, the CLA isomers could be desaturated and elongated, then further metabolised to produce various CLA-derived eicosanoids, such as conjugated-arachidonic acid, and other novel mediators that would exhibit biological activities in their own right.

Arachidonic acid is the precursor for prostaglandin (PG) synthesis, in particular $PGE_2$, which suggests that CLA affects the synthesis of $PGE_2$ also. Structurally, the way of elongation and desaturation of c9, t11-CLA and t10, c12-CLA is similar to that of linoleic acid, hence provides precursors for putative CLA-derived eicosanoids (Sebedio et al, 1997).

Pariza and coworkers reported that the change in body composition brought out by conjugated eicosadienoic acid in mice was similar to that of CLA. Modification of the cell membrane has implications for subsequent eicosanoid production and cell signalling events. Cell-to-cell contact is critical during the development of T and B cell effector functions. Therefore, it seems likely that the mechanisms of the CLA isomers effect is involved, at least in part, in both eicosanoid signalling, as well as possibly unique signalling of CLA-derived eicosanoids. **Altered eicosanoid signalling** could, in turn, affect a range of biological activities, such as cytokine synthesis and immune functions, including antigen presentation.

2. An alternative hypothesis is a **peroxisome proliferator-activated receptors (PPARs) dependent mechanism**. PPARs, including PPARα, PPARδ/β and PPARγ, are fatty acid receptors that modulate the expression of genes involved in energy homeostasis and immune function (Bassaganya-Riera et al, 2002). PPARs bind to the PPAR-response element and induce or suppress the transcription of target genes, which result in changes in lipid metabolism, energy balance, thermogenesis, glucose metabolism and atherosclerotic and carcinogenic processes. PPARγ has also been implicated in the regulation of immune cell differentiation and function (Tontonoz et al, 1998).

CLA has structural and physiological characteristics similar to the PPAR ligand peroxisome proliferators. CLA is a potent activator of PPAR (Belury et al, 1997), which can reduce the production of pro-inflammatory cytokines in macrophages by PPARγ (Yu et al, 2002). Dietary CLA enhanced the expression of PPARγ in porcine spleen and thymus tissues and both c9, t11-CLA and t10, c12-CLA isomers enhanced PPARγ activation and gene expression in cultured porcine peripheral blood mononuclear cells (PBMC).

In functionally similar action to that of CLA, synthetic PPARγ agonists are known to suppress the production of pro-inflammatory cytokines, including TNF-α in monocytes, in addition to affecting the differentiation of monocytes and macrophages. Antigen presentation is one of the principal functions of these cells. Therefore, modification of this function has implications in the development of subsequent effector functions in the Th1 or Th2 response. Therefore, regulation of cells at the antigen presentation amount by CLA can affect subsequent cellular and humoral responses to antigen challenge, thus affecting aspects of both innate and adaptive responses.

## OMEGA-3 AND ω-6: TWO CLASSES OF ESSENTIAL PUFA

### Mechanisms Underlying the Cardioprotective Effects of Omega-3 PUFA

*Essential Fatty Acids, Inflammation and Immunity*

Essential fatty acids and their metabolites such as eicosanoids, lipoxins, resolvins, protectins, maresins and nitrolipids are biologically active molecules that regulate gene expression and enzyme activity, modulate inflammation, immune response. They also regulate gluconeogenesis by direct and indirect pathways, function directly as agonists of a number of G-protein-coupled receptors (GPCRs) and thus regulate several cellular processes (Undurti N. Das, 2011).

Enhanced production of arachidonic acid (n-6 FA)-derived eicosanoids, such as $PGE_2$, is also associated with trauma and burns. The inflammatory effects of infection can be mimicked by administration of endotoxin (bacterial lipopolysaccharide, LPS).

The n-3 PUFAs are believed to possess the most potent immunomodulatory activities and among them, EPA and DHA are more biologically potent than α-linolenic acid. Total parenteral nutrition using fish oil as the lipid source has been found to prevent the endotoxin-induced reduction in blood flow to the gut and to reduce the number of viable bacteria in mesenteric lymph nodes and liver following exposure to live bacteria. With this brief on n-3 and n-6, now let us know about them.

### Essential PUFA: Structure and Biochemistry

Two classes of essential PUFA exist: n-3 and n-6. The difference between the two essential PUFA is based on the location of the first double bond of the molecule counting from the methyl end of the FA. The first double bond of the n-3 PUFA is between the third and fourth carbon atoms, while the first double bond of the n-6 PUFA is between the sixth and seventh carbon atoms (Fig. 7.1). These two classes of fatty acids are essential because animals lack the Δ12- and Δ-15-desaturases and hence must be obtained from the diet.

The parent fatty acids of the long-chain n-3 and n-6 PUFAs are alpha linolenic acid (ALA; 18:3 n-3) and linoleic acid (LA; 18:2 n-6), respectively (Figs 7.1 and 7.2). Linoleic acid is found in the nuts, seeds and vegetable oils such as maize, sunflower, safflower, canola and soya bean oil, while ALA is found in seeds of flax, rape, walnuts and chia and also in chloroplasts of leafy green vegetables.

## Imbalanced Ratio of Dietary n-6 and n-3 Fatty Acids

Consumption of high amounts of saturated fatty acid (SFA), trans fatty acid (FA) and omega-6 (n-6) PUFA and low amounts of n-3 PUFA (approx n-6:n-3 PUFA ratio of 16:1) is a pattern often observed in a typical Western diet. It is reported that fatty acid pattern found in the diets of our ancestors presumably had a n-6:n-3 PUFA ratio of ~1. Consequently, cells must adapt to this surplus n-6 and deficient n-3 fatty acids. An imbalance of dietary n-6:n-3 PUFA ratio may result in altered gene

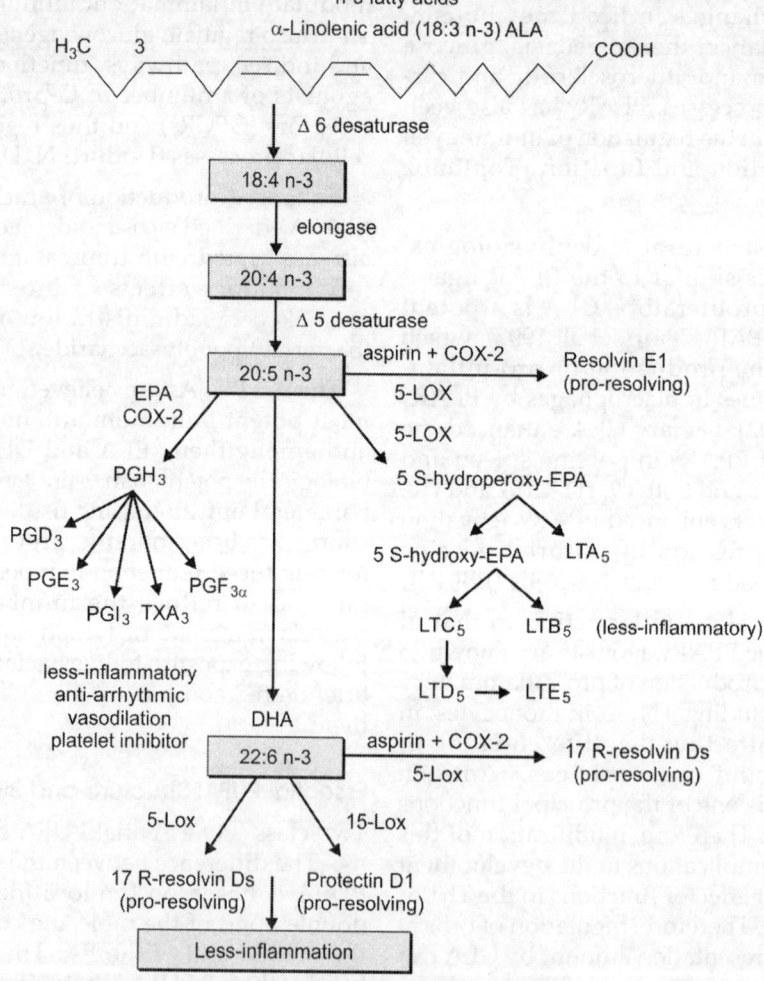

**Fig. 7.6:** Metabolism of n-3 PUFA and the biosynthesis of their respective eicosanoid and pro-resolving mediators. The n-3 PUFAs are generally less-inflammatory. The n-3 PUFA-derived eicosanoids have different physiological potencies than n-6 PUFA-derived eicosanoids. *Source*: Adkins and Kelley (2010)

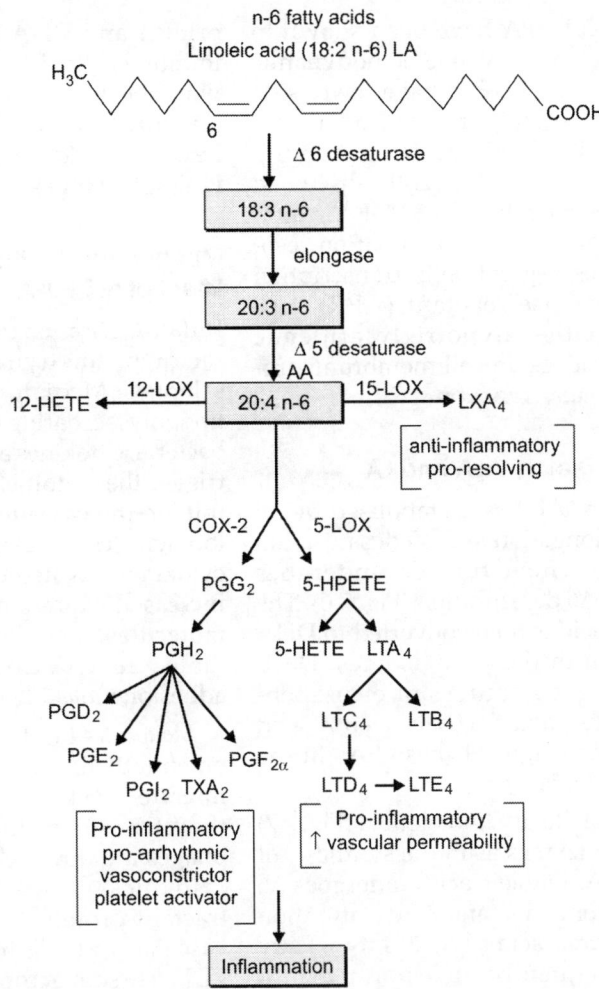

**Fig. 7.7:** Metabolism of n-6 PUFA and the biosynthesis of their respective eicosanoid and pro-resolving mediators. The n-6 PUFA are inflammatory. However, $PGE_2$ derived from n-6 PUFA can have an anti-inflammatory effect by decreasing $LTB_4$ production by the inhibition of 5-LOX and increasing production of lipoxin ($LXA_4$) by stimulating 15-LOX. *Source:* Adkins and Kelley (2010). Abbreviations: HPETE, hydroperoxyeicosatetraenoic acid; $LTA_4$, leukotriene $A_4$; $LXA_4$, lipoxin $A_4$.

regulation and expression in downstream pathways resulting in altered protein expression and activity that can negatively affect cell membrane composition and fluidity and organ function.

Omega-3 (n-3) and n-6 PUFAs regulate a number of transcription factors and interact with nuclear receptors such as peroxisome proliferator-activated receptors (PPARs), liver X receptor (LXR), hepatocyte nuclear factor-4α, nuclear factor κB (NFκB) and sterol regulatory element binding protein (SREBP), all of which influence inflammatory responses and lipid metabolism.

Cardiovascular disease (CVD) is one of the leading causes of death in humans. Many large-scale studies have concluded that consumption of fatty fish, fish oils or individual n-3 PUFA is an effective dietary strategy to lower CVD morbidity, mortality.

In addition, n-3 PUFA have been shown to improve a number of cardiac hemodynamic factors. Further, n-3 PUFAs have fewer side effects and are generally recognised as safe (GRAS) by the US Food and Drug Administration. Adkins and Kelley (2010) discussed the cardioprotective roles of n-3 PUFA in anti-inflammatory processes, inflammation resolving capabilities, regulation of transcription factors, acute-phase reactant (APR) suppression capacities, hypotriglyceridemic effects and influence on cell membrane properties and vascular function.

## Metabolism of Dietary ALA and LA

Once consumed, ALA is metabolised by Δ6 desaturation, elongation and Δ5 desaturation to yield EPA, which further undergoes elongation and Δ6 desaturation (Fig. 7.6). The resulting fatty acid is then converted to DHA via β-oxidation in the peroxisomes. Deep ocean fish are good sources of eicosapentaenoic acid (EPA) and docosahexaenoic acid (DHA) since the origin of these FAs in the aquatic ecosystem is algae.

Metabolism of dietary linoleic acid (Fig. 7.7) uses the same enzymes as in the synthesis of DHA from ALA. Linoleic acid undergoes Δ6 desaturation, elongation and Δ5 desaturation to form arachidonic acid (AA; 20:4 n-6). Fatty acids are subsequently incorporated into triglycerides (TGs; three FAs attached to a glycerol backbone), phospholipids (PL; two FAs on a phosphatidic acid backbone) and cholesteryl esters (one FA affixed to free cholesterol). Because metabolism of LA and ALA to longer chain PUFA shares the same pathway, the two compete for the same enzymes. High intakes of LA would preferentially shift the pathway to elongation of n-6 PUFA to increase arachidonic acid production and concurrently inhibit desaturation of ALA and reduce EPA and DHA formation.

Supplementation with dietary EPA ethyl esters resulted in an increase in plasma and serum phospholipid EPA, but DHA concentrations did not increase because of its inefficient conversion to DHA. The incorporation

of EPA and DHA into the phospholipid of immune cells (i.e neutrophils, monocytes, T lymphocytes and B lymphocytes) increased as a result of fish oil consumption. Docosahexaenoic acid concentration in human heart is about 10 times that of EPA (5.1% vs. 0.5%).

## Mechanisms for the Anti-inflammatory Effect of n-3 PUFA on Cardiovascular Health

Inflammation of the vascular wall is a key factor in the dynamic process of atherosclerosis. Mediators such as oxidised LDL, lipopolysaccharide (LPS) from gram-negative bacteria, cytokines and free radical species can trigger the endothelium of the arterial wall to initiate the cascade of atherosclerosis development. The local inflammatory response by cytokine-activated endothelium results in an **increased expression of leukocyte adhesion molecules,** including vascular cell adhesion molecule 1 (VCAM-1), intracellular cell adhesion molecule 1 (ICAM-1) and E-selectin.

*Monocytes* bind to the adhesion molecules on endothelial cells and subsequently transmigrate into the subendothelial space where they transform into *macrophages*. Macrophages are directed toward chemoattractant cytokines, such as macrophage chemoattractant protein-1 (MCP-1) secreted by the vascular wall cells in response to the oxidised LDL. These macrophages scavenge oxidised LDL, become lipid-laden and convert into *foam cells*. In the early stages of atherosclerosis, the accumulation of foam cells evolves into *fatty streak*. Lesion complications occur when smooth muscle cells in the intima divide and produce extracellular matrix molecules, such as collagen and the smooth muscle cells in the media migrate to the intima and contribute to the formation of a *fibrous cap*. Thrombosis is triggered when this fibrous cap ruptures.

n-3 PUFAs have the ability to respond to inflammation in atherogenesis through direct and indirect mechanisms. A direct mechanism through which n-3 PUFA decrease inflammation includes its rapid effect on the regulation of transcription factors and indirect modes of actions include the production of three-series prostaglandin and thromboxane and five-series leukotriene eicosanoids (Fig. 7.6) and inflammation-resolving lipid mediators and suppression of APRs.

### Antithrombotic and Anti-inflammatory Roles of n-3 PUFA

n-3 PUFA also decreased the production of several inflammatory cytokines. Eicosanoids are derived from 20-carbon PUFA, such as AA and EPA, which are physiologically active compounds that act locally as signalling molecules through G-protein-linked receptors (Figs 7.6 and 7.7). The phospholipase $A_2$ ($PLA_2$) releases AA from the membrane phospholipids in response to external stimuli, such as an injury or acute or chronic infection. Free AA serves as a substrate (Fig. 7.7) for the enzymes cyclooxygenases (COX) to produce two-series prostaglandins ($PGE_2$), prostacyclins ($PGI_2$) and thromboxanes ($TXA_2$), while 5-lipoxygenases (5-LOXs) catalyses the oxygenation reaction of free AA to four-series leukotrienes and hydroxyl eicosatetraenoic acids (HETEs).

Generally, the n-6 PUFA-derived eicosanoids are pro-inflammatory (Fig. 7.7). Depending upon which enzyme catalyses the oxygenation (COX or LOX), these signalling molecules elicit a wide range of responses, including vasoconstriction, vasodilation, activation of leukocytes, stimulation of platelet aggregation and generation of reactive oxygen species. 12-HETE formed from AA in the presence of 12-LOX increase inflammatory cytokine production tumour necrosis factor α (TNF-α), IL-1 and IL-6. In a study with healthy men, arachidonic acid (AA) supplementation significantly increased $PGE_2$ and $LTB_4$ production. $PGE_2$ at low concentration is pro-inflammatory by eliciting fever, pain and vasodilation and increase vascular permeability and edema. But at a higher concentration, $PGE_2$ is anti-inflammatory as it decreases $LTB_4$ production via inhibition of 5-LOX and stimulates lipoxin ($LXA_4$) synthesis through 15-LOX. $PGE_2$ can also stimulate COX-2 and stimulate its own production in fibroblasts and IL-6 by macrophages. Lipoxins are anti-inflammatory as it can inhibit NFκB activation, leukocyte migration, as well as decrease expression of cytokines and adhesion molecules (Fig. 7.6).

Eicosanoids produced from DHA and EPA are generally less inflammatory than their AA-derived eicosanoid counterparts, serve as vasodilators and inhibit platelet aggregation. n-3PUFA can reduce the production of AA-derived eicosanoids by competing with AA for incorporation into cell membrane phospholipid, by release of free AA by $PLA_2$ or by inhibiting the enzymes COX-2 and 5-LOX (Fig. 7.6). This would shift the production of inflammatory eicosanoids derived from n-6 PUFA to n-3 PUFA.

i. Eicosapentaenoic acid (EPA) can suppress COX-2, thereby decreasing two-series PG and TX production and increasing the three-series PG, PGI and TX. Eicosapentaenoic acid can also inhibit 5-LOX, which decreases production of four-series LT but increases five-series LT

ii. Docosahexaenoic acid on the other hand inhibited only COX-2 activity *in vitro*. However, supplementation of DHA to healthy men decreased production of both $PGE_2$ and $LTB_4$ (Kelley et al, 1999). Docosahexaenoic acid also decreased the *ex vivo* secretion of inflammatory cytokines, TNF-α and IL-1β by the peripheral blood mononuclear cell (PBMC) stimulated by LPS. Overall, there is plenty of information indicating that n-3 PUFAs decrease the production of inflammatory cytokines.

NOD-like receptor family, pyrin domain-containing 3 (NLRP3) senses non-microbial danger signals and forms an inflammasome, leading to a sterile inflammatory response in heart ailments (myocardial infarction, ischemia reperfusion injury, and pressure overload-induced cardiac remodelling). Omega-3 PUFAs prevented NLRP3 inflammasome-dependent inflammation and metabolic disorder in HFD-induced diabetic mice (Yan et al, 2013).

*Inflammation-resolving Effects of n-3 PUFA*

Impairment in the resolution of vascular inflammation can promote atherosclerosis development. Resolution of inflammation is a programmed normal response that enables the body to control inflammation and minimise tissue damage by limiting neutrophil and eosinophil infiltration. Most macrophages exit injured/infected sites via lymphatics and the inflammation subsides; however, under certain pathological conditions, inflammatory responses do not subside and lead to tissue injury. Using lipidomics and informatics with liquid chromatography-mass spectrometry (LC-MS)-based analysis, inflammation-resolving mediators $LXA_4$ derived from arachidonic acid (Fig. 7.7) and resolvins, protectins and maresins derived from EPA and DHA (Fig. 7.6) were identified and characterised. Lipoxin ($LXA_4$) is anti-inflammatory and pro-resolving. Resolvins, protectins and maresins are pro-resolving.

*Regulation of Transcription Factors by n-3 PUFA*

PUFA can affect gene expression by modulating gene transcription, mRNA processing and decay and stimulating post-translational protein modifications (Jump, 2002). When nonesterified FAs (NEFAs) enter the cell, they are immediately converted by acyl-CoA synthetases to fatty acyl CoA thioesters (*FA-CoAs*). The FA-CoAs can then be esterified to TG, PL and cholesterol esters or used to synthesise secondary signalling molecules (prostanoids and leukotrienes). PUFA in the cell can bind to nuclear receptors or transcription factors involved in lipid metabolism. PUFA also have the ability to regulate the expression of genes involved in inflammation.

a. **Nuclear factor κB:** Activation of NFκB transcription factor plays a key role in the regulation of the expression of genes involved in inflammatory responses. n-3 PUFA can decrease the expression of target genes involved in inflammation through NFκB.

b. **Peroxisome proliferator-activated receptors:** Peroxisome proliferator-activated receptors, which include the isoforms PPARα, PPARγ and PPARδ, are a group of nuclear receptors encoded by different genes. The PPAR isoforms are ligand-regulated nuclear transcription factors that form heterodimers with retinoid X receptor (RXR) and bind to peroxisome proliferator response elements in the promoter region of target genes involved in lipid metabolism and inflammation and subsequently modulate their expression. Peroxisome proliferator-activated receptor α and γ activation has the ability to inhibit expression of pro-inflammatory genes by inhibiting NFκB activation. Peroxisome proliferator-activated receptor α(PPARα) activators can improve cardiovascular risk factors and are antiatherosclerotic through anti-inflammatory effects in vascular smooth muscle cells (VSMCs) by inhibiting cytokine-induced VCAM-1 expression, and PPARγ has antiatherogenic and anti-inflammatory properties in monocyte/macrophages, endothelial cells, adipocytes and VSMCs through its ability to decrease IL-1β, IL-6 and TNF-α release into circulation when activated.

   Eicosapentaenoic acid and DHA have been implicated as PPARα/γ agonists and inhibit NFκB binding activity. n-3 PUFA also can activate PPARα, thereby increasing expression of FA oxidation genes and resulting in a decrease in hepatic and plasma TG, which would have an overall beneficial cardioprotective effect for hypertriglyceridemic patients.

c. **Toll-like receptor 4:** Inflammatory responses as a result of chronic and unresolved infection lead to epithelial barrier dysfunction. This results in low level endotoxemia that can contribute to the progression of atherosclerosis. Chronic inflammation is also a contributor for atherosclerotic plaque rupture, which is the leading cause of fatal coronary thrombi. Circulating endotoxins, such as LPS from gram-negative bacteria, bind and activate toll-like receptor 4 (TLR4) on immune cells, including macrophages infiltrating atherosclerotic lesions, VSMCs, adipose tissue and coronary artery endothelial cells. Furthermore, it has been proposed to be a key receptor in the development of atherosclerosis. Toll-like receptor 4 generates downstream signalling cascades that lead to NFκB activation and expression of COX-2, inflammatory cytokines and adhesion molecules. However, DHA and EPA can interfere with TLR4 activation by LPS or free saturated fatty acid.

### Effect of n-3 PUFA on Acute-phase Reactants (APRs)

During injury or inflammatory states certain proteins increase or decrease by 25%. Such proteins are called acute-phase reactants. Chronic activation of APR can have adverse consequences on health. These APRs include ceruloplasmin, C3 component of complements, haptoglobin, ferritin, α-1 antitrypsin, albumin, transferrin, apolipoprotein CIII (ApoCIII), C-reactive protein (CRP), fibrinogen and serum amyloid A (SAA). Among these APRs, elevated levels of fibrinogen, Apo CIII, CRP and SAA are considered predictors of CVD risk. n-3 PUFA supplementation has been shown to have no or modest effects on fibrinogen levels in humans. The ApoCIII-lowering effects of n-3 PUFA has been shown in hypertriglyceridemic men, but not in normolipidemic adult subjects.

The mode of action by which n-3 PUFA decreases APR concentration has mostly focused on its effect on CRP. C-reactive protein is a stronger predictor of cardiovascular events than LDL cholesterol. The major source of CRP is the hepatocytes and its synthesis is regulated by IL-6 and IL-1. Increased circulating concentrations indicate pathogenesis of atherosclerosis and inflammation. The mechanisms by which n-3 PUFA decreases CRP may also be through the inactivation of TLR4 and NFκB and IL-6/IL-1 expression.

Another possibility is through the farnesoid X receptor (FXR), the nuclear receptor for bile acids. This FXR functions as a ligand-activated transcription factor. When activated, FXR can inhibit VSMC inflammation and migration through downregulation of IL-1-induced iNOS and COX-2 expression. Docosahexaenoic acid, as well as AA and LA, are ligands for FXR.

Other nuclear receptors to which EPA and DHA are ligands include LXRα and LXRβ. Liver X receptor (LXR) ligands have been shown to delay atherosclerotic development in mouse models and inhibit atherosclerotic lesion progression. Liver X receptors are involved in cholesterol and FA metabolism. Activated LXRs have the potential to decrease atherosclerotic risk because they can inhibit intestinal cholesterol absorption, promote bile acid synthesis in the liver and stimulate cholesterol efflux in macrophages.

### Effect of n-3 PUFA on Cell Membrane Properties

A physicochemical mechanism by which n-3 PUFAs prevent CVD starts with the changes in the properties of the cell membrane as a result of n-3 PUFA incorporation because the type and amount of dietary FAs can directly affect cell membrane properties, such as fluidity (Stillwell and Wassail, 2003).

The cell membrane is composed of phospholipids that contain various types of fatty acids. The length and saturation of the fatty acids in these phospholipids is thought to affect the properties of cell membranes by altering the microdomain "rafts" and "caveolae" that concentrate membrane proteins and lipids and function as signalling platforms. Omega-3 PUFAs have many double bonds and long-chain carbons; their incorporation into the phospholipids within a membrane can alter its properties and influence the function of various membrane proteins, including the suppression of protein kinase C theta signalling and interleukin (IL)-2 production (Fan et al, 2004) and the disruption of dimerisation and recruitment of toll-like receptor 4 (Wong et al, 2009). Hence it has been found that alteration of the lipid microenvironment in cardiomyocytes through the inclusion of omega-3 PUFAs can modulate ion channel function, leading to anti-arrhythmic effects.

### Effect of n-3 PUFA on Vascular Endothelial and Smooth Muscle Cells

Omega-3(n-3) PUFAs have beneficial effects on vascular endothelial function by decreasing endothelial activation. Endothelial cells express ICAM-1, VCAM-1, E-selectin and P-selectin that are involved in leukocyte recruitment and platelet adhesion during thrombosis and inflammation and also contribute to early phases of atherogenesis. Cytokine-induced endothelial activation has been shown to increase the expression of genes for ICAM-1, VCAM-1 and E-selectin, and n-3 PUFA have been shown to inhibit the production of inflammatory cytokines that activate the endothelium. Treatment with n-3 PUFA also decreased the expression of adhesion molecule in human monocytes and murine macrophages. A decrease in expression of adhesion molecules by n-3 PUFA would decrease adhesion and migration of monocytes to the endothelium thereby mitigating atherosclerosis development and inflammation.

A balance between the concentrations of *vasoconstrictors* (TXA$_2$, PGH$_2$, endothelin-1) and vasodilators (NO, endothelium-derived hyperpolarising factor, PGI) that are produced by the endothelium determines the vascular tone. The vasorelaxant effect of DHA has been attributed to the decreases in Ca$^{2+}$ influx in vascular smooth muscle cells (VSMCs). As discussed earlier n-3 PUFA can modify eicosanoid production to favour vasodilation and antithrombotic actions. It has also been suggested that n-3 PUFAs increase endothelium-dependent relaxation through an enhancement of NO release (Abeywardene and Head, 2001). Nitric oxide inhibits platelet aggregation and adhesion, leukocyte adhesion and smooth muscle cell proliferation.

Another n-3 PUFA antiatherosclerotic mechanism is its effect on VSMC. Exaggerated VSMC growth results in arterial damage and is an important component in the patho-genesis of atherosclerosis. Eicosapentaenoic acid and DHA to a lesser extent, can affect vascular function through the inhibition in VSMC growth and proliferation at various steps of the signal transduction pathway of growth factors.

### Effects of n-3 PUFA on Blood Triglycerides (TGs)

Elevated fasting and postprandial plasma TG levels increase inflammation and are independent risk factors for cardiovascular diseases. n-3 PUFA supplementation decreased concentration of TGs and of inflammatory markers. Thus, DHA supplementation reduced both the fasting and postprandial TGs by more than 25% in hypertriglyceridemic men (Kelley et al, 2007). Furthermore, DHA also decreased the concentrations of atherogenic small dense LDL particles, total LDL particles and the remnant chylomicron particles (Kelley et al, 2008; Kelley et al, 2007). As discussed earlier, DHA supplementation decreased the circulating concentrations of ApoCIII. It inhibits the activity of lipoprotein lipase (LPL) that controls TG clearance from blood. Thus, a reduction in the concentration of ApoCIII means increased activity of LPL and hence increased clearance of plasma TG. ApoCIII-rich lipoproteins also enhance monocyte adhesion to vascular endothelial cells (Kawakami et al, 2006). Plasma concentration of Apo CIII is, therefore, considered another emerging lipoprotein-associated marker for CVD risk. n-3 PUFA also regulate ApoCIII through their effects on PPARα, which downregulates ApoCIII expression, and NFκB, which upregulates Apo CIII expression.

n-3 PUFA can also decrease TG concentration through the inhibition of hepatic very low-density lipoprotein (VLDL)-TG synthesis and secretion that is secondary to a decrease in TG synthesis. This decrease in VLDL-TG secretion may be due to the decrease in the expression of hepatic gene transcription factor, SREBP-1c, which is the key switch in controlling lipogenesis. This in turn would diminish the synthesis of acetyl-CoA carboxylase and FA synthase. The net effect is a decrease in FA synthesis.

The TG lowering effect may also be due to the simultaneous increase in mitochondrial and/or peroxisomal β-oxidation, which may be a direct result of increased PPARα-induced increase in acyl-CoA oxidase gene expression and therefore lead to reduced FA substrate for TG synthesis (Harris et al, 2008). Another nuclear receptor with TG lowering potential is farnesoid X receptor (FXR). Docosahexaenoic acid is an FXR ligand and has been shown to suppress the expression of hepatic lipase and Apo CIII and increase Apo CII and VLDL-receptor gene expression in HepG2 cells.

Another TG lowering mechanism by n-3 PUFA include the decreased activity of key enzymes in TG biosynthesis, such as phosphatidic acid phosphohydrolase diacylglycerol (DG) acyltransferase that catalyses phosphatidate to DG and DG to TG, respectively. **An overall decrease in TG production by n-3 PUFA in adipose tissue would ultimately lead to decreased serum NEFA transport.**

## Cardioprotective effects and ω-3 PUFA

Based on the results from cellular and molecular studies, Adkins and Kelley (2010) concluded that the cardioprotective effects of n-3 PUFA appear to be due not through a single mode of action but to a synergism between multiple, intricate mechanisms that involve TG lowering, anti-inflammatory, inflammation-resolving, regulation of transcription factors and gene expression, membrane fluidity and antiarrhythmic and antithrombotic effects. n-3 PUFAs inhibit inflammatory signalling pathways (nuclear factor κB activity) and downregulate fatty acid synthesis gene expression SREBP-1c (sterol regulatory element binding protein-1c) and upregulate gene expression involved in fatty acid oxidation (peroxisome proliferator-activated receptor α, PPARα).

Eicosapentaenoic acid and DHA have similar yet very distinctive cardioprotective properties. Only DHA seems to decrease

blood pressure, heart rate and the number of total and small dense LDL particles. Docosahexaenoic acid also has higher potency to regulate the activity of several transcription factors than EPA. Scientific knowledge regarding the cardioprotective benefits of n-3 PUFA has the potential to be used for the improvement or resolution of other inflammatory diseases, apart from cardiovascular health in lumens.

## THE INTERACTIVE EFFECT OF DIETARY N-6:N-3 FATTY ACID RATIO AND VITAMIN E LEVEL ON TISSUE LIPID PEROXIDATION AND GUT MORPHOLOGY IN CHICKENS

Lipids are one of the most unstable feed components, as they are highly susceptible to oxidation, leading to damage of various tissues. It is reported that the minute changes occurring in the intestinal mucosa is potentially, the first target for free radicals formed during oxidative reactions. All the more this is important, since it has been shown that broiler chickens are particularly exposed to oxidative stress due to the genetic selection (Sihvo et al, 2014). Thus, the activity of vitamin E, the major lipid-soluble chain-breaking antioxidant, appears to be of great significance.

### Elevated n-3 PUFA Accelerate Lipid Oxidation

Studies have been conducted for at least 3 decades on beneficial activities of n-3 long-chain polyunsaturated fatty acids (PUFA) in key biological processes. A simple dietary intervention with n-3 PUFA may affect chicken immunity (Swiatkiewicz et al, 2015) and enriches poultry products with these fatty acids (FA) to provide health benefits for humans. However, elevated dietary levels of n-3 fatty acids lead to accelerated lipid oxidation.

### Chicken Jejunal Epithelial Cells as an Indicator of Gut Health Status

Konieczka et al (2018) have investigated the effect of the dietary PUFA ratio (PUFAn-6:

n-3) and vitamin E level on DNA damage and morphological changes in the gut epithelium of broiler chickens. Maize oil (linoleic acid) is the source of n-6 and linseed oil (alpha linolenic acid) for n-3 fatty acids. The vitamin E doses are 50 mg (basal level) and 300 mg (increased level; beyond the recommended dose) per kg diet. High dose of vitamin E has been kept to have a protective role against oxidised lipids in the intestinal mucosa.

The duodenum and upper jejunum are the major sites of lipid digestion and absorption in chickens (Tancharoenrat et al, 2014) and the intestinal epithelium is highly sensitive to oxidative damage. It has been reported that lipids are the most susceptible nutrients to oxidative reactions, leading to the increased generation of free radicals and consequently may contribute to oxidative damage of macromolecules such as DNA. DNA damage has been measured more frequently in colonocytes due to its importance in colon cancer development. But it has also been analysed in chicken jejunal epithelial cells, as an indicator of gut health status.

## Oxidised Lipids Exert more Deleterious Effect on DNA of Jejunal Epithelial Cells

The induction of oxidative stress was a natural consequence of the increased incorporation of n-3 FA into the tissue lipids of birds fed high dietary n-3 fatty acids. The study showed that dietary n-3 FA increased DNA damage in gut epithelial cells. It was found that their effect depended on the intestinal segment. For instance, DNA damage in epithelial cells was greater in the jejunum than in the duodenum (Konieczka et al, 2018). There are 2 likely reasons for that. Firstly, the jejunum, compared to the duodenum, is the predominant site of fat digestion and absorption in birds. Therefore, oxidised lipids can exert more deleterious effect on DNA of epithelial cells in jejunum. Secondly, the passage of the digesta through the duodenum is significantly shorter than through the jejunum (Tancharoenrat et al, 2014) thus, the time of contact between oxidised lipids and the duodenal epithelium is shorter.

Overall, n-3 FA increased DNA damage in epithelial cells probably by inducing apoptosis. This phenomenon was documented in rats fed a high n-3 FA diet, in which EPA and DHA induced apoptosis and increased the count of differentiating cells in the colonic mucosa (Calviello et al, 1999). The effect of the dietary fatty acid ratio (n-6:n-3) on DNA damage in intestinal epithelial cells may also result from cellular protein oxidation. Lipid peroxidation may initiate protein carbonylation by chemical modifications of side chains of susceptible amino acids. As proteins (histones) play a key role in DNA packaging and chromatin organisation, oxidation may lead to changes in their properties and in consequence, to DNA fragmentation.

## What is the Effect of High Dose of Vitamin E?

It is known that vitamin E protects cell membranes by promoting bilayer integrity. Vitamin E is mainly hydrolysed and absorbed by the gut epithelium (Khan et al, 2012) and is readily incorporated into mucosal cells. Thus, vitamin E was expected to exert the greatest protective effect on this structure. Villaverde et al (2008) suggested that vitamin E, before it is absorbed, may play a protective role against oxidised lipids in the chicken gastrointestinal tract. However, the dose of 300 mg per kg diet, which is above the physiological requirements to maintain the redox balance in the intestinal mucosa, might have induced oxidative stress. The pro-oxidative activity of vitamin E on cellular DNA may involve the formation of malondialdehyde (MDA) and 4-hydroxynonenal. MDA is toxic and because it binds DNA, mutagenic adducts may be formed; 4-hydroxynonenal triggers apoptosis and consequently leads to cell death (Nair et al, 1999; Corpet, 2011). It is also possible that a high dose of vitamin E caused DNA damage through histone oxidation, but confirmation of this hypothesis would require further research (Konieczka et al, 2018).

The liver plays a key role in the metabolism and distribution of vitamin E and it is also the first organ of its accumulation. It was shown in rats that 45 minutes after intravenous injection of α-tocopherol, more than 50% of the injected dose was recovered in the liver. The product of α-tocopherol oxidation in the liver (α-tocopheryl quinone) was eventually excreted in the bile thus, the hyperactivity of hepatocytes could have led to liver enlargement. Similarly, it was documented earlier (Konieczka et al, 2017a) that feeding diets with the increased vitamin E level (300 mg/kg diet; higher than the recommended level) over a period of 42 days caused the enlargement of the bursa, suggesting a pro-oxidative activity of high vitamin E doses in broilers.

### Effect of High n-3 dietary PUFA (low n-6: n-3 Ratio)

The study of Konieczka et al (2018) indicated that feeding birds with high n-3 FA diets had a minor but undesirable influence on the gut structure and consequently, on the bird performance during the early growth period. The gut epithelium is organised into villus-crypt units to provide maximal mucosal surface area for nutrient absorption. Therefore, nutrient uptake and absorptive efficiency depend on the integrity of the gut mucosa (Zeitz et al, 2015). Overall, longer villi provide more mucosal surface, while deeper crypts indicate more rapid enterocyte turnover. In conclusion, feeding broilers with diets low in the PUFA n-6:n-3 ratio (0.5 to 1.0) might have negatively affected the bird performance, but predominantly in younger birds. In contrast, diets high in vitamin E had a positive effect on birds' performance indices but this effect varied in different growth periods.

Dietary n-3 FA effectively got incorporated into meat lipids increased the oxidative processes in different tissues, whose intensity might have been reduced, to some extent, by vitamin E supplementation. The effect of the PUFA n-6: n-3 ratio and vitamin E level on the extent of DNA damage in epithelial cells appeared to be depended on the chicken growth stage and intestinal segment. The study provides direct evidence that diets with a low PUFA n-6: n-3 ratio supplemented with higher vitamin E levels increase DNA damage, whereas diets low in PUPA n-6: n-3

ratios, regardless of the vitamin E level, may also negatively affect gut morphology.

## THE ROLE OF OMEGA-3 PUFA ON EXERCISE PERFORMANCE, INFLAMMATION AND IMMUNE RESPONSE

The effects of n-3 or omega-3 PUFA on health are mainly derived from its immunomodulatory and anti-inflammatory properties and its influence on immune function (Calder, 2015).

### Exercise Performance and Immune Function

Exercise training and competition are physiologically demanding for athletes and as such they can face a temporary reduction in immune function. This information may be useful and applicable in case of horses that are employed in similar feats.

High levels of endurance exercise are more susceptible to the development of upper respiratory tract infections (URTI) (Peters and Bateman, 1983) and this can interfere with performance during training and in competition. Furthermore, after a single bout of high intensity long-duration endurance exercise, there is clear evidence of an immuno-suppression (Gleeson and Bishop, 2005; Ostowski et al, 1999).

In the study of Boit et al (2016), it was found that n-3 PUFA supplementation resulted in a marked improvement in post-exercise lung function and reduced concentrations of sputum immune cell (eosinophil and neutrophil) count, pro-inflammatory eicosanoid ($LTC_4$-$LTE_4$, and $PGD_2$) concentrations and cytokine (IL-1β and TNF-α) concentrations.

### Inflammatory Properties of Omega-3 and Omega-6 Fatty Acids

PUFA of n-6 and n-3 series can alter the functioning of immune cells considerably. Omega-3 fatty acids have anti-inflammatory properties when provided in optimal proportions with omega-6 fatty acids. Both ω-3 and ω-6 fatty acids are precursors of eicosanoids, including prostaglandins, thromboxanes and leukotrienes. The ω-6 fatty acids produce eicosanoids that have inflammatory properties, while the eicosanoids synthesised from the ω-3 series of fatty acids (EPA, DHA) have anti-inflammatory properties (Simopoulos, 2002).

The (pro-)inflammatory properties of ω-6 fatty acids are attributed to arachidonic acid. EPA competitively inhibits the production of inflammatory prostaglandins and leukotrienes by competing as a substrate for COX enzymes and 5-lipoxygenase (Simopoulos, 2002). In dogs, ω-3 fatty acids are used as dietary supplements to control inflammatory responses (Wander et al, 1997; Kearns et al, 1999). Dietary supplements of cod liver oil (a source of ω-3 fatty acids) reduce the severity of rheumatoid arthritis in humans (Galarraga et al, 2008).

He et al (2017) investigated the effect and underlying mechanisms of the effects of DHA on LPS-stimulated primary bovine mammary epithelial cells (bMEC). The results indicated that DHA can reduce the mRNA levels of pro-inflammatory cytokines such as tumour necrosis facor-$\alpha$ (TNF-$\alpha$), interleukin-6 (IL-6) and interleukin-1$\beta$ (IL-1$\beta$). Further it may attenuate **LPS-stimulated inflammatory response in bMEC by suppressing NF$\kappa$B activation through a mechanism partly dependent on PPAR$\gamma$ activation.**

## Oxidative Stress

It is possible that due to the high number of double bonds present, an increase in n-3 fatty acid intake may lead to an increase in lipid peroxidation and the generation of a state of oxidative stress (Aruoma, 1998), which has been linked to many disease states such as Parkinson's (Jenner, 2003) and cardiovascular disease (Madamanchi et al, 2005). However, an optimal level of reactive oxygen species (ROS) production has a positive signalling role (Barbieli and Sestili, 2012). Indeed, there is evidence that this ROS production is important in modulating skeletal muscle contractile function, promoting mitochondrial biogenesis and for normal skeletal muscle remodelling in response to exercise (Madamanchi et al, 2005).

## DIETARY OMEGA-3 FATTY ACIDS AS A SOURCE OF ANTI-INFLAMMATORY BIOACTIVE METABOLITES

### Fatty Acids and Insulin Sensitivity

In general, high fat-diets promote obesity, insulin resistance (insulin insensitivity) and fatty liver. Saturated fatty acids (SFA) such as palmitic acid (C-16) causes insulin resistance and increases inflammatory biomarkers in adipose tissue, while monounsaturated fatty acid (MUFA) such as oleic acid (19:1n-9) improves insulin sensitivity and thereby reduces the risk of breast cancer in humans. Omega-3 fatty acids also improve insulin sensitivity.

### Omega-3 Fatty Acids

Omega-3 (n-3) polyunsaturated fatty acids (PUFA) are considered essential fatty acids [linoleic acid (n-6) is also essential] because they cannot be synthesised in the body and must be supplemented from diet. They are key components of the phospholipid bilayer membrane and lipid rafts, functioning to protect cell membrane integrity, fluidity and structure. Alpha linolenic acid, is the precursor to the two major classes of n-3 PUFA: eicosapentaenoic acid (EPA-20:5n-3) and docosahexaenoic acid (DHA-22:5n-3).

### Supplementary Effect of Omega-3 Fatty Acids During Cancer Therapy

Dietary n-3 PUFA are incorporated into cell membrane phospholipids in a dose-dependent manner and modify host fatty acid profiles by decreasing the proportion of n-6 PUFA such as arachidonic acid. Such alteration of membrane composition influences membrane fluidity, receptor activity, signalling molecule production and lipid mediator production (Calder and Yaqoob 2009) to evoke alterations in metabolism at the cellular and tissue levels.

### Potential Mechanisms of Action-Inflammation and Immune Responses

Omega-3 PUFA modulate the pattern of eicosanoid production and both the intensity and duration of inflammatory responses (Calder and Yaqoob 2009). n-6 PUFA-derived eicosanoids are well-characterised as pro-inflammatory molecules, while n-3 PUFA such as EPA are typically associated with the production of less inflammatory lipid mediators (Calder, 2008). Thus, increasing the amount of dietary EPA and DHA decreases the amount of substrate for n-6 PUFA-derived eicosanoids, while increasing the substrate for n-3 PUFA-derived eicosanoids and reducing the inflammatory profile of the host (Calder, 2008).

Omega-3 (n-3) PUFA are also known ligands for peroxisome proliferator activated receptor gamma (PPARγ; Deckelbaum et al, 2006). This nuclear receptor plays a role in a variety of physiological processes including immune function (Sertznig et al, 2007). n-3 PUFA decrease production of pro-inflammatory cytokines such as tumour necrosis factor-α, interleukin-1β and interleukin-6 (Sertznig et al, 2007).

## Modulation of Neurological Functions

Docosahexaenoic acid (DHA) is a major dietary n-3 PUFA in fish oil and has been reported to possess a number of biological properties, such as anti-inflammatory, anti-tumour and immune-regulatory properties. DHA is a major component of neuronal phospholipids that regulates signal transduction, neurotransmission and membrane fluidity (Rapoport, S.I., 2001).

## n-3 Fatty Acids are a Source of Anti-Inflammatory Bioactive Metabolites

Several studies have shown that n-3 PUFA have many beneficial health effects such as improving insulin sensitivity, reducing inflammation, lowering cardiovascular disease and reducing cancer by decreasing tumour growth and metastasis. EPA specifically suppresses adipose tissue inflammation by inhibiting production of inflammatory eicosanoids and pro-inflammatory cytokines. In contrast to n-3 PUFA, n-6 PUFA possess opposing physiological effects such as increasing inflammation, vasoconstriction and cell proliferation.

Both EPA and DHA are precursors to a series of bioactive metabolites such as resolvins, protectins and maresins, which act as anti-inflammatory and resolving agents, thereby altering cell signalling. In addition to producing anti-inflammatory metabolites, they also reduce the production of pro-inflammatory prostaglandin $E_2$ metabolites by inhibiting arachidonic acid (AA) synthesis, subsequently leading to reduced aromatase activity and estrogen synthesis and estrogen signalling thereby reducing breast cancer (AL-Jawadi et al, 2018).

# Selenium and Immunity

## SELENIUM AND ANIMAL PRODUCTION

### Brief History

The specific biological functions of selenium were first discovered in microorganisms in 1954, though selenium has numerous applications in electronics. It was shown to be essential for mammalian life in 1957. In 1973, it was found to be present in antioxidant enzyme, glutathione peroxidase. This was followed by the characterisation of selenoproteins, leading to further understanding of the role of selenium in nutrition and health. Most recently, the role of selenium in gene expression and maternal programming was proven.

### Occurrence and Availability

Selenium is naturally present in the soil. It can be found in several different forms including: selenide, selenite, selenate and organic selenium, as well as in the metallic form. Plants absorb selenium from the soil and their ability to do so is dependent on its mineral composition, pH, rainfall and rate of fertilisation as well as the particular plant species and its physiological stage.

Certain plants are selenium accumulators, storing high levels in leaves and stems when they are grown in selenium rich soils. However, typical cereal, oilseed and forage species are non-accumulators. They incorporate selenium into proteins within the plant, which ensures that they do not accumulate toxic amounts. Animals and humans would naturally consume selenium in the form of selenoamino acids, most commonly selenomethionine. If the soils are poor, the levels in crops are also low leading to a reduced selenium status of animal and human populations. Therefore, in most areas of the world it is necessary to add selenium to animal feed.

### Absorption and Metabolism of Selenium

Selenium (Se) is an essential trace element in animal nutrition and exerts multiple actions related to animal production, fertility and disease prevention. If animals' requirements are not met, it reflects in their poor performance, health and fertility issues. Selenium intake is affected by the amount of plant and animal food sources consumed. Certain vegetables and some nuts are rich in selenium, while the most concentrated sources are meat, milk and eggs. Inorganic or organic forms of selenium can be used to supplement animal feed. Historically sodium selenite and selenate were added to vitamin and mineral premixes. More recently organic sources including selenium yeast and pure forms of selenium (SeMet and OH-SeMet) have become popular.

Selenium absorption and metabolism take place in the gastrointestinal tract. There are intrinsic biochemical differences in the way selenium is absorbed, depending on whether it is inorganic or organic (mainly seleno-methionine). Inorganic selenium (selenite) is passively absorbed and little is stored; its absorption is lesser than selenomethionine. Organic selenium is actively transported through intestinal membranes and accumulated in tissues such as liver and muscle.

Inorganic selenium is mostly found in the metabolic tissues of the liver and kidney. Here it is metabolised into selenocysteine and is available for the synthesis of selenoproteins, which are needed for the antioxidant system. If there is no need of selenoproteins, seleno-cysteine gets excreted, as it cannot be stored. Selenomethionine is incorporated into proteins and stored in muscle tissues. This 'reserve selenium' can be utilised for synthesis of selenoproteins when it is required, e.g. under stress conditions.

**Dietary selenium absorption is lower in ruminants compared to non-ruminants.** The site of absorption is the duodenum in both ruminants and nonruminants. Selenium availability of ruminants varies from 11 to 35%, while in nonruminants its utilisability varies from 77 to 85% of dietary selenium intake (Koenig et al, 1991; Groff et al, 1995).

## Selenocysteine and Selenomethionine

Selenocysteine is the active form of selenium utilised by the body. Selenocysteine is considered to be the 21st amino acid, since it is the functional selenium. Animals need to consume enough selenium to ensure that sufficient selenocysteine can be synthesised in order to meet the requirements for all the selenoproteins. Replacing selenocysteine by cysteine dramatically reduces the oxidoreductive ability of selenoenzymes (Driscoll and Copeland, 2003). Ingested selenium is incorporated into specific selenoproteins such as the selenoenzyme, selenocysteine; selenite is reduced to selenate and later to selenophosphate, the only precursor of selenocysteine. However, selenomethionine is 'a source of

available reduced metabolic selenium' to generate selenocysteine (Allan et al, 1999; Behne and Kyriakopoulos, 2001).

Selenocysteine (SeCys) has also helped scientists to understand the genetic code. In mammals and birds UGA is both a terminal codon and a SeCys codon. This discovery brought about the identification of novel selenoprotein genes. It is the only amino acid, which contains an essential dietary micronutrient, selenium. This uses a tRNA-dependent process for its synthesis, delivery and insertion.

In chicken tissues selenium availability and stress are the main drivers for selenoprotein expression. The synthesis of selenoproteins requires SeCys to be inserted into the primary protein structure during translation. Its incorporation at UGA codons requires SeCys specific tRNA as well as other specific factors and proteins.

## Selenoproteins—Prioritisation in the Organs

Most of the selenium in the animal is tied to proteins. Since, the discovery of glutathione peroxidase in 1973, more than 30 proteins have been known and most of them are enzymes. More than 80% of protein-bound selenium is selenocysteine.

If selenium is limited, the system gives priority to the central organs (brain, pituitary, thyroid, adrenals) for the synthesis of selenoenzymes and the blood GSH-Px is the last priority (Driscoll and Copeland, 2003; Schomburg et al, 2007). In this way the regulation and synthesis of these proteins and its behaviour in the different organs and tissues are highly dependent on selenium supply. In rats, with extreme selenium deficiency, prioritisation in organs determines that selenium concentrations in the liver, muscle or blood are below 1% of normal, whereas in the brain it is 60% of normal. In this hierarchy, the brain is followed by the spinal cord, pituitary, thyroid, ovaries and adrenal gland. In these tissues, the synthesis of selenoenzyme, phospholipid hydroper-oxidase (PH-GSH-Px) is a priority against plasmatic and cellular GSH-Pxs (Behne and Kyriakopoulos, 2001).

A great body of available information related to the role and function of enzyme GSH-Px (described in 1973 as a selenoprotein) has been put this enzyme at the top of the selenoprotein list. However, thioredoxin reductase (TR) and methionine sulfoxide reductase B (MSR-B) (described as a seleno-proteins in 1996 and 2003, respectively) have changed that view on the importance of different selenoproteins. TR is involved in regulation of such processes as DNA synthesis, cell proliferation and apoptosis as well as participates in vitamin E recycling. At the same time understanding the functions of MSR is going to change our perception to lipid peroxidation.

Other selenoproteins are responsible for many different physiological and biochemical processes including regulation of thyroid hormones, maintenance of the endoplasmic reticulum and repairing proteins. It is these functions that explain the role of selenium in animal health and performance. Still a third of the selenoproteins have unknown functions. Their discovery may further reveal the importance of selenium.

### Stress in Animals Tilt the Delicate Balance Between Antioxidant Defence and Free Radical Generation

In intensive animal/poultry production, commonly encountered stresses are due to nutrients, environment and farm management. Presence of mycotoxins, toxic metals (lead, cadmium, mercury, etc.), oxidised fat account for nutritional stresses, changes in temperature to extremes (environmental stresses), stress due to vaccinations, increased stocking density, transport of animals/birds, poor hygiene (farm management) can all lead to stress in animals. It is these stresses that cause an increase in free radical levels, which cause oxidative stress.

The supply of natural and synthetic anti-oxidants can influence the effectiveness of the antioxidant system. Supplementation of optimal levels of micronutrients helps to maintain efficient levels of endogenous antioxidants. Offering of balanced diet allows dietary antioxidants to be effectively absorbed and metabolised. A delicate balance exists within the body between antioxidant defence and free radical generation. When there is imbalance, it leads to tissue damage within the body.

Under stressful situations, organisms increase energy expenditure and respiration within cells. This results in greater production of reactive oxygen species (ROS). ROS can damage membranes, proteins as well as DNA. Because of damage to cell membranes, cells' integrity is reduced, absorption and balance of nutrients is affected, performance, reproduction, immunity and end product quality are affected.

Stress also increases susceptibility to infections with production of acute phase proteins (APP) by pro-inflammatory cyto-kines. These APP cause anorexia, fever and decreased growth in the animals. To meet increased demands for the production of APP, lysine requirements increase by sixfold. Hence lysine, under normal physiological conditions used for growth is diverted for mounting immune responses (Klasing, 2004). Because of these reasons, immune responses in birds have significant energetic cost and can decrease BW gain. All these lead to decrease in overall productivity of animals. Cells can adapt by increasing the synthesis of anti-oxidants, in order to restore redox balance. However, there are limitations for the anti-oxidant system can cope with.

### Selenoproteins Help Maintain Antioxidant Defence

The importance of selenium in animal physiology was first reported in 1957, when its deficiency was associated with that of vitamin E, which resulted in white muscle disease (WMD) (Muth et al, 1958). However, its biological significance as a structural part of "selenoenzymes/selenoprotein" was understood in the year 1973 with the discovery of glutathione peroxidase (GSH-Px). This enzyme was the first proven selenoenzyme that can prevent oxidative damage of the cellular membrane due to free radical species released to kill pathogens. Hence, selenium deficiency especially damages cellular and mitochondrial membranes.

Twenty-six selenoproteins have been identified in birds and half of them are important for antioxidant protection within the body. They all contain a selenocysteine (SeCys) at their catalytic site. Three of them (GSH-Px, TR, MSR) are key enzymes that are able to breakdown ROS. Other selenoproteins are able to reduce oxidised methionine residues in proteins. The thiol redox system consists of the thioredoxin and glutathione systems, which together control the redox status of cells. Thioredoxin reductases (TR) are selenocysteine dependent and can directly reduce pro-oxidants and free radicals, as well as being involved in antioxidant recycling.

Glutathione peroxidases (GSH-Px) of four types are found in avian species (GSH-Px 1-4): The first two offer protection against antioxidants, the third maintains cellular redox status and the fourth detoxifies lipid hydroperoxides that are found in feed. Selenium supplementation has been shown to directly increase the activity of TR and GSH-Px in animals.

In animals the different forms of GSH-Px are located in different parts of the cell, in different tissues and (in some cases) are differently regulated. It seems likely that this is an adaptive mechanism to more effectively deal with free radical production. For example, selenoenzyme (1) phospholipid hydroxyperoxidase (PH-GSH-Px) is specifically located in membranes and is able to deal with lipid peroxides directly without necessity to release them from membranes by phospholipases. (2) GI-GSH-Px is considered to be the most important defensive mechanism against lipid hydroperoxide absorption. It maintains antioxidant-prooxidant balance in the GI tract. In fact, GI-GSH-Px destroys lipid peroxides in GI tract preventing them from absorption. However, low GI-GSH-Px activity could potentially fail to destroy all peroxides and some of them can be absorbed and incorporated into lipoproteins. This incorporation could be a tiggering mechanism of the lipid peroxidation in LDL leading to changes related to cardiovascular disease (CVD) development. Similarly, (3) sperm nuclear GSH-Px is of great importance for sperm quality maintenance.

**Methionine sulphoxide reductase:** Indeed, free radicals induce oxidation of not only PUFAs but also oxidise proteins and DNA. It is generally accepted now that methionine sulfoxide reductase (MSR) is an antioxidant enzyme responsible for prevention of protein oxidation. Indeed, methionine molecules located in active centre of various enzymes are considered to be "bodyguards" for active cysteine molecules. When free radicals attack proteins, methionine would be oxidised first protecting cysteine from oxidation and in this way enzymatic activity is maintained. MSR is responsible for reducing oxidised methionine back to an active form.

Living organisms would not be able to survive in our oxygen-rich environment without the natural antioxidants. The main players in the antioxidant system are: fat-soluble antioxidants (e.g. vitamin E), water-soluble antioxidants (e.g. vitamin C), antioxidant enzymes (e.g. GSHPx, MSR-B), and the thioredoxin system. Together they work as a team to protect the body, with selenium as the chief executive.

**Selenium is the chief executive of the antioxidant system:** The antioxidant system of mammals and birds has three levels of defence, all of which involve selenium:

1. Prevention of free radical formation using GSH-Px, superoxide dismutase (SOD) and catalase.

2. Restriction of propagation, which specifically requires vitamin E.

3. Repair or removal of damaged molecules (DNA, lipids, proteins)—utilising a variety of antioxidant enzymes including methionine sulfoxide reductase B (MSR-B).

Taking into account the possible role of all the known selenoproteins, it is suggested that selenium is "the chief executive of the antioxidant system". This means selenium is responsible for regulation of major antioxidant protections via direct antioxidant activities of GSH-Px, TR or MSR or indirectly via vitamin E recycling or other important interactions.

## Consequences of Selenium Deficiency in Animals

In selenium deficiency many important physiological functions could be compromised as a result of the detrimental changes in the antioxidant defence system. The lack of selenium seriously affected productive efficiency and animal health, with high mortality in the offspring as a result of degenerative lesions in the myocardium. Selenium deficiency symptoms on productive efficiency are lower weight gains, lower milk and wool production, reduced fertility and litter size and low seminal quality.

The lowest activity of GSH-Px results in direct damage from peroxides on cell membranes, especially mitochondrial membranes. It also increases the erythrocyte fragility consistent with anaemia and damage to the endothelium membrane resulting in general oedema.

Selenium deficiency has been originally recognised as a health problem due to the damage that occurs to the cell membranes including mitochondrial membrane structures: **white muscle disease (WMD) or nutritional muscular dystrophy (NMD),** with degenerative changes in skeletal muscle and in the myocardium of young animals. It is characterised by difficulty in walking and abnormal postural positions in adult animals. Degenerative changes in the skeletal muscle fibres with greater growth potential (indicating a probable need for higher requirement), as well as in cardiac muscle fibres, results in sudden death of the offspring in the first week of life (Silva et al, 2000). The presence of NMD remains as the central component in the suspected selenium deficiency, where its level or GSH-Px activity cannot be determined. Muscle fibres are swollen and fragmented and the characteristic injury is that affected muscles are paler than the rest of the musculature (Ramirez et al, 2004), prompting it named "white muscle disease".

**Ruminants appear to be more susceptible to the selenium deficiency disease,** with more severity in small ruminants (sheep and goats), though selenium deficiency can occur in all the animal species. This has been associated with degenerative changes in the myocardium of lambs and kids and muscular dystrophy in adults. This increased susceptibility in ruminants is attributed to (1) lower dietary absorption compared to nonruminants, (2) conversion of a proportion of selenium to insoluble forms (elementary Se and selenurs) and (3) another portion is incorporated into bacterial proteins with the formation of seleno amino acids by rumen microorganisms (Harrison and Conrad, 1984a,b).

Whanger (2002) reported that the concentration of selenium in rumen flora of adult sheep was 46 times greater than its concentration in the diet they consumed. This microbial selenium would be of high digestibility for the ruminant, except that its dominant form probably reflects selenomethionine of low metabolic efficiency. This could explain the lower dietary selenium absorption in ruminants compared to non-ruminants making ruminants more susceptible to selenium deficiency.

### Diagnosis of Selenium Deficiency

There are clear correlations between the presence of selenium in soil, plants and animal tissues. In soils with adequate levels of selenium, the presence of other minerals such as calcium, sulphur, copper and arsenic can interfere with its utilisation by the plant. The dietary presence of these same elements or of polyunsaturated fat and nitrates could also reduce their absorption in the small intestine (Combs and Combs, 1986). Deficiency occurs when soil is poor in selenium or contains high levels of other minerals competing for usage by plants.

The concentration of selenium in forage and soil is important to know the selenium status in a particular region. Several factors affect the concentrations of minerals in forages, such as soil type, the presence of antagonistic elements and contaminants, fertilisation, forage species, weather and season and plant maturity.

The **selenium concentration** in tissues appears to act as a reservoir for the element, with the lowest change of selenium concentration in liver, therefore being preferable to measuring selenium **in blood**. It should be considered that lambs have a digestive activity similar to non-ruminants, in which selenium utilisation from the diet is greater than that of adult sheep.

There is a high correlation between GSH-Px activity and selenium level in blood. Hence this enzyme is used as an indicator of deficiencies (Ammerman and Miller, 1975). However, when a response to supplementation is being evaluated in a short period of time, a direct determination of selenium is preferred (Stowe and Herdt, 1992).

### Supplementation of Selenium

Selenium deficiency should be prevented by supplementation in deficient regions and in deficient animals considering the serious impact on the productive efficiency of animals. Supplementation of the pregnant females is a key strategy to reduce these losses (Abd El-Ghany et al, 2007, 2008). Selenium supplementation of animals can be accomplished by incorporating the element in the diet (premixes), water, mineral supplements, intraruminal bolus, or injectable solutions. Selenium can be lost when food is processed or refined, due to its volatility.

### Selenium Sources and Availability

Sources of selenium include inorganic salts (selenates and selenites) and selenomethionine or less purified forms as selenoyeast, in which this amino acid is abundant. Any of these forms can be used in the diet. But for an injectable form or bolus, only inorganic salts can possibly achieve adequate concentrations (Revilla et al, 2008). The chemical form affects the injectable salt absorption; sodium selenite administered subcutaneously is more rapidly absorbed than barium selenate (Kuttler et al, 1961).

Availability of supplemental selenomethionine is greater than that of sodium selenite (Xia et al, 2005). Additionally, selenomethionine is rapidly incorporated into proteins (Nicholson et al, 1991). Mixtures with selenomethionine or selenoyeast are more expensive than selenites and selenates and supplemented inorganic selenium salts are converted to selenomethionine by the rumen microflora in ruminants (Kim et al, 1997). It is important to consider that organic forms of selenium can be better absorbed from the gut in comparison to inorganic forms (Mahima et al, 2012) and thus more efficient in the reduction of oxidative stress (Ahmad et al, 2012).

### Selenium Transfer and Availability

Pregnant animals at the end of gestation and during lactation transfer selenium to foetuses (placental transfer) and offspring (colostrum and milk). In ruminants, placental transfer happens even in deficient females, who sacrifice their own condition to provide selenium to the foetus (Koller et al, 1984; Abd El-Ghany et al, 2007, 2008). In animals and human beings, there is a reduction of maternal plasma levels, as gestation progresses and products increase in size and weight. Supplemented ewes have selenium levels in the allantoic fluid, milk and colostrum and their lambs have better weight gain in the first two weeks of life (Abd El-Ghany et al, 2008). Newborns obtain it through the colostrum and milk, thus selenium availability of the mothers is critical in lactation.

## Benefits on Animal Performance

Selenium is essential to maintain animal performance in view of the challenging situations of their rearing. Organic selenium helps in building reserves that are important in the effective fight against oxidative stress. Supplementation also helps to ensure the efficacy of the antioxidant system, as well as improving gut health and immunity.

In poultry production, a combination of these effects means that selenium improves both growth rate and feed conversion. Organic selenium supplementation increases its levels in chicken muscle and antioxidant status. When chicken meat is stored, drip loss and lipid peroxidation are reduced, improving the quality and the yield.

A reduction in mortality is also observed, explained in part by enhanced immuno-competence. Supplementation with organic selenium has also been shown to have an anti-viral effect, as well as protecting against damage to the intestine by pathogens. By increasing resistance to disease, energy for the immune system is spared. All these reflect in improving the feed conversion.

In layers organic selenium has been shown to maintain egg production during the peak period. The quality of both table and hatching eggs are enhanced by dietary selenium supplementation. The increase in Haugh units has been shown to help maintain albumin quality/freshness during storage. Egg weight is increased while feed consumption is reduced.

Through its implication in antioxidant processes, selenium is involved in various aspects of broiler breeder efficacy, from male fertility to hatchability, embryogenesis and chick early performance. As selenium is transferred from breeders to offspring, day-old-chicks (whose parents are fed organic selenium) benefit higher selenium availability, superior antioxidant capacities and thus exhibit a better start.

**Selenium and thyroid function:** Thyroid gland contains a larger amount of selenium per gram of tissue than any other organ in humans (Beckett and Arthur, 2005). Selenium is critical to thyroid hormone synthesis through the enzyme thyroid peroxidase. It is also very important for converting $T_4$ (thyroxin inactive form) to $T_3$ (active form) via thyroid deiodinases for the activation process. Thyroid peroxidase has a role in the process of iodisation of globulin avoiding thyroid epithelial cell membranal damage. **Thyroid deiodinases and thyroid peroxidases are selenoenzymes**. These relationships between selenium and thyroid function explain the negative effects of selenium deficiency in animal production.

## Benefits on Human Health

In humans selenium deficiency is associated with a number of disorders including cardio-vascular disease, diabetes, certain cancers and poor fertility. It is also important for the population's general immunity and anti-oxidant defences, particularly to counteract the stressors they encounter. However, depending on their diet and where they live, selenium requirements may not be met.

Selenium enriched animal products (milk, meat and eggs) are a good way of fulfilling human requirements. When organic selenium (in the form of OH-SeMet) is fed to laying hens, the level of selenium in eggs increases significantly. Supplementing broilers with organic selenium rather than inorganic selenium doubles its concentration in muscles. By feeding OH-SeMet, selenium levels in muscle are increased even further.

## SELENIUM AND IMMUNITY

### Introduction

Selenium is an important micronutrient and is fed either in organic (**selenocysteine, seleno-methionine)** or inorganic forms (selenite, selenate; $SeO^{2-}_3/SeO^{2-}_4$) in poultry rations, with organic selenium known to be more bioavailable (Delezie et al, 2014). Organic selenium supplementation has been shown to enhance performance and antioxidant activity (as determined by reduced lipid peroxidase and increased superoxide dismutase activities) in broiler chickens during heat stress (Rao et al, 2016). **Selenium is found in high** concentrations in the liver, spleen and lymph nodes.

## Selenium and Immune Response

**Selenium modulates immunity.** Immune enhancing activities of selenium are largely attributed to its role as an antioxidant. Selenium essentially regulates the function of glutathione peroxidise, e.g. an enzyme with antioxidant activity that neutralises ROS, to reduce oxidative stress and protect the integrity of cells, including cells of the immune system. Optimum selenium intake boosts immunity and high selenium intakes lead to toxic effects and suppression of immunity. Studies over the past 30 years have demonstrated that an adequate selenium intake is essential for both cell-mediated and humoral (antibody-mediated) immunity.

The selenium-dependent glutathione peroxidases (GSH-Px), methionine sulfoxide reductase (MSR) and thioredoxin reductases (TR) are important examples of antioxidant enzymes representing a potentially important molecular link for the action of selenium in the immune system. These enzymes are up-regulated during monocyte differentiation and are under the influence of vitamin D. Thioredoxin reductases are involved in antioxidant recycling. MSR is responsible for prevention of protein oxidation.

In the context of viral or bacterial infections, selenium supplementation has been shown to influence T helper (Th1/Th2) responses (Steinbrenner et al, 2015).

**Effects of selenium deficiency:** Selenium deficiency impairs immunity. Deficiency especially damages cellular and mitochondrial membranes. Selenium deficiency in laboratory animals decreases a range of immune functions and increases susceptibility to bacterial, viral, fungal and parasitic challenges (Stabel and Spears, 1993; McKenzie et al, 1998). Selenium deficiency affects blood levels of IgG and T cell function and this determines a higher prevalence and severity of present diseases in animal populations (John et al, 2003). The activity and lifespan of neutrophils, macrophages and lymphocytes diminishes, perhaps because of a decrease in the activity of GSH-Px. This condition would limit further the antigen processing and antigen presentation, thus limiting the humoral response (Awadeh et al, 1998).

**Effects of selenium supplementation:** Selenium supplementation has a positive impact on the immune response and quality of the colostrum (Jendryczko, 1994). Neutrophils from selenium-supplemented cows show greater phagocytic and bactericide activities against *Staphylococcus aureus* and *Candida albicans* and increase the production of leukotrienes (Grasso et al, 1990; Jukola et al, 1996). The production and activity of the chemotactic factors and migration of white blood cells is reduced in selenium-deprived animals (Jukola et al, 1996).

Positive correlations between blood selenium levels and increased concentrations of IgG in serum and colostrum have been reported in cows, which have been associated with higher serum IgG levels in their calves (Swecker et al, 1995; Awadeh et al, 1998).

## Effects of Selenium on Respiratory Burst and Microbe Killing

The respiratory burst is a microbicidal reaction that takes place in the animal body as a defence to protect it from the microbes that gain entry. It is an increase in the production of reactive oxygen species (ROS) to kill the pathogens. Therefore, macrophages as well as other phagocyte leukocytes (e.g. neutrophils, monocytes and eosinophils) can synthesise ROS and reactive nitrogen species (RNS) such as superoxide anion, hydroxyl radical, singlet oxygen, hydrogen peroxide, nitric oxide, peroxinitrite, hypochlorus acid (HOCl) and chloramines that kill bacteria during the respiratory burst (Zhao et al, 1998).

In general, the production of ROS and RNS is a characteristic for both mammalian and avian macrophages. As a defence mechanism, it is extremely effective, but the host must be able to remove the peroxides that are generated in the process, otherwise host cell damage will result. Superoxide anion radical is converted by superoxide dismutase to $H_2O_2$. Hydrogen peroxide can decompose to the extremely reactive hydroxyl radical ($OH^\bullet$), which is a deadly weapon able to damage any biological molecule.

Selenium deficiency situation leads to decreased GSH-Px, TR and MSR activity and an inability to produce a respiratory-burst reaction that is effective at killing microbes (Spallholz et al, 1990). This loss of respiratory-burst reaction impairs effective killing of bacteria and results in granuloma formation (a mass of activated, but ineffective, leukocytes) and an inability of the host to eliminate microbes. Furthermore, nitric oxide (NO) is used by a variety of host cells to destroy bacteria and viruses. Reaction of NO with $O_2^{\bullet-}$ leads to the formation of peroxynitrite ($ONOO^-$) and this is responsible for oxidative damage to lipids, proteins and DNA.

## Effects of Selenium on Eicosanoid Metabolism

Potent lipid modulators of inflammation are synthesised from arachidonic acid cleaved from membrane phospholipids by the action of phospholipases $A_2$ and C, followed by the action of cyclooxygenase (Fig. 8.1). This family of metabolites of arachidonic acid has both pro-inflammatory and immuno suppressive properties. Readers may refer 'Fatty acids and Immunity' Chapter 7 for further information. Cyclooxygenase is a key enzyme in eicosanoid synthesis, while GSH-Px is an activator of cyclooxygenase. Furthermore, the excessive generation of hydroperoxides formed by the lipoxygenase and cyclooxygenase enzymes in circulating leukocytes can lead to oxidative damage to endothelial cells.

High levels of peroxides inactivate cyclooxygenase. $PGG_2$ and $PGH_2$ are unstable

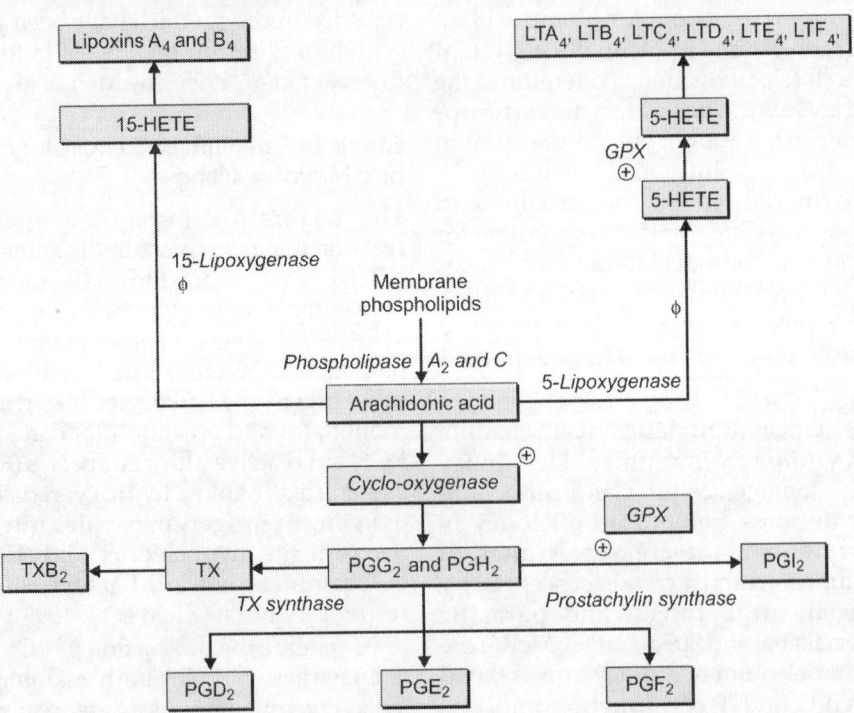

**Fig. 8.1:** The effects of selenium (Se) on the production of eicosanoids (*Adapted from* R.C. Mckenzie et al, 2002);⊕ Stimulated by Se;∅ Inhibited by Se; GSH-Px (GPX) indicates either a GSH-Px or phospholipid hydroperoxide PH-GSH-Px. TX, thromboxanes; PGI₂, prostacyclins; PG, prostaglandins; HETE, hydroxyeico-satetraenoic acid; LT, leukotriene

endoperoxides; these are converted to thromboxanes (TX), prostacyclins ($PGI_2$) or prostaglandins (PG). The leukotrienes (LTs), such as $LTB_4$, are pro-inflammatory compounds. Some, like $LTB_4$, are important chemoattractants for neutrophils (essential for neutrophil chemotaxis), bringing them into the inflamed tissue. Since leukotrienes are involved in regulation of cell proliferation, activation and maturation, they regulate immune responses. The $LTB_4$ synthase enzyme requires reduction of 12-hydroperoxyeicosatetraenoic acid (12-HPETE) by the PH-GSH-Px or other GSH-Px enzymes.

Selenium deficiency results in decreased $LTB_4$ synthesis and impaired neutrophil chemotaxis. Diminished peroxidase capacity in selenium deficiency also leads to a decrease in the synthesis of prostacyclins (Cao et al, 2000). These mediators prevent arterial thrombosis and platelet aggregation. Instead, selenium deficiency promotes the synthesis of thromboxanes (TX), which cause platelet aggregation. Platelet degranulation results in the release of pro-inflammatory mediators, including vasoactive amines, eicosanoids and pro-inflammatory cytokines. Thromboxane synthesis and platelet aggregation and activation are decreased by selenium (Zbikowska et al, 1999).

## Mechanisms of Immunomodulating Properties of Selenium

Selenium modulates immunity. It is believed that several mechanisms are involved in antioxidant-stimulation of immune system (Wu and Meydani, 1998; Surai, 2002):

### Protection of Cell Membranes and Receptors

Antioxidants prevent oxidative stress-induced damage to immune cells, since the immune cells are rich in PUFAs that are very susceptible to free radical attack. It is well-recognised that antioxidant defences directly and indirectly protect the host against the damaging effects of cytokines and oxidants. Antioxidants reduce activation of NF kappa B

(NFκB), and thereby indirectly prevent up-regulation of cytokine production by oxidants. On the other hand, cytokines increase both oxidant production and anti-oxidant defences, thus minimising damage to the host.

Cellular integrity is very important for receiving and responding to the messages needed to coordinate an immune response. Phagocytosis is the major mechanism for pathogen removal from the body. The immune system generates ROS as part of its defence function and these ROS are an important weapon to kill pathogens. However, chronic overproduction of ROS can cause damage to immune cells and compromise their function.

It is well-recognised that many immunological functions are membrane-dependent. These are antigen recognition, receptor expression, secretion of antibodies and cytokines, lymphocyte transformation and contact cell lysis (Wu and Meydani, 1998). In particular, the receptors are important for antigen recognition and the secretion of various chemical mediators such as interferon, tumour necrosis factor, prostaglandins and interleukins. Lipid peroxidation can change membrane structure and properties (e.g. fluidity, permeability, flexibility, etc.) that would affect immune cell functions, while antioxidants are able to prevent those damaging effects of ROS and maintain immune function. For example, $H_2O_2$ depressed lymphocyte proliferation, while vitamin E decreased $H_2O_2$ formation by polymorphonuclear lymphocytes (PMNL). It was found that $H_2O_2$ injured the lymphocytes immunocompetence deeply and administration of selenium counteracts this damage.

It is well known **that macrophage activation and phagocytosis of foreign particles are regularly accompanied by "respiratory burst"**, an increase in the production of ROS, exerted by the enzyme complex NADPH oxidase. A number of selenoproteins is expressed at the same time to protect the cells from the cytotoxic effects of ROS directed against engulfed microorganisms. Selenoproteins participating in antioxidant defences (GSH--Px, TR, MSR-B) are able to protect neutrophils from oxygen-derived radicals that are produced to kill ingested foreign organisms. Therefore, as a constituent of selenoproteins, selenium is needed for the proper functioning of neutrophils, macrophages, NK cells, T lymphocytes and some other immune mechanisms.

### Effect on Immunomodulator Production

There is a range of regulatory molecules produced by immune cells. For example, IL-2, a lymphocyte growth factor, is recognised as an important immunomodulatory molecule. Oxidative stress suppresses IL-2 production and antioxidants can help to overcome this suppression. Therefore, selenium up-regulates the expression of the T cell high affinity IL-2 receptor and provides a vehicle for enhanced T cell responses. Binding of IL-2 by the IL-2 receptor induces proliferation of T lymphocytes.

### Prostanoid Synthesis Regulation

Antioxidants alter the production of immuno-modulatory molecules such as prostaglandins and leukotrienes altering a ratio between immunosuppressive and immunostimulating

eicosanoids. The relationship between antioxidants and inflammatory reactions is shown in Fig. 8.2.

Good antioxidant status means nuclear transcription factor, NF kappa B (NFκB) activity is normal. NFκB is required for maximal transcription of many inflammatory cytokines. Poor antioxidant status due to selenium deficiency, e.g. activates NFκB. It is clear that poor antioxidant defence is associated with enhanced inflammation, overproduction of $PGE_2$ resulting in sup-pression of lymphocyte activity (Thimble, 1997). For example, at low concentrations, $PGE_2$ is essential for cellular immunity. However, increased $PGE_2$ concentration is associated with a suppression of cellular and humoral immunity, including antibody formation, DTH, lymphocyte proliferation and cytokine production.

Lymphocytes derived from selenium-deficient cows produced significantly less 5-hydroxyeicosatetraenoic acid (5-HETE) and leukotriene $B_4$ (Fig 8.1) ($LTB_4$ is essential for neutrophil chemotaxis) than those obtained from selenium-supplemented cows (Cao et al, 1992).

Dietary selenium status determines tissue selenium concentration. This plays an impor-tant role in the regulation of arachidonate

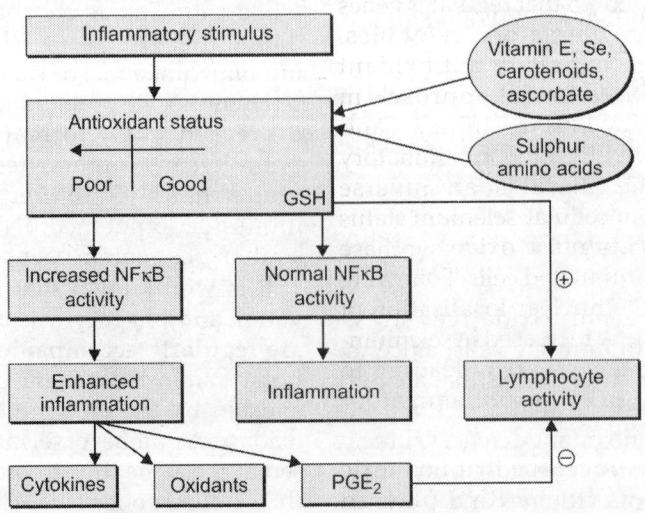

**Fig. 8.2:** Antioxidants and inflammation (*adapted from* Grimble, 1997)

metabolism affecting the 5-lipoxygenase pathway (Fig. 8.1). This may be one of the biochemical mechanisms underlying the inhibition of lymphocyte proliferation and the decrease in resistance to infectious diseases observed in selenium deficient animals (Cao et al, 1992). 5-Lipoxygenase (5-LO; a key enzyme in the biosynthesis of pro-inflammatory cytokines) is regulated by the cellular redox status with a requirement in hydroperoxides (Worz et al, 2000). In fact, granulocyte-derived ROS can activate B-lymphocyte 5-LO. Leukotrienes are involved in regulation of cell proliferation, activation and maturation. Thus they regulate immune responses.

## Effect on Signal Transduction

Natural antioxidants such as selenium and vitamin E may protect against oxidant-mediated inflammation and tissue damage by virtue of their ability to scavenge free radicals and by their ability to inhibit the activation of NFκB (and possibly other oxidant-sensitive transcription factors).

In fact, NFκB is required for maximal transcription of many inflammatory cytokines and adhesion molecules (Hughes, 1999). Furthermore, selenium at physiological levels mediates inhibition of the activation of the transcription factor NFκB that regulates genes those encoding inflammatory cytokines. Thus, maintaining adequate antioxidant status may provide a useful approach in attenuating the cellular injury and dysfunction observed in some inflammatory disorders. In fact, there is an inverse relationship between cellular selenium status and inducible form of nitric oxide synthase expression in LPS-stimulated cells. Following LPS stimulation, the nuclear localisation of NFκB was significantly increased in selenium-deficient macrophages, thereby leading to increased expression of pro-inflammatory enzyme cyclooxygenase-2.

It is necessary to underline that non-toxic concentration of ROS and RNS play an important role in regulating the expression of genes involved in the inflammatory response and in modulating apoptosis. At the same time an immune response requires extensive communication between a wide range of cell types (Klasing, 1998) and special cell receptors are of great importance in this communication. Therefore protective effect of antioxidants in prevention of membrane and receptor damages due to peroxidation could provide an important way of enhancing the immune system.

## Apoptosis Regulation

Antioxidants are considered to prevent apoptosis caused by oxidative stress. This could have a great effect on immune cell apoptosis preventing immunosuppression. Antioxidants selenium and vitamin E deficiency in chickens significantly increased caspase-like activity suggesting that cell death associated with exudative diathesis can follow the apoptotic pathway (Nunes et al, 2003). Immunomodulating properties of selenium could be mediated via prevention of apoptosis of immune cells in the case of mycotoxicoses. Indeed, many mycotoxins are immunosupressive and they can cause apoptosis (Surai, 2002), Therefore, selenium supplementation of the mycotoxin-contaminated feed could potentially have a beneficial effect.

## Adhesion Molecules Expression and Production of Soluble Mediators of the Immune Response

Jahnova et al (2002) reported that selenium was able to affect the adhesion molecules expressions that are crucial in the inflammatory process.

## Effect of Selenium Supplementation on Antiviral Immunity

Several studies have demonstrated the beneficial effects of dietary selenium in immunity to viruses including influenza, HIV and Coxsackie viruses (Gill and Walker, 2008). For example, infection with influenza virus in mice is shown to decrease GPx activity resulting in an increased oxidative stress in T cells leading to impaired immune response and reduced virus clearance (Beck et al, 2001). It has also been found that selenium deficient mice and rats infected with influenza virus has macrophages, NK cells and CD8+T cells with impaired functions.

There is little information available as to how selenium acts at the molecular level in host immunity and inflammation (Shrimali et al, 2008). To determine the effects of selenium supplementation in feed on the immune system, Shojadoost et al (2019) conducted a study in chickens (challenged with low pathogenic avian influenza virus subtype H9N2) and evaluated the expression of interferon stimulated genes (ISG) and interferon (IFN) genes in caecal tonsils and spleen tissues. Results demonstrated that selenium supplementation of chicken diets increased the expression of antiviral response genes, which could lead to reduction of virus shedding from infected birds.

# 9

# Vitamin D and Immunity

## VITAMIN D AND IMMUNITY

### Vitamin D

Vitamin D is a pleiotropic lipid soluble vitamin. Vitamin D is a collective term that encompasses both cholecalciferol (vitamin $D_3$) derived from the metabolism of cholesterol and vitamin $D_2$ (ergocalciferol), obtained from the plant steroid ergosterol. Both vitamin $D_2$ (ergocalciferol) and $D_3$ (cholecalciferol) are hydroxylated in the liver (enzyme is 25-hydroxylase or hepatic mitochondrial cytochrome p450 [CYP27A1]) to the two respective $25(OH)D_3$ metabolites, which collectively are measured in serum to determine vitamin D status of an individual.

Vitamin D is critical in the regulation of calcium (Ca) and phosphorus (P) homeostasis. It circulates throughout the bloodstream as 25-hydroxycholecalciferol ($25(OH)D_3$). **Vitamin D plays a beneficial role through both the direct activation of vitamin D receptor (VDR) and indirect action of regulating calcium and phosphorus. In simple terms,** this fat soluble vitamin has skeletal and extra-skeletal functions. The immune responses of vitamin D are dealt here.

### Vitamin D Requirement is Related to Dietary Ca and P Levels

Vitamin D requirement is estimated to be higher than the recommended values for the first two weeks of a broiler chicken's life and is heavily dependent on the concentrations of calcium and phosphorus in the diet. There are data indicating the beneficial effect of higher vitamin D levels on performance and overall health of the chickens highlighting its extra-skeletal roles. Indeed, higher concentrations of vitamin D have been shown to prevent tibial dyschondroplasia (TD) and vitamin D requirement of broiler chickens up to 14-day of age has been reported to be in the range of 35 to 50 μg/kg at optimal Ca and P concentrations in the diet (Whitehead et al, 2004).

In chickens the effect of varying levels of vitamin D metabolite [$25(OH)D_3$] on bone, kidney and intestinal health has been studied extensively. When Ca and P are deficient in the diet, vitamin D acts on the kidney and bone for new mineralisation; but when Ca and P levels in the diet are sufficient, vitamin D acts on the intestine as a result of suppressed parathyroid hormone due to the actions of both Ca and $1,25(OH)_2D_3$ in the parathyroid gland thereby conserving bone resorption and bone Ca (Plum and DeLuca, 2009).

### The Immune Responses of Vitamin D

The $25(OH)D_3$ metabolites of ergocalciferol and cholecalciferol are further hydroxylated principally within the kidneys (and immune cells) to form the biologically active hormonal forms of vitamin D, ercalcitriol (1,25-dihydroxy ergocalciferol) and calcitriol (1,25-dihydroxy cholecalciferol), which are collectively referred to as 1,25-dihydroxy vitamin $D_3$, or $1,25(OH)_2D_3$ (enzyme is 1-$\alpha$-hydroxylase or renal mitochondrial cytochrome p450 [CYP27B1]) (Fig. 9.1).

## Vitamin D Binding Protein (DBP)

Vitamin $D_3$ is bound to vitamin D binding protein (DBP) and is transported to the liver for subsequent steps of hydroxylation and activation. Vitamin D binding protein is a carrier protein found in the plasma and responsible for transport of cholecalciferol from plasma to liver, 25-hydroxy cholecalciferol to kidneys and 1,25-dihydroxy cholecalciferol to the target organs. Metabolites of vitamin D, 25-hydroxycholecalciferol and 1,25-dihydroxy-cholecalciferol, are lipophilic and penetrate cell membranes with relative ease and translocate to nucleus.

Vitamin D form, 25 $(OH)D_3$ is its storage form in the body, while the form $1,25(OH)_2D_3$ is its biologically active form with endocrine actions. Calcitriol or 1,25-dihydroxy vitamin $D_3$ is a naturally synthesised fat soluble vitamin shown to have immunomodulatory, anti-inflammatory and cancer prevention properties in human and animal models (Boodhoo et al, 2016). Calcitriol can act both in an autocrine and a paracrine manner on immune cells.

## Primary Purpose of the Hormone and its Pleitropic Nature

The secosteroid [a secosteroid (a latin word secare means "to cut") is a type of steroid with a "broken" ring; the prototypical secosteroid is cholesterol] hormone l$\alpha$,25-dihydroxyvitamin $D_3$ [$(1,25(OH)_2D_3)$] is a major calcitropic hormone. The primary purpose of this hormone is to keep the plasma $Ca^{2+}$ concentration within narrow limits. The renal production of $1,25(OH)_2D_3$ is, therefore, tightly regulated by two hormones: parathyroid hormone (PTH) secreted by parathyroid gland and FGF23 (fibroblast growth factor, the major phosphaturic hormone) secreted by osteoclasts (Fig. 9.2).

This pleiotropic hormone [pleiotropy occurs when one gene influences two or more seemingly unrelated phenotypic traits] exerts a variety of biological effects including the regulation of bone and mineral metabolism as well as the modulation of the immune

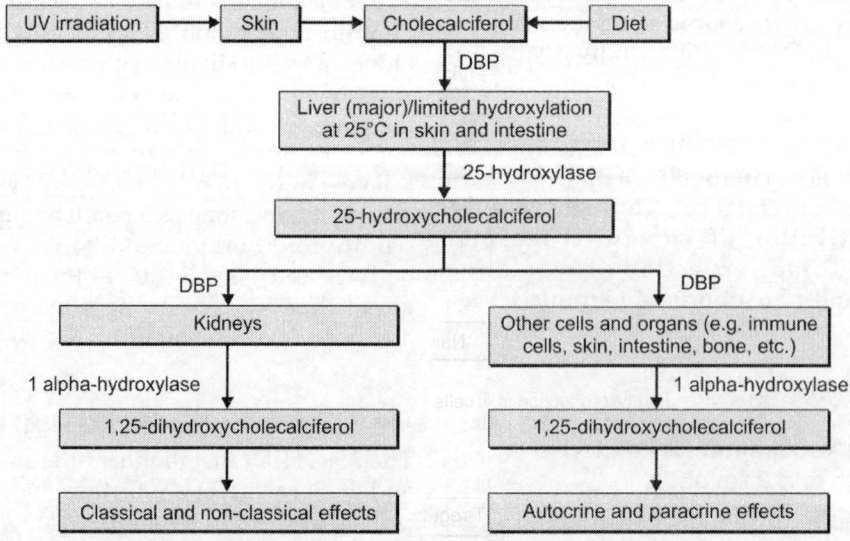

**Fig 9.1:** General overview of vitamin D synthesis. DBP, vitamin D binding protein

response (Schwarz et al, 2012). 1-α-hydroxylase is also expressed by different immune cells such as macrophages and dendritic cells, in addition to kidneys and high concentrations of 1,25(OH)$_2$D$_3$ can be found in lymphoid microenvironments (Chen et al, 2007). Hereby its specific action is increased and the potentially undesirable systemic effects such as hypercalcaemia and increased bone resorption are limited (Rodriguez-Lecompte et al, 2016). Higher circulating 25-(OH)D$_3$ levels are likely required for optimal intracrine actions of 1,25-(OH)$_2$D$_3$, whereas insufficient vitamin D$_3$ hormone levels may be linked to dysregulated immune function and possibly infectious diseases (Pae and Wu, 2017).

## Natural Ligand for the Vitamin D Receptor (VDR)

Inside the nucleus 1,25(OH)$_2$D$_3$ binds to a family of receptors called nuclear hormone receptors. The D$_3$ hormone [1,25(OH)$_2$D$_3$] is the natural ligand for the vitamin D receptor (VDR), a member of the nuclear receptor superfamily. Upon binding of the ligand, the vitamin D receptor heterodimerises with the retinoid X receptor (RXR) and binds to vitamin D response elements (VDREs) in the promoter region of target genes to induce/repress their expression (Verstuyf et al, 2010). This VDR, RXR and 1,25(OH)$_2$D$_3$ heterodimer complex stably binds to VDREs and performs its job. A large number of microarray studies have been performed to identify new key genes that are regulated by D$_3$ hormone. The variety of target genes identified reflects the pleitropic action of this hormone in different cellular processes next to cell-cell progression.

## Universal Presence of Vitamin D Receptors—Classical and Nonclassical Target Tissues

The VDR receptors have been shown to be present not only in classical target tissues such as bone, kidney and intestine, but also in many other nonclassical tissues in the immune system (T and B cells, macrophages and monocytes), in the reproductive system (uterus, testis, ovary, prostate, placenta and mammary glands), in the endocrine system (pancreas, pituitary, thyroid and adrenal cortex), in muscles (skeletal, smooth and heart muscles) and in brain, skin and liver. Besides

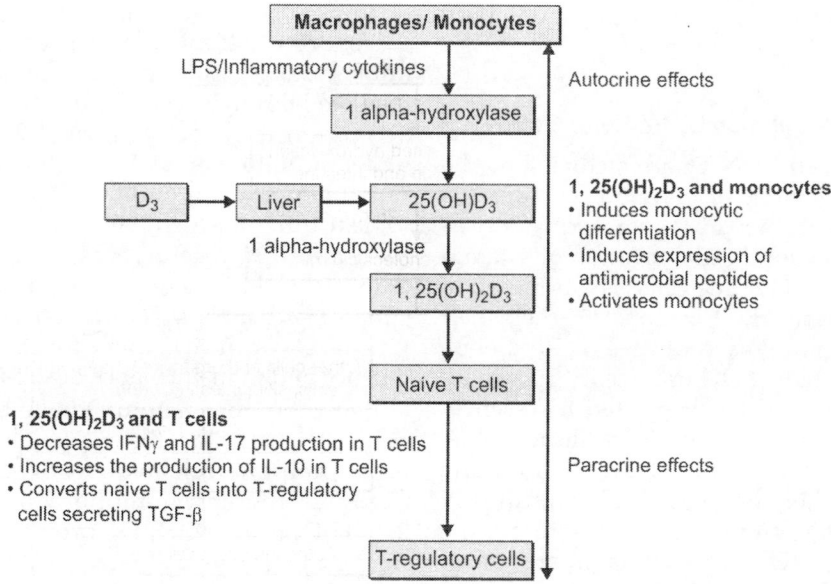

**Fig. 9.2:** Vitamin D and immune system

the almost universal presence of vitamin D receptors, different cell types such as keratinocytes, monocytes, bone, placenta are capable of metabolising 25-hydroxyvitamin $D_3$ to $1,25(OH)_2D_3$ by the enzyme 25(OH)$D_3$-1α-hydroxylase, encoded by CYP27B1. The combined presence of CYP27B1 and the specific receptor in several tissues introduced the idea of a paracrine/autocrine role for $1,25(OH)_2D_3$ (Fig. 9.2).

In humans, 1,25-dihydroxy cholecalciferol has converted dendritic cells into tolerogenic dendritic cells, which have decreased inflammatory cytokine production. Tolerogenic dendritic cells induce naive CD4+CD25-T cells into CD4+CD25+T regulatory cells. $1,25-(OH)_2D_3$ inhibited the production of inflammatory cytokine IFN-γ and IL-17 and upregulated the production of IL-10, the anti-inflammatory cytokine in CD4+ T cells. 1,25-dihydroxy cholecalciferol also upregulated the production of CTLA-4 and FoxP3 in CD4+ T cells a marker of T-regulatory cells. T cells have limited expression of 1α-hydroxylase enzyme and rely on extrinsic sources of 1,25-dihydroxy cholecalciferol. Production of 1,25-dihydroxy cholecalciferol by activated-monocytes or dendritic cells could act in a paracrine manner on CD4+ T cells and convert them to a regulatory phenotype (Jeffery et al, 2012).

## Hormone Regulation by Immune Cells

Endocrine actions of $D_3$ are mediated by the VDR. As majority of immune cells possess VDR and some of them express 1α-hydroxylase, localised activation of vitamin $D_3$ can act on immune cells. The presence of VDR and $1,25(OH)_2D_3$ in monocytes help their maturation into macrophages (DiRosa et al, 2012). Secretion of $D_3$ hormone [$1,25(OH)_2D_3$] by immune cells is regulated differently compared to its secretion by kidney cells. Immune cells (monocytes) use immune stimuli rather than calcaemic stimuli (by kidney) and immune stimuli regulate the levels of $1,25(OH)_2D_3$ in inflammatory foci. That is TLR4 (see page 273 for description on

TLR) stimulation by LPS increases 1α-hydroxylase expression and the biosynthesis of $1,25(OH)_2D_3$ from 25-OH cholecalciferol. 1,25-dihydroxy cholecalciferol acts in an autocrine manner and increases microbicidal activity in monocytes.

A crucial immune stimulus in the regulation of the final hydroxylation step (1α-hydroxylation by CYP27B1) is interferon-γ (IFN-γ). In addition to interferon-γ, macrophage activators/differentiators such as lipopolysaccharide (LPS) or tumour necrosis factor-α need to be present simultaneously to activate network of signalling pathways necessary for CYP27B1 induction.

As aforementioned, TLR signalling pathways are involved in the induction of 1α-hydroxylase. Blocking the key mediators of the TLR signalling pathway using inhibitors for MAPK, JAK or NFκB completely blocked the IFN-γ and TLR4 mediated induction of 1α-hydroxylase enzyme expression.

## Vitamin D as Immune Modulator

Absorption of UVB by 7-dehydrocholersterol present in keratinocytes initiates the pathway of vitamin D production. UV Radiation-exposed keratinocytes can be responsible for up to 80% of the body's vitamin D production. Exposure of skin to UV-B rays results in immunosuppression and part of this effect is mediated through synthesis of vitamin D and activation to its active form $1,25(OH)_2D_3$ under the influence of UV-B (Lehmann, 2005). This phenomenon hints toward a physiological function for vitamin D in immune regulation. In recent years, an increasing amount of data have become available to support such a physiological function for the vitamin D system in immune function, both in defence and in maintenance of self-tolerance.

Receptors for vitamin D have been described in most cells of the immune system and many immune cells express hydroxylase enzymes thereby immune cells activate 25(OH)$D_3$ to $1,25(OH)_2D_3$, providing within the immune system a paracrine presence of $1,25(OH)_2D_3$. In its biologically active form, vitamin $D_3$ has multiple effects on both the innate and adaptive-immune systems.

Adaptive immune system cells such as T and B cells have been shown to express VDR and constitutively transcribe the $1\alpha$-hydroxylase enzyme required for producing the active vitamin $D_3$ molecule (Chen et al, 2007; Sigmundsdottir et al, 2007). Therefore vitamin D can directly modulate T cell effector function. However, vitamin D may also indirectly affect avian T cell function via generation of immunomodulatory antigen presenting cells (APCs) (Shojadoost et al, 2015).

The physiological serum vitamin D [25(OH)$D_3$] concentration in healthy chickens (Kuhn et al, 2014) has been estimated to range between 60–100 nM, while the levels of serum $1,25(OH)_2D_3$ are significantly lower. It has been shown that APCs and T cells are able to convert 25(OH)$D_3$ to $1,25(OH)_2D_3$ at physiologically relevant concentrations and respond to this in an autocrine fashion, which can justify the supra-physiological concentration of $1,25(OH)_2D_3$ used by several groups (e.g. Boodhoo et al, 2016) to analyse the effects of vitamin D on T lymphocytes (Kongsbak et al, 2014).

## Toll-like Receptors (TLRs)

During the early stages of an infection, innate immunity serves as the first barrier against infection and sets the stage for the adaptive phase of the immune response. Upon infection, pathogen/microbial-associated molecular patterns (P/MAMPs) on pathogens trigger pattern recognition receptors (PRRs) called toll-like receptors (TLRs) in the host. The toll-like receptors (TLRs) are essential transmembrane signalling receptors of the innate immune system that alert the host to the presence of a microbial invader (bacteria, viruses and fungi). TLRs are key players in the innate immune response to pathogens by early detection of pathogen/microbial-associated molecular patterns (P/MAMPs) followed by a cascade of events resulting in clearance of infection and subsequently

activating the adaptive immune response (Opal and Huber, 2002).

Each toll-like receptor is specific to a unique pathogen associated molecular pattern. In general, TLRs can be divided into two subgroups depending on their cellular location and the PAMPs they recognise. TLR1, TLR2, TLR4, TLR5, TLR6 and TLR11 are localised on cell surfaces and recognise outer microbial cell wall components such as LPS, lipoproteins and proteins. The other group of TLRs (TLR3, TLR7, TLR21, TLR8 and TLR9) recognises microbial components such as nucleic acids located in intracellular compartments like endosomes, lysosomes and the endoplasmic reticulum (Kawai and Akira, 2010). In chickens, 8 TLRs have been identified including a unique TLR15, which is not found in mammals.

## Vitamin D-Innate Immunity

In the context of innate immunity, vitamin D may influence the type and magnitude of antigen presenting cell responses and their retrospective ability to modulate T lymphocyte function. It has been recently demonstrated that chicken macrophages exposed to 25(OH)$D_3$ have a 5-fold increase in nitric oxide production (Morris and Selvaraj, 2014). Stimulating nitric oxide production enhances phagocytic activity of macrophages and induces cytostatic or cytotoxic action against viruses, bacteria, fungi and tumour cells (MacMicking et al, 1997). In addition, low dose vitamin $D_3$ treatment may restore human macrophage proliferative ability (Ohta et al, 1985) and increase antimicrobial peptide production such as cathelicidin and $\beta$-defensin in response to stimuli (Wang et al, 2004).

## Vitamin D-Adaptive Immunity

In the context of adaptive immunity, defence against intracellular pathogens is mediated in part by CD4+ and CD8+ T lymphocytes. Vitamin D alters naive and effector T cell activation and their cytokine secretion patterns (Staeva-Vieira and Freedman, 2002).

This pleiotropic lipid soluble vitamin may be important for potentiating induction of naive T cells via an alternative mitogen-activated protein kinase (MAPK) pathway (von Essen et al, 2010). The latter is involved in establishing intracellular PLC-γ1 protein that plays a central role in classical T cell receptor (TCR) signalling pathway.

## Modulating Function of Vitamin D on Avian T lymphocytes

Macrophages have been shown to express both CYP27A1 and CYP27B1 (Gottfried et al, 2006) enzymes required to produce $1\alpha,25$ $(OH)_2D_3$ from vitamin $D_3$, whereas T cells can only perform the final metabolic step, i.e. from $25(OH)D_3$ to $1\alpha,25(OH)_2D_3$ (Shanmugasundaram and Selvaraj, 2012). Therefore, immune system cells may be able to use vitamin D in an autocrine and paracrine manner.

The immune modulatory functions of $1\alpha,25(OH)_2D_3$ have been linked to genomic effects mediated by vitamin D receptor (VDR) found in most immune cells (Di Rosa et al, 2011) such as macrophages, dendritic cells, B cells and T cells. The integrated effect of $D_3$ hormone on dendritic cells (DC) and T lymphocytes provides a unique potential to generate regulator cells (T regs).

It has been demonstrated that vitamin D reduces chicken T lymphocyte proliferation as well as the frequency of IFN-γ producing cells (Boodhoo et al, 2016). IFN-γ is an antiviral cytokine and has an important role in the generation of antiviral innate and adaptive immunity in both mammalian and avian systems. Lymphoid cells such as NK cells, γδ T cells, CD4+ T cells and CD8+ T cells are able to produce IFN-γ in response to the stimulation. The expression of IFN-γ significantly influences the initiation of antiviral adaptive immunity, including the generation of effector Th1 cells (Malmgaard, 2004).

## Vitamin D-Respiratory Infections

Respiratory infections are the major problems in poultry farms, with many possible causes including viral, bacterial and fungal. In humans, the peak incidence of respiratory tract infection coincides with the time of the year when there is insufficient UV-B light to produce vitamin D resulting in low serum vitamin D levels in the population (Cannell et al, 2006 and 2008). Verstuyf et al (2010) also has indicated that vitamin D deficiency is associated with an increased risk for nearly all major human diseases such as cancer, auto-immune diseases, cardiovascular and metabolic diseases.

Based on these aforementioned epidemiological assessments, indoor housed chickens may be at greater risk for respiratory infections and this might be explained by many mechanisms including variation in the levels of vitamin D (Kuhn et al, 2014). It is now believed that the effects of vitamin D on innate and adaptive immunity may play an important role in controlling seasonal respiratory infections (Hansdottir and Monick, 2011).

In conclusion, Boodhoo et al (2016) demonstrated that vitamin D can modulate the function of avian T lymphocytes by reducing T cell proliferation, cytokine production and a reduction in phosphorylation of non-stimulated T lymphocytes. However, vitamin D treatment did not alter the ability of T lymphocyte to undergo degranulation and did not suppress ERK1/2 phosphorylation in response to the stimuli. This may be due to differential effects of vitamin D on the functional abilities of T lymphocytes, which can inhibit immunopathology that leads to exhaustion of T lymphocytes without inducing general immunosuppression.

## Immune Functions of Vitamin $D_3$

Extraskeletal functions of vitamin D have been revealed along with the discovery of the VDR in tissue and cells because it regulates immune function through the VDR. These are as follows:

1. As the majority of immune cells possess VDR and some of them express 1α-hydroxylase, localised activation of

vitamin $D_3$ can act on immune cells with VDR in an autocrine or paracrine manner. Thus, higher circulating 25-(OH)$D_3$ levels are likely required for optimal intracrine actions of 1,25-(OH)$_2D_3$, whereas insufficient vitamin $D_3$ levels may be linked to dysregulated immune function and possibly infectious diseases (Pae and Wu, 2017).

2. Many *in vitro* studies have demonstrated significant importance of vitamin $D_3$ as an important modulator in both innate and adaptive immunity (Pae and Wu, 2017). For example, 1,25-(OH)$_2D_3$ stimulates differentiation of precursor monocytes to mature phagocytic macrophages. In addition, human macrophages are able to synthesise 1,25(OH)$_2D_3$ when stimulated with IFN-$\gamma$. Furthermore, both VDR and CYP27B1 mRNAs were induced when monocytes were stimulated with LPS or *M. tuberculosis-derived* lipopeptide. In particular, 1,25-(OH)$_2D_3$ supplementation can enhance the production of the **antimicrobial peptides cathelicidin** by macrophages (Liu et al, 2006) and **β-defensin** by endothelial cells.

3. T cells can also upregulate VDR upon antigenic activation. However, 1,25-(OH)$_2D_3$ inhibits T cell proliferation, in particular Th1 cells, which are a subset of CD4+ effector T cells capable of producing IL-2 and IFN-$\gamma$ and activating macrophages. Therefore, vitamin $D_3$ may help to limit the potential tissue damage associated with Th1 cellular immune response. It appears that other CD4+ effector cells can also be modulated by vitamin $D_3$. Studies reported that 1,25-(OH)$_2D_3$ can suppress pro-inflammatory Th17 cells, while increasing regulatory T cells. This may be a pivotal mechanism for the reported potential of vitamin D in mitigating autoimmune disorders.

4. Vitamin D regulates immune function through the VDR. Hence genetic variants in VDR could affect the function of VDR, which would modulate the biological effects of vitamin D. Indeed, VDR genetic variants have been implicated in several infectious diseases, including tuberculosis, rhinovirus lower respiratory tract infections and pneumonia. More studies are needed to address how epigenetic regulation of VDR and VDR-related genes affects plasma vitamin $D_3$ levels and an individual's response to vitamin $D_3$ supplementation, which can be linked to the host's susceptibility to infection (Pae and Wu, 2017).

## THE IMMUNOMODULATORY EFFECT OF VITAMIN D IN CHICKENS

Data on the role of higher vitamin D levels on the innate immune response of chickens are limited. Knowledge about how the chicken immune system responds to vitamin D and its metabolite [25(OH)$D_3$] is far from complete. Therefore, Rodriguez-Lecompte et al (2016) examined the effect of higher doses of vitamin D supplementation on the innate immune response in broiler chickens receiving optimal or calcium and phosphorus-deficient diets.

### Relation Between Dietary Vitamin D Level and TLRs with Different Dietary Ca and P Levels

Rodriguez-Lecompte et al (2016) evaluated the influence of vitamin D on the gene expression of TLRs, cytokines, a chemokine and cathelicidins in peripheral blood mononuclear cells (PBMCs), spleen and bursa of Fabricius of broiler chickens under non-challenged conditions and with different levels of Ca and P in the diet. Supplementation of the control diet with a high concentration of vitamin D resulted in downregulation of TLR4 expression in spleen tissue, while TLR2b expression was not affected. This is in agreement with other studies that have shown that 1,25-(OH)$_2D_3$ exerts its effect by downregulating TLR2 and TLR4 thereby inducing a hyporesponsive effect to MAMPs (Sadeghi et al, 2006).

However, supplementation of the Ca/P reduced diet with the same dose of vitamin D resulted in an upregulation of TLR2b expression and to a lesser extent TLR4 in spleen tissue. Activation of both TLR2 and

TLR4 has been shown to increase the expression of VDR and 1-α-hydroxylase. Thus, additional examination is warranted to further elucidate the relationship between Ca and P homeostasis and TLR2 and TLR4 expression.

Studies of Lemire et al (1995) and Boonstra et al (2001) suggested that the main immuno-modulatory property of vitamin D would be to inhibit pro-inflammatory cytokine production, while enhancing the expression of anti-inflammatory cytokines by acting directly on T lymphocytes or antigen presenting cells.

Reduction of dietary Ca and P levels resulted in overall enhanced cytokine expression in spleen, but with an IL-12/IL-10 ratio in favour of an anti-inflammatory status (Rodriguez-Lecompte et al, 2016). At the highest dose, vitamin D supplementation of the low Ca and P diet resulted in higher Th1 (IL-12, IFN-γ and IL-18) and Th2 (IL-4, IL-10 and IL-13) cytokines in the spleen and bursa of Fabricius and a higher CXCLi2 in the spleen. The more pronounced Th2 cytokine response in spleen suggests a more anti-inflammatory mode of action of vitamin D in this organ.

Results of the study showed that vitamin D or its derivative [25(OH)D$_3$] both have a robust immunomodulatory property with a more favourable Th2 response, while at the same time enhancing observed Th2 cytokine responses under both optimal and lower Ca and P inclusion levels in the diets of broiler chickens.

### Cathelicidin Peptides and their Functions

The term 'cathelicidin' was proposed in 1995 to acknowledge the evolutionary relationship of the novel protein family to cathelin (Zanetti et al, 1995) and it is used to denote holo-proteins that contain a cathelin-like sequence and a cationic antimicrobial domain. The cathelicidin family has gained increased recognition as their role, both as **endogenous antibiotics** and as **effector molecules of the innate immune system**.

The cathelicidin peptides comprise one of several families of antimicrobial peptides that are **found in neutrophils and epithelia as components of the early host defences of mammals against infection.** All cathelicidin family members are synthesised and stored in cells as two-domain proteins. These are split on demand to produce a cathelin protein and an antimicrobial peptide. Accumulating evidence indicates that both the cathelin portion and the C-terminal peptide exert biological activities connected with host protection.

Newly discovered cathelicidin family members are designated after the putative C-terminal antimicrobial domain, by using acronyms (e.g. CRAMP for 'cathelin-related antimicrobial peptide' or BMAPs for 'bovine myeloid antimicrobial peptides'), one-letter symbols of key amino acid residues followed by the number of residues of the antimicrobial domain (e.g. LL-37), or referring to other specific peptide features.

Cathelicidins are a group of host defence peptides (HDPs), multifunctional peptides with both antimicrobial and immuno-modulatory functions. Among the diverse functions described for mammalian cathelicidins are chemotaxis, stimulation of phagocytosis, activation and differentiation of immune cells and inhibition of LPS mediated effects (Zanetti, 2005).

The antimicrobial peptide LL-37 belongs to the group of membrane-active, amphipathic α-helical peptides with wide spectrum activity. This peptide inhibits the growth (*in vitro*) of a variety of gram-negative (*P. aeruginosa, S. typhimurium, E. coli*) and gram-positive (*S. aureus, S. epidermidis, L. monocytogenes* and vancomycin—resistant enterococci) species in the micromolar and submicromolar range of peptide concentrations (Turner et al, 1998).

### Vitamin D Mediated Modulation of Cathelicidin Expression

In the study of Rodriguez-Lecompte et al (2016), the three chicken cathelicidins were found to respond differently to vitamin D. Zhang et al (2011) reported increased bursal expression of CATH1 and upregulation of CATH1 expression in the thymus, but not examined in spleen tissue, where Rodriguez-Lecompte et al (2016) observed the strongest increase. Interestingly, in contrast to the considerable upregulation of CATH1 and CATHB1 in spleen by vitamin D supplementation of the low Ca/P diet, Rodriguez-Lecompte et al (2016) found a downregulation of CATH3 in this organ for all treatment groups relative to the control diet. This might point to a negative feedback loop within the cathelicidin cluster. As it is still mostly unclear in which cells the chicken cathelicidins are expressed, the observed increased mRNA expression could indicate induction of local gene expression as well as an influx of cathelicidin expressing cells.

Immunohistochemistry studies with cathelicidin specific antibodies could answer this question. The overall effect of increased cathelicidin expression cannot easily be predicted because of the multitude of effects these peptides possess. However, augmentation of immunity against bacterial pathogens may be expected. In fact, evidence is accumulating that vitamin D mediated modulation of cathelicidin expression may play a pivotal role in the outcome of some bacterial infections, such as tuberculosis. It has been shown that $25(OH)_2D_3$ modulates the expression of human cathelicidin LL-37 in monocytes when challenged with *M. tuberculosis* (Rivas-Santiago et al, 2008).

## Vitamin D Induced Expression of Both Pro- and Anti-inflammatory Cytokines

In chickens, the spleen acts both as reservoir and activation site for leukocytes and, therefore, splenic gene expression reflects systemic immune function (Redmond et al, 2010). In general, while vitamin D induced expression of both pro- and anti-inflammatory cytokines was upregulated, the **increased expression levels for anti-inflammatory cytokine IL-10 and the Th2 cytokine IL-4 were far greater** than those of the pro-inflammatory cytokines. Furthermore, the most profound effects of dietary vitamin $D_3$ supplementation were observed for spleen tissue of birds fed a low Ca/P diet. Under these circumstances vitamin D supplementation will result in the induction of Ca-binding protein in the intestine and increase calcium absorption and retention.

The simultaneously augmented TLR2b and TLR4 expression levels reflect an increased sensory status of the innate immune system and may in part have to do with an attempt to maintain an immunological balance. However, this could also result in an exaggerated immune response and not benefit the birds overall health. In conclusion, it has been shown (Rodriguez-Lecompte et al, 2016) that the presence of high doses of vitamin $D_3$ or its derivative 25-OH-$D_3$ above the recommended concentrations has a **robust systemic influence in shifting the immune system from Th1 towards Th2 response** and that this is most evident in the spleen particularly when dietary levels of calcium are low.

# Ageing and Immune System

## AGEING AND IMMUNE SYSTEM—NUTRIENTS' ROLE FOR IMPROVEMENT

### Ageing Process

Ageing is a complex process with an impact on essentially all organs. Declined cellular repair causes increased damage at genomic and proteimic levels upon ageing. This can lead to systemic changes in metabolism and pro-inflammatory cytokine (PIC) production, resulting in low-grade inflammation. Tissue macrophages are gatekeepers of parenchymal homeostasis and integrity. They are the prime inflammatory cytokine producers, as well as initiators and regulators of inflammation. Ageing-associated impairment in the immune system is a main factor contributing to the increased morbidity and mortality associated with infection in the elderly.

### Age-associated Changes to the Immune System

Frailty, sarcopenia and immunosenescence are commonly described in older adults.

- **Frailty** is a common negative consequence of ageing. Frailty is the condition of being weak (easily broken) in health.
- **Sarcopenia** is the syndrome of loss of muscle mass, quality and strength. It is more common in older adults and has been considered a precursor syndrome or the physical manifestation of frailty.

- **Immunosenescence** is a process of decline in immune function with age. Immunosenescence includes inflammageing.

Thus ageing is characterised by increased levels of inflammation markers in the blood. These age-related inflammatory responses can additionally be aggravated by excess calorie consumption due to metabolic stress. Age-associated changes to the immune system and inflammageing have been suggested as contributors to sarcopenia and frailty.

### Inflammageing

The process of ageing is associated with the appearance of low-grade subclinical inflammation. This is termed inflammageing. It is characterised by increased levels (2–4 times in elderly compared to healthy young ones) of pro-inflammatory cytokines such as interleukin 1β (IL-1β), interleukin 6 (IL-6) and tissue necrosis factor alpha (TNFα) as well as C-reactive protein (CRP) and a reduced serum level of anti-inflammatory cytokines including interleukin 10 (IL-10) and IL-1ra. These increased levels of circulating pro-inflammatory factors (hallmarks of inflammageing) have been associated with the development of a wide range of age-related pathologies and with higher risk of mobidity and mortality.

## Factors Responsible for Inflammageing

Many factors are responsible for inflammageing. They include (1) reduced physical activity with age, (2) increased adiposity leading to production of pro-inflammatory adipokines [leptin] and reduced anti-inflammatory adipokines [adiponectin] and (3) increased output of pro-inflammatory cytokines by resting monocytes, reduced level of anti-inflammatory cytokine [IL-10] production by regulatory lymphocytes.

## Immunosenescence

The immune system undergoes some adverse alterations during ageing. Immunosenescence is the age-associated dysregulation of immune function. Both arms of the immune system, i.e. innate and adaptive are affected by ageing, though the impact is not equal; certain components of the immune system are more dramatically affected than others with advancing age.

### Innate Immune System

The innate immune system provides the first barrier to infection and disease through various processes including activation of inflammation. Upon recognising molecular patterns of pathogens (pathogen-associated molecular pattern PAMP), the innate immune system initiates an immediate immune response, mainly through neutrophil granulocytes, monocytes/macrophages and natural killer (NK) cells. These cells directly attack pathogens and also secrete cytokines and chemokines that stimulate the cellular reaction of innate immunity, resulting in a process called inflammation.

**Neutrophils:** Neutrophils have a fundamental role in the defence against bacterial infections and in older adults many aspects of their function such as phagocytosis, superoxide production and neutrophil extracellular trap (NET) generation are impaired with age (Hazeldine and Lord, 2015). After an invasion of pathogens, neutrophils, the most abundant polymorphonuclear (PMN) leukocytes (also referred to as granulocytes), migrate into the infected sites and provide the first line of host defence by phagocytosis and oxidative burst.

**Chemotaxis is reduced in older adults:** Neutrophils migrate from the blood to a site of infection or tissue damage in response to chemoattractants, moving through tissue by releasing proteases such as neutrophil elastase at their leading edge and damaging healthy tissue in the process resulting in inflammation (Cepinskas et al, 1999). Earlier published work (Sapey et al, 2014) has shown that chemotaxis (directional movement in response to a gradient of a stimulus) is reduced in older adults making migration inefficient, leading to greater tissue damage and secondary systemic inflammation.

**Monocytes/macrophages:** Monocytes represent another important cell type in innate immunity. They migrate into the infected tissue shortly after neutrophils where they differentiate into macrophages. They mediate host defence not only by engulfing the pathogens and generating reactive oxygen species (ROS) and cytokines but also by serving as antigen-presenting cells (APCs). Although the number of monocytes is mostly unchanged in older adults, increased prostaglandin $E_2$ ($PGE_2$) production and cyclooxygenase-2 (COX-2) expression with ageing have been reported in mouse and rat macrophages (Wu et al, 2003).

**NK cells—Decreased function with ageing:** Natural killer (NK) cells are lymphocytes that are essential for maintaining the innate immune response and host defence against viral infections and tumours. They are characterised by the expression of CD56 and/or CD16 on the surface. Decreased function of NK cells (as manifested by decreased cytotoxicity) has been found in both aged mice and older adults (Panda et al, 2009), although the number or percentage of NK cells was reserved or even increased with age. Published research findings suggest that a potential approach for countering high-risk of infection in the elderly is to develop strategies to prevent, delay, or reverse NK cell immuno-senescence.

**Dendritic cells serve to bridge innate immune system and adaptive immune system:** Dendritic cells (DCs) are considered professional APCs because of their ability to capture, process and present antigen to T cells, thus serving to bridge innate and adaptive immune systems. DCs can be divided into 2 subsets: (1) myeloid (mDCs) and (2) plasmacytoid (pDCs) dendritic cells. (1) mDCs (also known as conventional DCs) facilitate adaptive T cell responses, in part through toll-like receptor (TLR)-induced interleukin (IL) - 12 production; (2) pDCs are the main producers of type I interferon (IFN) in response to viral infection (Panda et al, 2009). It appears that cytokine production upon activation is reduced in mDCs or pDCs, whereas basal cytokine production is increased with ageing (Shaw et al, 2013).

## Adaptive Immune System

The adaptive immunity or acquired immunity is carried out by T lymphocytes (T cells) and B lymphocytes (B cells). These cells recognise and distinguish different antigens and are responsible for specificity and memory. B cells are so-called because they are bone marrow-derived lymphocytes. B cells produce anti-bodies, which are proteins called immuno-globulins (Igs). The antibodies circulate in the bloodstream and permeate other body fluids, where they bind to the foreign antigens for neutralisation **(humoral immune response).** Although the number of peripheral B cells remains relatively constant during ageing, B cells from elderly individuals are less effi-ciently responsive to stimulation compared to those from young subjects. Further, age-associated defects in T cells significantly influence the decline of B cell-specific func-tions and reduce intact antibody response.

T cells also originate from the bone marrow, but they migrate to the thymus (T for thymus), where they become mature cells. T cells can either help other cells to eliminate microbes (CD4+ T cells) or kill the infected cells (CD8+ T cells) to fulfill the cell-mediated immune responses.

**T cells profile during ageing—decreased naive cells and increased memory cells:** The most significant change occurs in T cells during ageing process. A consistently observed change during ageing in the T cell profile is decreased naive cells and increased memory cells. The size of the naive T cell pool is governed by output from the thymus and not by replication and thus **thymic involution** with ageing decreases the output of naive T cells. There is a shift toward a greater number of antigen-experienced memory T cells and a smaller proportion of naive T cells (Aspinall and Andrew, 2000). In addition, T cells from aged animals and elderly individuals have decreased proliferation and production of IL-2 in response to mitogens. This decline in T cell function is in part attributed to alterations in the signalling pathways including a defect in forming the effective immune synapse. These age-associated changes in T cells are more specific to naive T cells.

Notably, aged CD4+ T cells contribute significantly to the impaired humoral response by promoting low-affinity antibody production as well as producing less IL-2 and expressing less CD4OL, critical for T-B cell interaction. CD8+ T cell responses specific to influenza virus are diminished with ageing in both mice and humans. It is obvious that intrinsic defects occur within T cells, but studies with macrophages from old mice suggest that extrinsic factors such as $PGE_2$ also contribute to the decline of T cell function with ageing.

**How to counteract ageing-associated decline in immune function and resistance to infections?** Optimal immune function depends on a normal, well-balanced nutri-tional status. Nutritional intervention may have a promising potential in mitigating negative impact of advanced age on immune function. The following nutrients are needed to improve immune function and resistance to infections to counteract ageing.

## Zinc

Zinc is a trace element essential for membrane integrity, DNA synthesis and cell proliferation. It plays an important role in maintaining immune cell homeostasis. Thus, it is a particularly important nutrient for cell functions in the immune system (Ibs and Rink, 2003). There is no specialised zinc storage system in the body. Zinc deficiency, therefore, can rapidly impair zinc supply to immune cells resulting in compromised immune function (Rink and Gabriel, 2001). Zinc deficiency can profoundly alters immunohomeostasis that involves both innate and adaptive immunity causing (1) impaired phagocytosis and intracellular killing activity of phagocytes, (2) decreased NK cell activity, (3) thymus involution and decreased thymic output and (4) decreased lymphocyte proliferation, IL-2 production, delayed-type hypersensitivity (DTH) response and antibody response to vaccines (Fraker and King, 2004; Mocchegiani et al, 2009).

**Mechanisms for zinc's immunomodulating effect:** Zinc can impact expression of hundreds of gene in immune cells and functions of different types of cells in immune system. Hence, the mechanisms for its immunomodulating effect are believed to be multifaceted. The most recognised factor in understanding the mode of zinc's action is **its role as a signalling ion. Free intracellular zinc can reversibly bind to regulatory sites in signalling proteins to affect immune cell signal transduction.** Upon stimulation, intracellular zinc increases within minutes and this response is known to control the regulation of T cell receptor signalling and thus T cell activation. Therefore, it is conceivable that zinc deficiency would reduce availability of intracellular zinc ion causing impaired intracellular signalling events and immune cell activation.

There are several **age-associated defects** in T cell activation. Hence, one-way in which zinc could affect T cell mediated immunity in the aged is to serve as a cofactor of thymulin. Thymulin is a hormone secreted by thymic epithelial cells and critical for differentiation and function of T cells. Thymulin exists in two forms: a zinc-bound active form and a zinc-free inactive form. Zinc-deficient mice had lower levels of active thymulin in circulation, and **zinc supplementation enhanced thymulin activity.**

**The intracellular concentration of free zinc is regulated by two main classes of proteins:** (a) zinc transporters and (b) metallothioneins.

a. **Zinc transporters include two families, Zip and ZnT.** Zip transporters increase cytosolic zinc bioavailability by increasing zinc influx, while ZnT transporters function by decreasing cytosolic zinc, e.g. zinc influx is mediated by zinc transporter Zip6, and Zip6 gene silencing is found to inhibit T cell activation. Recent study showed that compared with young, aged mice had lower intracellular zinc levels in immune cells, which were associated with less Zip6 mRNA levels upon activation.

b. **Metallothionein is a major storage protein for zinc.** Lower intracellular zinc levels (plasma zinc and intracellular zinc ion availability) may occur during ageing because of increased expression of metallothioneins resulting in increased sequestration of zinc. Therefore, age-associated dysregulation in zinc transporter and metallothioneins may in part contribute to reduced intracellular zinc levels, leading to immune dysfunction.

**Genetics may also influence an individual's response to zinc supplementation.** Mocchegiani et al (2008) proposed that single nucleotide polymorphism (SNP) at IL-6 gene is associated with zinc bioavailability and immune function. Elderly subjects carrying GG genotypes (C– carriers) in IL-6-174G/C locus had higher metallothioneins, low zinc status (plasma zinc and intracellular zinc ion availability) and impaired innate immune response (NK cell cytotoxicity) compared with those carrying GC and CC genotypes (C+ carriers). It is likely that old C– carriers benefit from zinc supplementation to a larger extent than old C+ carriers. Thus, genetic background is a factor to be considered for achieving the best outcome of zinc supplementation.

## Vitamin E

As a lipid-soluble antioxidant, **vitamin E (tocopherols and tocotrienols) plays a central role in protecting the integrity of cell membranes** from oxidative damage. α-tocopherol is the major form of vitamin E found in diet and it has the highest bioavailability and tissue concentrations. However, it has been suggested that tocotrienols may be superior regarding antioxidant activity and possess distinct biological properties not shared by tocopherols.

Vitamin E is particularly enriched in the membrane of immune cells. Hence, vitamin E deficiency impairs both humoral and cell-mediated immune functions. Thereby, vitamin E supplementation has a beneficial effect on the immune system, particularly in the aged individuals who have compromised immune function. It has been shown that vitamin E supplementation increased lymphocyte proliferation, IL-2 production and DTH response in old mice (Meydani et al, 1986).

**Working mechanisms underlying the immunomodulating effect of vitamin E:** It has been observed that vitamin E is efficient in restoring cell-mediated immunity as well as improving innate immunity in the aged animals. Studies conducted by S.N. Meydani and coworkers indicated that vitamin E supplementation improved T cell-mediated immunity. The working mechanisms underlying the immunomodulating effect of vitamin E have been studied mainly with experiments in cell cultures and animal models. Overall, vitamin E can enhance T cell-mediated function directly by influencing membrane integrity and signal transduction in T cells or indirectly by reducing production of suppressive factors such as $PGE_2$ by macrophages (Meydani et al, 2005; Wu and Meydani, 2008). Vitamin E supplementation can enhance resistance of aged mice to

bacterial pneumonia by modulating the innate immune response. From several research findings, it appears that vitamin E intake higher than the recommended levels has a beneficial effect on the immune function and reduces the risk of upper respiratory infections, particularly the common cold in the elderly, though vitamin E deficiency is rare.

## Vitamin D

With reference to vitamin $D_3$, it may be vitamin $D_3$ insufficiency rather than its deficiency. Vitamin D is a lipid-soluble vitamin, i.e. primarily produced in the skin during sun exposure rather than absorbed from the diet. Synthesised or ingested vitamin $D_3$ is transported to the liver where it is hydroxylated to 25-hydroxyvitamin $D_3$ [25-(OH)$D_3$] and further metabolised majorly in the kidney to the active functional form 1,25-dihydroxyvitamin D3 [1,25-(OH)$_2D_3$]. 1,25-(OH)$_2D_3$ circulates to various target tissues to exert its endocrine actions that are mediated by the vitamin D receptor (VDR). A long-recognised role of 1,25-(OH)$_2D_3$ involves calcium homeostasis and bone health. See "Vitamin D and Immunity" Chapter 9 for more information.

**Mechanisms underlying the immuno-modulating effect of vitamin D:** Vitamin D has extensive influences on multiple aspects of immune system, enabled by the expression of the VDR and the enzyme 1α-hydroxylase present in most immune cells (Liu et al, 2006). Vitamin D has been shown to enhance several innate immune functions necessary for fighting against microbial infections. Local synthesis of 1,25(OH)$_2D_3$ plays a critical role in respiratory infection. Both airway epithelial cells and lung macrophages express VDR and contain 1α-hydroxylase. Upon infection, pathogen-associated molecular patterns (PAMP) on pathogens trigger pathogen recognition receptors (PRRs) called toll like receptors (TRLs) in host. TLRs when triggered result in induction of the gene for 1α-hydroxylase (CYP27B1), which in turn induces local production of 1,25-$(OH)_2D_3$. Notably, 1,25-$(OH)_2D_3$ **is a direct inducer of antimicrobial peptide (cathelicidin) gene expression** (Liu et al, 2006).

For example, TLR activation in human macrophages has been shown to upregulate expression of VDR and vitamin D-1α-hydroxylase genes leading to increased 1,25$(OH)_2D_3$ production and its binding to VDR, which promotes synthesis of the antimicrobial peptide cathelicidin and killing of intracellular *M tuberculosis* (Liu et al, 2006). Cathelicidin has direct antiviral activity against several major respiratory viruses including influenza, respiratory syncytial virus and rhinovirus.

Furthermore, it can be suggested that **vitamin D's beneficial effect in infection may be related to its anti-inflammatory property.** Excessive and dysregulated inflammatory response is known to worsen the disease symptoms and mitigate pathogen clearance in infections. Vitamin D has been shown to inhibit production of pro-inflammatory cytokines (IL-6, IL-8, IL-12, IFN-γ, TNF-α) in the innate immune response. In the adaptive immune response, vitamin D inhibits T cell activation and modulates CD4+ T cell differentiation by favouring polarisation toward Th2 and regulatory T cell phenotypes, while suppressing Th1 and Th17 differentiation.

Taken together, the interaction of ageing, immunity, infection and nutrition is a dynamic area of research. Based on what we have known, nutrition is a modifiable factor that may allow us to mitigate age-associated defects in the immune system leading to improved defence against infection.

## A ROLE FOR NUTRITIONAL INTERVENTION TO COUNTERACT AGE-RELATED NEUROMUSCULAR DYSFUNCTION

### Healthy Ageing is Accompanied by a Decline in Physical and Neurocognitive Abilities

Normal, healthy ageing in humans is accompanied by a decline in physical and neurocognitive abilities. In ageing physical abilities (e.g. frailty) tend to decline more rapidly and to a greater extent. Within the neuromuscular system many factors contribute to the age-related decline in physical function. These include the structural, physiological and functional diminution of neural and muscular tissue, as well as systemic changes, like mitochondrial dysfunction, augmented oxidative stress and inflammation and diminished levels of anabolic hormones (Fig. 10.1).

But the neurocognitive decline is still common in ageing and it is difficult to manage. In regard to treatment strategies much emphasis has been laid on certain lifestyle factors like physical activity, while proper nutrition plays critical role in normal healthy ageing. With increasing evidence of dietary influences on healthy functional living in ageing (Parrott and Greenword, 2007), specific dietary nutrients have been shown to positively affect cognitive and musculoskeletal function in older adults. Hence, Kougias et al (2018) conducted a review on the effects of dietary supplements that promote healthy neuromuscular ageing by potentially counteracting age-related changes, which contribute to neuromuscular dysfunction.

### Features of Neuromuscular Dysfunction

Many systemic changes, like mitochondrial dysfunction, augmented oxidative stress and inflammation and reduced levels of anabolic hormones, are implicated in the age-related degeneration of the neuromuscular system. Altogether, these age-related changes result in neuromuscular dysfunction.

### *Mitochondrial Dysfunction*

Oxidative stress has been implicated in neuromuscular dysfunction (Baumann et al, 2016) and is mediated by reactive oxygen and nitrogen species, like free radicals, which are largely a byproduct of mitochondrial oxidative phosphorylation. In ageing, production of these reactive species increases due to

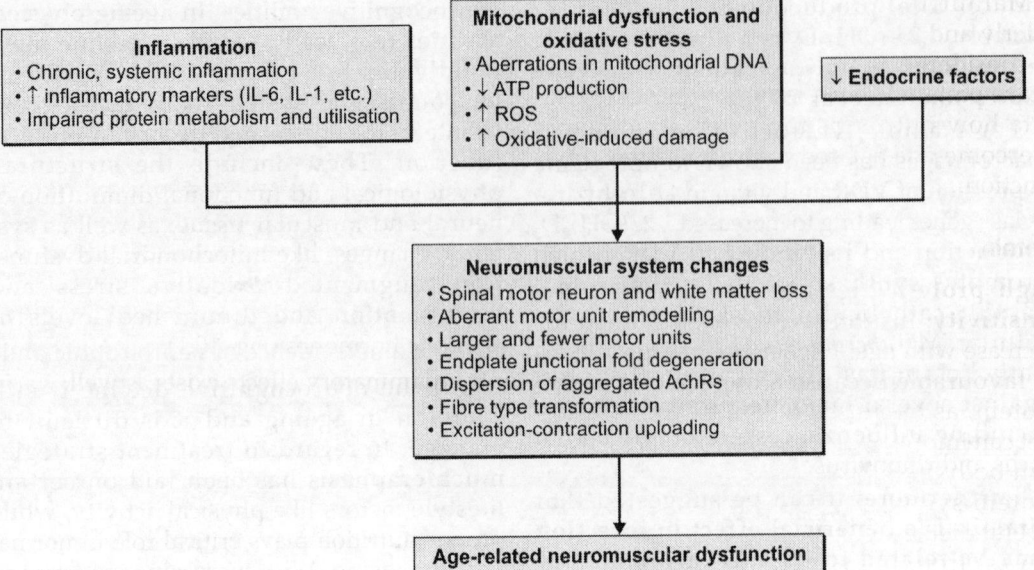

**Fig. 10.1:** A summary of the contributing factors to age-related neuromuscular dysfunction. *Source:* Kougias et al (2018); ↑indicates increased;↓decreased; ROS, reactive oxygen species; AchRs, acetylcholine receptors

mitochondrial dysfunction caused in part by age-related aberrations in mitochondrial DNA. If these reactive species are not neutralised by endogenous or exogenous antioxidants, they can induce oxidative damage to cellular infrastructure and subsequently impair function.

*Inflammation*

Inflammation is a biological process whereby immune cells, including macrophages respond to the tissue damage due to injury and/or disease and work together to eliminate it. Chronic or sustained inflammation, however, can be detrimental to the health and growth of animals.

Ageing is also accompanied by chronic, mild inflammation, which is marked by an elevated amount of circulating pro-inflammatory cytokines and has been demonstrated to be a risk factor for accelerated decline in muscle mass and strength.

*Endocrine Factors*

Normal, healthy ageing is accompanied by changes in circulating endocrine factors that

are implicated in neuromuscular dysfunction. Given that muscle atrophy partly contributes to the age-related functional deficits, the well-documented decline in circulating anabolic hormones, like testosterone, growth hormone and IGF-1, is of particular interest. Although IGF-1 has compelling anabolic effects on muscle, it also has potent neurotrophic effects that promote dendritic arborisation and synaptogenesis, as well as facilitate in the myelination of axons, prevention of motor neuron apoptosis, stimulation of axonal sprouting and restoration of damaged axons (Grounds, 2002).

**Targeted Nutritional Intervention**

Dietary supplements that include both nutrients and ingredients such as protein, vitamin D, omega-3 fatty acids, β-hydroxy-β-methylbutyrate (HMB), creatine and dietary phospholipids can positively affect neuromuscular output. Therefore, they are beneficial in counteracting the age-related changes, which contribute neuromuscular dysfunction.

Malnutrition is not uncommon in the elderly and dietary supplementation should be considered as an adjunct to usual dietary intake patterns. Now, let us go nutrient-wise data how nutrient supplementation helps overcome age-related neuromuscular dysfunction.

## Protein

**High protein diet can improve insulin sensitivity:** Insulin sensitivity is known to decrease with age. Higher-protein diets may be favourable because a hypocaloric high-protein, as opposed to high-carbohydrate, diet can improve insulin sensitivity and spare lean body mass (Piatti et al, 1994). Muscle protein synthesis (MPS) is modulated by several dietary factors. Essential amino acids (EAAs) from protein are the most efficient activators.

In fact, EAA supplementation in aged adults with sarcopenia has been shown to improve not only lean body mass (Borsheim et al, 2008) but also insulin sensitivity and insulin-like growth factor-1 (IGF-1) serum concentrations, as well as decrease serum concentrations of tumour necrosis factor $\alpha$, a systemic inflammatory marker (Solerte et al, 2008). It should be mentioned that IGF-1 also activates mTOR signalling (Fig. 10.2).

## Vitamin D

Vitamin D likely plays a beneficial role through both the direct activation of vitamin D receptor (VDR) and indirect action of regulating calcium and phosphorus. Ageing in humans is associated with decreased VDR expression in muscle, regardless of muscle location or serum 25(OH)D levels. From both animal and *in vitro* studies, it is known that VDR activation regulates gene expression that is involved in muscle cell development, differentiation and growth.

Moreover, a nonnuclear or membrane-associated VDR is presumably responsible for rapid, non-transcriptional signalling that mediates the actions of calcium influx and contraction, as well as involves pathways downstream of IGF-1 that regulate growth. Insulin-like growth factor 1 signalling is further implicated as vitamin D activates a specific tyrosine kinase, which can then activate the IGF-1 receptor. Lastly, myoblasts and myotubes have been shown to have functionally active l$\alpha$-hydroxylase (Srikuea et al, 2012), indicating that muscle may be a target tissue for 25(OH)D because it can be converted to biologically active vitamin D.

Aside from the effects of vitamin D in muscle, some evidence of neurotrophic and anti-inflammatory effects exists as well.

## Fortified Dairy Products

The (fortified) dairy products are rich in nutrients that are essential for good bone health. They contain protein, vitamin D, calcium, zinc, vitamin $B_{12}$, potassium and phosphorus.

## Omega-3 fatty acids

The essential omega-3 fatty acid $\alpha$-linolenic acid only can be converted into eicosapentaenoic acid (EPA) and docosahexaenoic acid (DHA). The latter two omega-3 polyunsaturated fatty acids (PUFAs) are known to be associated with many healthy effects and are found in fish, phytoplankton, marine algae and animal products (e.g. egg yolks).

In fact, fish oil supplements are generally taken for these beneficial health effects and as an inexpensive source of the PUFAs. In regard to its beneficial effects on the neuromuscular system, just 21 days of supplementation with 5 ml of seal oil (0.38 EPA and 0.51 g DHA) daily in young athletic adults has been shown to improve peripheral neuromuscular function, energy and overall performance (Lewis et al, 2015). These beneficial effects seem to extrapolate to the ageing population, too. For instance, higher plasma PUFA levels in older adults are associated with greater muscle size and strength, whereas lower levels are predictive of a greater age-related decline in peripheral nerve function.

The beneficial effects of omega-3 PUFA supplementation to neuromuscular function in ageing is corroborated by evidence at the molecular level. Dietary fish oil supplementation has been shown to regulate the muscle transcriptome in older adults. In particular, pathways involved in mitochondrial function and extracellular matrix organisation were increased,whereas pathways involved in proteolysis and inhibition of the main anabolic regulator, mTOR, were decreased (Yoshino et al, 2016). The impact on mitochondrial function can lead to a decrease in reactive species production and thus indirectly contributes to good health.

## Beta-hydroxy-β-methylbutyrate (HMB)

A minor leucine metabolite, HMB, is an ingredient commonly used to maintain muscle in elderly populations. A recent systematic review and meta-analysis has substantiated that HMB supplementation preserves muscle mass in older adults (Wu et al, 2012). Since it crosses the blood–brain barrier in rats, the effect of HMB in the brain is being explored. The beneficial effects of HMB have been proposed to be mediated through inhibiting proteolysis and upregulating the growth hormone/IGF-1 axis, mTOR signalling and presumably cholesterol biosynthesis (Zanchi et al, 2011). Mammalian target of rapamycin signalling is known to regulate autophagy, which is a dysregulated pathway recently implicated in age-related neuromuscular dysfunction. Overall, HMB seems to be promising for the ageing neuromuscular system.

## Creatine

Creatine is a nonessential nutrient naturally synthesised in the mammalian body from glycine, arginine and methionine that helps to supply cellular energy. It is stored as phosphocreatine in tissues. This high-energy phosphate group can be used to resynthesise ATP from ADP. Considering the high-energy needs of muscle and nervous tissue, creatine plays a vital role, especially in ageing when there is mitochondrial dysfunction.

Creatine is also found in meat and additively contributes to circulating creatine and its storage. Creatine supplementation, generally in the form of creatine monohydrate, seems to be beneficial for cognition and muscle performance.

Moon et al (2013) suggests that creatine supplementation, even without resistance training, in the elderly can potentially delay muscle atrophy and improve muscular endurance, muscular strength and bone strength. Dietary incorporation of guanidinoacetic acid (a natural precursor to creatine) is currently being investigated as a performance-enhancing supplement.

## Dietary Phospholipids

Dietary milk fat globule membrane (MFGM), composed of macronutrients and a substantial amount of phospholipids (e.g. phosphatidylcholine, phosphatidylserine, and sphingomyelin), may be beneficial for the neuromuscular system in ageing adults. The dietary phospholipids support in developing the nervous system of rodents. Because of this, it is unsurprising that MFGM supplementation with exercise in mice has been shown to improve age-related deficits in muscle function.

## Amino Acids are the most Potent Activators of mTOR

**Leucine is a potent stimulator of MPS:** Among the EAAs, branched-chain amino acids seem to be the most responsible for directly stimulating MPS. Leucine, one particular branched-chain amino acid, has been acknowledged to be a potent stimulator of MPS by mechanisms that involve mammalian target of rapamycin (mTOR) signalling and improved lean body mass (Fig. 10.2). It has been suggested that leucine is responsible for enhancing the ability to stimulate muscle protein anabolism in older adults when combined with physical activity (Dewansingh et al, 2018). Milk protein consists of whey with a high amount of leucine.

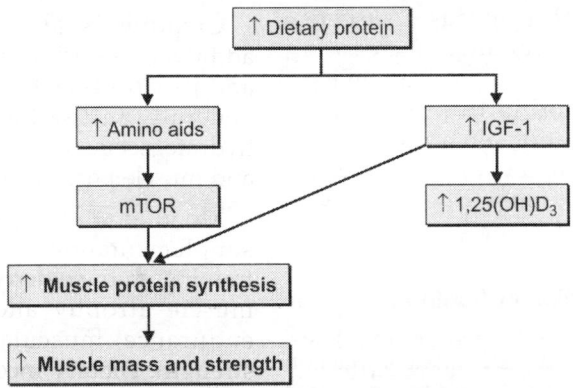

**Fig. 10.2:** Dietary protein increases serum levels of amino acids and IGF-1. IGF-I, insulin like growth factor-1; mTOR, mammalian target of rapamycin. *Adapted from* Bonjour et al (2013) and Rizzoli et al (2014)

However, considering that an age-related deficit in the muscle anabolic response to nutritional stimuli exists, a higher proportion of leucine is required for optimal stimulation of MPS in the elderly. With reference to the impaired response to anabolic stimuli in aged muscle, it has been suggested that a defect in activating an mTOR signalling protein (S6K1) that targets a ribosomal component to stimulate MPS is likely responsible.

The European Society for Clinical and Economic Aspects of Osteoporosis and Osteoarthritis has stated that the pathways through which dietary protein influences muscle synthesis are either via the activation of mammalian/mechanistic target of rapamycin (mTOR) and aromatic amino acids or via an increase in serum IGF-1. In other words amino acids are the most potent activators of mTOR, which stimulate muscle protein synthesis and consequently muscle strength. IGF-1 can directly affect both muscle synthesis, but also indirectly via vitamin D, as increases in serum IGF-1 also stimulate the renal production of 1,25-dihydroxyvitamin-D$_3$ [1,25(OH)$_2$D$_3$] (Fig. 10.2).

In addition to appropriate dietary calcium intake, sufficient serum vitamin D levels are important for skeletal health. Vitamin D also stimulates gene expression by involvement in cell development, differentiation and growth as well as stimulating muscle protein synthesis. 1,25-dihydroxyvitamin-D$_3$ contributes to improved balance and physical function via the vitamin D receptors in muscle tissue.

## Physical Activity-cum-Nutrient Supplementation Promote Healthy Neuromuscular Ageing

Physical activity is important for healthy neuromuscular ageing. Further, nutritional supplementation may be beneficial for promoting healthy neuromuscular ageing because they target precise mechanisms that are affected during the ageing process:

1. Vitamin D can promote myotrophic, neurotrophic and anti-inflammatory effects.
2. Omega-3 fatty acids can positively affect muscle transcriptome, specifically with pathways involved in mitochondrial function, muscle integrity and anabolism.
3. HMB can be neurotrophic, anticatabolic and indirectly anabolic.
4. Creatine can improve cellular bioenergetics.
5. Dietary phospholipids may have both neurotrophic and myotrophic effects.

## LOW GRADE INFLAMMATION IN AGEING AND DIETARY INTERVENTIONS TO CONTROL INFLAMMAGEING

### Ageing and Immunosenescence

One common characteristic of ageing is immunosenescence. Immunosenescence refers to decline in innate and acquired

immune function and it increases susceptibility to infection. With continued increase in
life expectancy, many older people are living
with one or more morbidities. Ageing is
associated with alterations in a number of
physiological systems and with a generalised
decline in function. Some individuals age
without showing these features.

## Low Grade Inflammation in Ageing

Inflammageing is the ageing process that has
been associated with the presence of low-
grade subclinical inflammation. The inflammatory response is beneficial as an acute,
transient reaction to limit the harmful
conditions. This response facilitates the
defence, repair, turnover and adaptation of
many tissues. However, chronic and low
grade inflammation is likely to be detrimental
for many tissues and for normal functions.
This is from two sources: (1) chronic antigenic
overload and an inability of immune cell
output, e.g. from thymus, to keep up with the
demand for naive cells (2) increased serum
levels of several inflammatory mediators in
the aged people.

These pro-inflammatory mediators in the
bloodstream include acute phase proteins
(CRP and serum amyloid A), cytokines (TNF-
α, IL-6 and IL-8) and adhesion molecules
(sICAM-1 and sVCAM-1), amongst others.
Based on the research studies, it is indicated
that inflammageing does not simply reflect an
increase of pro-inflammatory markers but an
overall activation of inflammatory systems
that probably also promotes a concomitant
rise in the levels of anti-inflammatory
mediators.

## Central Role of Inflammageing in Chronic Conditions of Ageing

This low grade inflammation (LGI) is seen to
contribute many of the common declines in
function, health and well-being that accom-
pany ageing (Fig. 10.3). Indeed, there are
many studies reporting strong links between
inflammation, morbidity and mortality. Thus,
it is highly relevant to healthy ageing and to

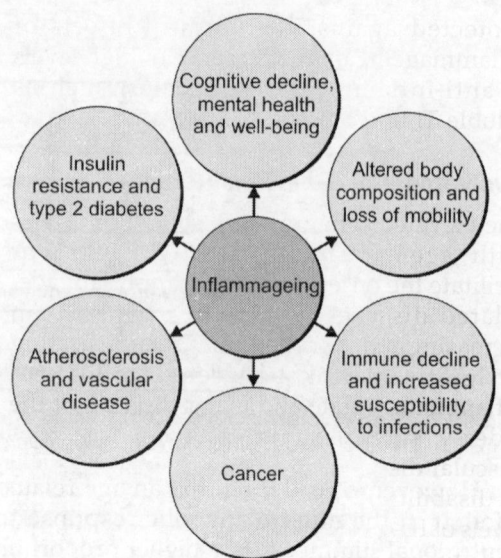

**Fig. 10.3:** Central role of inflammageing in chronic conditions of ageing. *Source:* Calder et al (2017)

improving well-being to prevent, slow or
reverse the process of inflammageing. Calder
et al (2017) has provided an overview of low
grade inflammation (LGI) and determine the
potential drivers and the effects of the "inflamed" phenotype observed in the elderly.
They have discussed the role of gut microbiota and host immune system crosstalk, the
gut-brain axis and some of the major health
complications associated to LGI in the elderly,
including susceptibility to infections and
cancers (Fig. 10.3). The possibility of manipulating LGI through nutritional interventions also has been dealt with.

The term "immunobiography" has been
recently suggested in an effort to capture the
lifelong exposure to antigens and inflammatory stimuli (Grignolio et al, 2014).
Overall, these data suggest that it is the
balance between pro- and anti-inflammatory
mediators that matters and this idea is
consistent with the hypothesis that human
longevity is paradoxically compatible with a
certain degree of inflammageing, likely
optimally counter-balanced by the concomitant increase/upregulation of anti-
inflammatory responses (Franceschi et al,
2007). Thus, long living persons may be

protected against the harmful effects of inflammageing by the presence of high levels of anti-inflammatory molecules, such as soluble TNF receptors.

### Involvement of LGI in Poor Health

The elevated inflammatory state that occurs with ageing can potentially trigger or facilitate the onset of the most important age-related diseases (Fig. 10.3). There are an increasing number of studies demonstrating a significant link between a mild pro-inflammatory state and major diseases of the elderly such as atherosclerosis, cardio-vascular diseases and type II diabetes, as well as disability and mortality. High circulating levels of IL-6 can predict the onset of disability and are positively associated with higher risk of mortality; IL-1β with angina, congestive heart failure and dyslipidemia; fibrinogen with type 2 diabetes.

Many possible triggers of LGI have been proposed, ranging from dysfunctional mitochondria (and consequent oxidative stress) to an imbalance in gut microbiota (termed dysbiosis) to excess of nutrients, e.g. free fatty acids and glucose (Calder et al, 2017). **Common triggers for LGI are debris arising from cellular damage and an imbalance in gut microbiota.** The terminal activators of the inflammatory response where most of the potential stimuli converge are (i) the nuclear factor kappa B (NFkB) pathway and (ii) the inflammasome platform.

 i. **The nuclear factor kappa B (NFκB):** The NFκB is a multimeric transcription factor that modulates gene expression by binding to specific DNA sequences (known as κB response elements) in gene promoters and enhancers (Lenardo and Baltimore, 1989; Hoffmann and Baltimore, 2006). In mammalian cells, there are five NFκB family members, RelA (p65), RelB, c-Rel, p50/p105 (NFκB1) and p52/p100 (NFκB2), and different NFκB complexes are formed as homo- and hetero-dimers.

NFκB can be activated by over 150 different stimuli, including cytokines, ultraviolet irradiation and bacterial or viral antigens. Moreover, it has a unique sensitivity to oxidative stress, as many of the agents activating NFκB are either modulated by oxidative stress or are pro-oxidants themselves (Chung et al, 2002) or are oxidised molecules, such as oxidised low density lipoprotein (oxidised LDL).

In turn, there is evidence that active NFκB participates in the control of transcription of more than 400 genes, the majority of them being involved in cell survival and inflammation (including cytokines such as IL-2, TNF-alpha and beta, IL-1β and IL-6, chemokines and their modulators, immunoreceptors, proteins involved in antigen presentation, cell adhesion molecules, acute phase proteins, stress response proteins, cell-surface receptors, regulators of apoptosis, growth factors).

 ii. **Inflammasomes** are cytoplasmatic platforms that trigger the maturation and release of pro-inflammatory cytokines such as IL-β.

Finally, different pro- and anti-inflammatory stimuli may be derived from the intestinal microbiota. Individuals capable of reaching the extreme limit of human life such as centenarians are characterised by an exceptionally healthy phenotype, i.e. a low number of diseases, low blood pressure, optimal metabolic and endocrine parameters and increased diversity in the gut microbiota and they are epigenetically younger than their chronological age. Such a remarkable phenotype is largely similar to that found in adults following a calorie-restricted diet (Franceschi et al 2018). The chronic inflammatory status of centenarians is peculiar, likely adaptable and less detrimental than that in younger people. Specific aspects of cross-talk between gut microbiota and the host seem to be involved in inflammageing.

### Immune-mediated Disorders and Gut Microbiota—host Crosstalk

In all the immune-mediated disorders ranging from inflammatory or metabolic diseases to neuropsychiatric disorders, the common features reported are an altered gut microbiota (often called dysbiosis). Dysbiosis is characterised by a reduced diversity with fewer butyrate-producing Firmicutes and more gram-negative pathobionts, together with a low grade to overt inflammatory status of the host. Evidence of microbiota-gut-brain axis (gut-brain signalling) interactions comes from the association of dysbiosis with central nervous disorders (i.e. autism, anxiety-depressive behaviours) and functional gastrointestinal disorders (i.e. irritable bowel syndrome). Further, such dysbiosis has been identified in the contexts of frailty in the elderly.

The very frequent association of dysbiosis with an altered inflammatory tone suggests an alteration in the crosstalk between commensal bacteria on the one side and intestinal epithelium including immune cells of the gut associated lymphoid tissue (GALT) on the other side. The interplay between the gut microbiota and the host immune system appears highly relevant in the elderly. Minor infections, nutritional or therapeutic stressors and immunosenescence can induce changes in the inflammatory tone that will inevitably alter the physicochemical conditions of the intestine.

Arboleya et al (2016) reviewed the current knowledge of the age-related changes in the gut microbiota phylogenetic composition. The emerged ones are: (1) larger variability of gut microbiota composition among the elderly with a concomitant reduced biodiversity and compromised stability, (2) with an increase in pathobionts and (3) a decrease in health-promoting bacteria such as bifidobacteria (Arboleya et al, 2016).

### How Does Gut Microbiota Affects Host Intestinal Epithelium, Immune-Inflammatory Response and Brain?

**Generation of catecholamines:** Intestinal microbiota activity results in the generation of catecholamines in the gut with an impact on gut physiology. Catecholamines such as

norepinephrine and dopamine are utilised in the central and peripheral nervous systems. These catecholamines regulate various types of body functions, such as cognitive abilities, mood and gut motility. Strong evidence suggests that gut microbiota has an important role in bidirectional interactions between the gut and the nervous system.

The epithelial layer consists of a single layer of epithelial cells that are sealed by tight junction proteins preventing paracellular passage. The lamina propria (connective tissue close to the epithelial cells) contains a large number of immune cells belonging to the innate immune system (e.g. macrophages, dendritic cells, mast cells) and the adaptive immune system (e.g. T cells, antibody-producing B cell derived plasma cells). Cells of the central and enteric nervous system are also innervated in the lamina propria.

When activated by immune modulators, lymphocytes release anti- and/or pro-inflammatory cytokines that trigger or regulate an inflammatory response. Further, the released cytokines signal the brain to activate immunomodulatory mechanisms like the cholinergic anti-inflammatory pathway, the hypothalamo-pituitary-adrenal (HPA) axis as well as the sympathetic nervous system (SNS). Furthermore, intestinal neurotransmitters or their precursors may modulate functions of the central nervous system. The neuronal efferent activation may also impact directly, the epithelium and the gut microbiota composition.

**Factors leading to chronic low grade inflammation:** Factors affecting intestinal barrier function include food-derived allergens, bacteria (pathogenic and commensal) and microbial compounds (lipopolysaccharides), metabolites such as short chain fatty acids (SCFAs), tryptophan-related metabolites, neurotransmitters and peptides, as well as drugs such as non-steroidal anti-inflammatory drugs (NSAIDs) and proton pump inhibitors (PPIs). SCFAs affect the intestinal mucosa as well as peripheral tissues. Intestinal barrier function may get impaired. Further, alterations in the gut microbial population and changes in gut permeability may contribute directly to chronic low grade inflammation.

For example, increased gut permeability has been shown to lead to the diffusion of lipopolysaccharide (LPS; endotoxin) into the circulation, thus promoting the development of chronic low-grade endotoxaemia and the activation of inflammatory processes. An important discovery has been the link between the gut microbiota and host behaviour via gut-brain signalling.

## LGI Mediated Alteration of Brain, Immune and Metabolic Functions

Pro-inflammatory cytokines (e.g. IL-6, IL-1β, TNF-α) released peripherally by activated immune cells have access to the brain through non-exclusive humoral, neural and cellular pathways (Capuron and Miller, 2011). Within the brain, pro-inflammatory cytokines are responsible for a large number of neurochemical and neurobiological changes impacting different systems. Moreover, the gut and the brain are highly connected through endocrine, immune and neural pathways (Collins et al, 2012) (Fig. 10.4).

Indeed the interactions of the gut microbiota with the host extend beyond the immune system and its inflammatory component and include metabolic organs such as the adipose tissue and liver and also the brain. Many of these interactions are bidirectional. Now strong evidence is available for a role of this gut-brain axis in the regulation of major brain functions, including mood and cognitive functions. The result of this is poor health and impaired well-being associated with ageing.

Pro-inflammatory cytokines potently modulate the activity of the neuroendocrine system. Under normal conditions, the activation of inflammatory signals is associated with the stimulation of the hypothalamic-pituitary-adrenal (HPA) axis, leading to the production of corticoid hormones, including cortisol, with strong immunoregulatory/anti-inflammatory effects necessary to counteract and resolve inflammation. However, with low grade inflammation (e.g. ageing), dysregulation of the HPA axis may occur, thus leading to an exacerbation of inflammation.

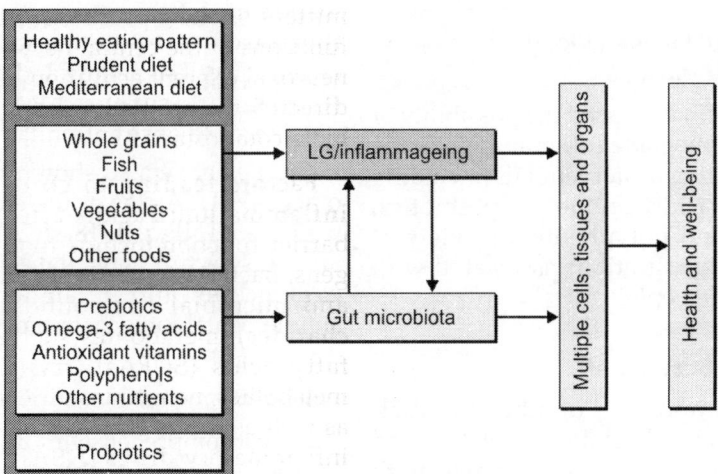

**Fig. 10.4:** Dietary ingredients and supplements are linked to health and well-being through modulation of gut microbiota and low grade inflammation. *Source:* Calder et al (2017)

## The Rationale for Targeting LGI to Improve Health in the Elderly

The National Institute on Ageing (NIA) launched the Interventions Testing Programme (ITP) in the year 2000 to evaluate prolongevity drugs in genetically heterogeneous mice (Warner et al, 2000) to extend longevity (lifespan and health span) by using non-steroidal anti-inflammatory drugs (NSAIDs). For primary prevention of cardiovascular diseases, particularly in 'at risk diabetic' patients, initial evidence also supported use of low dose NSAIDs classically with aspirin in a range of 75–325 mg/day for cardioprotection.

Long-term use (defined as > 24 months) of anti-inflammatory and/or antiplatelet treatment with NSAIDs demonstrate some efficacy in reducing the risk or severity of some age-related diseases. For instance, it is shown that long-term use of NSAIDs in arthritis patients has a protective effect against Alzheimer's disease (AD).

A concept of dietary low-dose aspirin fortification was even proposed as a cost-effective public health intervention (Mohapatra and Hota, 2013). Thus, the notion to lower LGI as way of improving health in the elderly is attractive to reduce incidence or severity of age-related functional decline and disease.

## Manipulating LGI in the Elderly by Nutritional Interventions

Calder et al (2017) discussed the possibility of manipulating **low grade inflammation** in the elderly by nutritional interventions (including omega-3 fatty acids, probiotics, prebiotics, antioxidants and polyphenols) in view of major health complications associated with LGI in the aged people.

## Plant Products Based Diet

Among the components of a healthy diet, higher intake of whole grains, vegetables and fruits, nuts and fish are all associated with lower inflammation (Calder et al, 2011). Magnesium is present in the centre of the chlorophyll molecule, with plants being a major dietary source. Magnesium is required to convert vitamin D to its active steroid hormone form (Rosanoff et al, 2016). Healthy diets are associated with lower concentrations of the inflammatory mediators like CRP and TNF-$\alpha$.

## Omega-3 Fatty Acids

Increased intake of long-chain omega-3 polyunsaturated fatty acids (PUFAs) results in increased proportions of those fatty acids in inflammatory cell phospholipids (Calder, 2015). DHA/EPA are present in high levels in the central nervous system and both are important for brain and retinal structure and function. DHA/EPA are important for vitamin D steroid hormone effectiveness (Patrick and Ames, 2015). Low blood levels of DHA/EPA are shown to be associated with a faster rate of telomere shortening, a marker of cell ageing.

The incorporation of eicosapentaenoic acid (EPA) and docosahexaenoic acid (DHA) into human inflammatory cells is partly at the expense of arachidonic acid resulting in less substrate available for synthesis of the classic inflammatory eicosanoids like prostaglandin $E_2$. Through this altered eicosanoid production omega-3 PUFAs could affect inflammation and inflammatory processes, although they also exert non-eicosanoid mediated actions on cell signalling and gene expression (Calder, 2015). Thus, EPA and DHA are considered to have anti-inflammatory effects.

Studies have also shown that long-chain omega-3 PUFAs lower the concentrations of CRP, IL-6, TNF-$\alpha$, IL-18, sICAM-1, sVCAM-1, and sE-selectin. Thus, there is quite a lot of evidence for anti-inflammatory effects of supplemental long chain omega-3 PUFAs.

## Probiotics

The most comprehensive study conducted by Moro-Garcia et al (2013) indicated that probiotic consumption (*Lactobacillus delbrueckii* subspp. bulgaricus 8481) over 6 months could counteract some hallmarks of immuno-senescence related to T cell immunity (i.e. increased number of recent thymus emigrant CD31+ T cells, decreased number of CD8+ CD28 null T cells and prevented cyto-megalovirus reactivation).

## Prebiotics

Prebiotics are best defined as dietary com-pounds that promote favourable intestinal colonisation by bacteria and/or bacterial release of anti-inflammatory fermentation products (Slavin, 2013). Calder et al (2017) summarises the details of studies in which prebiotics or fibres have been investigated in groups of adults (most of these interventions were conducted in an "at risk" population (i.e. type-2 diabetic and/or obese individuals). The interventions consistently lower the concentrations of several inflammatory markers and particularly C-reactive protein (CRP). Therefore, it is highly plausible that microbiota modulation by prebiotic fibres reduces LGI.

## Antioxidants

i. **Vitamin E:** Vitamin E supplementation to adults (mean age 56 years) had signi-ficantly lowered plasma CRP concen-trations compared with non-users (Schwab et al 2015). Vitamin E admini-stered at 200 mg/day together with fish oil for three months was able to blunt the inflammatory response of stimulated blood mononuclear cells (PMBCs) in elderly subjects (> 65 years).

iii. **Lycopene:** Administration of 5.7 mg/day of lycopene as part of a formulated soft drink significantly lowered TNF-α production in healthy humans aged about 26 years (Riso et al, 2006). Similarly administration of lycopene (6 or 15 mg/day) for eight weeks to healthy men aged 22–57 years significantly decreased plasma concentrations of the adhesion proteins sICAM-1 and sVCAM-1 and the higher dose also decreased CRP concen-tration (Kim et al, 2011).

iii. **Astaxanthin:** Astaxanthin administration at 2 mg daily for eight weeks to healthy young adult females significantly lowered the plasma CRP concentration (Park et al, 2010).

iv. **(Poly)phenols:** Plant (poly)phenols have been suggested as anti-inflammatory molecules (Calder et al, 2009). Immune modulating functional plant compounds such as 6-gingerol and resveratrol may be used as safe and natural feed additives to control inflammation and disease. The most common dietary sources of (poly) phenols and their anti-inflammatory actions are mentioned here.

Tea is rich in (poly)phenolic molecules, most of which are catechins. There is strong evidence in experimental models and in animals that suggest anti-inflammatory effects of tea and tea components, particularly epigallocatechin gallate (EGCG) (Deka and Vita, 2011). Neyestani et al (2010) reported a decrease in CRP concentration following consumption of black tea extract for four weeks in 46 patients with type-2 diabetes mellitus. Steptoe et al (2007) also reported a decrease in CRP concentration and in pro-inflammatory monocyte-platelet aggregates following four weeks of black tea con-sumption in healthy men aged 18–55 years. The anti-inflammatory effects of green tea were similar to those of cocoa and the former also lowered fibrinogen concentration (Stote et al, 2012).

Cocoa components have healthful effects. Cocoa and its products appear to exert anti-inflammatory effects in humans. These include inhibitory effects on leukocytes activation, reduced CRP concentration, anti-inflammatory effects in terms of lower concentration of adhesion molecules and reduced plasma biomarkers of endothelial dysfunction and inflammation.

Olives and their derivatives, such as extra virgin olive oil, olive oil and olive mill waste water (OMWW) are rich in phenolic com-pounds, which other vegetable oils do not contain. *In vitro*, hydroxytyrosol has been shown to have anti-inflammatory properties, via its inhibition of cyclo- and lipoxygenase enzymes. *In vivo*, OMWW was shown to lower circulating concentrations of CRP in adults with osteoarthritis. Bogani et al (2007) reported significantly lower leukotriene $B_4$ (LTB$_4$) accumulation in plasma in the extra virgin (i.e. phenol-rich) olive oil diet as compared with olive oil (i.e. phenol poor) and corn oil (i.e. phenol devoid) diets in humans (Bogani et al, 2007).

## Vitamin D

Vitamin D is not an antioxidant. It performs more than just its initially assigned function of maintaining bone health. It is included here because of its emerging multiple roles in a number of disorders involving inflammation. Indeed, the biochemical bases of immune-modulatory and anti-inflammatory roles of vitamin D are quite strong, in that macrophages can synthesise the active form of vitamin D and possess a vitamin D receptor (VDR) (Yin and Agrawal, 2014). Extensive evidence shows that vitamin D deficiency directly causes (or indirectly it has been associated with) a large number of diseases that affect healthy ageing, such as all cause mortality, cancer, cardiovascular disease (CVD), diabetes, brain function and so forth (Ames, 2018). Since, the elderly are often vitamin D deficient, its supplementation needs warranted. Newer evidence overrules the toxicity of vitamin D.

Calder and coworkers concluded that slowing, controlling or reversing low grade inflammation (LGI) is likely to be an important way to prevent, or reduce the severity of this inflammageing. One of the important triggers for LGI is an imbalance in gut microbiota. Since dietary components contribute to determining gut microbiota composition and diversity, nutrition has a key role in influencing health and well-being through microbiota-mediated effects. Hence healthful nutrients/feedstuffs that are associated with lower inflammation help healthy ageing.

## FREE RADICALS—MITOCHONDRIAL MUTATIONS—AGEING PROCESS

Free radicals are implicated in various diseases via generation of oxidative stress. Free radical production is unavoidable. Therefore, a comprehensive antioxidant defence system is present within the body to counteract the free radicals and their products and to keep them in check, which is essential for healthy life.

Mitochondrion is a membranous structure and is the 'power plant' of the cell. Mitochondrial membranes are rich in unsaturated fatty acids and hence are more susceptible to lipid peroxidation. **Mitochondria are the only sites outside the nucleus that contain DNA.** Mitochondria tend to be more prevalent in tissues requiring energy, including the central nervous system, heart, skeletal muscles, kidneys, liver, retina and pancreas.

### Free Radicals—Mitochondrial Mutations

Free radicals produced during oxygen processing are corrosive and can damage the vulnerable mitochondrial DNA and mitochondrial membranes. It is reported that **mitochondrial DNA** normally mutates 5 to 10 times faster than **nuclear DNA.** Such mutations may be inherited or acquired, due to environmental exposure to heavy metals, etc. It is suggested that mutations in the mitochondrial DNA may cause impaired oxygen processing. Consequently, the changes in cell's energy production somehow contribute to the ageing process and the development of degenerative diseases.

### Telomeres

Telomeres are repetitive noncoding DNA components (TTAGGG in vertebrates) located at the end of chromosomes to protect from degradation of coding sequences (Blackburn et al, 2006). Telomere is a segment of DNA located at the end of chromosome tip. The DNA that forms the telomere consists of the sequence 5'-TTAGGG-3', which is referred to as "telomeric repeat" since, it is randomly repeated. It reads as TTAGGG. TTAGGG.

TTAGGG... and so on. Although the bulk of telomeric DNA is double-stranded, the extreme terminus is single-stranded. Thus telomeres are composed of long strings of GT-rich hexanucleotide repeats that cap the ends of eukaryotic chromosomes.

## Telomeres are Hypothesised to Serve as a Countdown Clock for Somatic Cells

The primary function of telomeres is to protect the ends of chromosomes from recombination and degradation, without loss of essential genetic material and thus telomere is involved in replication and stability. A second function of telomeres is to provide some disposable DNA to accommodate the wastage that occurs when linear DNA molecules are replicated. Thereby a portion of telomeric material at the end of a DNA strand is lost during cell division rather than important coding DNA. Hence, the telomeres at the end of eukaryotic chromosomes progressively shorten (each strand will generally fall 100 bp or more) with each cycle of replication. Once telomeres shorten to a critical length, the cell encounters a proliferation block where it either ceases to divide (cellular senescence) or undergoes programmed cell death (apoptosis). That is why telomeres are hypothesised to serve as a countdown clock for somatic cells.

## Telomerase

The telomeres shorten each time a cell divides not only because of the end replication problem, but also by oxidative stress and lengthened by the enzyme telomerase and DNA exchange during mitosis. Telomerase is a reverse transcriptase enzyme responsible for elongating the telomeres to maintain their function. Most somatic cells in adult organisms do not express telomerase. Enzyme telomerase is active only in germ cells during embryogenesis, in adult stem cells and in activated immune cells (Kim et al, 1994). In addition, telomeric DNA is capped by a shelterin protein complex to protect from all aspects of DNA damage response and several

forms of double-strand break repair (Zhang et al, 2016).

The enzyme telomerase is important for long-term cell proliferation and genome stability, because it elongates telomeric DNA. Organisms are able to generate progeny that contain full length telomeres thanks to the intervention of the enzyme telomerase. Telomerase is less active in cells that divide less often. Using an RNA template, telomerase adds GT-rich hexanucleotide repeat sequences up to several thousand nucleotides in length (in humans) to the ends of linear DNA molecules to restore their telomeres to full length. In adult somatic cells, the absence or insufficient amount of telomerase results in telomere length attrition, which is associated with ageing.

## Telomere Length Reduction—Normal Ageing

Telomere shortening is a marker of cell ageing. See later for information on the telomere and its length reduction along with the related (Fig. 10.5), in normal ageing process and ageing with healthy and unhealthy lifestyles (P.J. Kenneelly, 2015).

Each time a somatic cell divides and the DNA within the cell is copied, the telomeres shorten. This process continues until the telomeres reach a critical length called the Hayflick limit (after the scientist who discovered it) at which point the cell stops dividing. When a cell stops replicating, it enters into a period of decline known as **cellular senescence**, which is the cellular equivalent of ageing. Moreover, disruption of the shelterin can uncap telomeres and induce cellular senescence (Liu et al, 2018; Zhang et al, 2016). It is hence proposed that both telomere length shortening and shelterin disruption are causes of cellular senescence (Liu et al, 2018).

As more and more cells within the body enter senescence, it progressively loses the capacity to replace lost or damaged cells Fig. 10.5, which depicts telomere length reduction in the normal ageing process in human beings, while Figs 10.6 and 10.7 show

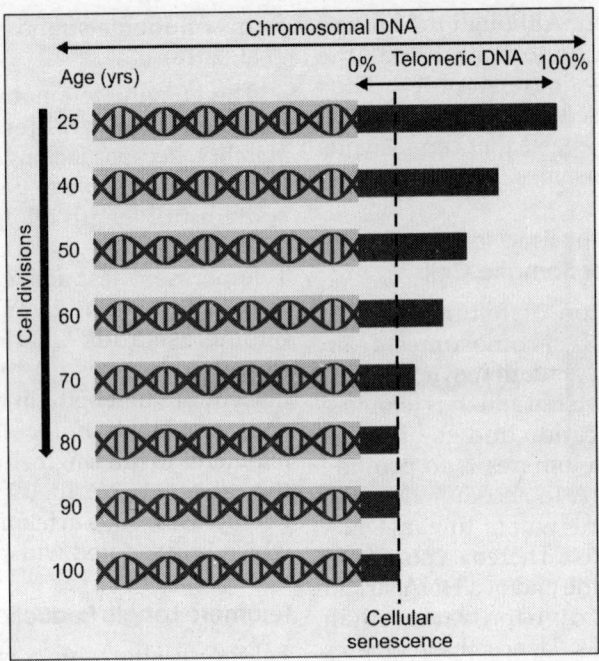

**Fig. 10.5:** Telomere length reduction - normal ageing. The critical telomere length limit for cellular senescence is seen at age 80 years (arbitrary)

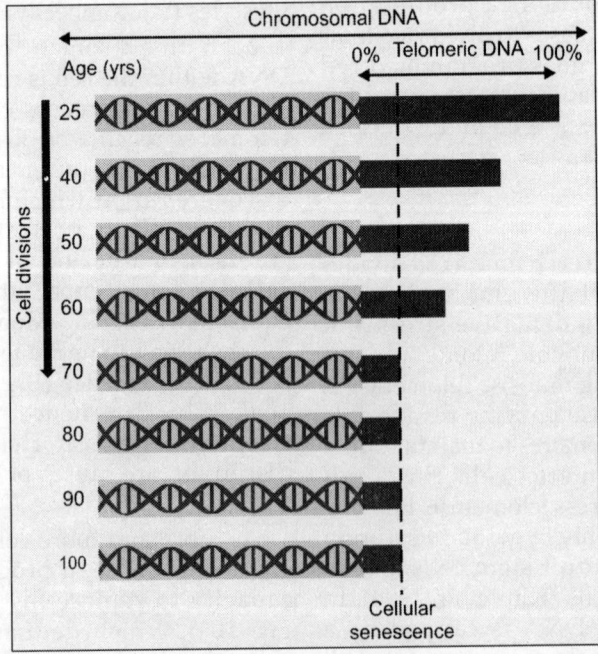

**Fig. 10.6:** Telomere length reduction - normal ageing with unhealthy lifestyle. The critical telomere length limit for cellular senescence is seen at age 70 years (arbitrary)

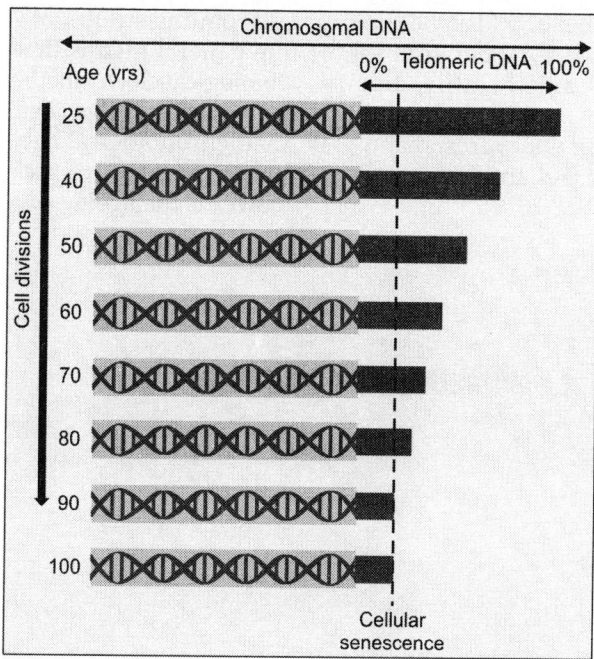

**Fig. 10.7:** Telomere length reduction—normal ageing with healthy lifestyle. The critical telomere length limit for cellular senescence is seen at age 90 years (arbitrary)

telomere length reduction with unhealthy and healthy lifestyles, respectively.

### Healthy and Unhealthy Lifestyles— Telomere Length Reduction

Telomere shortening can be influenced by genetic factors (e.g. single nucleotide polymorphisms [SNPs] in the genes important for telomeric maintenance), epigenetic factors, and other factors such as sex, body mass index, ethnicity, inflammation level, tobacco smoking, alcohol consumption and physical activity.

Mitochondria are the site of the electron transport chain, by far the largest source of reactive oxygen species (ROS) in the cell. ROS are highly reactive, often participating in chain reactions that multiply their impact and are continually generated as a byproduct of the complex network of redox reactions taking place in the electron transport chain. Unhealthy lifestyle, which manifests in the form of generation of large number of ROS, inflicts greater damage to the cells over time.

Unhealthy lifestyle hasten the process and the somatic cells enter a state of 'cellular senescence' at earlier age (Fig.10.6), while healthy lifestyle reverses the trend and thereby enhances the lifespan (Fig. 10.7) of the individual.

Telomere is considered a sort of biological clock that measures the lifespan of a cell and an organism. Shorter telomeres are associated with decreased life expectancy and an increased rate of developing age related chronic diseases (Heidinger et al, 2012).

Systemic exposures that contribute to oxidative stress and age-related disease, e.g. smoking, obesity and chronic stress, have been associated with shorter telomere in white blood cells. Additionally, an accelerated telomere shortening in humans has been linked with increased intake of red meat, processed meat, sweetened carbonated beverages, sodium and white bread.

On the otherhand, healthy lifestyle choices such as tobacco abstinence, moderate physical activity, lower BMI and healthy dietary patterns (grains, fruits, vegetables and nuts) promote more stable telomere presumably via enhanced antioxidant and anti-inflammatory activities (Davinelli et al, 2019).

From the studies of Cawthon et al (2003), the general idea is that telomeres may be a "biological clock" that reflects an individual's physiological age/health more accurately than chronological age. In other words, the longer the telomere, the healthier the cells and slower is the ageing process.

# 11

# Transition Phase and Immune System

## IMMUNITY AND INFLAMMATION IN TRANSITION DAIRY ANIMALS

### Immunosuppression in Early Lactation

World-wide dairy herd records' analysis indicated that transition cow problems account for more than 50% of mature animal health problems on a typical dairy farm. There is also a well-documented publication indicating an alteration in immune function during the weeks around calving (Kerhli, 2015). In particular, the function of innate immune cells seems to be consistently impaired. Innate immune cells are those involved in quick recognition and clearance of pathogens, independent of pathogen-specific memory (antibodies).

### Why is the Immune System of Transition Dairy Animals Suppressed?

There is no simple answer to this question. However, studies with mastectomised cows suggest that the primary driver is lactation and the metabolic changes that come with it (Nonnecke et al, 2003). Many studies have demonstrated that metabolic diseases (e.g. ketosis) put cows at higher risk of contracting clinical infections; likewise, cows with infectious diseases (e.g. metritis) are also at higher risk of subsequent metabolic disorders. The inter-dependent nature of the immune and metabolic systems in the animal are only

now becoming clear, but high blood ketone and non-esterified fatty acid (NEFA) concentrations as well as hypocalcaemia are known to limit the responsiveness of immune cells to pathogenic signals. It is likely that the high rate of infections in early lactation can be attributed in part to immunosuppression.

### Inflammation and the Immune System

Animal producers need to pay close attention to inflammation and the immune system. While inflammation is necessary, it has visible impact on the animal performance. When an animal is sick, its feed intake decreases. At the same time, the nutrients meant for growth are redirected to immune cell function for its protection during an acute inflammatory response. When the immune response persists, the inflammation is termed chronic inflammation; nutrients and energy are diverted away from animal performance (including growth, production and reproduction) ultimately decreasing profitability.

### What is inflammation?

Inflammation is a normal biological response to stress involving a complex network of cells, intra- and extra-cellular stimuli, organs and tissues to maintain homeostasis. In healthy individuals, inflammation is a two step process where, initially, pro-inflammatory and anti-inflammatory mediators exert precise control in signalling leukocyte infiltration into the damaged area. This is followed by resolution—a return to and persistence of homeostasis. Eicosanoid class switching occurs during the transition between stages. As high levels of pro-inflammatory leukotrienes (LTs) or prostaglandins (PGs, $PGE_2$) are detected, there is a shift in production to pro-resolving lipoxins (LXs) and resolvins (Rvs) [LXs and Rvs are more potent anti-inflammatory molecules], which is consequential for inflammation resolution in diseases (Jain et al, 2018).

## Multiple Phenotypes of Inflammation

In other words, inflammation is the most prevalent manifestation of host defence in reaction to alterations in tissue homeostasis. It is elicited by innate immune receptors that recognise and detect infection, host damage and danger signalling molecules that activate a highly regulated network of immunological and physiological events for the purpose of maintaining homeostasis and restoring functionality. There are multiple phenotypes of inflammation based on the type of trigger or stimuli namely **physiological, pathological, metabolic, sterile inflammation** (Kogut et al, 2018). These stimuli can be of microbial (e.g. microbe-associated molecular patters [MAMPs]) or non-microbial (e.g. host metabolites).

Sterile and metabolic inflammations are, typically, chronic, low-grade inflammatory states resulting from innate immune system stimulation by non-infectious cellular components and metabolites. Features of modern animal production (e.g. increased feed intakes and nutrient excesses) are more likely to predispose these animals to, particularly chronic, inflammatory triggers/states, which may be minimised by thoughtful dietary strategies, including the use of enzymes (e.g. mannanase) to reduce dietary components (e.g. mannans) that may be recognised by PRRs.

**Common sources of inflammation:** There are several common inflammation sources. Two of the most common sources are poor gut integrity and heat stress.

**Poor gut integrity:** The gastrointestinal (GI) tract lining serves as an important barrier to prevent bacteria, pathogens and their toxins from passing through the intestinal lining and into the bloodstream. When a breakdown in the barrier occurs, this can lead to a condition called leaky gut. When a prolonged inflammatory response occurs in the GI tract, this decreases feed intake and animal performance.

**Heat stress:** When animals are under heat stress, blood flow is diverted away from the tissues that line the blood vessels within the stomach, digestive tract and other internal organs to the skin, which facilitates the heat dissipation process. However, the reduction in blood flow causes a decrease in the amount of oxygen and energy available to the epithelial layer of cells lining the gastrointestinal tract, allowing pathogens and their toxins to enter the bloodstream, due to leaky gut.

## Inflammation in Postpartum Dairy Animals

Inflammation is a key component of the immune response to infection or tissue-damage. Immune cells that first sense pathogens or signs of traumatised cells release signals that activate pain sensors, promote blood flow to the local tissue and cause fever, accounting for the traditional signs of inflammation. Additionally, the systemic effects of inflammation include an alteration of liver function, typically called the acute phase response (APR). Most of these responses are beneficial for recruiting innate immune cells to the site of immune activation and for inhibition of bacterial growth, but they come at a cost to the animal.

The presence of an APR in postpartum dairy cows is well-established (Bradford et al, 2015). The process of parturition requires the initiation of a non-infectious inflammation, which is coupled with an intense oxidative stress due to galactopoiesis, marked reduction in feed intake and endotoxin overload. Numerous studies conducted during the past ten years have demonstrated that inflammatory and acute-phase mediators are elevated in the days after parturition, even in apparently healthy animals.

Dairy animals orchestrate an adaptive homeorhetic process, inducing insulin resistance in peripheral tissues to spare glucose for the mammary gland, potentially sacrificing nutrient supply to immune cells to some degree. Hence, as insulin resistance is associated with inflammation, it is possible that endogenous inflammation is an adaptive mechanism of dairy cows to regulate partitioning of nutrients and energy balance. Although the process of parturition is initiated by a 'sterile inflammation', dairy animals with a higher degree of inflammation after parturition have greater incidence of diseases, lower milk yields and poorer reproductive efficiency. These associations of inflammation imply a subsequent or parallel inflammation with infectious origin.

## Inflammatory Responses to Infection

During infections such as mastitis or metritis, immune cells in the body recognise invading pathogens and become activated. When the infection is caused by gram-negative bacteria, endotoxin released by the bacteria also activates immune cells. The activated immune cells release several inflammatory mediators such as nitric oxide, prostaglandins and cytokines (e.g. tumour necrosis factor alpha (TNFα), interleukin 1β, and interleukin 6). The pro-inflammatory cytokine tumour necrosis factor alpha (TNFα) has been implicated in several metabolic disorders, including fatty liver disease and insulin resistance in dairy cattle. Bradford and coworkers conducted several studies to confirm that TNFα-induced inflammation alters metabolic function in dairy cows. For cows in late lactation, TNFα infusion promoted hepatic triglyceride (TG) accumulation, with changes in hepatic mRNA profiles consistent with a shift from lipid oxidation to storage (Bradford et al, 2009).

One effect of cytokines is to activate production of acute phase proteins (APP) by the liver. The positive APPs include haptoglobin, serum amyloid A and C-reactive protein. These are regarded as markers of inflammation and thus mammary and uterine infections result in both local and systemic inflammation. In periparturient cows, TNFα increased circulating haptoglobin, reduced dry matter intake and milk yield, albeit without altering liver TG content (Yuan et al, 2013). Growing evidence suggests that inflammation may be a key factor in the development of many transition disorders and it results in suppressed immune function and altered nutrient metabolism; ultimately result in decreased productivity and productive life of dairy animals.

## Magnitude of this Inflammatory Condition on Animal Production

Although most transition dairy cows apparently experience a period of inflammation, the magnitude of this inflammatory condition varies greatly between dairy animals. Bertoni et al (2008) assessed the importance of this variation by measuring a panel of inflammatory markers (e.g. elevated haptoglobin [a positive acute phase protein, posAPP]) and separating the transition cows into quartiles for degree of inflammation. Cows in the highest quartile had (high haptoglobin) significantly lower milk yields than those in the lowest quartile (had high paraoxonase) throughout the first month of lactation, differing by 20% on day 28 of lactation (Bertoni et al, 2008). A variety of inflammatory stimuli suppress paraoxonase, a plasma biomarker (see below). Transition cows with high paraoxonase concentrations produced more milk. Such cows have lower concentrations of APPs and reactive oxygen metabolites (ROMs). Plasma concentrations of haptoglobin (posAPP) greater than 1.1 g/L were associated with a 947 L decrease in 305-day mature equivalent milk yield and elevated haptoglobin was also associated with a 19% decreased risk of conception. Abnormally high markers of inflammation are associated with poor production, health and fertility.

## Paraoxonases

The paraoxonases (PON1, PON2 and PON3) are antioxidant enzymes that have lactonase activity and degrade lipid peroxides in lipoproteins and cells. As such they have a role in protection against oxidation and inflammation. Infectious diseases are often associated with oxidative stress and an inflammatory response. Infection and inflammation trigger a cascade of reactions in the host and this is referred to as APR. This response is associated with dramatic changes in serum proteins and lipoproteins, including a decrease in serum paraoxonases.

## Factors that Promote Strong Immunity

With the growing interest in animal characteristics influencing infection risk, a number of factors have emerged as important for supporting strong immunity (Bradford, B.J., 2018). Data currently available suggest that cows have improved transition immune function when:

1. They are not exposed to significant heat stress during the dry period.

2. They calve with a body condition system between 2.5 and 3.5.

3. They are supplemented with antioxidants during the dry period.

4. Total serum calcium concentrations are maintained near 9 mg/dL.

5. Blood BHBA and NEFA concentrations stay below 1 mM during the transition.

Hence, it is important to manage the dairy animals well during dry period to prevent heat stress (if any), provide balanced feed, manage body condition, support calcium homeostasis and monitor oxidative balance.

Further, vaccines and dietary agents (e.g. dietary yeast product) are useful tools in promotion of adaptive immunity, while pharmacological tools are useful for promotion of innate immunity. The granulocyte colony-stimulating factor (GCSF) treatment, prior to the period of immunosuppression, stimulates the development and maturation of neutrophils, resulting in a fairly dramatic increase in the population of these key innate immune cells in circulation. In conditions favourable to environmental mastitis, the administration of GCSF significantly decreases the incidence of clinical mastitis (Hassfurther et al, 2015).

## CHANGES AND FUNCTIONALITY OF IMMUNE SYSTEM DURING THE TRANSITION PERIOD

### Critical Points in the Transition Period of Dairy Cows

The transition period is the most critical phase in the life of high yielding dairy cows. Cows are considered to be immunosuppressed in late lactation and available data suggest that the immune system is dysregulated around parturition. Trevisi and Minuti (2018) identified five critical points of the transition period:

i. Reduction of immune competence.

ii. Negative energy balance (NEB), resulting in mobilisation of adipose and muscle tissue.

iii. Hypocalcaemia, as a consequence of the delayed availability of calcium in the blood for the sudden and huge demand of the mammary gland for milk synthesis.

iv. An overt systemic inflammatory response around the time of calving, which commonly occurs immediately after calving even in the absence of signs of microbial infections or other pathologies.

v. A situation of oxidative stress (OS), due to the unbalanced availability of antioxidants in presence of phenomena that increase the production of potent pro-oxidant molecules.

Figure 11.1 reports the evolution of these five critical phenomena that characterise the transition period of healthy animals. Trevisi and Minuti (2018) pictorially depicted these imminent changes based on the available literature.

Most of the changes are concentrated at the time immediately after calving, except few modifications of the immune system occurring days before parturition. A comprehension of the origin of these modifications and the time of their appearance with respect

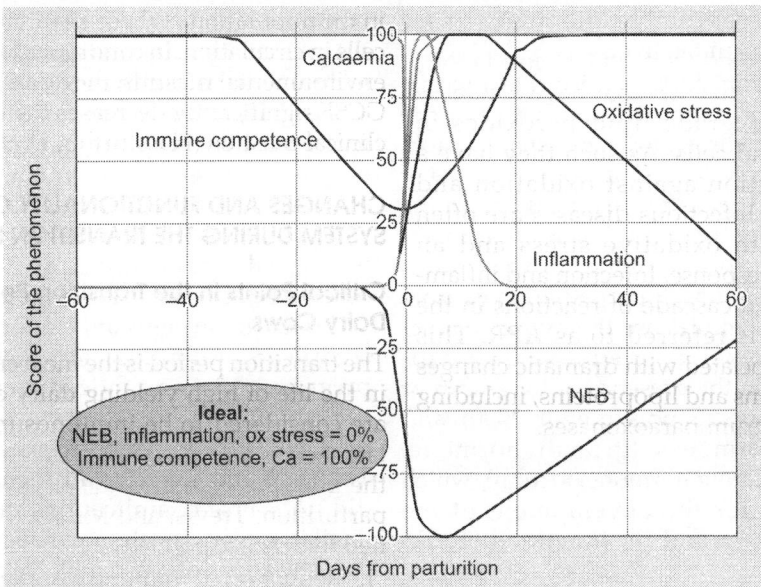

**Fig. 11.1:** Theoretical pattern of changes in healthy subjects during the transition period. Ideally, the NEB, inflammation and OS would be close to zero, whereas the immunocompetence and the calcaemia would be close to 100% of their optimal level. *Source:* Trevisi and Minuti, 2018

to calving appears pivotal to initiate a corrective follow-up action for the betterment of the transition cow/buffalo.

### Changes of the Immune System During the Transition Period

The immune system is an interactive network of lymphoid organs, cells and humoral factors, such as cytokines, that is organised to recognise, resist and eliminate contaminants (biotic or abiotic) that penetrate the body membranes (Bertoni et al, 2015). Conventionally, the system is divided into two components (innate and adaptive) on the basis of the speed and specificity of the reactions, but in reality the two parts are highly integrated and in continuous interplay (Daha, 2011). Recent evidence suggests that the innate component also has a memory-like behaviour (Bordon, 2014) and this concept may deeply modify the current understanding of many immune functions.

Innate immunity encompasses the physical, chemical and cellular elements of the immune system which provide immediate non-specific defence to the host against both biotic and abiotic inducers. Daha (2011) suggests that approximately 95% of infectious challenges are resolved by the response of the innate system, through a coordinated action of cells (neutrophils, monocytes, macrophages), humoral factors (i.e. complement, lysozyme) and the network of cytokines. Cells recognise specific molecules (e.g. pathogen associated molecular patterns and damage-associated molecular patterns, [PAMPs and DAMPs]) through receptors (pattern-recognition receptors, [PRRs]), which induce two types of responses: inflammation and phagocytosis (by neutrophils and macrophages) (Trevisi et al, 2016). The responses occur even if the host has never previously been exposed to these agents and are driven by the synthesis of several biochemical mediators. Among them, vasogenic compounds (such as histamine) and pro-inflammatory cytokines (PIC, for instance TNF$\alpha$, IL1$\beta$, IL6) attract immune cells into the damaged area and induce local inflammation, by the activation of the nuclear factor kappa B (NF$\kappa$B) signalling pathway. At a systemic level PIC also promote the acute-phase response (APR) in the liver.

It is important to recognise that there is bidirectional communication between the immune and neuroendocrine systems (Taub, 2008). The two systems share a common set of hormones and receptors. Thus, the immune system is under the control of sex hormones, which play a role as modulators of auto-immune disease onset/perpetuation (Cutolo et al, 2004). Examples are the hypothalamic-pituitary-adrenal axis, which has a suppressive role in the presence of long-term or chronic stressors (Sapolsky et al, 2000), and metabolic hormones (growth hormone, thyroid stimulating hormone, insulin), which are essential for the development of the immune system and its functions (Taub, 2008).

Variations occur in pro-inflammatory cytokine secretion around parturition. In the last part of pregnancy, the functionality of the immune system should remain active to counteract infectious agents and any possible injury. Nevertheless, several pieces of data suggest a reduction in the immunocompetence of mammals at this stage (Lacetera et al, 2005; Orsi et al, 2006; Raghupathy et al, 2000). The ratio among Th1 and Th2 (T helper cells which produce cytokines with opposite pro- and anti-inflammatory effects, respectively) is low during pregnancy (Raghupathy et al, 2000). It has been suggested that this low ratio is useful for a successful parturition because it optimises the foetomaternal immune interaction and vascularisation. Under these conditions, the concentration of PIC in plasma before parturition should be low, because they are mainly released by Th1 cells. At parturition, the ratio of Th1/Th2 should increase rapidly in the uterus, switching from a condition that provides tolerance for the foetus (high Th2) to a condition that offers protection against infectious agents (high Th1).

Moreover, Saito et al (2010) suggest that the T cell paradigm in pregnancy should also include Th17 and regulatory T (T reg) cells. These latter cells play central roles in immunoregulation, but their activity can be suppressed by immunoregulatory cytokines, including transforming growth factor (TGF)-β and IL10, or by cell-to-cell interaction. An imbalance between T reg and Th17 cells could be the pathogenic mechanism involved in preterm labour and pre-eclampsia, both associated with exaggerated systemic inflammatory changes (Saito et al, 2010). On the other hand, Orsi et al (2006) indicated that the Th1-Th2 dichotomy only poorly describes complex immunological process, such as pregnancy in mice. Indeed, very high concentrations of TNF-α during pregnancy of mice, which indicates an imbalance of Th1 and Th2 ratio and suggests a pregnancy at risk, did not cause complications in pregnancy. Similarly, cows in late pregnancy had higher concentrations of plasma PIC relative to those measured after parturition or in clinically healthy cows. Thus, in cows, a high concentration of PIC in plasma during the dry period does not seem to be critical for the maintenance of pregnancy (Trevisi et al, 2015) and may not even reflect the ratio of Th1 to Th2 cells.

Interestingly, relatively high and stable values of plasma PIC occurring in late pregnancy can nevertheless signal an immuno suppression status weeks before calving (Kehrli et al, 1989a; Kehrli et al, 1989b). This apparent contradiction suggests that the immune system remains active during late pregnancy, despite some functions of leukocytes being impaired or suppressed. However, besides immune cells, PIC can be released by many type of cells in the periphery, as well as by glial cells and neurons within the brain. The contribution of leukocytes is most important only when the immune system is challenged by pathogens or antigens. Cows in the transition period have a higher probability of experiencing events which challenge the immune system and promote the release of PIC. These events have biotic (i.e. pathogen, virus, parasites) and abiotic (i.e. climate, nutritional, social, metabolic) causes (Trevisi et al, 2016). Non-infectious sources are numerous and are particularly relevant in this critical physiological period. These include psychological stresses such as isolation, overcrowding, grouping, nutritional aspects, oxidative stress and environmental conditions.

The topic of immunosuppression during the transition period requires special mention. Some functions of the immune system are depressed before calving, such as the phagocytosis of neutrophils, the ability of lymphocytes to respond to mitogens and to produce antibodies, DNA synthesis in peripheral blood mononuclear cell (PBMC) and concentrations of relevant components in plasma, such as immunoglobulins, IFNγ, complement and lysozyme. In some of these studies, the alteration of immunity has been associated with various pathologies, including the recrudescence of existing intra-mammary infections or appearance of new mammary infections, postpartum uterine diseases such as retained placenta or metritis and also with obesity.

Hammon et al (2006) suggested that the negative energy status in late pregnancy can account for changes in neutrophil functions in Holstein cows and, in turn, can cause uterine disorders. Indeed, severe reduction of feed intake prior to parturition is an important factor for the impairment of immunity peripartum as discussed by Rukkwamsuk et al (1999) and Bertoni et al (2009).

Research to date suggests that immune dysfunctions before calving are due to a combination of endocrine and metabolic factors, but it is not clear if the reduced immunocompetence is a physiological condition of dairy cows or an early signal of disease induced by other events. In any case, the effects of this impairment become evident mainly after calving. With the purpose of clarifying the reason for the immune impairment, it is necessary to understand the actual onset of the alteration in immune functions during pregnancy.

More or less at the same time, cows present an overt systemic inflammatory response (Bertoni and Trevisi, 2013; Bionaz et al, 2007; Sordillo and Mavangira, 2014), which can be confirmed by a peak of actue phase proteins (APP) a few hours after calving, occurring in almost all cows independently of the appearance of full-blown infection at the uterine level. In other research, cows showed a peak of haptoglobin (one of the most specific positive acute phase proteins [posAPPs] of ruminants) within 24 hours of calving. Therefore, healthy cows appear to maintain functionality of the immune system until a few days before calving and then various functions such as diapedesis are depressed and others such as inflammation are strengthened.

## Are Dairy Cows Truly Immunosuppressed in Late Pregnancy?

The general paradigm that cows are immunosuppressed in the last part of the dry period seems to falter when the recent literature is taken into account along with the healthy (clinical and subclinical) conditions of the animals. Some functions are reduced, but the susceptibility to inflammation (one of the most important mechanisms of defence for the innate immune system) is increased. Transcriptomic data (Minuti et al, 2018) mainly indicates an increase in immune system activities and functions in circulating cells and supports the idea, also shared by Sordillo and Mavangira (2014) that the functions of the immune system are not suppressed, but merely dysregulated around calving. Thus, immunosuppression in periparturient cows represents an oversimplification that may cover a variety of conditions and factors.

## Why Should the Immune System be Dysregulated in Late Pregnancy?

Heyland et al (2006) have hypothesised that multiple external insults that could occur during the transition from dry off to calving are able to induce a systemic inflammatory response that is capable of attenuating the cellular immune response. Trevisi and Minuti (2018) has applied Heyland's hypothesis to the transition period, during which many immuno-challenging events occur that can determine the release of PIC (as presented in

Fig. 11.2) and an inflammatory response. The number and the severity of these challenging events may progressively reduce immuno-competence and increase susceptibility to inflammation, which reaches a maximum level at calving. Thus, the dysfunctional or unregulated inflammatory responses could represent the link between an increased incidence of metabolic and infectious diseases during the transition period (Sordillo and Raphael, 2013). Interestingly, many of the critical points of the transition period previously mentioned have strict interactions with the innate immune system (and inflammation). Specifically:

i. The severe body fat mobilisation alters immunocompetence (Lacetera et al, 2005).

ii. The production of reactive oxygen species (ROS) induces inflammation (Sordillo and Aitken, 2009; Sordillo and Mavangira, 2014).

iii. The presence of ketosis immediately after calving is exacerbated by the presence of inflammatory events (clinical or subclinical) in late pregnancy (Bertoni et al,

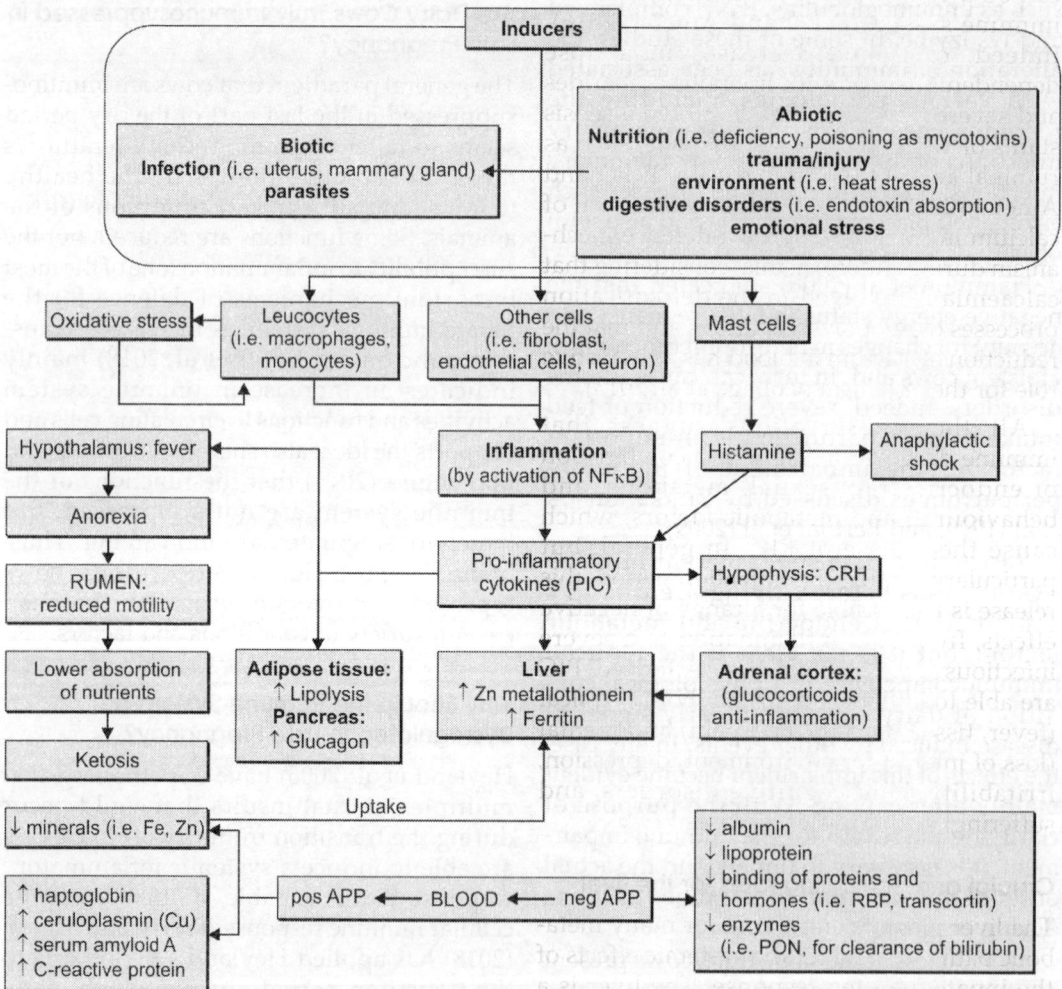

**Fig. 11.2:** Potential inducers of immune system response and of the activation of the inflammatory response and the main consequences in the dairy cow. *Source:* Trevisi and Minuti, 2018

2009). Indeed, the occurrence of inflammation before calving accentuates the peripartum reduction of feed intake, anticipates the mobilisation of body reserves and, thus, promotes ketosis, which is secondary to inflammation.

The concentration of calcium (Ca) in the plasma is a key mediator in several cell processes, including those related to immune system responses. A low concentration of calcium in the first two weeks postpartum is associated with decreased neutrophil functions (Martinez et al, 2012). Hypocalcaemia can be a consequence of challenges to the immune system (Eckel and Ametaj, 2016). Indeed, calcaemia decreases in a dose dependent manner with lipopolysaccharides and severe hypocalcaemia occurs in a sepsis status or with severe tissue damage, such as ruminal acidosis. For this reason, Eckel and Ametaj (2016) suggested that a decrease of calcium in plasma could be a defence mechanism during endotoxaemia, considering that calcaemia is involved in the detoxification processes of lipopolysaccharides and that the reduction of calcium in blood has a protective role for the organism (Collage et al, 2013).

All these observations suggest that immune dysfunction is due to a combination of endocrine (i.e. sexual, metabolic, and behavioural) and metabolic factors, which cause the release of PIC. In general, but particularly during the transition period, this release is responsible for a range of negative effects, from light inflammation to a severe infectious and metabolic disease. Indeed, PIC are able to initiate and sustain both physical (fever, tissue damage, and pain) and mental (loss of interest for environment, depression, irritability, mild cognitive disorders, and suffering) symptoms of diseases.

### Crucial and conflicting roles for the liver

The liver plays a central role for many metabolic pathways and for the systemic effects of the innate immune response. The liver is a vital organ that fulfills several functions in the metabolism of carbohydrates, proteins and lipids, the clearance of toxins and pathogens, and the regulation of immune responses. The activity of aspartate-aminotransferase (AST), gamma-glutamyl-transferase (GGT), glutamate dehydrogenase (GLDH) measured in blood is suitable for assessing liver cell integrity (Bertoni and Trevisi, 2013). It has been reported that elevated activities of AST and GGT are linked to fatty liver.

Regarding the immune response, the liver is involved in two main ways: it responds to PIC produced in other cells with the so-called acute phase response (APR) (Ceciliani et al, 2012) and it can also react against antigens that are metabolised locally and could lead to local tissue damage. The latter function is relevant in cases of severe toxicosis, but is less important in healthy, well-fed subjects. On the other hand, the APR is a prominent systemic reaction of the organism to local or systemic disturbances to its homeostasis that have many causes, i.e. infection, tissue injury, trauma or surgery, neoplastic growth or immunological disorders. Thus, APR is a common experience in animals whichever event triggers the innate immune system.

During the acute phase response, liver is activated and impaired at the same time (Fig. 11.2). The synthesis of several proteins, specifically positive acute phase proteins (posAPPs, i.e. C-reactive protein [CRP], serum amyloid A, haptoglobin, ceruloplasmin) are increased. The posAPPs have a protective role against pathogens, e.g. (1) in opsonisation and trapping of microorganisms and their products. (2) in activating complements, (3) in binding cellular remnants such as nuclear fractions, (4) in neutralising enzymes, scavenging free haemoglobin and radicals, and (5) in modulating the host's immune response. Some posAPPs are capable of capturing minerals (e.g. Fe, Zn) from the blood to reduce pathogen survival.

In addition, other functions of the liver are impaired due to the synthesis of common proteins being reduced, likely because of competition for substrates (Trevisi et al, 2016; Zhou et al, 2016). These proteins are called negative acute phase proteins (negAPP) and include albumin, enzymes (i.e. paraoxonase, enzymes for the clearance of bilirubin), apolipoproteins, carriers of lipophilic molecules (i.e. hormones such as cortisol and vitamins such as vitamin A) (Bernabucci et al, 2004; Trevisi et al, 2016). Several of these parameters are commonly used to interpret metabolic status, without considering the relationship with liver functionality.

**Monitoring liver functionality:** When APR occurs the liver is not damaged, but the profile of produced proteins is changed. It is possible to monitor liver functionality on the basis of the haematic variations in the posAPPs, negAPPs and other parameters related to APR. The plasma concentrations of these biomarkers fluctuate in accordance with the severity and duration of the inflammation. For a long time, the posAPPs were investigated as biomarkers of disease in ruminants (Ceciliani et al, 2012). Nevertheless, variation in the negAPPs, mainly during the transition period, can better describe the inability to maintain homeostasis for the innate immune response when challenged by various agents, which can in turn suggest the onset of a subsequent disease (Trevisi et al, 2016). Indeed, the functions of negAPPs are essential for the maintenance of the metabolic integrity of the whole body. When their concentrations are markedly reduced (albumin, paraoxo-nase) or exhibit a slow increase (cholesterol, retinol binding protein) after calving, the cows manifest health problems, reduced feed intake and performance, increased body reserves mobilisation and impaired nutrient utilisation.

## Assessment of the Severity of an Inflammatory Event in the Transition Period

Inflammation is not a negative process per se, but causes concerns if occurring in excess, because it produces many side effects, or if the response is repeated. The measurement of posAPPs is not an index of the consequences of damage caused by the inflammation because correlation with the severity of the process is poor. Rather, the reduction in negAPPs after the inflammatory events occurring around calving has demonstrated a more consistent relationship with the health status and performance of cows (Bionaz et al, 2007). The negAPPs and some related biomarkers include parameters that reflect various functions of the liver (digestive tract-related, metabolic and immune state). The use of only one parameter to identify cows at risk of developing disease conditions is not prudent and could reflect the peculiar conditions of a restricted population. Therefore, Trevisi and Minuti (2018) have developed some aggregate indices (supplementing their

**Table 11.1:** Some aggregate indices to assess the health of early lactating cows around calving: liver activity index (LAI), liver functionality index (LFI), and postcalving inflammatory response index (PIRI)

| Aggregate index | LAI | LFI | PIRI |
|---|---|---|---|
| Meaning of biomarkers | negAPPs or related parameters | negAPPs or related parameters | posAPPs, negAPPs, Oxidative stress |
| Biomarkers | Albumin, cholesterol (indirect measure of lipoproteins), vitamin A (indirect measure of the retinol binding protein) | Albumin, cholesterol (indirect measure of lipoproteins), bilirubin (indirect measure of liver enzymes responsible for its clearance) | Haptoglobin, reactive oxygen metabolites (ROM), cholesterol and paraoxonase (PON) |

posAPPs = positive acute phase proteins; negAPPs = negative acute phase proteins. *Source:* Trevisi and Minuti, 2018

earlier proposal) that include a combination of negAPPs or related parameters. These are the liver activity index (LAI), the liver functionality index (LFI), and the postcalving inflammatory response index (PIRI). These indices allow the identification of inadequate physiological conditions in the absence of clinical signs. Measuring them helps in more accurate diagnosis of the condition and its cure (Table 11.1).

## Biomarkers of a Risky Transition Period in Late Pregnancy

It is not at all uncommon for cows to show no clinical symptoms of disease during late pregnancy, but then to become clinically ill in early lactation, sometimes with disastrous consequences. This coincides with a sudden change of metabolism (Fig. 11.1). It seems probable that some pathways start to be altered during late pregnancy and, thus, some indicators in biological fluids might signal these events in advance. Indeed, potential candidates have been proposed in the literature (Table 11.2). Most of these biomarkers are indices of the immune response or consequent adaptation of some components (e.g. PIC, haemolytic complement, lysozyme, posAPPs, and negAPPs). The suggestion has been made that many of these adaptations may be associated with suboptimal environmental conditions (mainly poor hygiene, nutritional mistakes, mentally stressful situations) and exert negative imprinting on the innate immune system (Trevisi et al, 2016). In this context, some common and harmless opportunistic bacteria could pose a threat in this period and the control over the inflammatory response may not be adequate around calving.

The most interesting biomarkers that show important changes in the last 3–4 weeks of the dry period are:

• Ceruloplasmin is a posAPP which remains at high concentrations in the plasma for weeks after an inflammatory stimulus. Often, the ceruloplasmin concentration is correlated with markers of oxidative stress

**Table 11.2:** Candidate biomarkers in late pregnancy for the identification of cows with a risky transition period. The concentrations have been determined in plasma samples collected in the morning before the meal, from 4 to 2 weeks before calving

| Candidate biomarkers | Suggested risky threshold |
|---|---|
| Interleukin 6 (IL6) (pg/ml) | > 450 |
| Interleukin 1β (IL1β) (pg/ml) | > 140 |
| Lysozyme (mg/ml) | < 1.0 |
| Complement, haemolytic (U 50%/μl) | < 25 |
| Sialic acid (g/L) | > 0.45 |
| Globulin (g/L) | > 38 |
| Ceruloplasmin (μmol/L) | > 2.7 |
| Albumin (g/L) | < 35 |
| Bilirubin, total (μmol/L) | > 2.0 |
| Vitamin A (RBP) (μg/100 ml) | < 35 |
| Paraoxonase (U/ml) | < 60 |
| NEFA (mmol/L) | > 0.35 |
| Reactive oxygen metabolites (ROM) (mg $H_2O_2$/100 ml) | > 11.5 |

*Source:* Trevisi and Minuti, 2018

(positively with ROM), inflammation (positively with total bilirubin and negatively with albumin) and the innate immune system (negatively with lysozyme).

• lysozyme is an enzyme present in many body fluids, has bactericidal properties and participates in homeostatic regulation of the inflammatory response. In late pregnancy, lysozyme in the plasma of cows with risky transition period has been shown to be present at a lower concentration in comparison with healthy cows. At low concentration (<1 mg/ml), lysozyme may reduce its role in the homeostatic regulation of the inflammatory response and may contribute to increased susceptibility of an inflammatory response.

• PIC (e.g. IL1β and IL6) are mediators of the immune response that remain almost stable in the plasma of cows in late pregnancy, but have been shown to be hugely variable (Trevisi et al, 2015). Subjects with the highest PIC concentrations showed the greatest prevalence of diseases, higher mobilisation of lipid and a lower milk yield in early lactation. Amadori et al (2015) have confirmed these results and suggested that the elevated serum concentrations of IL6, measured 4–5 weeks before calving, seems to be a promising prognostic biomarker of a risky transition period.

Overall the available information suggests that one or several events occur between the end of one lactation and the start of the next lactation, repeatedly challenging the immune system. These repeated responses to infectious and noninfectious stressors may determine a negative imprinting in cows and may worsen homeostatic reactions (Trevisi et al, 2016). Therefore, depression of the immune system can result in an excessive overload of its activity, something which is not necessarily a peculiar adaptation of late pregnancy. The variations of various humoral components (from the innate immune response or metabolic status) can be used as biomarkers to measure the increased susceptibility to new stressors and may be used to predict which cows are at risk in the peripartum period.

## TRANSITION PERIOD AND IMPAIRED IMMUNE FUNCTION IN MULTIPAROUS COWS

### Dysfunctional Immune Response and Immunosuppression

Research has shown that transition phase (3 wk before until 3 wk after calving) goes along with increased inflammation, oxidative stress and a dysfunctional immune response. During the transition period dairy cows are subjected to various endocrinological and metabolic changes. These changes are accompanied by a decreased immune response. Neutrophil function, lymphocyte responsiveness to mitogen stimulation, antibody responses and cytokine production

by immune cells are components of the cow's host defence that are altered during the transition period.

Causes for altered immune cell function and consequently immunosuppression are manifold.

1. **Endocrinological:** At parturition the concentration of glucocorticoids is increased. Glucocorticoids like the stress hormone cortisol, is reported to impair neutrophil migration as well as lymphocyte proliferation and development.

2. **Negative energy balance:** After parturition, transitional dairy cows are in a state of a negative energy balance (NEB) due to the onset of lactation and a decreased dry matter intake (DMI). This NEB is accompanied by lipid mobilisation, leading to elevated blood concentrations of non-esterified fatty acids (NEFA). Due to a relatively small amount of oxaloacetate, fatty acids can only partly be metabolised by the liver and, consequently, ketone bodies are produced. Over-conditioned cows are more prone to lipomobilisation leading to higher NEFA concentrations and ketone bodies.

   Elevated beta-hydroxy butyrate (BHB) and NEFA concentrations play important role in the disruption of immune functions around calving. It was discovered that the function of neutrophils and leukocytes might be impaired due to increased concentrations of fatty acids and ketone bodies (Contraras and Sordillo, 2011). As a consequence, production diseases (ketosis, milk fever, etc.) show the highest incidence in early lactation (Goff and Horst, 1997); especially over-conditioned cows are prone to immune suppression eventually leading to health disorders like mastitis, metritis, and retained placenta.

3. **Oxidative stress:** The oxidative stress the animals experience in the transition phase is also a significant factor leading to dysfunctional host immune and inflammatory responses and consequently increasing cows' susceptibility to health disorders

(Sordillo and Aitken, 2009). Impairment of immune function caused by calving was more severe in cows in $\geq$ 3rd parity than in younger cows. The reasons for oxidative stress are many. It may be due to the enhanced metabolic activity in consequence of the increased energy demands, a reduced antioxidant capacity, increased reactive oxygen species (ROS) production in the fight against invading organisms.

### Primiparous Versus Pluriparous Dairy Cows with Reference to Immune Function

Peripheral blood mononuclear cells (PBMC), haptoglobin (one of the most specific positive acute phase proteins [posAPPs]), aspartate-aminotransferase, red blood cell count and leukocyte percentage and populations are influenced by parity.

A. **Blood concentrations of PMNL and PBMC are higher in primiparous cows**

- Primiparous and pluriparous cows have different blood concentrations of polymorphonuclear leukocytes (PMNL) and PBMC and this is also evident during the periparturient period. Primiparous animals do have higher numbers of PMNL and PBMC. Additionally, it was shown that the viability of PMNL had been higher in primiparous cows and they exhibited higher numbers of circulating immature PMNL.

- Primiparous cows have higher growth hormones due to the ongoing growth during pregnancy and first lactation. Growth hormone is known to influence blood cell maturation in the bone marrow and this may explains the different numbers in the circulating blood cells.

- The calculated blood concentrations of phagocytosing PMNL and PBMC were higher in primiparous cows (Buhler et al, 2018). However, the percentage of phagocytosing PBMC was higher in pluriparous cows. This may be due to more mature blood leukocytes in

pluriparous animals that are able to better phagocytose. However, Schafers et al (2018) concluded that the ability of PMNL to elicit an oxidative burst reaction might be impaired in older cows compared with younger cows.

- As the oxidative burst of granulocytes is an important defence mechanism against pathogens, older cows might be more sensitive to infections. Older cows might be more susceptible to inflammatory events due to their impaired ability to produce liver proteins in the state of inflammation caused by the event of parturition. Thus immune function of older cows is more sensitive to the event of calving.

The effect of high levels of BHB and insulin on PBMC activity was studied by Wang et al (2018). They conducted an *in vitro* study to examine the ability of important immune modulators [βhydroxy-butyrate (BHB), cortisol, prolactin, isoproterenol and insulin] to influence the responsiveness of peripheral blood mononuclear cells (PBMC) from multiparous transition dairy cows (29 $\pm$ 2 days before and 14 $\pm$ 3 days after calving). Mitogen used was phytohaemagglutinin. The concentration of BHB and insulin in postpartum cows (early lactation) and antepartum (dry) cows were 2 and 0.5 mmol/L and 0.7 and 0.2 ng/ml, respectively. The results indicated that in early lactation higher BHB reduced PBMC activation and proliferation, while the higher insulin enhanced PBMC proliferation. In dry cows, the low concentrations of BHB and insulin and both concentrations of prolactin (20 vs 300 ng/ml) and isoproterenol (70 vs 130 ng/L) enhanced activation, but not proliferation compared to cultures without immune modulator addition. In postpartum cows, the high BHB concentrations and the high insulin concentrations seem to act as negative and positive signals for PBMC, respectively, to utilise nutrients for activation and proliferation.

B. **Pluriparous cows need more antioxidants:** Pluriparous cows exhibit an increased need for anti-oxidative capacity during the periparturient period compared to primiparous animals because of higher DM intake and milk yield in pluriparous animals and consequently higher cell respiration. Therefore, the higher basal ROS (reactive oxygen species) production in pluriparous cows might be an output of this increased respiration rate.

## Influence of Vitamin E supplementation

Vitamin E has been proven to elicit antioxidant activities by reacting with peroxyl radical and thereby protecting polyunsaturated fats. According to Rimbach et al (2002), vitamin E influences different inflammatory cell signalling pathways and acts as a ligand at the peroxisome proliferator activating receptor (PPAR)γ, whereby it is involved in the expression of different antioxidative enzymes (Nakamura and Omaye, 2010).

Schafers et al (2018) investigated the effects of treatment with conjugated linoleic acid (CLA) or vitamin E or a combination thereof on biochemical, haematological and immunological variables of dairy cows during the critical transition phase. It was found that the supplemented dose of vitamin E was not sufficient to counteract the immunesuppression caused even in healthy cows by the event of parturition.

## Niacin Supplementation

Niacin (the vitamin $B_3$) is found as nicotinic acid and as nicotinamide in the vertebrates' body. Nicotinic acid is readily transformed into nicotinamide and it is a precursor of the coenzymes nicotinamide adenosine dinucleotide (NAD+) and nicotinamide adenosine dinucleotide phosphate (NADP+). As such, it participates in many redox reactions including anabolic and catabolic pathways. Niacin's anti-lipolytic effect in the animal is variable (See Buhler et al, 2018).

Niacin is also known to have anti-oxidative and anti-inflammatory effects. It acts as cytoprotectant in blocking inflammatory cell activation and has immune modulating properties (Maiese et al, 2009; Yu and Zhao, 2007). Hence, niacin is an interesting supplementary substance to test in the periparturient cow, where metabolic and oxidative stress as well as increased inflammation occur and are associated with a dysfunctional immune response.

## HOW TO IMPROVE RESISTANCE TO METABOLIC AND INFECTIOUS DISEASES DURING THE TRANSITION PERIOD?

### Prevalence of Metabolic and Infectious Diseases in Dairy Animals and its Consequences

The incidence of metabolic and infectious diseases varies greatly during the lactation cycle. Most new cases of clinical mastitis, many other infectious diseases become clinically apparent during the first 2 weeks of lactation. During this time, cows are in a negative energy balance (NEB) and must mobilise body reserves to balance the deficit between feed energy intake and energy required for milk production. This NEB results in lower blood glucose levels. Mobilisation of body reserves to provide additional energy leading to elevated blood concentrations of non-esterified fatty acids (NEFA) and β-hydroxybutyric acid (BHBA). Now, there is good evidence that the increase in circulating NEFA impairs immune cell functions during the transition period.

Calcium and phosphorus are also mobilised for milk synthesis leading to a decrease in their blood concentrations. All of these metabolic changes can lead to hypocalcaemia, ketosis, displaced abomasum and hepatic lipidosis. Improving the energy balance in the immediate postpartum period should greatly reduce the incidence of periparturient diseases in dairy cows.

Dairy cows experience a natural state of immunosuppression, which can increase their susceptibility to uterine and mammary infections. Parturition is associated with a decrease in the number of polymorpho-nuclear leukocytes (PMNL), along with a weakening of those cells' phagocytosis capacity and a decrease in their ability to fight bacteria. This period is also marked by a decreased responsiveness of blood lymphocytes to stimulation with mitogenic agents and by decreased immunoglobulin production by B cells.

## Links Between Metabolic Perturbations and Immune Functions

**Intact cows versus mastectomised cows:** Impairment of immune functions around the time of calving has become an established fact. Various hypotheses have been put forward attributing this to endocrine or metabolic changes. To establish the relative contribution of these two types of changes, studies evaluated neutrophil and lymphocyte functions during the peripartum period in intact cows and in mastectomised cows. As expected, mastectomy prevented metabolic perturbations such as hypocalcaemia and the increase in blood NEFA (Goff et al, 2002), since there was no milk production. Lymphocyte functions were reduced in milk producing cows, especially close to calving, but remained stable in mastectomised cows (Nonnecke et al, 2003).

The myeloperoxidase activity of neutrophils declined in both intact and mastectomised cows as calving approached. However, that activity returned to normal within a week after parturition in mastectomised cows and was still depressed at 20 day of lactation in milk-producing cows (Kimura et al, 1999). Mastectomy also reduced the decrease in the percentage of T lymphocytes in the peripheral blood mononuclear cells (PBMC), a change that had previously been shown to be associated with immunosuppression in periparturient cows (Kimura et al, 2002). These results indicate that the **physiological demands placed on the cows by milk production play an important role in periparturient immunosuppression.**

The increases in blood NEFA and BHBA concentrations during the transition period are proportional to the degree of fat mobilisation necessary to support milk production. Studies identified high blood concentrations of metabolities, notably (NEFA and) BHBA, as risk factors for mastitis and uterine diseases. The results of studies of Ster et al (2012) and Hammon et al (2006) indicate that the increase in circulating NEFA impairs PBMC and PMNL functions. Therefore, management approaches that reduce the NEB and increase in NEFA at the beginning of lactation are likely to improve resistance to infection. Hence improving the nutrient supply through periparturient nutritional management is imperative to improve resistance to metabolic and infectious diseases during the transition period.

**Strategies to decrease metabolic perturbations and immune function perturbations during the transition period:** The peripartum period is characterised by a negative energy balance (NEB) associated with transient immunosuppression and a higher incidence of diseases in dairy cows. There are strong indications that the increase in circulating NEFA impairs PBMC functions. Although PMNL are less sensitive to NEFA, they can also be affected by those fatty acids at very high levels. Lacasse et al (2018) tried several strategies to limit the NEB.

**Inhibition of milk fat synthesis:** Fat is the most energetically expensive component of milk to synthesise, accounting for about 50% of the total milk energy. Fat is also the milk component whose concentration is most easily modified by management. Therefore, reducing fat content during the postpartum period could be a valuable strategy to improve the energy balance during the transition period (Lacasse et al, 2018). Of course, this is only purely academic as milk pricing in India is based on fat content of the milk.

It has been known for a long-time that feeding cows a high-concentrate, low-fibre diet can cause milk fat depression (MFD). Although feeding such a diet during the transition period would be detrimental, MFD can be safely induced by feeding a small amount of rumen-protected fish oil or trans-10, cis-12 conjugated linoleic acid (CLA). Both lipid supplements cause MFD by inhibiting the mammary gene expression of several lipogenic enzymes (Ahnadi et al, 2002). While fish oil also depresses milk protein content and feed intake, CLA appears to have few side effects and has been proposed as a tool to improve the energy balance during the transition period (Bernal-Santos et al, 2003).

Several experiments tested the usefulness of rumen-protected CLA during the transition period. Unexpectedly, doses of CLA that cause MFD in established lactation failed to inhibit milk fat synthesis immediately postpartum (Bernal-Santos et al, 2003; Sigl et al, 2010). When a much larger amount of CLA was fed, milk fat concentration decreased within the first week of lactation, but maximum MFD occurred during the second or third week of lactation.

Overall, it appears that feeding rumen-protected CLA might be a useful strategy to increase milk and milk protein yield during established lactation. However, in view of the large amount of CLA required and its limited effect on metabolite levels, the usefulness of feeding CLA during the transition period remains to be proven.

Among all the strategies evaluated to reduce metabolic perturbations and immunosuppression during the transition period, limiting the milk production during the first week of lactation by way of milking cows incompletely twice daily appears to be the most promising. Indeed, this strategy is an effective way of limiting the NEB, metabolic perturbations and immunosuppression without compromising the rest of the lactation. In addition, this strategy does not involve extra costs or the use of pharmacological compounds (Lacasse et al, 2018).

# IMMUNE FUNCTION IN TRANSITION COW/ BUFFALO AND INTERACTION WITH METABOLIC DISEASES

## Potential Interventions to Overcome the Transition Disorders

### Introduction

The multitude of disorders (metabolic diseases) that dairy bovines (buffaloes and cows) face during the transition to lactating is a perennial source of concern for dairy farmers, nutritionists and veterinarians. Some of the common disorders are high rates of mastitis, metritis, milk fever, displaced abomasum, ketosis and fatty liver. Most of the metabolic diseases of dairy bovines (milk fever, ketosis, retained placenta and displacement of the abomasum) and majority of infectious diseases (in particular mastitis) becomes clinically apparent during the first 2 weeks of lactation. The aetiology of many of those metabolic diseases can be traced back to insults that occurred in early lactation.

### Power of Immunity of Dairy Animal at Calving

At calving, the animal's reproductive tract is exposed to bacteria, even in the cleanest of environments. The cow survives because her white blood cells provide protection from infection. (1) Neutrophil provides the first line of defence, moving out of the blood whenever and wherever bacteria invade body tissue. Once in the infected tissue, the neutrophils ingest the bacteria and release enzymes and free radical compounds onto the bacteria to kill them. Occasionally, the neutrophils do not succeed in killing the intruder. (2) The immune system then calls on macrophages and lymphocytes, which work together to produce antibodies and other antibacterial factors. Production of these factors takes a little more time but will eventually eliminate most infections that the neutrophils cannot handle.

### Oxidative Stress and Immunity

Imagine the immune system is an army and the immune cells are soldiers fighting against the invasive organisms. To perform their function effectively, major immune cells (macrophages, neutrophils/heterophils, T and B lymphocytes) have receptors on their surface. These receptors are extremely sensitive to communicating molecules, but they are also sensitive to free radicals and can be easily damaged. Hence all those huge armies of immune cells need proper communication for effective functioning. They also can start fighting with each other, eventually destroying immunocompetence and causing autoimmune reactions. Therefore, immune cells need protection and it is provided by natural antioxidants as major defences, e.g. Se-GSH-Px, thioredoxin reductases and other selenoproteins.

Indeed, if not properly protected, macrophage functions could be compromised including initial overproduction of free radicals with consecutive damages to specific enzymatic systems resulting in decreasing efficiency of oxidative burst and apoptosis. Therefore, it is clear that antioxidant defence is a crucial factor of immune defence in the body. It has been proven that oxidative stress affects all stages of the immune/inflammatory response. Pattern recognition receptors (PRRs) present on innate immune cells, such as toll-like receptors (TLRs), recognise specific molecular patterns and signal an immune response. Some TLRs are also receptors for endogenous biomolecules such as saturated NEFAs. That means PRRs are sensing not only invading pathogens but also recognise endogenous nonmicrobial danger or stress signals. Interestingly, receptors play a major role in signalling leading to apoptosis, a major cause of immune cell number reduction in stress conditions.

In fact, pathogen recognition receptors (PRRs) are responsible for the activation of signalling pathways leading to an inflammatory, antimicrobial response. A growing body of evidence demonstrates a link between the innate PRRs and the activation of the adaptive immune response responsible for building an effective defence against invasive organisms (Fritz et al, 2007). Activation of TLRs and other PRRs elicits downstream signalling cascades, activating pro-inflammatory gene transcription [including nuclear factor kappa-light-chain-enhancer of activated B cells (NFκB) and TNF-α, resulting in the transcription of pro-inflammatory proteins] and suppressing anti-inflammatory genes. Peroxisome proliferator-activated receptor gamma (PPAR-γ) ligands are anti-inflammatory as they inhibit NFκB activation.

## Oxidative Stress and Incidence of Infectious and Metabolic Disorders

Increased incidence of health problems observed during the periparturient period can be partly attributed to suboptimal immune responses due to milk production and environmental stresses. This is a transition from non-lactating pregnant status to non-pregnant lactation status. Most infectious diseases and metabolic disorders including retained placenta, metritis and mastitis take place during this time. The physical and metabolic stresses of pregnancy, calving and lactation may contribute to this decrease in host resistance and the subsequent increase in disease incidence (Goff and Horst, 1997). Substantial evidence indicates that innate and acquired defence mechanisms are lowest from 3-week precalving to 3-week postcalving (transition period).

The immunosuppression leads to the increased incidence of peripartum diseases including retained placenta, increased somatic cell count (SCC) and mastitis (Surai, 2006). It was suggested that immunosuppression at calving is related to problems of expulsion of foetal membranes. It seems likely that impaired neutrophil function causes retained placenta. For example, neutrophils isolated from blood of cows with retained placenta had significantly lower immune function before calving and this impaired function lasted for 1 to 2 weeks after parturition (Kimura et al, 2002). A loss in neutrophil-chemoattraction for foetal membrane tissue after parturition and decreased superoxide radical production by neutrophils were observed in metritic-cows due to retention of placenta. It is well-accepted that neutrophils are the primary mechanisms of uterine and mammary immune defence (Surai and Kochish, 2018).

## Inflammatory Responses to Infection— Inflammatory Mediators

Recent research has highlighted the role of inflammation in infectious diseases and has suggested that inflammation is involved in metabolic diseases as well. During infections such as mastitis or metritis, immune cells in the body recognise invading pathogens and become activated. When the infection is caused by gram-negative bacteria, endotoxin released by the bacteria also activates the immune cells.

The activation of local and systemic host defence mechanisms requires crosstalk between numerous types of immune cells. One component of this response is inflammation. The host of signalling molecules released by activated immune cells include inflammatory mediators such as **nitric oxide, prostaglandins and cytokines**. While many of these molecules promote local inflammation and increased blood flow, inflammatory cytokines play a key role in stimulating systemic inflammatory responses, including increased body temperature, increased heart rate and decreased feed intake (Dantzer and Kelley, 2007).

**Cytokines:** Key inflammatory cytokines include tumour necrosis factor alpha (TNFα), interleukin 1β and interleukin 6. One effect of cytokines is to activate production of acute phase proteins (APPs). Primarily produced by the liver, this class of proteins includes haptoglobin, serum amyloid A and C-reactive protein (CRP). Proteins that participate in the acute phase response to infection are generally found in very low abundance in the bloodstream, but are greatly elevated during systemic activation of the immune system. These are positive APPs (posAPPs).

## Role of Inflammation in Transition Disorders

Inflammation has been proposed as a missing link in the pathology of metabolic disorders in transition cows (Drackley, 1999). The metabolic effects of acute systemic inflammation include adipose tissue mobilisation, breakdown of liver glycogen and liver triglyceride accumulation, all of which occur during the transition period. More specifically, cytokines promote the breakdown of fat stores through decreased feed intake, impaired insulin sensitivity and direct stimulation of lipolysis. All of these conditions are associated with ketosis and fatty liver in dairy cattle. Even more intriguing is the evidence that TNFα decreases liver glucose production (Kettelhut et al, 1987) and promotes triglyceride accumulation once mobilised NEFA reach the liver (García-Ruiz et al, 2006).

Abrupt dietary shifts during the transition period can also contribute to systemic inflammation. High roughage diets are transitioned to high concentrate diets to meet the energy demands at the onset of lactation. When the change (of diet) is sudden, it can result in ruminal production of endotoxin and subsequent transfer of endotoxin into the bloodstream.

Furthermore, monocytes are known to become more responsive to inflammatory stimulants during the transition period, resulting in greater secretion of inflammatory cytokines when stimulated (Sordillo et al, 1995). Mastitis, metritis and acute acidosis can, therefore, result in systemic inflammation, elevated cytokine concentrations and altered liver metabolism.

## Relationship between Inflammatory Mediators and Metabolic Disorders

Recent findings have supported previous speculation regarding the relationships between inflammatory mediators and metabolic disorders. The direct effects of cytokines on liver metabolism may play a key role in promoting metabolic disorders in transition cows, especially those already combating infectious disorders or with excessive body condition (Barry Bradford, 2009). Ametaj and coworkers reported that plasma concentrations of a number of inflammatory markers were increased in cows that developed fatty liver (Ametaj et al, 2005). Similar findings were reported by Ohtsuka and colleagues, who observed increased serum TNFα activity in cows with moderate to severe fatty liver (Ohtsuka et al, 2001). Most recently, endotoxin-induced mastitis was shown to alter expression of metabolic genes in the liver, including decreased expression of genes important for glucose production (Jiang et al, 2008). In lactating cows, impaired glucose production would likely lead to increased adipose tissue mobilisation, elevated plasma NEFA and increased ketone production by the liver.

## Relationships between Oxidative Stress and Inflammation

Although the importance of inflammation in transition disorders is becoming clear, the pathways that cause this inflammation are less clear. Infections certainly initiate the process in some cows, but this is not likely the cause of metabolic disorders in all cows. In particular, the dramatically higher incidence of transition disorders in cows with excessive body condition (Morrow, 1976) is difficult to attribute exclusively to infections.

High-yielding dairy animals mobilise excess body fat (to meet energy requirements of milk production while such animals experience depressed feed intake) resulting in an augmented hepatic mitochondrial oxidative metabolism (Schaff et al, 2012) and production of toxic ROS. The ROS induce oxidative stress. All the more, cows with excessive body condition experience severe oxidative stress. Mounting evidence indicates that mitochondrial function and oxidative stress are closely related to innate immune response (West et al, 2011) and inflammation (Lopez-Armada et al, 2013). However, immune system's response to an infection is reflected by a way of inflammation. The following also furnishes further reasoning.

## Adipokines

In addition to acute inflammatory events, chronic low-grade inflammation may play a role in transition disorders. In the early 1990's, it was discovered that adipose tissue is capable of producing inflammatory cytokines such as TNFα. With the extensive list of "adipokines" discovered in the ensuing 15 years, human metabolic disorders are increasingly being viewed as products of low-grade adipose tissue inflammation induced by obesity (Barry Bradford, 2009). Adipose tissue is now recognised as an important source of circulating TNFα and plasma TNFα concentrations are increased in obese individuals in a number of species, including sheep (Daniel et al, 2003). Based on these findings, infection is no longer a required component of an inflammation-based aetiology for metabolic disorders in the transition period. Low-grade inflammation associated with obesity may help to explain "fat cow syndrome" (Morrow, 1976).

## Lipid Peroxides

Lipid peroxides are also emerging as likely mediators linking plasma lipids to inflammation (Pessayre et al, 2004). Lipid peroxides are produced when intracellular lipids encounter ROS such as hydrogen peroxide. Some ROS are always produced in the liver. The events occurring in early lactation do likely contribute to enhanced ROS production as explained above.

**Peroxisomal oxidation and mitochondrial oxidation:** The transition from late gestation through early lactation in dairy cows is associated with a substantial mobilisation of body reserves, in particular fat, leading to a marked increase in circulating concentrations of fatty acids (NEFA), which are oxidised by hepatic and extrahepatic tissues as an energy source. However, the oxidative capacity for NEFA and for exporting fatty acids via VLDL is limited and fatty liver is the consequence.

One adaptation to increasing delivery of NEFA to the liver in early lactation is an increase in the capacity of peroxisomal oxidation (Grum et al, 1996), an alternative pathway for fatty acid oxidation. Enhanced peroxisomal oxidation increases total oxidative capacity of the cell, but the first step in this pathway produces hydrogen peroxide rather than NADH (Drackley, 1999), and therefore, it contributes to ROS production to a greater extent than mitochondrial oxidation.

Increased ROS production in early lactation cows, coupled with increased NEFA concentration, increases lipid peroxide formation. Thus, both the transition to lactation and high body condition are associated with increased plasma markers of lipid peroxidation.

Lipid peroxides activate inflammatory cascades, which in turn alter nutrient metabolism (Pessayre et al, 2004). In addition, ROS are especially harmful to immune cells and can decrease the ability of the immune system to respond to infections (Spears and Weiss, 2008).

## How do you Explain the Development of Transition Cow Disorders?

A combination of insults, including infection, chronic inflammation in obese cows and lipid peroxide formation promotes systemic inflammation during the transition period. Inflammation impairs immune function, making cows more susceptible to infectious disorders and causes maladaptive shifts in metabolism, increasing the risk of metabolic disorders (Barry Bradford, 2009). Neutrophil and lymphocyte function is diminished in the periparturient period, especially in the dairy cow. The onset of milk production imposes tremendous challenges to the mechanisms responsible for energy, protein and mineral homeostasis in the cow. Negative energy, protein, and/or mineral balance and hormonal fluxes associated with the onset of lactation may be responsible for the immunosuppression observed in periparturient dairy cattle.

## Prevention of Metabolic Diseases

Three basic physiologic functions must be maintained during the periparturient period

if disease is to be avoided (Goff, 2008). These are: (1) A strong immune system (2) Normocalcaemia and (3) Maintaining feed intake during the days before and after calving. Both metabolic disease and infectious disease incidence are greatly increased whenever one or more of these physiological functions is impaired. As explained earlier, immune system is compromised in transition animals. Immunosuppression is explained further in the following.

## Hypocalcaemia and Mastitis Susceptibility

**Milk fever cows are at increased risk of developing mastitis (Curtis et al, 1983). Why?** Calcium is necessary for proper contraction of muscle. Severe hypocalcaemia prevents skeletal muscle contraction to the point that the clinical syndrome known as milk fever occurs. Muscle contraction is reduced by any decrease in blood calcium concentration. However, it must be severe before we observe the "downer cow". Daniel et al (1983) demonstrated that contraction rate and strength of the smooth muscle of the intestinal tract is directly proportional to blood calcium concentration.

Hypocalcaemia reduces abomasal contraction which causes the abomasum to fill with gas and become displaced. Of course, lack of effective fibre is the other contributor to displacement of the abomasum.

While milk fever is associated with the day of calving, it has been demonstrated that many cows remain subclinically hypocalcaemic for the first week of lactation. Hypocalcaemic cows tend to spend more time lying down than do normocalcaemic animals, which could increase teat end exposure to environmental opportunists.

**Hypocalcaemia creates stress to the cow:** Cows typically exhibit a 3 to 4 fold increase in plasma cortisol as part of the act of initiation of parturition. However, subclinically hypocalcaemic cows may have 5 to 7 fold increases in plasma cortisol on the day of calving and the typical milk fever cow may exhibit plasma cortisol concentrations that are 10 to 15 fold higher than precalving plasma cortisol concentration. **Cortisol** is generally considered a powerful **immune suppressive agent** and likely exacerbates the immune suppression normally observed in the periparturient period. Immune suppression begins 1 to 2 weeks before calving and the cortisol surge is fairly tightly confined to the day of calving and perhaps the day after calving.

## How Does Hypocalcaemia Contributes to Periparturient Immune Suppression?

In a normal cow, when an immune cell (such as a lymphocyte) encounters a bacterial antigen at its surface, it triggers the release of calcium from organelles within the cell. This begins the process by which the lymphocyte will produce antibodies, bactericidal peptides, etc. to kill the bacteria. **A rise in intracellular calcium is a key early feature in immune cell activation.** But in hypocalcaemic cows, Kimura et al. (2006) reported the failure of immune cells to become activated when they encountered a stimulus such as bacteria. Hypocalcaemic cows had decreased intracellular calcium stores in peripheral mononuclear cells. This caused a blunted intracellular calcium release response to an immune cell activation signal and helps explain how hypocalcaemia contributes to periparturient immune suppression.

## Ketosis and Mastitis Susceptibility

Ketosis is diagnosed whenever there are elevated levels of ketones in the blood, urine, or milk of a cow/buffalo. The disease is always characterised by a decline in blood glucose as well. In lactation, the amount of energy required for maintenance of body tissues and milk production exceeds the amount of energy the cow/buffalo can obtain from its diet, especially in early lactation when dry matter intake is still low.

**Dairy animal in early lactation is comparable to humans with protein-calorie malnutrition:** The fresh dairy animal is also in negative protein balance shortly after calving, though this is not perceived to be as big a problem as the negative energy balance of early lactation. Much of this body protein is being used to support the amino acid and glucose requirements of milk production. Therefore, in many respects, the dairy animal in early lactation is in a physiological state comparable to that of humans and rodents with prolonged protein-calorie restriction (Goff, 2008). This shows it is certain that such animals have no resistance to infectious diseases.

## Immune Function and Retained Placenta, Metritis and Endometritis

**Retained placenta or retained foetal membranes:** Goff and coworkers confirmed studies begun by Gunnink (1984) that suggest the two disorders: mastitis and retained placneta are likely linked because both are due to immune suppression in affected cows. Gunnink's theory suggested that the foetal placenta must be recognised as "foreign" tissue and rejected by the immune system after parturition to cause expulsion of the placenta within 8–12 hours after calving. Retained placenta probably does not cause mastitis, but it is symptomatic of a depressed immune system.

**Metritis:** In the immune-compromised animals, the bacteria are not kept in check and grow to large numbers in the uterus, causing a condition known as metritis. Around 20 to 30% of cows will develop metritis, which is characterised by a foul-smelling, red-brown, watery discharge from the uterus within 10 to 14 days after calving. It is often, but not always, accompanied by a fever. Hammon et al (2006) demonstrated that neutrophils of cows with metritis are significantly less able to kill bacteria (measured by a neutrophil iodination assay) than neutrophils from cows without metritis. The surprise was that poor neutrophil function was evident in these cows on the day of calving—before lactation began and before any bacteria could have entered the uterus.

**Endometritis:** Endometritis is a uterine problem characterised by inflammation of the lining of the uterus, lasting more than 3 to 4 weeks after calving. Studies suggest 40 to 50% of cows can have endometritis at 4 weeks after calving. These cows are less likely to be successfully bred back (Goff, 2008).

## Potential Interventions to Overcome the Transition Disorders

### Nutritional Management to Avoid Metabolic Disorders

The transition from late gestation to early lactation dramatically increases requirements for energy, glucose, amino acids and other nutrients in dairy bovines. Simultaneously, feed intake is often depressed. The resulting negative energy balance (NEB) suppresses immune function and promotes metabolic disorders, potentially explaining relationships between infectious and non-infectious transition (metabolic) disorders. The most widely adopted practice to avoid metabolic disorders is the nutritional management of prepartum cows/dry cows to prevent excess body condition. This limits the pool of stored fat available for mobilisation. Restricting energy intake during the dry period limits the increase in plasma non-esterified fatty acid (NEFA) concentrations during the transition period, resulting in lower fat storage and ketone production in the liver (NRC, 2001).

Cows during the transition period are immunosuppressed. This predisposes the dairy cow to be susceptible to infections. Immune system gets activated; intracellular lipids react with ROS, lipid peroxides are generated; they are the cause of inflammation. The inflammatory events induced by an infectious agent, oxidative stress and/or their combination act directly on the liver through the pro-inflammatory cytokines (PIC) including IL-6, TNFα and IL-1.

The hepatocytes have intracellular proteins (receptors) that can sense these PIC, which upon binding to these receptors (e.g. NFκB) responds by altering the gene expression (mRNA) and subsequently synthesising

'acute phase proteins (APPs)'. The so-called 'positive APPs' are increased by inflammation, while the 'negative APPs' are decreased. The complex interactions of oxidative stress, inflammatory cascades and metabolic pathways give way for a broad array of potential treatments to prevent transition disorders. These potential interventions are briefed in the following.

### Antioxidants—Vitamin E

Dietary antioxidants, notably vitamin E and selenium, are important for their ability to contribute to ROS neutralisation, thereby impeding the progression toward inflammation. Interestingly, plasma concentrations of α-tocopherol (vitamin E) decrease through the transition period and low antioxidant status is associated with transition cow disorders. Supplementing vitamin E prepartum improves antioxidant status. Given the importance of antioxidants in modulating inflammation, it is not surprising that multiple studies have shown that supplementing vitamin E in excess of traditional recommendations decreases the incidence and severity of clinical mastitis.

Recently, a meta-analysis showed that supplemental vitamin E is also effective at preventing retained placenta. Low plasma vitamin E concentrations are associated with increased incidence of fatty liver and displaced abomasum. Given that supplemental vitamin E can decrease inflammatory cytokine production (Poynter and Daynes, 1998) and improve liver antioxidant status in mice with fatty liver (Soltys et al, 2001), supplemental vitamin E may improve liver function in transition cows. With its demonstrated effects on immune function and its potential to benefit liver function, it is recommended that vitamin E be supplemented at a rate of at least 1,500 IU/day for close-up dry cows (that is during the last three weeks before calving).

### Selenium

Selenium is the other most important dietary antioxidant in dairy rations. Responses to selenium are most dramatic when vitamin E status is marginal. Selenium has unique roles in ROS neutralisation and must be considered independently to achieve optimal health. The FDA restricts selenium supplementation in dairy rations to 0.3 ppm and most farms supplement it at that level, without paying the attention to its role in transition animals' health. Feeding **selenium yeast** rather than inorganic selenium sources is an effective means of increasing selenium status of animals that already receive the legal limit of selenium (Salman et al, 2009).

## Beta Carotene

Beta carotene, a precursor of vitamin A, can also function as an antioxidant. It has been found that concentrations of both vitamin A and β-carotene typically decrease during the transition period. Supplementing vitamin A at concentrations above the current recommendations has improved udder health in some studies (NRC, 2001). However, supplementation of β-carotene during the transition period significantly decreased incidence of both metritis and retained placenta compared to vitamin A supplementation. Cows fed 600 mg/day of β-carotene had equivalent plasma retinol concentrations to those supplemented with 120,000 IU/day of vitamin A (Michal et al, 1994). Replacing vitamin A supplements in transition rations with relatively high concentrations of β-carotene may be beneficial for transition cow health.

## Metabolic Modifiers—Methionine

The onset of lactation in dairy cows is characterised by high output of methylated compounds when sources of methyl group are in short supply. Methionine and choline are key methyl group donors and their availability during early lactation may be limiting for milk production, hepatic lipid metabolism and immune function. The work of Delbach et al (2011; Journal of Dairy Science 94: 3913-3927) demonstrated that it is feasible to increase serum concentration of methionine during the first 2 weeks postpartum by feeding rumen-protected methionine. Methionine is a well-established source of intracellular antioxidants glutathione and taurine and a source of methyl groups. Antioxidant enzyme glutathione peroxidase can be derived in part via methionine. Studies conducted by Zhou et al (2016; JDS 99:8716-8732) indicated that peripartal supplementation of rumen-protected methionine had improved overall performance and health of transition cows.

Cows fed the methionine-enriched diets during the transition period had higher concentration of carnitine (essential for the transport of NEFA from cytosol into mitochondria for subsequent fatty acid oxidation [FAO]) suggesting a greater potential for liver FAO and a better transport of fat out of the liver via the formation of VLDL (Osorio et al, 2014). Further, cows fed the methionine-enriched diets had lower blood concentrations of ceruloplasmine and serum amyloid A (posAPPs) indicating a reduced inflammatory response, an enhanced liver function and a greater antioxidant capability (higher glutathione). Such transition cows had higher DMI postpartum and produced more energy-corrected milk.

## Choline

Choline is crucial for normal function of all cells. The most common form of choline in biological systems is phosphatidylcholine (PC) that function to transport lipids through the circulatory system. Choline is a source of methyl groups, therefore, it can spare methionine and have interactions with other nutrients involved in one carbon metabolism (e.g. folate). Choline is also a component of acetylcholine, an important neurotransmitter.

## Why do Transition Dairy Bovines Develop Fatty Liver?

During early lactation when dairy bovines experience negative energy balance (NEB) there are hormonal changes that trigger an intense period of lipid mobilisation from adipose tissue and as a result, blood non-esterified fatty acid (NEFA) concentrations typically increase 5- to 10-fold (Grummer, 1993). Blood flow to the liver doubles as a cow transitions from the dry period to lactation (Reynolds et al, 2003).

As a result, daily fatty acid uptake by the liver increases 13-fold at calving, from approximately 100 to 1300 g/day (Reynolds et al, 2003). Drackely (2001) estimated that during peak blood NEFA concentration, approximately 600 g might be deposited in 24 hours which would correspond to an increase in liver fat of 6–7% by weight. As a reference, fat above 5% in the liver (wet basis) is considered to be moderate to severe fatty liver. Several studies have shown 50 to 60% of transition cows experience moderate to severe fatty liver (Bobe et al, 2004). The consistency amongst these studies suggests that development of fatty liver is a "normal" part of the cow's biology in transition phase. It is not restricted to fat cows, poorly fed cows, or cows housed in suboptimal environments.

The most desirable fate of fatty acids entering the liver would be complete oxidation to provide energy to the liver or re-esterification and export as triglyceride from the liver as part of a very low density lipoprotein (VLDL). Hepatic oxidation increases approximately 20% during the transition period (Drackley et al, 2001). It occurs because the liver becomes metabolically more active. Unfortunately, the increase in oxidation is not sufficient to cope with the increased load of fatty acid being presented to the liver.

It is known that ruminants have a "low capacity to export" triglyceride from the liver as VLDL as compared to nonruminants. This "low capacity to export" and the inability to markedly increase fatty acid oxidation are the two reasons why transition dairy cattle develop fatty liver when experiencing elevated blood NEFA.

### Evidence for a Choline Deficiency in Transition Dairy Bovines

It is now apparent that choline deficiency is a limiting factor for VLDL triglyceride export from the liver. It has been shown in many species, using a wide variety of experimental approaches, that rate of VLDL export is highly related to the rate of hepatic PC synthesis.

In addition to direct PC synthesis from dietary choline, there is endogenous hepatic synthesis of PC via methylation of phosphotidylethanolamine (PE). Sharma and Erdman (1988) demonstrated dietary choline is extensively degraded in the rumen of dairy cows and very little is available to the small intestine for absorption. Therefore, ruminants are more highly dependent (because of rumen degradation) than nonruminants on endogenous synthesis of PC from PE. The high proportion of transition cows developing moderate to severe fatty liver during the transition period suggests that endogenous synthesis is not sufficient in many cows.

The first piece of evidence that transition cows are deficient in choline is the development of fatty liver during the periparturient period (Grummer, 1993; Bobe et al, 2004). More compelling evidence is the alleviation of fatty liver when supplying cows with choline that is protected from ruminal degradation (Cooke et al, 2007; Zom et al, 2011). Dutch researchers (Goselink et al, 2013) recently demonstrated greater gene expression for microsomal triglyceride transfer protein (MTTP) in liver of transition cows supplemented with rumen-protected choline (RPC). MTTP is an important protein required for hepatic VLDL synthesis.

Recently, it was shown that choline, but not methionine, increases VLDL secretion from primary bovine hepatocytes (McCourt et al, 2015). This provided solid evidence that choline limitation is a causative factor for inadequate fat export out of the liver.

### Can Protected Methionine be a Substitute for Protected Choline?

Protected methionine has often been suggested as a possible alternative to protected choline for supplementation to transition dairy cows. Methionine and choline both serve as methyldonors. Methionine methyl groups can be used for endogenous synthesis of PC from PE. As an amino acid, methionine is needed for the synthesis of apolipoproteins. Therefore, there is a conceptual basis for methionine substitution for choline. The feeding trials that have been conducted to examine the effects of rumen-protected methionine or methionine analog on liver total lipid or triglyceride content revealed that it did not reduce the liver fat content.

The reason for methionine's failure to prevent fatty liver in transition cows is not known; it could be due to insufficient dose of protected methionine or methionine analog. Choline contains three methyl groups while methionine has only one methyl group. When differences in molecular weight between choline and methionine are accounted for, choline by weight is 4.3 times more "potent" than methionine as a methyl donor. Therefore, assuming equal bioavailability of the rumen-protected (RP) products being fed, one could speculate that one would need to feed 64.5 g/day of methionine during the transition period to obtain a similar amount of methyl groups as when feeding 15 g/day of choline. McCourt et al (2015) reported choline (but not methionine) increased VLDL secretion from primary bovine hepatocytes.

Since, the last NRC (2001) publication, a significant body of evidence has accumulated to support choline being a required but limiting nutrient in transition cow diets. There is overwhelming evidence that feeding transition dairy cows 15 g RP choline/day will alleviate choline's classic deficiency symptom and lead to improvements in health and performance.

## Transition Dairy Bovines are Insulin-resistant

Insulin is a key hormone that regulates nutrient metabolism in dairy cows. It is known as an anabolic hormone because it signals to tissues that the nutritional state is favourable and nutrients can be stored. Results from these signals include increasing glucose storage in the liver (as glycogen) and stimulation of fat synthesis and storage in adipose tissue and inhibition of fat mobilisation from adipose tissue.

During the transition period, cows become "insulin resistant". Simply defined, this means that insulin has less effect than normal. If insulin is less effective, it means that liver glucose storage is decreased and fat mobilisation from adipose tissue is increased. It is important to note that insulin resistance is not an all or nothing proposition. The magnitude of resistance is a sliding scale, so the degree of fat mobilisation can vary and does not only occur at a maximum rate or not at all. Mobilisation of fat helps support lactation. If mobilisation of fat is too extensive, metabolic disorders such as fatty liver and ketosis can result. Hence lipid mobilisation needs to be reduced during the transition period.

## Strategies to Manage Insulin Resistance

Agents such as niacin and propylene glycol reduce fat mobilisation. Choline enhances triglyceride export from the liver as part of very low density lipoproteins (VLDL). Strategies to manage insulin resistance include feeding controlled energy diets during the dry period (Janovick et al, 2011) to prevent excessive body condition, feeding protected niacin (Yuan et al, 2012) and drenching with propylene glycol (Studer et al 1993). Loss of milk or milk fat yield has been observed with these strategies. Feeding rumen-protected choline is the only proven strategy to assist the liver during times of elevated NEFA. Feeding rumen-protected choline to transition cows reduces severity of fatty liver and ketosis (Lima et al, 2012) and increases milk production and energy-corrected milk production (Grummer et al, 2012).

## Anti-inflammatory Agents

Direct inhibition of inflammation through the use of non-steroidal anti-inflammatory drugs (NSAIDs) has shown promise for treatment of metabolic disorders in laboratory animals. These findings suggest that NSAIDs may be useful in transition cows, which face low blood glucose and fatty liver related problems. It is motivated by evidence linking early lactation inflammation to decreased health and productivity. Sodium salicylate is a member of the NSAID class and is the parent compound of aspirin. Delivery of sodium salicilate via drinking water (2 g/L) responded by producing 21% more milk over the full lactation and 30% more milk fat in multiparous (those in parity 3 and greater) cows compared to primiparous cows (Farney et al, 2013).

Numerous NSAIDs have been evaluated for use in the treatment of mastitis and in general they are effective at reducing body temperature, but do not appear to decrease the severity of the infection. The use of NSAIDs to combat transition cow disorders has produced mixed results. Anyway the use of NSAIDS to treat nonspecific postpartum inflammation is not approved. Therefore, it is worthwhile to consider nutritional approach to limit inflammation.

Some polyphenols have been clearly shown to have anti-inflammatory effects. For example, feed supplement containing green tea and curcumin extract feeding to cows for the close-up period through 9 weeks in milk decreased plasma NEFA concentrations (after calving) and increased milk yield in weeks 4–8 of lactation (Winkler et al, 2015).

Feeding whole flaxseed (omega-3 FA source) increased plasma glucose and decreased plasma ketones in fresh cows; further circulating leukocytes exhibited greater phagocytic activity (due to anti-inflammatory activity of omega-3 FA) (Gandra et al, 2016).

## Conclusions

Growing evidence suggests that inflammation may be a key factor in the development of many transition disorders (Barry Bradford, 2009). Because it results in suppressed immune function and altered nutrient metabolism, inflammation may provide a novel link between infectious and metabolic disorders that are common during the transition period. This model suggests that dietary antioxidants in dry cow rations should be re-evaluated on farms struggling with transition cow disorders. Additional steps, such as the incorporation of β-carotene, omega-3 fatty acid sources, rumen-protected methionine or choline and niacin, may also help to prevent oxidative stress and subsequent inflammation. Future research may provide additional tools to directly combat inflammation to overcome the transition disorders in dairy bovines.

## INNOVATIVE NUTRITIONAL STRATEGY TARGETING MITOCHONDRIA TO OVERCOME METABOLIC STRESS AND THE CONSEQUENTIAL DYSFUNCTIONAL IMMUNE RESPONSE

The continuous increase in demand for animal products (milk, meat and eggs) is putting a constant pressure on animal agriculture. To remain competitive and economically profitable, it is imperative for animal agriculture to increase its productivity efficiency. Crossbreeding and upgrading the germplasm of cattle and buffaloes, respectively, for milk production, prolificacy or animal growth had already been implemented. Performance enhancement by genetic selection has been accompanied by undesired side effects such as decrease in conception rates and susceptibility to diseases. Moreover, these consequences are amplified by the actual withdrawal of antibiotics as prophylactic treatments after the antibiotic ban since 2006. This elimination (of the prophylactic use) of antibiotics is rather associated with an increase in health problems for the animals that require therapeutic use of antibiotics.

### Negative Energy Balance is the Common Metabolic Stress

This situation is especially evident when animals encounter metabolic stresses during the transition period for dairy cows, the gestation for gilts and the postweaning period for piglets. Negative energy balance

(NEB) is common during these periods. The NEB is related to a major risk factor for health. The energetic deficit coincides with dysfunctional immune responses, uncontrolled inflammation and oxidative stress conditions, which are associated with infections and diseases.

## Mitochondria are Dynamic Organelles for Energy Generation and Immune-cell Regulation

In all cells, mitochondria are remarkably dynamic organelles that are mainly known as the energy-generating system in the form of adenosine triphosphate (ATP). However, mitochondrial energy metabolism is associated with the production of toxic reactive oxygen species (ROS). They induce oxidative stress conditions in periods of high metabolic activity.

Mitochondria are now considered as central hubs of immune-cell regulation. Many studies have revealed that in immune cells, mitochondria participate in signalling through ROS production, metabolite availability and by physically acting as scaffolding for protein interaction (West et al, 2011, Weinberg et al, 2015). Mitochondrial signals appear to be necessary for the immune cell to fulfil its specific role in the immune response in both innate and adaptive settings to a variety of intruders. Mitochondrial signalling dictates macrophage polarisation and function, regulates T cell activation and controls CD8+ memory T cell formation (Leavy, 2013).

Mounting evidence indicates that mitochondrial function and oxidative stress are closely related to innate immune response (West et al, 2011), inflammation (Circu and Aw, 2012), programmed cell death (Circu and Aw, 2010) and bacterial pathogenesis (Arnoult et al, 2009).

As a result, mitochondria from metabolically-stressed animals require optimal conditions in terms of antioxidant protection and metabolic substrates availability in order to ensure adequate energetic status, gut health and resistance to diseases. Here, we will study mitochondria and energy production, toxic side-products of mitochondrial energy metabolism and optimising mitochondrial function with supplementation of 'mitochondrial nutrients' to improve their function and decrease oxidative damage.

**Mitochondria and energy production:** The mitochondria are the most efficient source of cellular ATP. In response to energy demands, various substrates such as carbohydrates, proteins and fatty acids are metabolised via several pathways including glycolysis, $\beta$-oxidation, the tricarboxylic acid (TCA) or Krebs cycle and electron transport through the respiratory chain to ultimately drive energy synthesis, in the form of ATP, by oxidative phosphorylation.

The oxidative phosphorylation process involves the action of the mitochondrial respiratory chain consisting of five complexes located at the inner mitochondrial membrane level. The reduced forms of nicotinamide-adenine dinucleotide (NADH) and flavin-adenine dinucleotide ($FADH_2$) transfer electrons to oxidised coenzyme $Q_{10}$ ($CoQ_{10}$) or ubiquinone, cytochrome C through complexes I, II, III and IV that will ultimately drive the reduction of molecular oxygen to form water. The final ejection of protons ($H^+$) from the matrix and the passage of protons into the intermembrane space create an electrochemical gradient that eventually drives the phosphorylation of ADP to ATP through complex V or ATPase when protons re-enter the matrix.

The ATP is then transferred out of the mitochondria by the adenine nucleotide translocase complex and the energy became available for all cellular processes. Mitochondria that fail to generate a mitochondrial membrane potential and produce energy are targeted for destruction through mitophagy process. Thus, when metabolic demands are elevated as it is for modern dairy cows and pigs, the mitochondrial respiratory chain is heavily solicited for answering all energetic needs by generating large amount of ATP. The physiologic state of an animal determines the nutrient requirements and energetic efficiency of mitochondrial function. Numerous factors, such as high metabolic activity and hypoxia can significantly affect substrate utilisation and activities of key mitochondrial enzymes.

## Reactive Oxygen Species (ROS) are the Toxic Side-products of Mitochondrial Energy Metabolism

ROS, including free radicals, are mainly generated as normal byproducts of aerobic respiration and energy metabolism by mitochondria. Oxygen reduction during mitochondrial electron transport is the main source of the superoxide radical ($O_2^{•-}$), which are turned into hydrogen peroxide ($H_2O_2$) and $O_2$ by mitochondrial superoxide dismutases (SODs). This caustic $H_2O_2$ is relatively stable and membrane-permeable and can diffuse out of the mitochondria into the cytoplasm (Veal et al, 2007). ROS can thus inflict serious damage to both mitochondrial and cytoplasmic macromolecules, such as lipids, nucleic acids and proteins.

Polyunsaturated fatty acids are one of the most sensitive oxidation targets for ROS because once lipid peroxidation is initiated, a damaging chain reaction takes place. DNA bases are also very susceptible to ROS attack and oxidation of DNA bases is believed to cause mutations and deletions in both nuclear and mitochondrial genomes. Almost all amino acid residues in a protein can be oxidised by ROS and lose their function (Ugarte et al, 2010). Exposure to ROS appears to be unavoidable for cells living in an aerobic environment and ROS toxicity is controlled by a complex network of non-enzymatic and enzymatic antioxidants, including the superoxide dismutases (SODs), the glutathione peroxidases (GPxs), the thioredoxin reductases (TRxs), the peroxiredoxins (PRxs), catalase and glutathione (GSH).

Mitochondrial energy production is associated with ROS production. Hence high producing transition cows, hyperprolific sows and post-weaned piglets need to handle substantive ROS amounts when the inherent protection invariably fails. Thus high producing transition cows and hyperprolific sows become susceptible to the ROS-induced oxidative damage, which likely perturbs reproductive processes, increase their vulnerability to various diseases and decrease their longevity.

## Mitochondria as Promising Nutritional Targets in Animal Production

Dairy cows encounter severe metabolic stresses during the transition period, as feed intake is too low to meet energy requirements for maintenance and milk production (Le Blanc, 2010). To meet these requirements, high-yielding dairy cows mobilise body fat resulting in an augmented hepatic mitochondrial oxidative metabolism (Schaff et al, 2012).

In mammary tissue, the rate of oxygen consumption increases dramatically with the onset of lactation and a significant increase in secretory cell mitochondrial number was observed (Hadsell et al, 2006). These observations support the hypothesis that during lactation, secretory epithelial cells within the mammary gland are exposed to increasing amounts of toxic ROS produced by mitochondria resulting in oxidative damage and programmed cell death. Taken together, these observations suggest that managing strategies for dairy cows during the transition period should be geared toward reducing NEB by feeding specially formulated diets to improve mitochondrial function.

Reproductive sows are known to have high energetic demands associated with growth and energy utilisation during critical periods such as gestation and lactation. Given the increase in litter size observed in recent times, aged sows and first parity gilts frequently fail to satisfy their energetic nutrient requirements even if voluntary feed intake usually increases with litter size. As a consequence, sows nursing large litters lose generally more body weight during lactation than sows nursing smaller litters. Thus, in order to adequately fulfil their cellular energetic needs throughout gestation and lactation processes, hyperprolific sows completely rely on the maintenance of functional mitochondria (Lapointe, 2014).

Weaning is known to impose tremendous stress on piglets and the period following weaning is characterised by a high incidence of intestinal disturbances, bacterial infections and energetic deficiencies that led to serious diseases. These weaning related issues are exacerbated in hyperprolific sows due to increased litter size leading to an increased number of low-birth weight piglets. Such piglets are more fragile to intestinal infectious diseases and energetic deficiencies (De Vos et al, 2014).

## Optimising Mitochondrial Function

Nutritional supplementation may be useful to support mitochondrial function in stressful conditions such as transition period, hyperprolific gilts and post-weaned piglets. Interestingly, increasing evidence now suggests that targeting mitochondria with specific nutrients from natural sources, now termed "mitochondrial nutrients" or "mitonutrients", could efficiently prevent and ameliorate various conditions associated with mitochondrial dysfunction (Lapointe, 2017).

## Antioxidant Nutrients

Several nutrients with antioxidant properties such as α-lipoic acid, coenzyme $Q_{10}$ ($CoQ_{10}$), vitamin E, selenium and B vitamin have been shown to positively affect mitochondrial-function.

Alpha lipoic acid (α-LA) is a powerful mitochondrial antioxidant and a coenzyme found naturally in mitochondria and involved in energy metabolism. Dietary supplemented α-LA is known to exert an anti-inflammatory action within cells.

Coenzyme $Q_{10}$ is a bioactive lipid which is principally known as an electron carrier in the mitochondrial respiratory chain. It is also recognised for its antioxidant, anti-apoptotic and anti-inflammatory properties and is incorporated within mitochondrial membranes when used as a nutritional supplement (Lapointe et al, 2012).

Vitamin E is a lipid soluble antioxidant present in mitochondrial membranes (Lauridsen and Jensen, 2012).

Selenium (Se) is a mineral that participates in the synthesis of selenoproteins with strong-antioxidant properties, such as glutathione peroxidases (GPxs) and thioredoxin reductases (TRxs) (Dursun et al, 2011).

B vitamins are especially important for supporting mitochondrial function because they directly act as cofactors for mitochondrial enzymes or as precursors of important cofactors. It is well-recognised that B vitamins play an essential role in mitochondrial aerobic respiration and energy production. Furthermore, mitochondrial integrity and functions are compromised by dietary deficiency of B vitamins (Depeint et al, 2006). Riboflavin (vitamin $B_2$) is a water soluble vitamin that is the major component of the flavin adenine dinucleotide (FAD) and flavin mononucleotide (FMN), which function as redox cofactors in the mitochondrial respiratory chain (Depeint et al, 2006).

## Energetic Enhancers

Other mitochondrial nutrients such as creatine and L-carnitine have the capacity to act as energetic enhancers. Creatine is actively incorporated in mitochondria to act as an energy-boosting compound by increasing creatine/phosphocreatine stores and consequently preventing ATP depletion. L-carnitine and its acetyl derivative (Acetyl-L-carnitine) transport long-chain fatty acids into mitochondria for β-oxidation and production.

**Combination of nutrients with complementary and synergistic effects:** It was shown that some combinations of nutrients may possess unique functions and be more efficient than the individual nutrients.

Several studies indicate that the antioxidant and/or the energetic potential of

CoQ$_{10}$ could be more efficient when acting with either α-tocopherol, α-lipoic acid or creatine (Marriage et al, 2003).

Similarly, it was shown that a combination of α-lipoic acid and L-carnitine significantly improve mitochondrial function and stimulate mitochondrial biogenesis (Tarnopolsky, 2008).

These strong synergistic effects between mitochondrial nutrients could be observed both in cell/tissue culture and at the whole animal level.

# Bibliography

## Chapter 1: Immune system, Nutrition and Animal Productivity

Aledo, J.C. (2004) Glutamine breakdown in rapidly dividing cells: waste or investment? Bioessays, 26:778–785.

Ardawi, M.S. and Newsholme, E.A. (1985) Metabolism in lymphocytes and its importance in the immune response. Essays Biochem., 21:1–44.

Bayyari, G.R., Huff, W.E., Rath, N.C., Balog, J.M., Newberry, L.A., Villines. J.D., Skeeles, J.K., Anthony, N.B. and Nestor, K.E. (1997) Poultry Science, 76:289–296.

Beck, M.A. (2000) American Journal of Clinical Nutrition, 71:1676S–1679S.

Berczi, I., Chow, D.A. and Sabbadini, E.R. (1998) Domestic Animal Endocrinology, 15:273–781.

BoaAmponsem, K., Yang, A., Praharaj, N.K., Dunnington, E.A., Gros, W.B. and Siegel, P.B. (1997) Journal of Applied Poultry Research, 6:123–127.

Calder, P.C. and Jackson, A.A. (2000) Undernutrition, infection and immune function. Nutrition Research Reviews, 13:3–29.

Calder, P.C. and Kew, S. (2002) The immune system: a target for functional foods? British Journal of Nutrition 88 (Supplement 2), S165–S177.

Chapkin, R.S., McMurray, D.N. and Jolly, C.A. (2000) In: Nutrition and Immunology: Principles and Practice (Gershwin, M.E., German, J.B. and Keen, C.L., eds.), pp. 121–134, Humana Press Inc., Totowa, NJ.

Chew, B.P. and Park, J.S. (2004) Carotenoid action on the immune response. Journal of Nutrition, 134:257S–261S.

Dantzer, R. (2001) Cytokine-induced sickness behaviour: mechanisms and implications. Annals of the New York Academy of Sciences, 933:222–234.

Elasser, T.H., Kahl, S., Steele, N.C. and Rumsey, T.S. (1997) Nutritional modulation of somatotropic axis-cytokine relationships in cattle: a brief review. Comparative Biochemistry and Physiology, 116A(3):209–221.

Erickson, K.L. and Hubbard, N.E. (2000) Probiotic immunomodulation in health and disease. J. Nutr., 130:403S–409S.

Fraker, P. (2000) Impact of Nutritional Status on Immune Integrity. Pp 147–156. In: Nutrition and Immunology: Principles and Practice, (eds.) Humana Press, Totowa, N.J.

Grimble, R.E. (1998) Nutrition, 14:634–640.

Galarraga, B., Ho, M., Youssef, H.M., Hill, A., McMahon, H., Hall, C., Ogston, S., Suki G. and Belch, J.J.F. (2008) Cod liver oil (n-3 fatty acids) as a non-steroidal anti-inflammatory drug sparing agent in rheumatoid arthritis. Rheumatology. Available at: rheumatology.oxfordjournals.org/cgi/content/abstract/ken024v1doi:10.1093/rheumatology/ken204.

Goldsby, R., Kindt, T., Osborne, B. and Kuby, J. (2003) Immunology, 5 ed. W. H. Freeman and Company.

Hammond, J. (1944) Physiological factors affecting birth weight. Proceedings of the Nutrition Society, 2:8–12.

Humphrey, B.D. and Klasing, K.C. (2004) Modulation of nutrient metabolism and homeostasis by the immune system. World's Poult. Sci. J., 60:90–100.

Janeway, C.A., Travers, P., Walport, M. and Sholmchik, M.J. (2005) Immunobiology: the Immune System in Health and Disease. Garland Publishing, New York.

Johnson, R.W. (1997) Inhibition of growth by pro-inflammatory cytokines: an integrated view. Journal of Animal Sciences, 75:1244–1255.

Johnson, R.W. (1998) Domestic Animal Endocrinology, 15:309–319.

Kearns, R.J., Hayek, M.G., Turek, J.J., Meydani, M., Burr, J.R., Greene, R.J., Marshall, C.A., Adams, S.M., Borgert, R.C. and Reinhart, G.A. (1999) Effect of age, breed and dietary omega-6 (n-6): omega-3 (n-3) fatty acid ratio on immune function, eicosanoid production, and lipid peroxidation in young and aged dogs. Veterinary Immunology and Immunopathology, 69:165–183.

Kelley, K.W., Kent, S. and Dantzer, R. (1996) Why sick animals don't grow: an immunological explanation. In: Growth of the Pig, pp 119–132. Edited by G.R. Hollis. Wallingford: CAB International.

Kim, H.W., Chew, B.P., Wong, T.S., Park, J.S., Weng, B.B., Byrne, K.M., Hayek, M.G., Reinhardt (2000) Dietary lutein stimulates immune response in the canine. Veterinary Immunology and Immunopathology, 74:315–327.

Klasing, K.C. (1988) Nutritional aspects of leukocytic cytokines. Journal of Nutrition, 118:1436–1446.

Klasing, K.C. (1988) Nutritional modulation of resistance to infectious diseases. Poultry Science, 77:1119–1125.

Klasing, K.C. and Johnstone, B.J. (1991) Poultry Science, 70:1781–1789.

Klasing, K.C. and Leshchinsky, T.V. (2000) In: Nutrition and Immunology: Principles and Practice (Gershwin, M.E., German, J.B. and Keen, C.L., eds.), pp. 363–373, Humana Press, Inc., Totowa, NJ.

Knight, C.D., Klasing, K.C. and Forsyth, D.M. (1983) Journal of Animal Science, 57:387–393.

Li, Z., Nestor, K.E., Saif, Y.M., Bacon, W.L. and Anderson, J.W. (1999) Poultry Science, 78:1532–1535.

Malmezat, T., Breuille, D., Capitan, P., Mirand, P.P. and Obled, C. (2000) Glutathione turnover is increased during the acute phase of sepsis in rats. J. Nutr., 130:1239–1246.

McCann, S.M., Kimura, M., Walczewska, A., Karanth, S., Rettori, V. and Yu, W.H. (1998) Domestic Animal Endocrinology, 15:333–344.

Niewold, T.A. (2007) The nonantibiotic anti-inflammatory effect of antimicrobial growth promoters, the real mode of action? A hypothesis. Poultry Science, 86:605–609.

Rastall, R.A. and Maitin, V. (2002) Prebiotics and synbiotics: towards the next generation. Curr Opin. Biotechnol., 13:490–496.

Rosales, F.J., Ritter, S.J., Zolfaghari, R., Smith, J.E. and Ross, A.C. (1996) Journal of Lipid Research, 37:962–971.

Sauber, T.E. and Stahly, T.S. (1996) Chronic immune system activation impairs lactational performance of sows. Feedstuffs, July 22.

Simopoulos, A.P. (2002) Omega-3 fatty acids in inflammation and autoimmune diseases. Journal of the American College of Nutrition, 21:495–505.

Spurlock, M.E. (1997) Regulation of metabolism and growth during immune challenge: an overview of cytokine function. Journal of Animal Science, 75:1773–1783.

Szabo, T., Kadish, J.L. and Czop, J.P. (1995) Biochemical properties of the ligand-binding 20-kDa subunit of the β-glucan receptors on human mononuclear phagocytes. J. Biol. Chem., 270:2145–2151.

Talvas et al. (2015) Immunonutrition stimulates immune functions and antioxidant defence capacities of leukocytes in radiochemotherapy-treated head and neck and esophageal cancer patients: A double-blind randomised clinical trial. Clinical Nutrition, 34:810–817.

Van der Stede, Y., Cox, E., Goddeeris, B.M. (2000) 1–25 Dihydroxyvitamine D3 role in het immuunsysteem., Vlaams Diergeneeskundig Tijdschrift, 69:229–234.

Waldron, M.R., Nonnecke, B.J., Nishida, T., Horst, R.L. and Overton, T.R. (2003) Effect of lipopolysaccharide infusion on serum macromineral and vitamin D concentrations in dairy cows. Journal of Dairy Science, 86:3440–3446.

Waldron, M.R., Kulick, A.E., Bell, A.W. and OVerton, T.R. (2006) Acute experimental mastitis is not causal toward the development of energy-related metabolic disorders in early postpartum dairy cows. Journal of Dairy Science, 89:596–610.

Wander, R.C., Hall, J.A., Gradin, J.L., Du, S.H. and Jewell, D.E. (1997) The ratio of dietary (n-6) to (n-3) fatty acids influence immune system function, eicosanoid metabolism, lipid peroxidation and vitamin E status in aged dogs. Journal of Nutrition, 127:1198–1205.

Webel, D.M., Mahan, D.C., Johnson, R.W. and Baker, D.H. (1998) Pretreatment of young pigs with vitamin E attenuates the elevation in plasma interleukin-6 and cortisol caused by a challenge dose of lipopolysaccharide. J. Nutr., 128:1657–1660.

Weinberg, E.D. (1998) Cancer Investigation, 16:291.

Williams, D.L., Mueller, A. and Browder, W. (1996) Glucan-based macrophage stimulators-A review of their antiinfective potential. Clin. Immunother., 5:392–399.

Wills, R.B.H., Bone, K. and Morgan, M. (2000) Herbal products: active constituents, modes of action and quality control. Nutrition Research Reviews, 13:47–77.

Wu, S.C., Chen, H.L., Yen, C.C., Kuo, M.F., Yang, T.S., Wang, S.R., Weng, C.N., Chen, C.M. and Cheng, W.T.K. (2007) Recombinant porcine lactoferrin expressed in the milk of transgenic mice enhances offspring growth performance. Journal of Agricultural and Food Chemistry, 55:4670–4677.

Yang, N., Larsen, C.T., Dunnington, E.A., Geraert, P.A., Picard, M. and Siegel, P.B. (2000) Poultry Science, 79:799–803.

## Chapter 2: Immune System and Nutrients for Immune cell Development

Alvarez-Curto, E. and Milligan, G. (2016) Metabolism meets immunity: the role of free fatty acid receptors in the immune system. Biochem. Pharmacol., 114:3–13.

Ananieva, E.A., Powell, J.D. and Hutson, S.M. (2016) Leucine metabolism in T cell activation: mTOR signalling and beyond. Adv. Nutr., 7:798S–805S.

Buck, M.D., O'Sullivan, D. and Pearce, E.L. (2015) T cell metabolism drives immunity. J. Exp. Med., 212:1345–1360.

Buck, M.D. et al. (2016) Mitochondrial dynamics controls T cell fate through metabolic programming. Cell, 166:63–76.

Cunningham-Rundles, S. (2002) Evaluation of the effects of nutrients on immune function. pp 21–39, In: Nutrition and Immune Function CABI 2002 (eds P.C. Calder, C.J. Field and H.S. Gill).

Devereux, G. (2002) 1. The Immune System: an overview. pp 1–20, In: Nutrition and Immune Function CABI 2002 (eds P.C. Calder, C.J. Field and H.S. Gill).

Forsberg, N.E., Wang, Y., Puntenney, S.B. and Carrol, J.A. (2010) chapter 23. Nutrition and Immunity in Ruminants. pp 290–297, In: Comparative Animal Nutrition and Metabolism CABI 2010 (eds P.R. Cheeke and E.S. Dierenfeld).

Johnson, M.O., Siska, P.J., Contreras, D.C. and Rathmell, J.C. (2016) Nutrients and the microenvironment to feed a T cell army. Seminars in Immunology, 28:505–513.

Lam, W.Y. and Bhattacharya, D (2018) Metabolic Links between Plasma Cell Survival, Secretion, and Stress. Trends in Immunology, 39:No.1 http://dx.doi.org/10.1016/j.it.2017.08.007

Powell, J.D., Pollizzi, K.N., Heikamp, E.B. and Horton, M.R. (2011) Regulation of immune responses by mTOR. Annu. Rev. Immunol.,

Rodriguez-Espinosa, Q., Rojas-Espinosa, O., Moreno-Altamirano, M.M.B., López-Villegas, E.O. and Sánchez-Garcia, F.J. (2015) Metabolic requirements for neutrophil extracellular traps formation. Immunology, 145:213–224.

Saho, A., Pattanaik, A.K. and Goswami, T.K. (2009) Immunobiochemical status of sheep exposed to periods of experimental protein deficit and realimentation. Journal of Animal Science, 87:2664–2673.

Surai, P.F. (2006) Selenium in Nutrition and Health. Published by Nottingham University Press, Nottingham.

Vinolo, M.A., Rodrigues, H.G., Hatanaka, E., Sato, F.T., Sampaio, S.C. and Curi, R. (2011) Suppressive effect of short-chain fatty acids on production of proinflammatory mediators by neutrophils. J. Nutr. Biochem., 22:849–855.

Walls, J., Sinclair, L. and Finlay, D (2016) Nutrient sensing, signal transduction and immune responses. Seminars in Immunology http://dx.doi.org/10.1016/j.smim.2016.09.001

Wang, R. and Green, D.R. (2012) Metabolic reprogramming and metabolic dependency in T cells. Immunol. Rev., 249:14–26.

Yan, Y., Jiang, W., Spinetti, T., Tardivel, A., Castillo, R., Bourquin, C., Guarda, G., Tian, Z., Tschopp, J. and R. Zhou (2013) Omega-3 fatty acids prevent inflammation and metabolic disorder through inhibition of NLRP3 inflammasome activation. Immunity, 38:1154–1163.

Zeng, H. and Chi, H. (2015) Metabolic control of regulatory T cell development and function. Trends Immunol., 36:3–12.

## Chapter 3: Prooxidants and Antioxidants

Celi, P. (2011) Oxidative stress in ruminants. pp. 191–231., In; 'Studies on veterinary medicine, Vol. 5'. (Eds L. Mandelker, P. Vajdovich) (Humana Press: Totowa, NJ).

Celi P. (2013) Yerba Mate *(Ilex paraguariensis)* as strategic supplement for dairy cows. In: Makkar HPS, editor. Enhancing Animal Welfare and Farmer Income Through Strategic Animal Feeding – Some Case Studies. Paper No. 175. Rome, Italy: FAO Animal Production and Health. P. 11–18.

Celi, P. and Gabai, G. (2015) Oxidant/antioxidant balance in animal nutrition and health: the role of protein oxidation. Front. Vet. Sci., 2:48.

Chauhan, S.S., Celi, P., Ponnampalam, E.N., Leury, B.J., Liu, F. and Dunshea, F.R. (2014a) Antioxidant dynamics in the live animal and implications for ruminant health and product (meat/milk) quality: role of vitamin E and selenium. Anim Prod Sci., 54 (10):1525–1536.

Chauhan, S.S., Celi, P., Fahri, F.T., Leury, B.J. and Dunshea, F.R. (2014b) Dietary antioxidants at supranutritional doses modulate skeletal muscle heat shock protein and inflammatory gene expression in sheep exposed to heat stress. J Anim Sci92(11):4897–4908.

Contreras, G.A. and Sordillo, L.M. (2011) Lipid mobilization and inflammatory responses during the transition period of dairy cows. Comp Immunol Microbiol Infect Dis.,34(3):281–289.

Farmer, C., Lapointe, J. and Palin, M.F. (2014) Effects of the plant extract silymarin on prolactin concentrations, mammary gland development, and oxidative stress in gestating gilts. J Anim Sci 92(7):2922–2930.

Leskovec, J., Levart, A., Svete, A.N., Peric, L., Stojcic, M.D., Zikic, D., Salobir, J. and Rezar, V. (2018) Effects of supplementation with α-tocopherol, ascorbic acid, selenium, or their combination in linseed oil-enriched diets on the oxidative status in broilers. Poultry Science, 97:1641–1650.

Makkar, H.P.S., Francis, G. and Becker, K. (2007) Bioactivity of phytochemicals in some lesser-known plants and their effects and potential applications in livestock and aquaculture production systems. Animal 1(09):1371–1391.

Mavangira, V. and Sordillo, L.M. (2018) Role of lipid mediators in the regulation of oxidative stress and inflammatory responses in dairy cattle. Research in Veterinary Science, 116:4–14.

Moini, H., Packer, L. and Saris, N. L. (2002) Antioxidant and prooxidant activities of α-lipoic acid and dihydrolipoic acid. Toxicology and Applied Pharmacology, 182:84–90.

Packer, L., Roy, S. and Sen, C.K. (1997) Alpha-lipoic acid: A metabolic antioxidant and potential redox modulator of transcription. Advance Pharmacology, 38:79–101.

Raphael, W. and Sordillo, L. (2013) Dietary polyunsaturated fatty acids and inflammation: the role of phospholipid biosynthesis. Int J Mol Sci., 14(10):21167–21188. doi:10.3390/ijms141021167

Rizzo, A., Roscino, M.T., Binetti, F. and Sciorsci, R.L. (2012) Roles of reactive oxygen species in female reproduction. Reproduction in Domestic Animals, 47:344–352.

Sabino, M., Capomaccio, S., Cappelli, K., Verini-Supplizi, A., Bomba, L., Ajmone-Marsan, P., Cobellis, G., Olivieri, O., Pieramti, C. and Trabalza-Marinucci, M. (2018) Oregano dietary supplementation modifies the liver transcriptome profile in broilers: RNASeq analysis. Research in Veterinary Science, 117:85–91.

Sohaib, M., Anjum, F.M., asir, M. Saeed, F., Arshad, M.S. and Hussain, S. (2018) Alpha-lipoic acid: An inimitable feed supplement for poultry nutrition. J Anim Physiol Anim Nutr., 102:33–40.

Sordillo, L.M. (2016) Nutritional strategies to optimize dairy cattle immunity. J. Dairy Sci., 99 (6):4967–4982.

Sordillo, L.M. and Raphael, W. (2013) Significance of metabolic stress, lipid mobilization, and inflammation on transition cow disorders. Vet Clin North Am., 29(2):267–278.

Sordillo, L.M. and Mavangira, V. (2014) The nexus between nutrient metabolism, oxidative stress and inflammation in transition cows. Anim Prod Sci.,54(9):1204–1214.

Srilatha, T., Reddy, V.R., Quadratullah, S. and Raju, M.V.L.N. (2010) Effect of alpha-lipoic acid and vitamin E in diet on the performance, antioxidation and immune response in broiler chicken. International Journal of Poultry Science, 9:678–683.

Talukder, S., Kerrisk, K.L., Gabai, G., Fukutomi, A. and Celi, P. (2015) Changes in milk oxidative stress biomarkers in lactating dairy cows with ovulatory and an-ovulatory oestrous cycles. Animal Reproduction Science, 158:86–95.

Yu, L., Peng, Z., Dong, L., Wang, S., Ding, L., Huo, Y. and Wang, H. (2018) Bamboo vinegar powder supplementation improves the antioxidant ability of the liver in finishing pigs. Livestock Science, 211:80–86.

Zebeli, Q. and Metzler-Zebeli, B.U. (2012) Interplay between rumen digestive disorders and diet-induced inflammation in dairy cattle. Res Vet Sci93(3):1099–1108.

Zhang, W., Xiao, S., Lee, E.J. and Ahn, D.U. (2011) Consumption of oxidized oil increases oxidative stress in broilers and affects the quality of breast meat. J Agric Food Chem., 59(3):969–974.

Zorov, D.B., Juhaszova, M. and Sollott, S.J. (2014) Mitochondrial reactive oxygen species (ROS) and ROS-induced ROS release. Physiological Reviews, 94:909–950.

## Chapter 4: Oxidative Stress Combating Potential of Plant Phenols

Alvarenga, L.d.A, Leal, V.d.O., Borges, N.A., Silva de Aguiar, A., Faxen-Irving, G., Stenvinkel, P., Lindholm, B. and Mafra, D. (2018) Curcumin – A promising nutritional strategy for chronic kidney disease patients. Journal of Functional Foods, 40:715–721.

Barnes, P.J. (1997) Nuclear factor-kappa B. International Journal of Biochemistry and Cell Biology, 29:867–870.

Barry, T.N., McNeill, D.M. and McNabb, W.C. (2001) Plant secondary compounds; their impact on nutritive value and upon animal production. In: Proceedings of the XIX International Grass. Conference, Sao Paulo, Brazil, pp. 445–452.

Beutler, B. (2004) Innate immunity: an overview. Mol Immunol., 40:845–859.

Bouwstra, R.J., Nielen, M., Newbold, J.R., Jansen, E.H., Jelinek, H.F. and van Werven, T. (2010b) Vitamin E supplementation during the dry period in dairy cattle. Part II: oxidative stress following vitamin E supplementation may increase clinical mastitis incidence postpartum. Journal of Dairy Science, 93:5696–5706.

Bouwstra, R.J., Nielen, M., Stegeman, J.A., Dobbelaar, P., Newbold, J.R., Jansen, E.H. and van Werven, T. (2010a) Vitamin E supplementation during the dry period in dairy cattle. Part I: adverse effect on incidence of mastitis postpartum in a double-blind randomized field trial. Journal of Dairy Science, 93:5684–5695.

Bradford, B. J., Yuan, K., Farney, J.K., Mamedova, L.K. and Carpenter, A. J. (2015) Invited review: Inflammation during the transition to lactation: new adventures with an old flame. Journal of Dairy Science, 98:6631–6650.

Ceciliani, F., Ceron, J. J., Eckersall, P.D. and Sauerwein, H. (2012) Acute phase proteins in ruminants. Journal of Proteomics, 75:4207–4231.

Gessner, D.K., Fiesel, A., Most, E., Dinges, J., Wen, G., Ringseis, R. and Eder, K. (2013) Supplementation of a grape seed and grape marc meal extract decreases activities of the oxidative stress-responsive transcription factors NF-KappaB and Nrf2 in the duodenal mucosa of pigs. Acta Veterinaria Scandinavica, 55:18.

Gessner, D.K., R. Ringseis and K. Eder (2017) Potential of plant polyphenols to combat oxidative stress and inflammatory processes in farm animals. Journal of Animal Physiology and Animal Nutrition, 101:605–628.

Halliwell, B. (1996) Antioxidants in human health and disease. Annual Review of Nutrition, 16:33–50.

Halliwell, B. (2007) Biochemistry of oxidative stress. Biochemical Society Transactions, 35:1147–1150.

Huang, Q., Liu, X., Zhao, G., Hu, T. and Wang, Y. (2018) Potential and challenges of tannins as an alternative to in-feed antibiotics for farm animal production. Animal Nutrition, in press.

Lopez-Andres, P., Luciano, G., Vasta, V., Gibson, T.M., Biondi, L., Priolo, A., et al. (2013) Dietary quebracho tannins are not absorbed, but increase the antioxidant capacity of liver and plasma in sheep. Br J Nutr, 14:1e8.

Luciano, G., Vasta, V., Monahan, F.J., Lopez-Andres, P., Biondi, L., Lanza, M., et al. (2011) Antioxidant status, colour stability and myoglobin resistance to oxidation of longissimus dorsi muscle from lambs fed a tannin-containing diet. Food Chem, 124:1036e42.

Mathew, D. and Hsu, Wei-Li. (2018) Antiviral potential of curcumin. Journal of Functional Foods, 40:692–699.

Mueller-Harvey, I. (2006) Unravelling the conundrum of tannins in animal nutrition and health. J. Sci. Food Agric., 86:2010–2037.

Park, M., Cho, H., Jung, H., Lee, H. and Hwang, K.T. (2014) Antioxidant and anti-inflammatory activities of tannin fraction of the extract from black raspberry seeds compared to grape seeds. J Food Biochem., 38(3):259e70.

Pathak, A.K., Dutta, N., Banerjee, P.S., Goswami, T.K. and Sharma K. (2016) Effect of condensed tannins supplementation through leaf meal mixture on voluntary feed intake, immune response and worm burden in *Haemonchus contortus*-infected sheep. J Parasit Dis., 40:100.

Patra, A.K. and Saxena, J. (2011) Exploitation of dietary tannins to improve rumen metabolism and ruminant nutrition. J Sci Food Agri., 91(1):24e37.

Provenza, F.D. and J.J. Villalba (2010) The role of natural plant products in modulating the immune system: An adaptable approach for combating disease in grazing animals. Small Ruminant Research, 89:131–139.

Sahin, K., Akdemir, F., Orhan, C., Tuzcu, M., Hayirli, A. and N. Sahin. (2010) Effects of dietary resveratrol supplementation on egg production and antioxidant status. Poult. Sci., 89:1190–1198.

Surai, P.F. (2014) Polyphenol compounds in the chicken/animal diet: from the past to the future. Journal of Animal Physiology and Animal Nutrition, 98:19–31.

Tizard, I.R., Carpenter, R.H., McAnalley, B.H. and Kemp, M.C. (1989) The biological activities of mannans and related complex carbohydrates. Mol. Biother., 1:290–296.

Villalba, J.J. Provenza, F.D. and Olson, K.C. (2006a). Terpenes and carbohydrate source influence rumen fermentation, digestibility, intake, and preference in sheep. J. Anim. Sci., 84:2463–2473.

Villalba, J.J. and Provenza, F.D. (2007) Self-medication and homeostatic behaviour in herbivores: learning about the benefits of nature's pharmacy. Animal, 1:1360–1370.

Yadav, R., Jee, B. and Awasthi, S.K. (2015) Curcumin suppresses the production of proinflammatory cytokine interleukin-18 in lipopolysaccharide stimulated murine macrophage-like cells. Indian Journal of Clinical Biochemistry, 30:109–112.

Zhang, C., Luo, J., Yu, B., Zheng, P., Huang, Z., Mao, X., He, J., Yu, J., Chen, J. and D. Chen. (2015b) Dietary resveratrol supplementation improves meat quality of finishing pigs through changing muscle fibre characteristics and antioxidative status. Meat Sci., 102:15–21.

Zhang, C., Wang, L., Zhao, X.H., Chen, X.Y., Yang, L. and Geng, Z. Y. (2017) Dietary resveratrol supplementation prevents transport-stress-impaired meat quality of broilers through maintaining muscle energy metabolism and antioxidant status. Poultry Science, 96:2219–2225.

## Chapter 5: Immunomodulatory Nutrients to Support Gut Health

Adams, C. A. (2010) The probiotic paradox: Live and dead cells are biological response modifiers. Nutrition Research Reviews, 23:37e46.

Allaire, J.M., Crowley, S.M., Law, H.T., Chang, S-Y., Ko, H.J. and Vallance, B.A. (2018) The Intestinal Epithelium: Central Coordinator of Mucosal Immunity. Trends in Immunology, September 2018, 39(9):677–696. https://doi.org/10.1016/j.it.2018.04.002

Andrade, M.E.R. et al., (2015) The role of immuno-modulators on intestinal barrier homeostasis in experimental models. Clinical Nutrition, 34:1080–1087.

Bachinger D, Mayer E, Kaschubek T, Schieder C, König J, Teichmann K. (2018) Influence of phytogenics on recovery of the barrier function of intestinal porcine epithelial cells after a calcium switch. J Anim Physiol Anim Nutr. 00:1–11. https://doi.org/10.1111/jpn.12997

Bauer, E., Williams, B.A., Smidt, H., Mosenthin, R. and Verstegen, M.W. (2006a) Influence of dietary components on development of the microbiota in single-stomached species. Nutrition Research Reviews, 19:63–78.

Bauer, E., Williams, B.A., Smidt, H., Verstegen, M.W. and Mosenthin, R. (2006b) Influence of the gastrointestinal microbiota on development of the immune system in young animals. Current Issues in Intestinal Microbiology, 7:35–52.

Bermudez-Brito, M., Plaza-Diaz, J., Mu-noz-Quezada, S., G_omez-Llorente, C., and Gil, A. (2012) Probiotic mechanisms of action. Annals of Nutrition and Metabolism, 61:160–174.

Celi, P., A.J. Cowieson, F. Fru-Nji, R.E. Steinert, A.M. Luenter and V. Verlhac (2017) Gastro-intestinal functionality in animal nutrition and health: New opportunities for sustainable animal production. Animal Feed Science and Technology, 234:88–100.

Clavijo, V. and Fl'orez, M.S.V. (2018) The gastrointestinal microbiome and its association with the control of pathogens in broiler chicken production: A review. Poultry Science, 97:1006–1021.

De Almada, C.N., Almada, C.N., Martinez, R.C.R. and Sant'Ana, A.S. (2016). Paraprobiotics: Evidences on their ability to modify biological responses, inactivation methods and perspectives on their application in foods. Trends in Food Science and Technology, 58:96–114.

De Lange, C.F.M., Pluske, J., Gong, J. and Nyachoti, C.M. (2010) Strategic use of feed ingredients and feed additives to stimulate gut health and development in young pigs. Livestock Science, 134:124–134.

Diaz-Sanchez, S., D'Souza, D., Biswas, D. and Hanning, I. (2015) Botanical alternatives to antibiotics for use in organic poultry production. Poult. Sci., 94:1419–1430.

FAO. (2016) Probiotics in animal nutrition – Production, impact and regulation by Yadav S. Bajagai, Athol V. Klieve, Peter J. Dart and Wayne L. Bryden. Editor Harinder P.S. Makkar. FAO Animal Production and Health Paper No.179. Rome.

Freimoser, F.M., Pelludat, C. and Remus-Emsermann, M.N.P. (2016) Tritagonist as a new term for uncharacterized microorganisms in environmental systems. ISME J., 10:1–3.

Gilani, S., Howarth, G.S., Kitessa, S.M., Forder, R.E.A., Tran, C.D. and Hughes, R.J. (2016) New biomarkers for intestinal permeability induced by lipopolysaccharide in chickens. Animal Production Science, http://dx.doi.org/10.1071/AN15725

Grashorn, M. (2010) Use of phytobiotics in broiler nutrition – an alternative to infeed antibiotics? J. Anim. Feed Sci., 19:338–347.

Han, G.G., Kim, E. B., Lee, J., Lee, J.-Y., Jin, G., Park, J., Huh, C.-S., Kwon, I.-K., Kil, D. Y., Choi, Y.-J. and Kong, C. (2016) Relationship between the microbiota in different sections of the gastrointestinal tract, and the body weight of broiler chickens. Springerplus. 5:911.

Ivanov, A. I. (2013) Structure and regulation of intestinal epithelial tight junctions. In C.Y. Cheng (Ed.), Biology and regulation of blood tissue barriers (pp. 132–148). New York, NY: Springer New York.

Jha, R. and Berrocoso, J.F.D. (2016) Dietary fibre and protein fermentation in the intestine of swine and their interactive effects on gut health and on the environment: a review. Anim. Feed Sci. Tech., 212:18–26.

Kim, J.C., Hansen, C.F., Mullan, B.P. and Pluske, J.R. (2012a) Nutrition and pathology of weaner pigs: Nutritional strategies to support barrier function in the gastrointestinal tract. Animal Feed Science and Technology, 173:3–16.

Kvidera, S.K., Horst, E.A., Al-Qaisi, M., Dickson, M.J., Rhoads, R.P. and L.H. Baumgard (2016) Leaky Gut's Contribution to Inefficient Nutrient Utilization. Proceedings of Four-State Dairy Nutrition and Management Conference June 15 and 16, 2016, Dubuque, Iowa.

Laxminarayan, R., Van Boeckel, T and Teillant, A. (2015) 'The economic costs of withdrawing antimicrobial growth promoters from the livestock sector.' OECD food, agriculture and fisheries papers, 78. (OECD Publishing: Paris)

Leonard, S.G., Sweeney, T., Bahar, B., Lynch, B.P. and O'Doherty, J.V. (2010) Effect of maternal fish oil and seaweed extract supplementation on colostrum and milk composition, humoral immune response, and performance of suckled piglets. Journal of Animal Science, 88:2988–2997.

Muanprasat, C., Wongkrasant, P., Satitsri, S., Moonwiriyakit, A., Pongkorpsakol, P., Mattaveewong, T., Pichyangkura, R. and Chatsudthipong, V. (2015) Activation of AMPK by chitosan oligosaccharide in intestinal epithelial cells: mechanism of action and potential applications in intestinal disorders. Biochem. Pharmacol., 96:225–236.

O'Doherty, J.V., Bouwhuis, M.A. and Sweeny, T. (2017) Novel marine polysaccharides and maternal nutrition to stimulate gut health and performance in post-weaned pigs. Animal Production Science, 57:2376–2385.

Patel, R.M. and Denning, P.W. (2013). Therapeutic use of prebiotics, probiotics, and postbiotics to prevent necrotizing enterocolitis. What is the current evidence? Clinics in Perinatology, 40:11–25.

Rakoff-Nahoum, S. et al. (2004) Recognition of commensal microflora by Toll-like receptors is required for intestinal homeostasis. Cell, 118:229–241.

Roselli, M., Pieper, R., Rogel-Gaillard, C., Vries, H., Bailey, M., Smidt, H. and Lauridsen, C. (2017) Immunomodulating effects of probiotics for microbiota modulation, gut health and disease resistance in pigs. Animal Feed Science and Technology, 233:104–119.

Seifi, K., Torshizi, M.A.K., Rahimi, S. and Kazemifard, M. (2017) Efficiency of early, single-dose probiotic administration methods on performance, small intestinal morphology, blood biochemistry, and immune response of Japanese quail. Poult. Science, 96:2151–2158.

Steiner, T. and Syed, B. (2015) Phytogenic feed additives in animal nutrition. In Á. Máthé (Ed.), Medicinal and aromatic plants of the world: Scientific production and commercial utilization aspects (pp. 403–423). Dordrecht, the Netherlands: Springer Netherlands.

Stoakes, S.K., Nolan, E.A., Abuajamieh, M., Sanz Fernandez, M.V. and L.H. Baumgard. (2015d) Estimating glucose requirements of an activated immune system in growing pigs. J. Anim. Sci., 93 (E-Suppl. S3):634.

Stoakes, S.K., Nolan, E.A., Valko, D.J., Abuajamieh, M., Mayorga, E.J., Seibert, J. T., Sanz Fernandez, M.V., Gorden, P.J. and Baumgard, L.H. (2015a) Estimating glucose requirements of an activated immune system in lactating Holstein cows. J. Dairy Sci., 98 (E-Suppl.2):509.

Stoakes, S.K., E.A. Nolan, D.J. Valko, M. Abuajamieh, M.V. Sanz Fernandez and L.H. Baumgard. 2015c. Estimating glucose requirements of an activated immune system in Holstein steers. J. Dairy Sci. 98 (E-Suppl.2):21.

Stoakes, S.K., Nolan, E.A., Valko, D.J., Abuajamieh, M., Seibert, J.T., Sanz Fernandez, M.V., Gorden, P.J., Green, H.B., Schoenberg, K.M., Trout, W.E. and L.H. Baumgard. (2015b) Characterizing the effect of feed restriction on biomarkers of leaky gut. J. Dairy Sci., 98 (E-Suppl.2):274.

Suryanarayana, M.V A.N. and Ramana, J.V. (2015) A review of the effects of dietary organic acids fed to swine. Journal of Animal Science and Biotechnology, 6:45.

Suzuki, T. (2013) Regulation of intestinal epithelial permeability by tight junctions. Cellular and Molecular Life Sciences, 70:631–659. https://doi.org/10.1007/s00018–012–1070-x.

Tran, T.H.T., Everaert, N. and Bindelle, J. (2017) Review on the effects of potential prebiotics on controlling intestinal enteropathogens *Salmonella* and *Escherichia coli* in pig production, Journal of Animal Physiology and Animal Nutrition, DOI:10.1111/jpn. 12666.

Vander Heiden, M.G., Cantley, L.C. and Thompson, C.B. (2009) Understanding the Warburg effect: the metabolic requirements of cell proliferation. Science, 324:1029–1033.

Vander Meer, Y., Lammers, A., Jansman, A.J., Rijnen, M.M. Hendriks, W.H. and Gerrits, W.J. (2016) Performance of pigs kept under different sanitary conditions affected by protein intake and amino acid supplementation. J. Anim. Sci., 94:4704–4719.

Wang, Y.Q., Puntenney, S.B., Burton, J.L. and Forsberg, N.E. (2009) Use of gene profiling to evaluate the effects of a feed additive on immune function in periparturient dairy cattle. Journal of Animal Physiology and Animal Nutrition, 93:66–75.

Wijtten, P.J., van der Meulen, J. and Verstegen, M.W. (2011) Intestinal barrier function and absorption in pigs after weaning: a review. British Journal of Nutrition, 105:967–981.

Yang, G., Bibi, S., Du, M., Suzuki, T. and Zhu, M.J. (2017) Regulation of the intestinal tight junction by natural polyphenols: A mechanistic perspective. Critical Reviews in Food Science and Nutrition, 57:3830–3839. https://doi.org/10.1080/10408398.2016.1152230

Zhao, J., Tian, F., Zhao, N., Zhai, Q., Zhang, H. and Chen, W. (2017) Effects of probiotics on D-galactose-induced oxidative stress in plasma: A meta-analysis of animal models. Journal of Functional Foods, 39:44–49.

## Chapter 6: Amino Acids and Immunity

Adedokun, S.A., Ajuwon, K.M., Romero, L.F. and Adeola, O. (2012) Ileal endogenous amino acid losses: Response of broiler chickens to fibre and mild coccidial vaccine challenge. Poult. Sci., 91:899–907.

Artis, D. (2008) Epithelial-cell recognition of commensal bacteria and maintenance of immune homeostasis in the gut. Nat Rev Immunol, 8:411–420.

Bauchart-Thevret, C., Stoll, B., Chacko, S. and Burrin, D.G. (2009) Sulfur amino acid deficiency upregulates intestinal methionine cycle activity and suppresses epithelial growth in neonatal pigs. Am J Physiol Endocrinol Metab, 296:E1239–E1250.

Bernard, A.C., Mistry, S.K., Morris, S.M. Jr., O'Brien, W.E., Tsuei, B.J., Maley, M.E., Shirley, L.A., Kearney, P.A., Boulanger, B.R. and Ochoa, J.B. (2001) Alterations in arginine metabolic enzymes in trauma. Shock, 15:215–219.

Blachier, F., Boutry, C., Bos, C. and Tome, D. (2009) Metabolism and functions of L-glutamate in the epithelial cells of the small and large intestines. Am J Clin Nutr., 90:814S–821S.

Bortoluzzi, C., Rochell, S.J. and Applegate, T.J. (2018) Threonine, arginine, and glutamine: Influences on intestinal physiology, immunology, and microbiology in broilers. Poultry Science, 97:937–945.

Brandtzaeg, P. (2009) Mucosal immunity: induction, dissemination, and effector functions. Scand. J. Immunol., 70:505–515.

Brisbin, J. T., Gong, J. and Shard, S. (2008) Interactions between commensal bacteria and the gut-associated immune system of the chicken. Anim. Health Res. Rev., 9:101–110.

Burkey, T.E., Skjolaas, K.A. and Minton, J.E. (2009) Board-Invited Review: Porcine mucosal immunity of the gastrointestinal tract. J Anim Sci, 87:1493–1501.

CABI (2002) Nutrition and Immune Function. Chapter 7. Sulphur Amino Acids, Glutathione and Immune Function R.F. Grimble, pp 133–150.

CABI (2002) Nutrition and Immune Function. Chapter 5. Arginine and Immune Function M.D. Duff and J.M. Daly pp 93–108.

Calder, P.C. (2006) Branched-chain amino acids and immunity. J Nutr, 136:288S–293S.

Calder, P.C. and Yagoob, P. (1999) Glutamine and the immune system. Amino Acids, 17:227–241.

Chen, Y. P., Cheng, Y. F., Li, X. H., Yang, W. L., Wen, C., Zhuang, S. and Zhou, Y. M. (2016) Effects of threonine supplementation on the growth performance, immunity, oxidative status, intestinal integrity, and barrier function of broilers at the early age. Poult. Sci., 96:405–413.

Cunningham-Rundles, S. (2002) Evaluation of the effects of nutrients on immune function. In: Calder PC, Field CJ, Gill HS (eds) Nutrition and immune function. CABI Publishing, Wallingford, UK, pp 57–92.

Ewaschuk, J.B., Murdoch, G.K., Johnson, I.R., Madsen, K.L. and Field, C.J. (2011) Glutamine supplementation improves intestinal barrier function in a weaned piglet model of *Escherichia coli* infection. Br J Nutr, 106:870–877.

Faure, M., Chone, F., Mettraux, C., Godin, J., Bechereau, F., Vuichoud, J., Papet, I., Breuille, D. and Obled, C. (2007) Threonine utilization for synthesis of acute phase proteins, intestinal proteins, and mucins is increased during sepsis in rats. J. Nutr., 137:1802–1807.

Fernandes, J.I.M. and Murakami, A.E. (2010) Arginine metabolism in uricotelic species. Acta Sci., 32:357–366.

Fernandez, S.R., Aoyagi, S., Han, Y., Parsons, C. M. and Baker, H. (1994) Limiting order of amino acid in corn and soybean meal cereal for growth of the chick. Poult. Sci., 73:1887–1896.

Gaskins, H.R. 2001. Intestinal bacteria and their influence on swine growth. Pages 585–608, In: Swine Nutrition. A. J. Lewis, and L.L. Southern, ed. CRC Press, Boca Raton, FL.

Grimble, R.F. (2001) Nutritional modulation of immune function. Proc Nutr Soc, 60:389–397.

Grimble, R.F. (2006) The effects of sulfur amino acid intake on immune function in humans. J Nutr, 136:1660S–1665S.

Johnsona, I.R., Ball, R.O., Baracos, V.E. and Field, C.J. (2006) Glutamine supplementation influences immune development in the newly weaned piglet. Dev Comp Immunol, 30:1191–1202.

Kidd, M.T. 2004. Nutritional modulation of immune function in broilers. Poult. Sci., 83:650–657.

Kidd, M.T. and Kerr, B. J. (1996) L-threonine for poultry: a review. J. App. Poult. Res., 5:358–367.

Kim, S.W., Mateo, R.D., Yin, Y.L. and Wu, G.Y. (2007) Functional amino acids and fatty acids for enhancing production performance of sows and piglets. Asian-Australas J Anim Sci, 20:295–306.

Konashi, S., Takahashi, K. and Akiba, Y. (2000) Effects of dietary essential amino acid deficiencies on immunological variables in broiler chickens. Br J Nutr, 83:449–456.

Laparra, J.M. and Sanz, Y. (2010) Interactions of gut microbiota with functional food components and nutraceuticals. Pharmacol. Res., 61:219–225.

Law, G.K., Bertolo, R.F., Adjiri-Awere, A., Pencharz, P.B. and Ball, R.O. (2007) Adequate oral threonine is critical for mucin production and gut function in neonatal piglets. Am J Physiol Gastrointest Liver Physiol, 292:G1293–G1301.

Le Floc'h, N. and Seve, B. (2007) Biological roles of tryptophan and its metabolism: potential implications for pig feeding. Livest Sci, 112:23–32.

Li, D.F., Xiao, C.H., Qiao, S.Y., Zhang, J.H., Johnsonb, E.W. and Thacker, P.A. (1999) Effects of dietary threonine on performance, plasma parameters and immune function of growing pigs. Anim Feed Sci Technol, 78:179–188.

Li, P., Yin, Y.L., Li, D.F., Kim, S.W. and Wu, G. (2007) Amino acids and immune function. Br. J. Nutr., 98:237–252.

Mani, V., Weber, T.E., Baumgard, L.H. and Gabler, N.K. (2012) Endotoxin inflammation and intestinal function in livestock. J Anim Sci., doi:10.2527/jas.2011–4627.

McBride, B.W. and Kelly, J.M. (1990) Energy cost of absorption and metabolism in the ruminant gastrointestinal tract and liver: A review. J. Anim. Sci., 68:2997–3010.

Newsholme, P. (2001) Why is L-glutamine metabolism important to cells of the immune system in health, postinjury, surgery or infection? J. Nutr., 131:2515–2522.

Opapeju, F.O., Rademacher, M., Blank, G. and Nyachoti, C.M. (2008) Effect of low-protein amino acid-supplemented diets on the growth performance, gut morphology, organ weights and digesta characteristics of weaned pigs. Animal, 2:1457–1464. doi:10.1017/S1751731 10800270X

Pluske, J.R., Kim, J.C. and Black, J.L. (2018) Manipulating the immune system for pigs to optimise performance. Animal Production Science, 58:666–680. https://doi.org/10.1071/AN17598

Rakhshandeh, A., Htoo, J.K. and de Lange, C.F.M. (2010) Immune system stimulation of growing pigs does not alter apparent ileal amino acid digestibility but reduces the ratio between whole body nitrogen and sulfur retention. Livest Sci, 134(1):21–23.

Reeds, P.J. and Jahoor, F. (2001) The amino acid requirement of disease. Clin Nutr, 20:15–22.

Rhoads, J.M. and Wu, G. (2009) Glutathione, arginine and leucine signalling in the intestine. Amino Acids, 37:111–122.

Ruth, M.R. and Field, C.J. (2013) The immune modifying effects of amino acids on gut-associated lymphoid tissue. Journal of Animal Science and Biotechnology, 4:27.

Scheppach, W., Dusel, G. Kuhn, T. Loges, C. Karch, H. and Bartram, H.P. (1996) Effect of L-glutamine and n-butyrate on the restitution of rat colonic mucosa after acid induced injury. Gut., 38:878–885.

Sinkora, M. and Butler, J.E. (2009) The ontogeny of the porcine immune system. Dev Comp Immunol, 33 (3):273–283.

Soares, A.D., Costa, K.A., Wanner, S.P., Santos, R.G., Fernandes, S.O., Martins, F.S., Nicoli, J.R., Coimbra, C.C. and Cardoso, V.N. (2014) Dietary glutamine prevents the loss of intestinal barrier function and attenuates the increase in core body temperature induced by acute heat exposure. Br. J. Nutr., 112:1601–1610.

Tan, B., Xie, M. and Yin, Y. (2013) Chapter 12, Amino Acids and Immune Functions, pp175–185. In: Nutritional and Physiological Functions of Amino Acids in Pigs, (Ed. F. Blachier et al.) Springer-Verlag Wien.

Tan, J., Applegate, T.J., Liu, S., Guo, Y. and Eicher, S. (2014a) Supplemental dietary L-arginine attenuates intestinal mucosal disruption during a coccidial vaccine challenge in broiler chickens. Br. J. Nutr., 112:1098–1109.

Tan, J., Liu, S., Guo, Y., Applegate, T. J. and Eicher, S.D. (2014b) Dietary L-arginine supplementation attenuates lipopolysaccharide induced inflammatory response in broiler chickens. Br. J. Nutr., 111:1394–1404.

Turner, J.R. (2009) Intestinal mucosal barrier function in health and disease. Nat Rev Immunol, 9:799–809.

Wang, J., Chen, L., Li, P., Li, X., Zhou, H., Wang, F., Li, D., Yin, Y. and Wu, G. (2008) Gene expression is altered in piglet small intestine by weaning and dietary glutamine supplementation. J. Nutr., 138:1025–1032.

Wang, X., Qiao, S. Y., Liu, M. and Ma, Y. X. (2006) Effects of graded levels of true ileal digestible threonine on performance, serum parameters and immune function of 10–25 kg pigs. Anim. Feed Sci. Technol., 129:264–278.

Wang, X.C., Yang, H. S., Gao, W., Xiong, X., Gong, M. and Yin, Y. L. (2016) Differential effects of dietary protein contents on jejunal epithelial cells along the villus-crypt axis in nursery piglets. J. Anim. Sci. 2016., 94:354–358.

Wu, G. (1998) Intestinal mucosal amino acid catabolism. J. Nutr. 128(8):1249–1252.

Wu, G. (2009) Amino acids: Metabolism, functions, and nutrition. Amino Acids, 37:1–17.

Wu, G. (2010) Functional amino acids in growth, reproduction and health. Adv. Nutr., 1:31–37.

Wu, G. (2013) Functional amino acids in nutrition and health. Amino Acids, 45:407–411.

Wu, G., Knabe, D.A., Yan, W. and Flynn, N.E. (1995) Glutamine and glucose metabolism in enterocytes of the neonatal pig. Am J Physiol, 268:R334–R342.

Wu, G., Meier, S.A. and Knabe, O.A. (1996) Dietary glutamine supplementation prevents jejunal atrophy in weaned pigs. J Nutr, 126:2578–2584.

Wu, G., Meininger, C.J., Knabe, D.A., Bazer, F.W. and Rhoads, J.M. (2000) Arginine nutrition in development, health and disease. Curr Opin Clin Nutr Metab Care, 3:59–66.

Wu, G., Fang, Y.Z., Yang, S., Lupton, J.R. and Turner, N.D. (2004) Glutathione metabolism and its implications for health. J Nutr, 134:489–492.

Wu, G.Y., Field, C.J. and Marliss, E.B. (1991) Glutamine and glucose metabolism in rat splenocytes and mesenteric lymph node lymphocytes. Am J Physiol, 260:E141–E147.

Xu, Y.Q., Guo, Y.W., Shi, B.L., Yan, S.M. and Guo, X.Y. (2018) Dietary arginine supplementation enhances the growth performance and immune status of broiler chickens. Livestock Science, 209:8–13.

Yang, H., X. Xiong, and Y. Yin. 2013a. Development and renewal of intestinal villi in pigs. pp. 29–47, In: F. Blachier, G. Wu, and Y. Yin, editors, Nutritional and physiological functions of amino acids in pigs. Springer, Vienna.

Yoneda, J., Andou, A. and Takehana, K. (2009) Regulatory roles of amino acids in immune response. Cuff Rheumatol Rev, 5:252–258.

Zhang, Q., Eicher, S. D. and Applegate, T. J. (2015) Development of intestinal mucin 2, IgA, and polymeric Ig receptor expressions in broiler chickens and Pekin ducks. Poult. Sci., 94:172–180.

Ziegler, T.R., Evans, M.E., Fernandez-Estivariz, C. and Jones, D.P. (2003) Trophic and cytoprotective nutrition for intestinal adaptation, mucosal repair, and barrier function. Annu Rev Nutr, 23:229–261.

## Chapter 7: Fatty acids and Immunity

Abeywardena, M.Y. and Head, R.J. (2001) Long chain n-3 polyunsaturated fatty acids and blood vessel function. Cardiovasc Res, 52:361–71.

Adkins, Y. And Kelley, D.S. (2010) Mechanisms underlying the cardioprotective effects of omega-3 polyunsaturated fatty acids. Journal of Nutritional Biochemistry, 21:781–792.

AL-Jawadi, A., Moussa, H., Ramalingam, L., Dharnmwardhane, S., Gollahon, L., Gunaratne, P., Rahman, R.L. and Moustaid-Moussa, N. (2018). Protective properties of n-3 fatty acids and implications in obesity-associated breast cancer. Journal of Nutritional Biochemistry, 53:1–8.

Alvarez-Curto, E. and Milligan, G (2016) Metabolism meets immunity: The role of free fatty acid receptors in the immune system. Biochemical Pharmacology, 114:3–13.

Aruoma O. (1998) Free radicals, oxidative stress, and antioxidants in human health and disease. J Am Oil Chem Soc, 75:199–212. http://dx.doi.org/10.1007/s11746-998-0032-9

Barbieri E and Sestili P. (2012) Reactive oxygen species in skeletal muscle signalling. J Signal Transduct, 2012:982794.

Bassaganya-Riera, J., Hontecillas, R., Zimmerman, D.R., and Wannemuehler, M.J. (2002) Long-term influence of lipid nutrition on the induction of CD8(+) responses to viral or bacterial antigens. Vaccine, 20:1435–1444.

Belury, M. A., Moya-Camerena, S. Y., Liu, L. L., and Vanden Heuvel, J.P. (1997) Dietary conjugated linoleic acid induces peroxisome-specific enzyme accumulation and ornithine decarboxylase activity in mouse liver. J. Nutr. Biochem., 8:579–584.

Boit, M.D., Hunter, A.M. and Gray, S.R. (2017) Metaboilsm, Fit with good fat? The role of n-3 polyunsaturated fatty acids on exercise performance. Metabolism Clinical and Experimental, 66:45–54, http://dx.doi.org/10.1016/i.metabol.2016.10.007

CABI (2002) Nutrition and Immune Function. Chapter 4. Fatty acids, Inflammation and Immunity by Calder and Field pp57–92.

Calder, P.C. (2002) Dietary modification of inflammation with lipids. Proc Nutr Soc, 1:345–358.

Calder, P.C. (2012) Mechanisms of action of (n-3) fatty acids. J. Nutr., 142:592S–599S.

Calder, P.C. (2013) Omega-3 polyunsaturated fatty acids and inflammatory processes: nutrition or pharmacology? Br. J. Clin. Pharmacol., 75:645–662.

Calder, P.C. (2015) Marine n-3 PUFA fatty acids and inflammatory processes: effects mechanisms and clinical relevance. Biochim Biophys Acta, 1851(4):469–484.

Calder, P.C. and Grimble, R.F. (2002) Polyunsaturated fatty acids, inflammation and immunity. Eur J Clin Nutr, 56 (Suppl 3):S14–19.

Calder, P.C. and Yaqoob, P. (2009) Understanding omega-3 polyunsaturated fatty acids. Postgrad Med, 121(6):148e57. http://dx.doi.org/10.3810/pgm.2009.11.2083.

Calviello, G., Palozza, P., Maggiano, N., Piccioni, E., Franceschelli, P., Frattucci, A., Di Nicuolo, F. and Bartoh, G.M. (1999). Cell proliferation' differentiation' and apoptosis are modified by n-3 polyunsaturated fatty acids in normal colonic mucosa. Lipids, 34:599–604.

Cook, M.E., Miller, C.C., Park, Y. and Pariza, M. (1993) Immune modulation by altered nutrient metabolism: nutritional control of immune-induced growth depression. Poult. Sci., 72:1301–1305.

Corino, C., Bontempo, V. and Sciannimanico, D. (2002) Effects of dietary conjugated linoleic acid on some aspecific immune parameters and acute phase protein in weaned piglets. Can. J. Anim. Sci., 82:115–117.

Corpet, D.E. (2011). Red meat and colon cancer: should we become vegetarians, or can we make meat safer? Meat Sci., 89:310–316.

Deckelbaum, R.J., Worgall, T.S. and Seo, T. (2006) n-3 fatty acids and gene expression. Am J Clin Nutr, 83(6 Suppl):1520S–1525S.

DeVoney, D., Pariza, M. W. and M.E. Cook. (1999) *Trans*-10 *Cis*-12 octadecadienoic acid increases lymphocyte proliferation. FASEB. J., 13:4565.

Fan, Y.Y., Ly, L.H., Barhoumi, R., McMurray, D.N., Chapkin, R.S. (2004). Dietary docosahexaenoic acid suppresses T cell protein kinase C theta lipid raft recruitment and IL-2 production. J Immunol., 173:6151–6160.

Gleeson M and Bishop NC. (2005) The T cell and NK cell immune response to exercise. Ann Transplant, 10 (4):43–48.

Hara, T., Kashihara, D., Ichimura, A., Kimura, I., Tsujimoto, G. and Hirasawa, A. (2014) Role of free fatty acid receptors in the regulation of energy metabolism, Biochim. Biophys. Acta., 1841:1292–1300.

Hara, T., Kimura, I., Inoue, D., Ichimura, A. and Hirasawa, A. (2013) Free fatty acid receptors and their role in regulation of energy metabolism. Rev. Physiol. Biochem. Pharmacol., 164:77–116.

Harris, W.S., Miller, M., Tighe, A.P., Davidson, M.H. and Schaefer, E.J. (2008) Omega-3 fatty acids and coronary heart disease risk: clinical and mechanistic perspectives. Atherosclerosis, 197:12–24.

He, X., Liu, W., Shi, M., Yang, Z., Zhang, X. and Gong, P. (2017) Docosahexaenoic acid attenuates LPS-stimulated inflammatory response by regulating the PPARy/NF-x13 pathways in primary bovine mammary epithelial cells. Research in Veterinary Science, 112:7–12

Hirasawa, A., Tsumaya, K., Awaji, T., Katsuma, S., Adachi, T., Yamada, M. et al., (2005) Free fatty acids regulate gut incretin glucagon-like peptide-1 secretion through GPR120, Nat. Med. 11 90–94.

Ichimura, A., Hirasawa, A., Hara, T. and Tsujimoto, G. (2009) Free fatty acid receptors act as nutrient sensors to regulate energy homeostasis. Prostaglandins Other Lipid Mediat., 89:82–88.

Ichimura, A., Hirasawa, A., Poulain-Godefroy, O., Bonnefond, A., Hara, T., Yengo, L. et al. (2012) Dysfunction of lipid sensor GPR120 leads to obesity in both mouse and human. Nature, 483:350–354.

Jenner P. (2003) Oxidative stress in Parkinson's disease. Ann Neurol, 53 (Suppl 3):S26–36 [discussion S36–8].

Jump, D.B. (2002) Dietary polyunsaturated fatty acids and regulation of gene transcription. Curr Opin Lipidol, 13:155–164.

Kawakami, A., Aikawa, M., Libby, P., Alcaide, P., Luscinskas, F.W. and Sacks, F.M. (2006) Apolipoprotein CIII in apolipoprotein B lipoproteins enhances the adhesion of human monocytic cells to endothelial cells. Circulation, 113:691–700.

Kelley, D.S., Siegel, D., Vemuri, M. and Mackey, B.E. (2007) Docosahexaenoic acid supplementation improves fasting and postprandial lipid profiles in hypertriglyceridemic men. Am J Clin Nutr, 86:324–333.

Kelley, D.S., Siegel, D., Vemuri, M., Chung, G.H. and Mackey, B.E. (2008) Docosahexaenoic acid supplementation decreases remnant-like particle-cholesterol and increases the (n-3) index in hypertriglyceridemic men. J Nutr, 138:30–35.

Kelley, D.S., Taylor, P.C., Nelson, G.J., Schmidt, P.C., Ferretti, A., Erickson, K.L. et al. (1999) Docosahexaenoic acid ingestion inhibits natural killer cell activity and production of inflammatory mediators in young healthy men. Lipids, 34:317–324.

Khan, R.U., Rahman, Z.U., Nikousefat, Z., Javdani, M., Tufarelli, V., Dario, C., Selvaggi, M. and Laudadio, V. (2012). Immunomodulating effects of vitamin E in broilers. World. Poult. Sci. J., 68:31–40.

Klasing, K.C. (1988) Nutritional aspects of leukocytic cytokines. J. Nutr., 118:1436–1446.

Klasing, K.C. and Johnstone, B.J. (1991) Monokines in growth and development. Poult. Sci., 70:1781–1789.

Konieczka, P., Barszcz, M., Chmielewska, M., Cie'slak, N., Szlis, M. and Smulikowska, S. (2017). Interactive effects of dietary lipids and vitamin E level on performance, blood eicosanoids, and response to mitogen stimulation in broiler chickens of different ages. Poult. Sci., 96:359–369.

Konieczka, P., Barszcz, M., Choct, M. and Smulikowska, S. (2018) The interactive effect of dietary n-6: n-3 fatty acid ratio and vitamin E level on tissue lipid peroxidation, DNA damage in intestinal epithelial cells, and gut morphology in chickens of different ages. Poultry Science, 97:149–158.

Lackey, D.E. and Olefsky, J.M. (2016) Regulation of metabolism by the innate immune system, Nat. Rev. Endocrinol., 12:15–28.

Lai, C.H., Li, D.F., Chen, X.L. and Ding, Y.H. (2006) Immunomodulatory effect of conjugated linoleic acid on baby pigs. Proceedings of international symposium on Recent advances in Animal Nutrition, September 20, 2006 at Busan, Korea, pp115–124.

Le Chatelier, E., Nielsen, T., Qin, J., Prifti, E., Hildebrand, F., Falony, G., et al., (2013) Richness of human gut microbiome correlates with metabolic markers. Nature, 500:541–546.

Lewis, G.P. (1983) Immunoregulatory activity of metabolites of arachidonic acid and their role in inflammation. Br. Med. Bull., 39:243–248.

Madamanchi, N.R., Vendrov, A. and Runge, M.S. (2005) Oxidative stress and vascular disease. Arterioscler Thromb Vase Biol, 25 (1):29–38.

Maslowski, K.M. and Mackay, C.R. (2011) Diet, gut microbiota and immune responses. Nat. Immunol., 12:5–9.

Maslowski, K.M., Vieira, A.T., Ng, A., Kranich, J., Sierro, F., Yu, D., et al., (2009) Regulation of inflammatory responses by gut microbiota and chemoattractant receptor GPR43. Nature, 461:1282–1286.

Miller, C. C., Park, Y., Pariza, M. W. and Cook, M.E. (1994) Feeding conjugated linoleic acid to animals partially overcomes catabolic responses due to endotoxin injection. Biochem. Biophys. Res. Commun., 198:1107–1112.

Morland, S.L., Martins, K.J.B. and Mazurak, V.C. (2016) n-3 polyunsaturated fatty acid supplementation during cancer chemotherapy. Journal of Nutrition and Intermediary Metabolism, 5:107–116.

Murray, P.J., J. Rathmell, and E. Pearce (2015) Snap Shot: immunometabolism, Cell Metab., 22,190.

Oh da, Y., Walenta, E., Akiyama, T.E., Lagakos, W.S., Lackey, D., Pessentheiner, A.R. et al. (2014) A GPR120-selective agonist improves insulin resistance and chronic inflammation in obese mice. Nat. Med., 20:942–947.

Oh, D.Y., Talukdar, S., Bae, E.J., Imamura, T., Morinaga, H. Fan, W. et al., (2010) GPR120 is an omega-3 fatty acid receptor mediating potent anti-inflammatory and insulin-sensitising effects. Cell, 142:687–698.

Ostrowski, K., Rohde, T, Asp, S., Schjerling, P. and Pedersen, B.K. (1999) Pro- and anti-inflammatory cytokine balance in strenuous exercise in humans. J Physiol, 515 (Pt 1):287–291.

Pariza, M.W., Park, Y. and Cook, M.E. (2000) Mechanisms of action of conjugated linoleic acid: evidence and speculation. Proc. Soc. Exp. Biol. Med., 223:8–13.

Romagnani, S. (1995) Biology of human TH1 and TH2 cells. J. Clin. Immunol., 15:121–129.

Rasoamanana, R., Darcel, N., Fromentin, G. and Tome, D. (2012) Nutrient sensing and signalling by the gut. Proc. Nutr. Soc., 71:446–455.

Roura, E. and Fu, M. (2017) Taste, nutrient sensing and feed intake in pigs (130 years of research: then, now and future). Animal Feed Science and Technology, 233:3–12.

Sebedio, J.L., Juaneda, P., Dobson, G., Ramilison, I., Martin, J.C., Chardigny, J. M. and Christie, W. W. (1997) Metabolites of conjugated isomers of linoleic acid (CLA) in the rat. Biochim. Biophys. Acta., 1345:5–10.

Stillwell, W. and Wassall, S.R. (2003) Docosahexaenoic acid: membrane properties of a unique fatty acid. Chem Phys Lipids, 126:1–27.

Suckow, A.T., Polidori, D., Yan, W., Chon, S., Ma, J.Y., Leonard, J. et al. (2014) Alteration of the glucagon axis in GPR120 (FFAR4) knockout mice: a role for GPR120 in glucagon secretion. J. Biol. Chem., 289:15751–15763.

Sugano, M. A., Tsujita, M., Yamasaki, K., Noguchi, M. and Yamada, K. (1998) Conjugated linoleic acid modulates tissue levels of chemical mediators and immunoglobulins in rats. Lipids, 33:521–527.

Swiatkiewicz, S., A. Arczewska-Wlosek, and D. Jozefiak. (2015) The relationship between dietary fat sources and immune response in poultry and pigs: An updated review. Livest. Sci., 180:237–246.

Takahashi. K., Kawamata, K., Akiba, Y., Iwata, T. and Kasai, M. (2002) Influence of dietary conjugated linoleic acid isomers on early inflammatory responses in male broiler chickens. Br. Poult. Sci., 43:47–53.

Tancharoenrat, P., V. Ravindran, F. Zaefarian, and G. Ravindran. (2014).Digestion of fat and fatty acids along the gastrointestinal tract of broiler chickens. Poult. Sci., 93:371–379.

Thorbum, A.N., Macia, L. and Mackay, C.R. (2014) Diet, metabolites and "western lifestyle" inflammatory diseases. Immunity, 40:833–842.

Tontonoz, P., Nagy, L., Alvarez, J.G., Thomazy, V.A. and Evans, R.M. (1998) PPAR gamma promotes monocyte/macrophage differentiation and uptake of oxidized LDL. Cell, 93:241–252.

Trompette, A., Gollwitzer, E.S., Yadava, K., Sichelstiel, A.K., Sprenger, N., Ngom-Bru, C. et al (2014) Gut microbiota metabolism of dietary fibre influences allergic airway disease and hematopoiesis. Nat. Med., 20:159–166.

Wong, S.W., Kwon, M.J., Choi, A.M., Kim, H.P., Nakahira, K., Hwang, D.H. (2009) Fatty acids modulate Toll-like receptor 4 activation through regulation of receptor dimerisation and recruitment into lipid rafts in a reactive oxygen species-dependent manner. J Biol Chem., 284:(273)84–92.

Villaverde, C., M.D. Baucells, E.G. Manzanilla, and A.C. Barroeta. (2008) High levels of dietary unsaturated fat decrease α-tocopherol content of whole body, liver, and plasma of chickens without variations in intestinal apparent absorption. Poult. Sci., 87:497–505.

Yan, Y., Jiang, W., Spinetti, T., Tardivel, A., Castillo, R., Bourquin, C., Guarda, G., Tian, Z., Tschopp, J. and Zhou, R (2013) Omega-3 fatty acids prevent inflammation and metabolic disorder through inhibition of NLRP3 inflammasome activation. Immunity, 38:1154–1163.

Yoshikawa, T., Shimano, H., Yahagi, N., Ide, T., Amemiya-Kudo, M., Matsuzaka, T., et al. (2002) Polyunsaturated fatty acids suppress sterol regulatory element-binding protein lc promoter activity by inhibition of liver X receptor (LXR) binding to LXR response elements. J Biol Chem, 277:1705–1711.

Yu, Y., Correll P.H., and Vanden Heuvel, J.P. (2002) Conjugated linoleic acid decreases production of proinflammatory products in macrophages: evidence for a PPAR gamma-dependent mechanism. Biochim. Biophys. Acta., 1581:89–99.

Zeitz, J.O., J. Fennhoff, H. Kluge, G.I. Stangl, and K. Eder. (2015) Effects of dietary fats rich in lauric and myristic acid on performance, intestinal morphology, gut microbes, and meat quality in broilers. Poult. Sci., 94:2404–2413.

Zhao, L.D., Yin, J.D., Li, D.F., Lai, C.H., Chen, X.J. and Ma, D. (2005) Conjugated linoleic acid can prevent tumour necrosis factor gene expression by inhibiting nuclear factor binding activity in peripheral blood mononuclear cells from weaned pigs challenged with lipopolysaccharide. Arch. Anim. Nutr., 59(6):429–438.

## Chapter 8: Selenium and Immunity

Ahmad, H., Tian, J., Wang, J., Khan, M.A., Wang, Y., Zhang, L. and Wang, T. (2012) Effects of dietary sodium selenite and selenium yeast on antioxidant enzyme activities and oxidative stability of chicken breast meat. J. Agric. Food. Chem., 60:7111–7120.

Beck, M.A. (1999) Selenium and host defence towards viruses. Proceedings of the Nutrition Society, 58:707–711.

Beck, M.A., 2001. Antioxidants and viral infections: host immune response and viral pathogenicity. J. Am. Coll. Nutr. 20 (Suppl. 5), 384S–388S.

Calder, P.C. (2001) Polyunsaturated fatty acids, inflammation, and immunity. Lipids, 36:1007–1024.

Delezie, E., Rovers, M., Van der Aa, A., Ruttens, A., Wittocx, S. and Segers, L. (2014) Comparing responses to different selenium sources and dosages in laying hens. Poult. Sci. 93:3083–3090.

Gill, H. and Walker, G. (2008) Selenium, immune function and resistance to viral infections. Nut. Diet. 65 (S3), S41–S47.

Hefnawy, A.E.G. and Tortora-Perez, J.L. (2010) The importance of selenium and the effects of its deficiency in animal health, Small Ruminant Research, 89:185–192.

Klasing, K.C. (1998) Nutritional modulation of resistance to infectious diseases. Poultry Science, 77:1119–1125.

Klasing, K. (2004) The costs of immunity. Acta Zoologica Sinica,50:961–969.

Nordberg, J. and Amer, E.S. (2001) Reactive oxygen species, antioxidants, and the mammalian thioredoxin system. Free Radical Biology and Medicine, 31:1287–1312.

Rao, S.V.R., Prakash, B., Raju, M.V., L.N. Panda, A.K., Kumari, R.K., Reddy, E.P., 2016. Effect of supplementing organic forms of zinc, selenium and chromium on performance, antioxidant and immune responses in broiler chicken reared in tropical summer. Biol. Trace. Elem. Res. 172:511–520.

Shojadoost, B., Kulkarni, R.R., Yitbarek, A., Laursen, A., Taha-Abdelaziz, K., Alkie, T.N., Barjesteh, N., Quinteiro-Filho, W.M., Smith,

T.K. and Sharif, S. (2019) Dietary selenium supplementation enhances antiviral immunity in chickens challenged with low pathogenic avian influenza virus subtype H9N2. Veterinary Immunology and Immunopathology 207:62–68.

Shrimali, R.K., Irons, R.D., Carlson, B.A., Sano, Y., Gladyshev, V.N., Park, J.M., Hatfield, D.L., 2008. Selenoproteins mediate T cell immunity through an antioxidant mechanism. J. Biol. Chem. 283 (29), 20181–20185.

Surai, P.F. (2002). Natural Antioxidants in Avian Nutrition and Reproduction. Nottingham University Press, Nottingham.

Wu, D.O. and Meydani, S.N. (1998) Antioxidants and immune function. pp.371–400. In: Antioxidant Status, Diet, Nutrition, and Health, Edited by Papas, A. M., CRC Press, Boca Raton.

## Chapter 9: Vitamin D and Immunity

Boodhoo, N., Sharif, S. and Behboudi, S. (2016) 1α,25(OH)$_2$ Vitamin D$_3$ modulates avian T lymphocyte functions without inducing CTL unresponsiveness. PLoS ONE 11(2):e0150134. doi:10.1371/journal.pone.0150134

Boonstra, A., Banat, F. J., Crain, C., Heath, V. L., Savelkoul, H. F. and O'Gaffa, A. (2001) 1-alpha,25-Dihydroxyvitamin D$_3$ has a direct effect on naive CD4(+) T cells to enhance the development of Th2 cells. J. Immunol. (Baltimore, Md. 1950), 167:4974–4980.

Chen, S., Sims, G.P., Chen, X.X., Gu, Y.Y., Chen, S. and Lipsky, P.E. (2007) Modulatory effects of 1,25-dihydroxyvitamin D$_3$ on human B cell differentiation. J Immunol, 179(3):1634–1647.

Di Rosa, M., Malaguarnera, M., Nicoletti, F. and Malaguarnera, L. (2011) Vitamin D$_3$: a helpful immuno-modulator. Immunology, 134(2): 123–139.

Di Rosa, M., Malaguarnera, G., De Gregorio, C., Palumbo, M., Nunnari, G. and Malaguarnera, L. (2012) Immuno-modulatory effects of vitamin D$_3$ in human monocyte and macrophages. Cell Immunol, 280:36–43.

Gottfried, E., Rehli, M., Hahn, J., Holler, E, Andreesen R and Kreutz M. (2006) Monocyte-derived cells express CYP27A1 and convert vitamin D$_3$ into its active metabolite. Biochemical and biophysical research communications, 349(1):209–213.

Jeffery, L.E., Wood, A.M., Qureshi, O.S., Hou, Gardner, Z., Briggs, Z., Kaur, S. Raza, and

Sansom, D. M. (2012) Availability of 25-hydroxyvitamin D3 to APCs controls the balance between regulatory and inflammatory T cell responses. J Immunol, 189:5155–5164.

Kawai, T. and Akira, S. (2010) The role of pattern-recognition receptors in innate immunity: update on Toll-like receptors. Nat Immunol, 11:373–384.

Kongsbak, M., von Essen, M.R., Levring, T.B., Schjerling, P., Woetmann, A., Odum, N., et al. (2014) Vitamin D-binding protein controls T cell responses to vitamin D. BMC immunology, 15:35.

Kuhn, J., Schutkowski, A., Kluge, H., Hirche, F. and Stangl, G.I. (2014) Free-range farming: a natural alternative to produce vitamin D-enriched eggs. Nutrition, 30(4):481–484.

Lemire, J.M., Archer, D. C., Beck, L. and Spiegelberg, H.L. (1995) Immunosuppressive actions of 1,25-dihydroxyvitamin D$_3$: preferential inhibition of Th1 functions. J. Nutr., 125:1704S–1708S.

MacMicking, J., Xie, Q.W. and Nathan, C. (1997) Nitric oxide and macrophage function. Annual review of immunology, 15:323–350.

Morris, A. and Selvaraj. R.K. (2014) *In vitro* 25-hydroxycholecalciferol treatment of lipopoly saccharide-stimulated chicken macrophages increases nitric oxide production and mRNA of interleukin-1beta and 10. Vet Immunol Immunopathol, 161(3–4):265–270.

Opal, S.M. and Huber, C.E. (2002) Bench-to-bedside review: Toll-like receptors and their role in septic shock. Crit. Care, 6:125–136.

Plum, L. and DeLuca, H. (2009) The functional metabolism and molecular biology of vitamin D action. Clin. Rev. Bone Miner. Metab., 7:20–41.

Redmond, S.B., Tell, R. M., Coble, D., Mueller, C., Palic, D., Andreasen, C.B. and Lamont, S.J. (2010) Differential splenic cytokine responses to dietary immune modulation by diverse chicken lines. Poult. Sci., 89:1635–1641.

Rivas-Santiago, B., Hernandez-Pando, R., Carranza, C., Juarez, E., Contreras J.L., Aguilar-Leon, D., Tones, M. and Sada, E. (2008) Expression of cathelicidin LL-37 during Mycobacterium tuberculosis infection in human alveolar macrophages, monocytes, neutrophils, and epithelial cells. Infect. Immun., 76:935–941.

Rodriguez-Lecompte, J.C., Yitbarek, A., Cuperus, T., Echeverry, H. and van Dijk, A. (2016) The immunomodulatory effect of vitamin D in chickens is dose-dependent and influenced by calcium and phosphorus levels, Poultry Science, 95:2547–2556.

Sadeghi, K., Wessner, B., Laggner, U., Ploder, M., Tamandl, D., Friedl, J., Zugel, U., Steinmeyer, A., Pollak, A., Roth E., Boltz-Nitulescu, G. and Spittler, A. (2006) Vitamin $D_3$ downregulates monocyte TLR expression and triggers hyporesponsiveness to pathogen-associated molecular patterns. Eur. J. Immunol., 36:361–370.

Shanmugasundaram, R. and Selvaraj, R.K. (2012) Vitamin D-1alpha-hydroxylase and vitamin D-24-hydroxylase mRNA studies in chickens. Poult Sci, 91(8):1819–1824.

Shojadoost, B., Behboudi, S., Villanueva, A.I., Brisbin, J.T., Ashkar, A.A. and Sharif, S. (2015) Vitamin $D_3$ modulates the function of chicken macrophages. Res. Vet. Sci., 100:45–51.

Sigmundsdottir, H., Pan, J., Debes, G.F., Alt, C., Habtezion, A., Soler, D. et al. (2007) DCs metabolise sunlight induced vitamin $D_3$ to 'program' T cell attraction to the epidermal chemokine CCL27. Nat Immunol, 8(3):285–93.

Staeva-Vieira, T.P. and Freedman, L.P. (2002) 1,25-dihydroxyvitamin $D_3$ inhibits IFN-gamma and IL-4 levels during *in vitro* polarisation of primary murine CD4+ T cells. J Immunol, 168(3):1181–1189.

Turner, J., Cho, Y., Dinh, N.N., Waring, A.J. and Lehrer, R.I. (1998) Activities of LL-37, a cathelin-associated antimicrobial peptide of human neutrophils. Antimicrob. Agents Chemother., 42, 2206–2214.

Verstuyf, A., Carmeliet, G., Bouillon, R. and Mathieu, C. (2010) Vitamin D: a pleiotropic hormone. Kidney International, (2010) 78:140–145.

von Essen, M.R., Kongsbak, M., Schjerling, P., Olgaard, K., Odum, N. and Geisler, C. (2010) Vitamin D controls T cell antigen receptor signalling and activation of human T cells. Nat Immunol, 11(4):344–349.

Wang, T.T., Nestel, F.P., Bourdeau, V., Nagai, Y., Wang, Q., Liao, J., et al. (2004) Cutting edge: 1,25-dihydroxyvitamin $D_3$ is a direct inducer of antimicrobial peptide gene expression. J Immunol, 173(5):2909–2912.

Whitehead, C. C., McCormack, H. A., McTeir, L. and Fleming, R. H. (2004) High vitamin $D_3$ requirements in broilers for bone quality and prevention of tibial dyschondroplasia and interactions with dietary calcium, available

phosphorus and vitamin A. Br. Poult. Sci., 45:425–436.

Zanetti, M., Gennaro, R. and Romeo, D. (1995) Cathelicidins: a novel protein family with a common proregion and a variable C-terminal antimicrobial domain. FEBS Lett., 374:1–5.

Zanetti, M. (2005) The role of cathelicidins in the innate host defences of mammals. Curr. Issues Mol. Biol., 7:179–196.

Zhang, G.W., Li, D.B., Lai, S.J., Chen, S.Y., Lei, R.P. and Zhou, D.G. (2011) Effects of Dietary Vitamin $D_3$ Supplementation on AvBD-1 and chCATH-1 Genes Expression in Chicken. J. Poult. Sci., 48:254–258.

# Chapter 10: Ageing and Immune System

Ames, B. N. (2018) Prolonging healthy ageing: Longevity vitamins and proteins. www.pnas.org/cgi/doi/10.1073/pnas.1809045115

Aspinall, R. and Andrew D. (2000) Thymic involution in ageing. J Clin Immunol, 20:250–256.

Baylis, D., Bartlett, D.B., Patel, H.P. and Roberts, H.C. (2013) Understanding how we age: insights into inflammageing. Longev. Healthspan 2, 1–8.

Bonjour, JP., Kraenzlin, M., Levasseur, R., Warren, M. and Whiting, S. (2013). Dairy in adulthood: from foods to nutrient interactions on bone and skeletal muscle health. J Am Coll Nutr., 32:251–263.

Cawthon, R.M., Smith, K.R., O'Brien, E. et al. (2003) Association between telomere length in blood and mortality in people aged 60 years or older. Lancet, 361:360.

Cepinskas, G., Sandig, M. and Kvietys, P.R. (1999) PAF-induced elastase-dependent neutrophil transendothelial migration is associated with the mobilisation of elastase to the neutrophil surface and localisation to the migrating front. J. Cell Sci., 112 (Pt. 12), 1937–1945.

Davinelli, S., Trichopoulou, A., Corbi, G., De Vivo, I. and Scapagnini, G. (2019) The potential nutrigeroprotective role of Mediterranean diet and its functional components on telomere length dynamics. Ageing Research Reviews, 49:1–10.

Dewansingh, P., Melse-Boonstra, A., Krijnen, W.P., van der Schans, C.P., Jager-Wittenaar, H. and van den Heuvel, E.G.H.M. (2018) Supplemental protein from dairy products increases body weight and vitamin D improves physical performance in older adults: a systematic review and meta-analysis. Nutrition Research, 49:1–22.

Fraker, P.J. and King, L.E. (2004) Reprogramming of the immune system during zinc deficiency. Annu Rev Nutr, 24:277–298.

Heidinger, B.J., Blount, J.D., Boner, W., Griffiths, K., Metcalfe, N.B. and Monaghan, P. (2012) Telomere length in early life predicts lifespan. Proc Natl Acad Sci, U S A., 109:1743–1748.

Ibs, K.H. and Rink, L. (2003) Zinc-altered immune function. J Nutr, 133:1452S–1456S.

Kougias, D.G., Das, T., Perez, A.B. and Pereira, S.L. (2018) A role for nutritional intervention in addressing the ageing neuromuscular junction. Nutrition Research, 53:1–14.

Liu, P.T., Stenger, S., Li, H., Wenzel, L., Tan, B.H., Krutzik, S.R, et al. (2006) Toll-like receptor triggering of a vitamin D-mediated human antimicrobial response. Science, 311:1770–1773.

Liu, Y., Bloom, S.I., Donato, A.J. (2018) The Role of Senescence, Telomere Dysfunction and Shelterin in Vascular Ageing. Microcirculation, e12487.

Meydani, S.N., Han, S.N. and Wu, D. (2005) Vitamin E and immune response in the aged: molecular mechanisms and clinical implications. Immunol Rev, 205:269–284.

Meydani, S.N., Meydani, M., Verdon, C.P., Shapiro, A.A., Blumberg, J.B. and Hayes, K.C. (1986) Vitamin E supplementation suppresses prostaglandin E1(2) synthesis and enhances the immune response of aged mice. Mech Ageing Dev, 34:191–201.

Mocchegiani, E., Giacconi, R., Cipriano, C. and Malavolta, M. (2009) NK and NKT cells in ageing and longevity: role of zinc and metallothioneins. J Clin Immunol, 29:416–25.

Moon, A., Heywood, L., Rutherford, S., Cobbold, C. (2013) Creatine supplementation: can it improve quality of life in the elderly without associated resistance training? Curr Aging Sci., 6:251–257.

Pae, M. and Wu, D. (2017) Nutritional modulation of age-related changes in the immune system and risk of infection. Nutrition Research, 41:14–35.

Panda, A., Arjona, A., Sapey, E., Bai, F., Fikrig, E., Montgomery RR, et al. (2009) Human innate immunosenescence: causes and consequences for immunity in old age. Trends Immunol, 30:325–333.

Piatti, P.M., Monti, F., Fermo, I., Baruffaldi, L., Nasser, R., Santambrogio, G., et al. (1994) Hypocaloric high-protein diet improves glucose oxidation and spares lean body mass: comparison to hypocaloric high-carbohydrate diet. Metab Clin Exp., 43:1481–1487.

Rink, L. and Gabriel, P. (2001) Extracellular and immunological actions of zinc. Biometals, 14:367–383.

Rizzoli, R., Stevonson, J.C., Bauer, J.M., van Loon, L.J.C., Walrand, S., Kanis, J.A., et al. (2014) The role of dietary protein and vitamin D in maintaining musculoskeletal health in postmenopausal women: a consensus statement from the European Society for Clinical and Economic Aspects of Osteoporosis and Osteoarthritis (ESCEO). Maturitas 79:122–132.

Sapey, E., Greenwood, H., Walton, G., Mann, E., Love, A., Aaronson, N., Insall, R.H., Stockley, R.A. and Lord, J.M. (2014) Phosphoinositide 3-kinase inhibition restores neutrophil accuracy in the elderly: toward targeted treatments for immunosenescence. Blood, 123:239–248.

Shaw, A.C., Goldstein, D.R. and Montgomery, R.R. (2013) Age-dependent dysregulation of innate immunity. Nat Rev Immunol, 13:875–887.

Srikuea, R., Zhang, X., Park-Sarge, O.K., Esser, K.A. (2012) VDR and CYP27B1 are expressed in C2C12 cells and regenerating skeletal muscle: potential role in suppression of myoblast proliferation. Am J Physiol Cell Physiol., 303:C396–405.

Tseng, C.W. and Liu, G.Y. (2014) Expanding roles of neutrophils in ageing hosts. Curr Opin Immunol, 29:43–48.

Viswanath Sardesai (2012) Introduction to Clinical Nutrition, 3rd edition, CRC Press Taylor and Francis Group, chapter 31.Gene - Nutrient Interaction - molecular Genetics, Epigenetics and Telomeres, pp 617–635.

Wang, T.T., Nestel, F.P., Bourdeau, V., Nagai, Y., Wang, Q., Liao J., et al. (2004) Cutting edge: 1,25-dihydroxyvitamin D3 is a direct inducer of antimicrobial peptide gene expression. J Immunol, 173:2909–2912.

Wilson, D., Jackson, T., Sapey, E. and Lord, J.M. (2017) Frailty and sarcopenia: The potential role of an aged immune system. Ageing Research Reviews, 36:1–10.

Wu, D., Marko, M., Claycombe, K., Paulson, K.E. and Meydani, S.N. (2003) Ceramide-induced and age-associated increase in macrophage COX-2 expression is mediated through upregulation of NF-κB activity. J Biol Chem, 278:10983–10992.

Wu, D. and Meydani, S.N. (2008) Age-associated changes in immune and inflammatory responses: impact of vitamin E intervention. J Leukoc Biol, 84:900–914.

Zanchi, N.E., Gerlinger-Romero, F., Guimaraes-Ferreira, L., de Siqueira Filho, M.A., Felitti, V., Lira, F.S., et al. (2011) HMB supplementation: clinical and athletic performance–related effects and mechanisms of action. Amino Acids, 40:1015–1025.

Zhang, J., Rane, G., Dai, X., Shanmugam, M.K., Arfuso, F., Samy, R.P., Lai, M.K., Kappei, D., Kumar, A.P., Sethi, G. (2016) Ageing and the telomere connection: An intimate relationship with inflammation. Ageing Res Rev., 25, 55–69.

# Chapter 11: Transition Phase and Immune System

Ahnadi, C.E., Beswick, N., Delbecchi, L., Kennelly, J.J. and Lacasse, P. (2002) Addition of fish oil to diets for dairy cows. II. Effects on milk fat and gene expression of mammary lipogenic enzymes. J. Dairy Res., 69:521–531.

Ametaj, B.N., Bradford, B. J., Bobe, G., Nafikov, R. A., Lu, Y., Young, J. W. and Beitz, D. C. (2005) Strong relationships between mediators of the acute phase response and fatty liver in dairy cows. Can. J. Anim. Sci., 85(2):165–175.

Amiridis, G.S., Leontides, L., Tassos, E., Kostoulas, P. and Fthenakis, G.C. (2001) Flunixin meglumine accelerates uterine involution and shortens the calving-to-first oestrus interval in cows with puerperal metritis. J. Vet. Pharmacol. Ther., 24(5):365–367.

Arnoult, D., Carneiro, L., Tattoli, I. and Girardin, S. E. (2009) "The role of mitochondria in cellular defence against microbial infection." Seminars in Immunology, 21(4):223–232.

Bauman, D.E. and Currie, W.B. (1980) Partitioning of nutrients during pregnancy and lactation: a review of mechanisms involving homeostasis and homeorhesis. J. Dairy Sci., 63:1514–1529.

Bernabucci, U., Ronchi, B., Lacetera, N. and Nardone, A. (2005) Influence of body condition score on relationships between metabolic status and oxidative stress in periparturient dairy cows. J. Dairy Sci., 88(6):2017–2026.

Bertoni, G., Trevisi, E., Han, X. and Bionaz, M. (2008) Effects of inflammatory conditions on liver activity in puerperium period and consequences for performance in dairy cows. J. Dairy Sci., 91(9):3300–3310.

Bertoni, G., Trevisi, E., Houdijk, J., Calamari, L. and Athanasiadou, S. (2016) Welfare is affected by nutrition through health (immune function and inflammation), In: Phillips, Clive J.C. (Ed.), Nutrition and the Welfare of Farm Animals. Springer International Publishing Switzerland, pp. 85–114.

Bobe, G., J. W. Young, and D. C. Beitz. 2004. Invited review: Pathology, etiology, prevention, and treatment of fatty liver in dairy cows. J. Dairy Sci. 87:3105–3124.

Bourne, N., Laven, R., Wathes, D C., Martinez, T. and McGowan, M. (2007) A meta-analysis of the effects of vitamin E supplementation on the incidence of retained foetal membranes in dairy cows. Theriogenology, 67(3):494–501.

Bradford, B. (2009) Inflammation and Transition Cow Disorders. The Proceedings of Four-State Dairy Nutrition conference, 2009.

Bradford, B.J. (2017) Immunity, inflammation and the transition cow. Department of Animal Sciences and Industry, Kansas State University.

Bradford, B.J., Mamedova, L.K., Minton, J.E., Drouillard, J.S., Johnson, B.J. (2009) Daily injection of tumor necrosis factor-α increases hepatic triglycerides and alters transcript abundance of metabolic genes in lactating dairy cattle. J Nutr., 139:1451–1456.

Bradford, B.J., K. Yuan, J.K. Farney, L.K. Mamedova, and A.J. Carpenter. (2015). Invited review: Inflammation during the transition to lactation: New adventures with an old flame. J. Dairy Sci. DOI:10.3168/jds.2015-9683.

Buhler, S., Frahm, J., Liermann, W., Tienken, R., Kersten, S., Meyer, U., Huber, K. and Danicke, S. (2018) Effects of energy supply and nicotinic acid supplementation on phagocytosis and ROS production of blood immune cells of periparturient primi- and pluriparous dairy cows. Research in Veterinary Science, 116:62–71.

Calabrese, V., Guagliano, E., Sapienza, M., Panebianco, M., Calafato, S., Puleo, E., PennisiI, G., Mancuso, C., Butterfield, D.A. and Stella, A.G. (2007) Redox regulation of cellular stress response in ageing and neurodegenerative disorders: role of vitagenes. Neurochem. Res., 32:757–773.

Circu, M. L. and Aw, T. Y. (2010) "Reactive oxygen species, cellular redox systems, and apoptosis." Free Radic Biol Med., 48(6):749–762.

Circu, M.L. and Aw, T. Y. (2012) "Intestinal redox biology and oxidative stress." Seminars in Cell and Developmental Biology, 23(7):729–737.

Contreras, G.A. and Sordillo, L.M. (2011) Lipid mobilisation and inflammatory responses during the transition period of dairy cows. Comp. Immunol. Microbiol. Infect. Dis., 34:281–289.

Cooke, R.F., Del Rio, N. S., Caraviello, D.Z., Bertics, S.J., Ramos, M.H., and Grummer, R.R. (2007) Supplemental choline for prevention and alleviation of fatty liver in dairy cattle. J. Dairy Sci., 90(5):2413–2418.

Daniel, J.A., Elsasser, T.H., Morrison, C.D., Keisler, D.H., Whitlock, B.K., Steele, B., Pugh, D. and Sartin, J.L. (2003) Leptin, tumour necrosis factor-$\alpha$ (TNF$\alpha$), and CD14 in ovine adipose tissue and changes in circulating TNF in lean and fat sheep. J. Anim Sci., 81(10):2590–2599.

Dantzer, R. and Kelley, K.W. (2007) Twenty years of research on cytokine-induced sickness behavior. Brain. Behav. Immun., 21(2):153–160.

Depeint, F., Bruce, W.R., Shangari, N., Mehta, R. and O'Brien, P.J. (2006) Mitochondrial function and toxicity: Role of the B vitamin family on mitochondrial energy metabolism." Chemico-Biological Interactions, 163(1–2):94–112.

De Vos, M., Che, L., Huygelen, V., Willemen, S., Michiels, J., Van Cruchten, S. and Van Ginneken, C. (2014)" Nutritional interventions to prevent and rear low-birthweight piglets." J Anim Physiol Anim Nutr (Berl)., 98(4):609–619.

Doepel, L., Lapierre, H. and Kennelly, J.J. (2002) Peripartum performance and metabolism of dairy cows in response to prepartum energy and protein intake. J. Dairy Sci., 85(9):2315–2334.

Drackley, J.K. (1999) ADSA foundation scholar award. Biology of dairy cows during the transition period: the final frontier? J. Dairy Sci., 82(11):2259–2273.

Drackley, J.K., T.R. Overton, and G.N. Douglas. (2001). J. Dairy Sci. 84(E. Suppl.):E100–112.

Drillich, M., Voigt, D. Forderung, D. and Heuwieser, W. (2007) Treatment of acute puerperal metritis with flunixin meglumine in addition to antibiotic treatment. J. Dairy Sci., 90(8):3758–3763.

Dursun, N., Taskin, E., Yerer Aycan, M.B. and Sahin, L. (2011) "Selenium-mediated cardioprotection against adriamycin-induced mitochondrial damage." Drug and chemical toxicology, 34(2):199–207.

Goff, J.P. (2008) Transition Cow Immune Function and Interaction with Metabolic Diseases. The Proceedings of the Tri-state dairy nutrition conference, 2008.

Goff, J.P. and Horst, R.L. (1997) Physiological changes at parturition and their relationship to metabolic disorders. J. Dairy Sci., 80:1260–1268.

Goselink, R., J. van Baal., A. Widaja, R. Dekker, R. Zom., M.J. de Veth, and A. van Vuuren. (2013) Regulation of hepatic triacylglycerol level in dairy cattle by rumen-protected choline supplementation during the transition period. J. Dairy Sci. 96:1102–1116.

Grummer, R.R. (1993) Etiology of lipid related metabolic disorders in periparturient dairy cattle. J. Dairy Sci. 76:3882–3896.

Hassfurther, R.L., T.N. TerHune, and P.C. Canning. (2015) Efficacy of polyethylene glycol–conjugated bovine granulocyte colony-stimulating factor for reducing the incidence of naturally occurring clinical mastitis in periparturient dairy cows and heifers. Am. J. Vet. Res. 76:231–238.

Jaguezeski, A.M., Perin, G., Bottari, N.B., Wagner, R., Fagundes, M.B., Schetinger, M.R.C., Morsch, V.M., Stein, C.S., Moresco, R.N., Barreta, D.A., Danieli, B., Defiltro, R.C., Ana Luiza B. Schogor, A.L. and Da Silva, A.L.S. (2018) Addition of curcumin to the diet of dairy sheep improves health, performance and milk quality. Animal Feed Science and Technology, 246:144–157

Hadsell, D., Torres, D., George, J., Capuco, A., Ellis, S. and Fiorotto, M. (2006) "Changes in secretory cell turnover, and mitochondrial oxidative damage in the mouse mammary gland during a single prolonged lactation cycle suggest the possibility of accelerated cellular ageing." Experimental Gerontology, 41(3):271–281.

Hammon, D.S., Evjen, I.M., Dhiman, T.R., Goff, J.P. and Walters, J.L. (2006) Neutrophil function and energy status in Holstein cows with uterine health disorders. Vet. Immunol. Immuno-pathol., 113:21–29.

Jain, R., C. Pickens, A. and Fenton, J.I. (2018) Reviews: current topics—The role of the lipidome in obesity-mediated colon cancer risk. Journal of Nutritional Biochemistry, 59:1–9

Kerhli, M. E. (2015) Immunological dysfunction in periparturient cows: evidence, causes and ramifications. Proc. Florida Nutr. Conf. pp 14–29. http://dairy.ifas.ufl.edu/rns/2015/02.%20Kehrli.pdf

Kehrli Jr., M.E., Nonnecke, B.J. and Roth, J.A. (1989) Alterations in bovine neutrophil function during the periparturient period. Am. J. Vet. Res., 50:207–214.

Kimura, K., Goff, J.P. and Kehrli Jr., M.E. (1999) Effects of the presence of the mammary gland on expression of neutrophil adhesion molecules and myeloperoxidase activity in periparturient dairy cows. J. Dairy Sci., 82:2385–2392.

Kogut,. M.H., Genovese, K.J., Swaggerty, C.L., He, H. and Broom, L. (2018) Invited Review Inflammatory phenotypes in the intestine of poultry: not all inflammation is created equal. Poultry Science 97:2339–2346.

Lacasse, P., Vanacker, N., Ollier, S. and Ster, C. (2018) Innovative dairy cow management to improve resistance to metabolic and infectious diseases during the transition period. Research in Veterinary Science, 116:40–46.

Lapointe, J. (2014) "Mitochondria as promising targets for nutritional interventions aiming to improve performance and longevity of sows." J Anim Physiol Anim Nutr (Berl) 98(5):809–821.

Lapointe, J., Wang, Y., Bigras, E. and Hekimi, S. (2012) "The submitochondrial distribution of ubiquinone affects respiration in long-lived Mclk1+/- mice." J Cell Biol., 199(2):215–224.

Lauridsen, C. and Jensen, S.K. (2012) "α-Tocopherol incorporation in mitochondria and microsomes upon supranutritional vitamin E supplementation." Genes and Nutrition, 7(4):475–482.

Leavy, O. (2013) "T cells: Mitochondria and T cell activation." Nat Rev Immunol., 13(4):224.

Marriage, B., Clandinin, M. T. and Glerum, D. M. (2003) "Nutritional cofactor treatment in mitochondrial disorders." J Am Diet Assoc., 103(8):1029–1038.

Molosse,V., Souza, C.F., Baldissera, M.D., Glombowsky, P., Campigotto, G., Cazaratto, C.J., Stefani, L.M. and da Silva, A.S. (2019) Diet supplemented with curcumin for nursing lambs improves animal growth, energetic metabolism, and performance of the antioxidant and immune systems. Small Ruminant Research, 170:74–81.

Nakamura, Y.K., and S.T. Omaye. (2010) Lipophilic compound-mediated gene expression and implication for intervention in reactive oxygen species (ROS)-related diseases: Minireview. Nutrients, 2:725–736. https://doi.org/10.3390/nu2070725.

Nonnecke, B.J., K. Kimura, J.P. Goff, and M.E. Kehrli. (2003) Effects of the mammary gland on functional capacities of blood mononuclear leukocyte populations from periparturient cows. J. Dairy Sci. 86:2359–2368.

Rahmani, M., Golian, A., Kermanshahi, H., Reza Bassami, M. (2018) Effects of curcumin or nanocurcumin on blood biochemical parameters, intestinal morphology and microbial population of broiler chickens reared under normal and cold stress conditions. J. Appl. Anim. Res., 46:200–209.

Rattan, S.I. (1998) The nature of gerontogenes and vitagenes. Antiageing effects of repeated heat shock on human fibroblasts. Ann. N.Y. Acad. Sci., 854:54–60.

Reynolds, C.K., P.C. Aikman, B. Lupoli, D.J. Humphries, and D. E. Beaver. (2003) Splanchnic metabolism of dairy cows during the transition from late gestation through early lactation. J. Dairy Sci. 86:1201–1217.

Rimbach, G., A.M. Minihane, J. Majewicz, A. Fischer, J. Pallauf, F. Virgli, and P.D. Weinberg. (2002) Regulation of cell signalling by vitamin E. Proc. Nutr. Soc., 61:415–425. https://doi.org/10.1079/PNS2002183.

Schaff, C., Borner, S., Hacke, S., Kautzsch, U., Albrecht, D., Hammon, H. M., Rontgen, M. and Kuhla, B. (2012) "Increased anaplerosis, TCA cycling, and oxidative phosphorylation in the liver of dairy cows with intensive body fat mobilisation during early lactation." J Proteome Res., 11(11):5503–5514.

Schafers, S., von Soosten, D., Meyer, U., Drong, C., Frahm, J., Tröscher, A., Pelletier, W., Sauerwein, H. and Danicke, S. (2018) Influence of conjugated linoleic acids and vitamin E on biochemical, hematological, and immunological variables of dairy cows during the transition period. J. Dairy Sci., 101:1585–1600.

Sigl, T., Schlamberger, G., Kienberger, H., Wiedemann, S., Meyer, H.H.D. and Kaske, M. (2010) Rumen-protected conjugated linoleic acid supplementation to dairy cows in late pregnancy and early lactation: effects on milk composition, milk yield, blood metabolites and gene expression in liver. Acta Vet. Scand., 52:16.

Sordillo, L.M. and Aitken, S.L. (2009) Impact of oxidative stress on the health and immune function of dairy cattle. Vet. Immunol. Immunopathol., 128:104–109.

Sordillo, L.M. and Raphael, W. (2013) Significance of metabolic stress, lipid mobilisation, and inflammation on transition cow disorders. Vet. Clin. Food Anim., 29, (2):267–278.

Surai, P.F. and Fisinin, V.I. (2016a) Vitagenes in poultry production. Part 2. Nutritional and Internal stresses. World's Poult. Sci. J., 72:761–772.

Surai, P.F. and Fisinin, V.I. (2016b) Vitagenes in poultry production. Part 3. Vitagene concept development. World's Poult. Sci. J., 72:793–804.

Surai, P.F. and Fisinin, V.I. (2016c) Natural antioxidants and stresses in poultry production: from vitamins to vitagenes. The Proceedings of XXV World's Poultry Congress 2016, Invited Lecture Papers, September 5–9, 2016, Beijin, China, p. 116–121.

Tarnopolsky, M.A. (2008) "The mitochondrial cocktail: Rationale for combined nutraceutical therapy in mitochondrial cytopathies." Advanced Drug Delivery Reviews, 60(13–14):1561–1567.

Taub, D.D. (2008) Neuroendocrine interactions in the immune system. Cell. Immunol., 252 (1–2), 1–6.

Trevisi, E. and Minuti, A. (2018) Assessment of the innate immune response in the periparturient cow. Research in Veterinary Science, 116:47–54.

Trevisi, E., Moscati, L. and Amadori, M. (2016) Chapter 9. Disease-Predicting and prognostic potential of innate immune responses to noninfectious stressors: human and animal models. In: Amadori, M. (Ed.) The Innate Immune Response to Noninfectious Stressors. Elsevier Inc., The Netherland, pp. 209–235.

Ugarte, N., Petropoulos, I. and Friguet, B. (2010) "Oxidised mitochondrial protein degradation and repair in ageing and oxidative stress." Antioxid Redox Signal, 13(4):539–549.

Veal, E.A., Day, A.M. and Morgan, B.A. (2007) "Hydrogen peroxide sensing and signalling." Mol Cell, 26(1):1–14.

Wang, S., Meese, S., Ulbrich, S.E., Bollwein, H., Röntgen, M., Gimsa, U. and Schwarm, A. (2018) Effect of immune modulators on *in vitro* activation and proliferation of peripheral blood mononuclear cells from multiparous Holstein cows peripartum. Journal of Animal Phisiology and Animal Nutrition, https://doi.org/10.1111/jpn.12972

Wang, X., Gao, J., Wang, Y., Zhao, Y., Zhang, Y., Han, F., Zheng, Z., Hu, D. (2018) Curcumin pretreatment prevents hydrogen peroxide-induced oxidative stress through enhanced mitochondrial function and deactivation of Akt/Erk signalling pathways in rat bone marrow mesenchymal stem cells. Mol. Cell. Biochem., 443:37–45.

Weinberg, S.E., Sena, L.A. and Chandel, N.S. (2015) "Mitochondria in the regulation of innate and adaptive immunity." Immunity, 42(3):406–417.

West, A.P., Shadel, G.S. and Ghosh, S. (2011) "Mitochondria in innate immune responses." Nature Reviews Immunology, 11(6):389–402.

Yarru, L.P., Settivari, R.S., Gowda, N.K., Antoniou, E., Ledoux, D.R., Rottinghays, G.E. (2009) Effects of turmeric (*Curcuma longa*) on the expression of hepatic genes associated with biotransformation, antioxidant, and immune systems in broiler chicks fed aflatoxin. Poult. Sci., 88:1620–2627.

Yuan, K., Farney, J.K., Mamedova, L.K., Sordillo, L.M., Bradford, B.J. (2013) TNFα altered inflammatory responses, impaired health and productivity, but did not affect glucose or lipid metabolism in early-lactation dairy cows. PLoS One., 8:e80316.

Zhou, Z., Valilati-Riboni, M., Trevisi, E., Drackley, J. K., Luchini, D. N. and Loor, J. J. (2016) J. Dairy Sci., 99:8716–8732.

Zom, R.L.G, van Baal, J., Goselink, R.M.A., Bakker, J.A., de Veth, M. J. and van Vuuren, A.M. (2011) Effect of rumen-protected choline on performance, blood metabolites, and hepatic triacylglycerols of periparturient dairy cattle. J. Dairy Sci. 94:4016–4027.

# Appendix

**Anaplerotic and cataplerotic biosynthetic pathways:** in addition to generating ATP, the tricarboxylic acid cycle generates biosynthetic precursors for fatty acids and several amino acids. This process of substrate exit from the tricarboxylic acid cycle to generate biosynthetic products is known as cataplerosis. Cataplerosis must be balanced by anaplerotic reactions which restore tricarboxylic acid intermediates.

**Anergy:** Lack of reaction by the body's defence mechanisms to foreign substances.

**Antibody:** Protein (i.e. immunoglobulin) produced on exposure to an antigen that neutralise the activity of the antigen.

**Antigen:** A molecule that induces a specific antibody or cell-mediated immune response.

**Autophagy:** A cellular process by which cellular proteins and organelles are degraded in double-membraned vesicular structures called auto-phagosomes. Once degraded, the component pieces of the cargo can be recycled and reused by the cell. Autophagy can be triggered by nutrient shortage, among other stimuli.

**Chemokine:** A protein secreted by cells, which induces directed chemotaxis or chemical attraction in responsive cells.

**Chemotaxis:** A process which causes cells to direct their movements due to the presence of certain chemicals in the environment.

**Complement system:** A biochemical cascade that amplified the effects that result in helping to clear a pathogen from the body.

**Cytokine:** A chemical that mediates communication between cells of the immune system.

**Gut-associated lymphoid tissue (GALT):** The immune system within the GIT located in the lymphoid tissue.

**Hexosamine pathway (HSP):** This metabolic pathway shunts the glucose catabolite fructose-6-phosphate away from glycolysis to produce N-acetyl glucosamine, and then into various glycosylation sugars. Through a complex set of subsequent enzymatic reactions, various glycosylation sugars such as mannose, galactose, fucose and sialic acids are added to proteins.

**Immune modulator:** A substance that modulates the immune response is known as immuno-modulator or immune modulator.

**Immunogens:** Immunogens are substances that elicit an immune response.

**Inflammation:** Local changes that characterise the tissue response to the entry of a foreign body or a pathogenic agent. It is a protective response to remove the injurious stimulus as well as to initiate the healing process.

**Interferon:** A protein released in response to the presence of a pathogen or tumour cell, which allows the communication between cells, to trigger the immune system to respond to eradicate the pathogen or tumour cell.

**Mammalian target of rapamycin complex 1 (mTORC1):** a complex made up of five proteins. mTORC1 positively regulates biosynthesis, cell growth and proliferation by phosphorylating specific enzymatic substrates, which then promote biosynthesis of proteins, lipids and organelles and limit autophagy.

**Mitogen:** A protein that encourages a cell to commence division by triggering mitosis.

**N-linked glycan and O-linked glycan:** A protein modification where sugar molecules or glycans are attached to the nitrogen atom of asparagines residues. By contrast, O-linked glycans are covalently added to serine or threonine residues.

**Opsonin:** A molecule that acts as a binding enhancer to facilitate phagositosis.

**Transcription:** Transcription is transfer of genetic code from DNA to produce RNA.

**Amino sugars**

The hydroxyl groups of monosaccharides can be replaced with other groups to form sugar derivatives. For example, glucose 6-phosphate (phosphorylated sugar) is an important metabolite in glycolysis. In amino sugars, one or more hydroxyl groups are each replaced by an amino group (which is often acetylated), e.g.

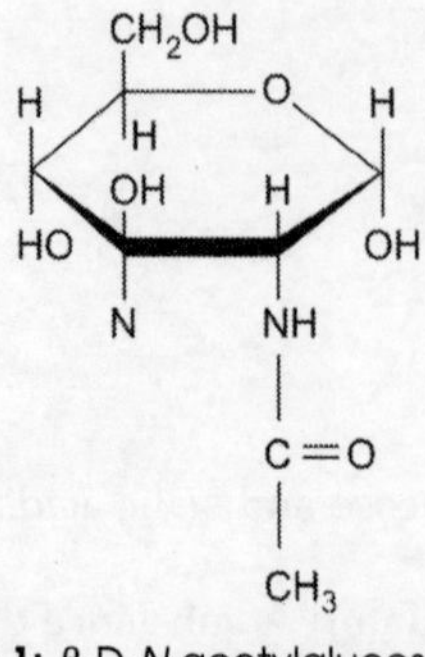

**Fig. A.1:** β-D-*N*-acetylglucosamine

β-D-*N*-acetylglucosamine (Fig. A.1). Simple sugars have three-letter abbreviations [e.g. Glc (glucose), Gal (galactose), Man (mannose), Fuc (fucose)]. Sugar derivatives can also be abbreviated, such as GlcNAc (*N*-acetylglucosamine), GalNAc (*N*-acetylgalactosamine).

**Oligosaccharides** are short chains of monosaccharides linked together by glycosidic bonds. In the case of oligosaccharides linked to proteins (glycoproteins) or lipids (glycolipids), the oligosaccharide is not a repeating unit but consists of a range of different monosaccharides joined by a variety of types of bonds.

Most proteins made by ribosomes on the rough endoplasmic reticulum (RER) contain short chains of carbohydrates (oligosaccharides). They are glycoproteins. The oligosaccharides are of two main types in this protein glycosylation:

1. **O-linked oligosaccharides** are commonly attached to the protein via O-glycosidic bonds to OH groups of serine or threonine side chains (Fig. A.2a). These are synthesised by the sequential addition of monosaccharides to the protein as it passes through the Golgi complex.

2. **N-linked oligosaccharides** are linked to the protein via N-glycosidic bonds, to the $NH_2$ groups of asparagine (Asn) side chains (Fig. A.2b).

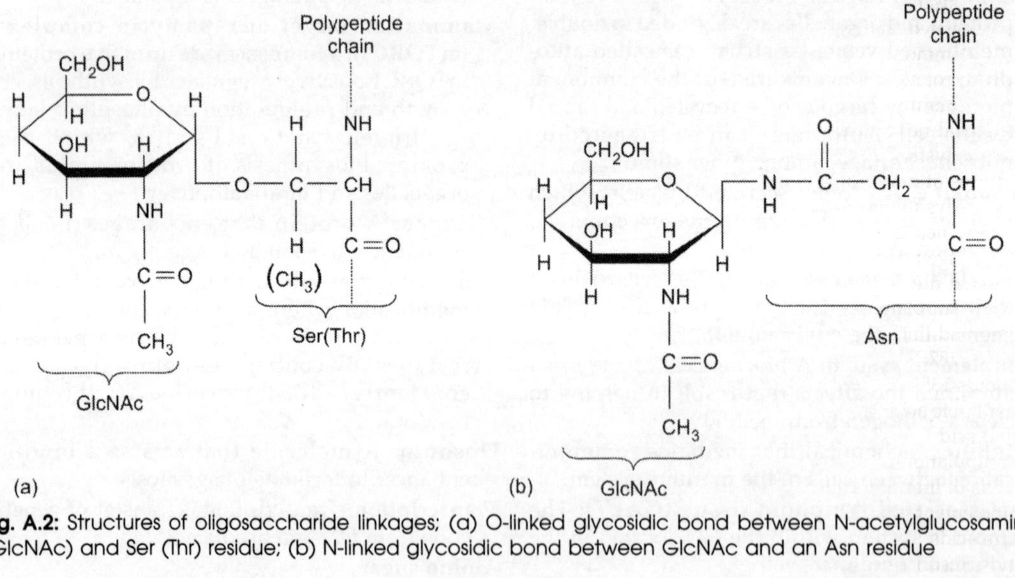

**Fig. A.2:** Structures of oligosaccharide linkages; (a) O-linked glycosidic bond between N-acetylglucosamine (GlcNAc) and Ser (Thr) residue; (b) N-linked glycosidic bond between GlcNAc and an Asn residue

# Index